Lecture Notes in Computer Science

# Lecture Notes in Artificial Intelligence 16748

Founding Editor

Jörg Siekmann

Series Editors

Randy Goebel, *University of Alberta, Edmonton, Canada*
Wolfgang Wahlster, *DFKI, Berlin, Germany*
Zhi-Hua Zhou, *Nanjing University, Nanjing, China*

AF183856

The series Lecture Notes in Artificial Intelligence (LNAI) was established in 1988 as a topical subseries of LNCS devoted to artificial intelligence.

The series publishes state-of-the-art research results at a high level. As with the LNCS mother series, the mission of the series is to serve the international R & D community by providing an invaluable service, mainly focused on the publication of conference and workshop proceedings and postproceedings.

Pavel Andreev · William Van Woensel ·
John Holmes · Antoine Sauré
Editors

# Artificial Intelligence in Medicine

## 24th International Conference, AIME 2026
## Ottawa, ON, Canada, July 7–10, 2026
## Proceedings, Part I

Springer

*Editors*
Pavel Andreev
University of Ottawa
Ottawa, ON, Canada

John Holmes
University of Pennsylvania
Philadelphia, PA, USA

William Van Woensel
University of Ottawa
Ottawa, ON, Canada

Antoine Sauré
University of Ottawa
Ottawa, ON, Canada

ISSN 0302-9743 ISSN 1611-3349 (electronic)
Lecture Notes in Artificial Intelligence
ISBN 978-3-032-30709-5 ISBN 978-3-032-30710-1 (eBook)
https://doi.org/10.1007/978-3-032-30710-1

LNCS Sublibrary: SL7 – Artificial Intelligence

© The Editor(s) (if applicable) and The Author(s), under exclusive license
to Springer Nature Switzerland AG 2027

This work is subject to copyright. All rights are solely and exclusively licensed by the Publisher, whether the whole or part of the material is concerned, specifically the rights of translation, reprinting, reuse of illustrations, recitation, broadcasting, reproduction on microfilms or in any other physical way, and transmission or information storage and retrieval, electronic adaptation, computer software, or by similar or dissimilar methodology now known or hereafter developed.
The use of general descriptive names, registered names, trademarks, service marks, etc. in this publication does not imply, even in the absence of a specific statement, that such names are exempt from the relevant protective laws and regulations and therefore free for general use.
The publisher, the authors and the editors are safe to assume that the advice and information in this book are believed to be true and accurate at the date of publication. Neither the publisher nor the authors or the editors give a warranty, expressed or implied, with respect to the material contained herein or for any errors or omissions that may have been made. The publisher remains neutral with regard to jurisdictional claims in published maps and institutional affiliations.

This Springer imprint is published by the registered company Springer Nature Switzerland AG
The registered company address is: Gewerbestrasse 11, 6330 Cham, Switzerland

If disposing of this product, please recycle the paper.

# Preface

AIME 2026 arrived at a pivotal moment—as artificial intelligence in medicine was moving from a research frontier to a clinical reality, bringing extraordinary promise but also profound responsibility. It is our honor to welcome readers to the proceedings of the 24th International Conference on Artificial Intelligence in Medicine, held at the University of Ottawa, Canada, from July 7 to 10, 2026.

Since its first edition in Pavia in 1985, AIME has provided an international forum for researchers working at the intersection of artificial intelligence, biomedicine, and healthcare. Over the last four decades, the field has moved from symbolic and knowledge-based systems to machine learning, deep learning, multimodal modeling, large language models, and increasingly agentic AI systems. Yet the central concern of the AIME community has remained consistent: how to design, develop, evaluate, and responsibly use AI to better support clinical decisions, improve health systems, and provide better care for patients.

AIME 2026 took place in Ottawa—Canada's capital city and home to federal health agencies, national research councils, research hospitals and institutes, and a vibrant technology sector. The conference was co-hosted by the Telfer School of Management and the Faculty of Medicine at the University of Ottawa—one of Canada's leading research universities and the world's largest bilingual university. uOttawa is a core partner of the Ottawa Academic Health Network (OAHN) linking it with affiliated hospitals and research institutes. Telfer is also one of the few business schools in North America where health research is a core strategic pillar, training professionals to navigate clinical decision making, healthcare delivery, and policy—precisely the challenges at the heart of AIME.

With 236 submissions from 53 countries, AIME 2026 became a record-setting North American edition and one of the most internationally diverse in the conference's history. Submissions originated from Asia, Europe, North America, South America, Africa, and Oceania, demonstrating the growing global reach of the AIME community and the increasing importance of AI across health systems.

For AIME 2026, the conference themes were organized into two broad areas: *AI Foundations and Methodological Innovations* and *Applications, Systems, and Health Impact*. Many submissions targeted subthemes of *Language, Imaging, and Signal Intelligence*, followed by *Clinical AI and Decision Support Systems*; *Deployment, Evaluation, and Governance*}; and *Patient-Centered and Population-Level Applications*. The volume and distribution of submissions covered the full spectrum of the field: clinical decision support, triage, and precision medicine; human-AI collaboration, trust, safety, and ethics; biomedical imaging and signal processing; and multimodal learning, generative AI, and foundation models.

To accommodate the record number of submissions spanning such a broad spectrum of topics, AIME 2026 introduced several changes to the review process. Reviewers indicated their expertise, and authors rated their papers against, the conference themes, improving reviewer matching; Senior Program Committee (PC) members took greater responsibility in overseeing the process. We followed a single-anonymous peer review process. Most papers received three reviews from the regular PC and one review from the Senior PC, who synthesized the reviews and provided a final recommendation. Of the 221 papers sent for peer review, 30 full papers (20% acceptance rate), 21 short papers (18% acceptance rate), and 82 poster and demo papers were accepted. Authors of full and short papers were invited to present their work orally; poster and demo papers were presented across six poster sessions. To increase their visibility and accessibility, AIME 2026 implemented fully digital poster presentations, including 60-second audio summaries. A final novelty was the introduction of a Journal-First track with presentations for recent journal papers, which exposed the AIME community to state-of-the-art results while also giving the authors broader visibility.

We had the privilege of hosting two invited keynote speakers: Tal Arbel of McGill University, whose address on equitable, personalized, and image-based medicine emphasized that clinical AI must be trustworthy before it can be useful; and Muhammad Mamdani of Ontario Health and the University of Toronto, who challenged the community to close the gap between algorithmic performance and real-world impact. Additionally, a panel discussion brought together clinicians, researchers, and policymakers to address a central challenge: that the successful application of AI in medicine depends not only on model performance, but also on clinical acceptability, professional accountability, workflow integration, patient trust, and institutional governance.

The tutorial and workshop programs complemented the main conference and covered interpretable, responsible, trustworthy, and privacy-preserving AI; imaging and signal-based AI methods; AI applications in nursing, oncology, and public health; and the practical evaluation and implementation of AI. The Doctoral Consortium continued AIME's commitment to doctoral training by providing feedback to six PhD students on their research programs in an informal setting.

We sincerely thank everyone who made AIME 2026 possible: the authors, the Program Committee and Senior Program Committee members, keynote speakers, panelists, tutorial and workshop organizers, Doctoral Consortium panelists, sponsors, institutional partners, volunteers, and the local organizing team.

The question before us is no longer focused on whether AI is able to perform a task, but also how it should be evaluated, deployed, and governed, and how this can meaningfully improve care. We hope that AIME 2026 contributed to these conversations and helped move AI in medicine from promising innovation toward responsible, trustworthy, and clinically meaningful practice.

The AIME community has always believed that better science leads to better care. We left Ottawa more convinced than ever that our work matters, and that how we do it matters just as much as what we do.

May 2026

Pavel Andreev
William Van Woensel
John Holmes
Antoine Sauré

# Organization

## General Chair

| | |
|---|---|
| Pavel Andreev | University of Ottawa, Canada |

## Scientific Chairs

| | |
|---|---|
| William Van Woensel | University of Ottawa, Canada |
| John Holmes | University of Pennsylvania, USA |

## Local Organization Chair

| | |
|---|---|
| Antoine Sauré | University of Ottawa, Canada |

## Program Committee Chairs

| | |
|---|---|
| Enea Parimbelli (*Doctoral Consortium*) | Università di Pavia, Italy |
| Daniel Amyot (*Tutorials*) | University of Ottawa, Canada |
| Christopher Sun (*Workshops*) | University of Ottawa, Canada |

## Senior Program Committee

| | |
|---|---|
| Syed Sibte Raza Abidi | Dalhousie University, Canada |
| Riccardo Bellazzi | Università di Pavia, Italy |
| Jaime Cardoso | University of Porto, Portugal |
| Carlo Combi | Università degli Studi di Verona, Italy |
| Arianna Dagliati | University of Pavia, Italy |
| Kerstin Denecke | Bern University of Applied Sciences, Switzerland |
| Barbara Di Camillo | University of Padua, Italy |
| Michel Dojat | INSERM, France |
| Peter Elkin | Ontolimatics, USA |
| Joseph Finkelstein | University of Utah, USA |
| Graciela Gonzalez-Hernandez | Cedars-Sinai Medical Center, USA |

| | |
|---|---|
| Milos Hauskrecht | University of Pittsburgh, USA |
| Pedro Henriques Abreu | University of Coimbra, Portugal |
| Zhengxing Huang | Zhejiang University, China |
| Jose Juarez | Universidad de Murcia, Spain |
| Elpida Keravnou-Papailiou | University of Cyprus, Cyprus |
| Nan Liu | Duke-NUS Medical School, Singapore |
| Peter Lucas | University of Twente, Netherlands |
| Mar Marcos | Universitat Jaume I, Spain |
| Martin Michalowski | University of Minnesota, USA |
| Wojtek Michalowski | University of Ottawa, Canada |
| Stefania Montani | University of Piemonte Orientale, Italy |
| Robert Moskovitch | Ben-Gurion University of the Negev, Israel |
| Barbara Oliboni | University of Verona, Italy |
| Panagiotis Papapetrou | Stockholm University, Sweden |
| Enea Parimbelli | University of Pavia, Italy |
| Silvana Quaglini | University of Pavia, Italy |
| Lucia Sacchi | University of Pavia, Italy |
| Aleksander Sadikov | University of Ljubljana, Slovenia |
| Brigitte Seroussi | Assistance Publique – Hôpitaux de Paris, France |
| Yuval Shahar | Ben-Gurion University of the Negev, Israel |
| Li Shen | University of Pennsylvania, USA |
| Myra Spiliopoulou | Otto-von-Guericke-University Magdeburg, Germany |
| Fabio Stella | University of Milano-Bicocca, Italy |
| Gregor Stiglic | University of Maribor, Slovenia |
| Stephen Swift | Brunel University of London, UK |
| Annette Ten Teije | Vrije Universiteit Amsterdam, Netherlands |
| Paolo Terenziani | Università del Piemonte Orientale, Italy |
| Allan Tucker | Brunel University of London, UK |
| Szymon Wilk | Poznań University of Technology, Poland |
| Migao Wu | Carleton University, Canada |
| Blaz Zupan | University of Ljubljana, Slovenia |
| Frank van Harmelen | Vrije Universiteit Amsterdam, Netherlands |

## Program Committee

| | |
|---|---|
| Samina Abidi | Dalhousie University, Canada |
| Syed Sibte Raza Abidi | Dalhousie University, Canada |
| Giuseppe Agapito | Università Magna Graecia Catanzaro, Italy |
| Alexander Alekseyenko | Medical University of South Carolina, USA |
| Rute Almeida | CINTESIS, Portugal |

| | |
|---|---|
| Amparo Alonso-Betanzos | University of A Coruña, Spain |
| Sanja Avramovic | George Mason University, USA |
| Hamed Ayoobi | University of Groningen, Netherlands |
| Luís Azevedo | University of Porto, Portugal |
| Hajer Baazaoui | ETIS, CY Cergy Paris University, France |
| Arriel Benis | Holon Institute of Technology, Israel |
| Balu Bhasuran | Florida State University, USA |
| Isabelle Bichindaritz | State University of New York at Oswego, USA |
| Alessio Bottrighi | Università del Piemonte Orientale, Italy |
| Dariusz Brzeziński | Poznań University of Technology, Poland |
| Marcos L. P. Bueno | Radboud University, Netherlands |
| Jorie Butler | University of Utah, USA |
| Jerzy Błaszczyński | Poznań University of Technology, Poland |
| David Calhas | University of Ljubljana, Slovenia |
| Francesco Calimeri | University of Calabria, Italy |
| Manuel Campos | University of Murcia, Spain |
| Ricardo Cardoso Pereira | University of Coimbra, Portugal |
| Rita Casadio | University of Bologna, Italy |
| Chuming Chen | University of Delaware, USA |
| Simone Ciccolella | Università degli studi di Milano-Bicocca, Italy |
| Kathleen Curran | University College Dublin, Ireland |
| Bernardo Cánovas Segura | University of Murcia, Spain |
| Gayo Diallo | University of Bordeaux, France |
| Georg Dorffner | Medical University Vienna, Austria |
| Mauro Dragoni | Fondazione Bruno Kessler, Italy |
| Adam Dunn | University of Sydney, Australia |
| Inês Dutra | University of Porto, Portugal |
| Lauren Erdman | University of Toronto/Hospital for Sick Children, Canada |
| Bjoern Eskofier | FAU Erlangen, Germany |
| Brígida Mónica Faria | Polytechnic Institute of Porto, Portugal |
| Jesualdo Tomás Fernández-Breis | Universidad de Murcia, Spain |
| Daniela Ferreira-Santos | University of Porto, Portugal |
| Joseph Finkelstein | University of Arizona, USA |
| Pedro Furtado | University of Coimbra/CISUC, Portugal |
| Roberto Gatta | Università Cattolica del Sacro Cuore, Italy |
| Ben Glicksberg | University of California, San Francisco, USA |
| Natalia Grabar | STL CNRS Université Lille 3, France |
| Vida Groznik | University of Ljubljana, Slovenia |
| Bertha Guijarro-Berdiñas | University of A Coruña, Spain |
| Milos Hauskrecht | University of Pittsburgh, USA |

| | |
|---|---|
| Morihiro Hayashida | National Institute of Technology, Matsue College, Japan |
| Zhe He | Florida State University, USA |
| Shenda Hong | Peking University, China |
| Zhengxing Huang | Zhejiang University, China |
| Xiayuan Huang | Yale University, USA |
| Kyu-Baek Hwang | Soongsil University, South Korea |
| Nevo Itzhak | Ben-Gurion University of the Negev, Israel |
| Filip Jagodzinski | Western Washington University, USA |
| Milica M. Jankovic | University of Belgrade, Serbia |
| Xiaoqian Jiang | UTHealth at Houston, USA |
| Jose Juarez | Universidad de Murcia, Spain |
| Rafał Jóźwiak | Warsaw University of Technology, Poland |
| Charles Kahn | University of Pennsylvania, USA |
| Eleni Kaldoudi | Democritus University of Thrace, Greece |
| Evangelia Katsoulakis | University of South Florida, USA |
| Sophie Kearney | University of Pennslyvania, USA |
| Denisse Kim | University of Murcia, Spain |
| Dokyoon Kim | University of Pennsylvania, USA |
| Jaebum Kim | Konkuk University, South Korea |
| Primoz Kocbek | University of Maribor, Slovenia |
| Haridimos Kondylakis | Institute of Computer Science, FORTH, Greece |
| Leon Kopitar | University of Maribor, Slovenia |
| Krzysztof Krawiec | Poznań University of Technology, Poland |
| Craig Kuziemsky | MacEwan University, Canada |
| Himabindu Lakkaraju | Harvard University, USA |
| Pedro Larranaga | University of Madrid, Spain |
| Nguyen Quoc Khanh Le | Nanyang Technological University, Singapore |
| Carson Leung | University of Manitoba, Canada |
| Chung-Sheng Li | PwC, USA |
| Michael Liebman | IPQ Analytics. LLC, USA |
| Aneta Lisowska | Vrije Univeriteit Amsterdam, Poland |
| Mei Liu | University of Florida, USA |
| Hao Liu | Montclair State University, USA |
| Enrico Longato | University of Padua, Italy |
| Beatriz Lopez | University of Girona, Spain |
| Antonio Lopez-Martinez-Carrasco | University of Murcia, Spain |
| Gang Luo | University of Washington, USA |
| Yves Lussier | University of Utah, USA |
| Hiroshi Mamiya | McGill Clinical and Health Informatics, Canada |
| Simone Marini | University of Florida, USA |
| Begoña Martinez-Salvador | Universitat Jaume I, Spain |

| | |
|---|---|
| Stan Matwin | Dalhousie University, Canada |
| Eneida Mendonca | Cincinnati Children's Hospital Medical Center, USA |
| Ana Maria Mendonça | INESC TEC, Portugal |
| Martin Michalowski | University of Minnesota, USA |
| Silvia Miksch | Vienna University of Technology, Austria |
| Diego Molla | Macquarie University, Australia |
| Irina Moreira | Center for Neuroscience and Cell Biology, Portugal |
| Robert Moskovitch | Ben-Gurion University of the Negev, Israel |
| Laura Moss | University of Glasgow, UK |
| Fleur Mougin | AHeaD, INSERM U1219 – Université de Bordeaux, France |
| Kenta Nakai | University of Tokyo, Japan |
| Loris Nanni | University of Padua, Italy |
| Ardalan Naseri | University of Texas Health Science Center at Houston, USA |
| Goran Nenadic | University of Manchester, UK |
| Denis Newman-Griffis | University of Sheffield, UK |
| Shu-Kay Ng | Griffith University, Australia |
| Tram Anh Nguyen | University of Pennsylvania, USA |
| Giovanna Nicora | University of Pavia, Italy |
| Anne Torill Nordsletta | Norwegian Centre for e-health Research, Norway |
| Arnau Oliver | University of Girona, Spain |
| Daniele Pala | University of Pavia, Italy |
| Laura Maria Peltonen | University of Turku and Turku University Hospital, Finland |
| Samantha Piekos | University of Pennsylvania, USA |
| Maciej Piernik | Poznań University of Technology, Poland |
| Luca Piovesan | Università del Piemonte Orientale, Italy |
| Ronald Piscotty | Oakland University, USA |
| Jędrzej Potoniec | Poznań University of Technology, Poland |
| Mattia Prosperi | University of Florida, USA |
| Lisiane Pruinelli | University of Florida, USA |
| Nisha Puthiyedth | Thompson Rivers University, Canada |
| Arya Rahgozar | University of Ottawa, Canada |
| Nadav Rappoport | Ben-Gurion University of the Negev, Israel |
| Je-Keun Rhee | Soongsil University, South Korea |
| Kirk Roberts | University of Texas Health Science Center at Houston, USA |
| Joseph Romano | University of Pennsylvania, USA |
| Simona E. Rombo | University of Palermo, Italy |

| | |
|---|---|
| Abdul Roudsari | University of Victoria, Canada |
| Luis Rueda | University of Windsor, Canada |
| Elisa Salvi | Norwegian Centre for e-health Research, Norway |
| Leonardo Sanna | Fondazione Bruno Kessler – FBK, Italy |
| Joana Cristo Santos | University of Coimbra, Portugal |
| Neil Sarkar | Brown University, USA |
| Abeed Sarker | Emory University School of Medicine, USA |
| Isabel Sassoon | Brunel University of London, UK |
| Michael Ignaz Schumacher | University of Applied Sciences Western Switzerland (HES-SO), Switzerland |
| Floriano Scioscia | Polytechnic University of Bari, Italy |
| Joao Setubal | University of São Paulo, Brazil |
| Arash Shaban-Nejad | University of California, Berkeley, USA |
| Wenqi Shi | UT Southwestern Medical Center, USA |
| Justyna Skibińska | University of Ljubljana, Slovenia |
| Neil Smalheiser | University of Illinois Chicago, USA |
| Wenyu Song | Brigham and Women's Hospital, USA |
| Giltae Song | Pusan National University, South Korea |
| Marco Spruit | Leiden University Medical Centre, Netherlands |
| Manuel Striani | University of Piemonte Orientale, Italy |
| Madhumita Sushil | University of California, San Francisco, USA |
| Baris Suzek | Muğla Sıtkı Koçman University, Turkey |
| Sing-Hoi Sze | Texas A\&M University, USA |
| Erica Tavazzi | University of Padua, Italy |
| César Teixeira | University of Coimbra, Portugal |
| Shubo Tian | National Center for Biotechnology Information, National Library of Medicine, National Institutes of Health, USA |
| Max Topaz | University of Columbia, USA |
| Ryan Urbanowicz | University of Pennsylvania, USA |
| Iacopo Vagliano | Amsterdam Universitair Medische Centra, Netherlands |
| Ágnes Vathy-Fogarassy | University of Pannonia, Hungary |
| Alfredo Vellido | Universitat Politècnica de Catalunya, Spain |
| Pierangelo Veltri | Università della Calabria, Italy |
| Maria-Esther Vidal | TIB–Leibniz Information Centre for Science and Technology, Germany |
| Giorgio Vinciguerra | University of Pisa, Italy |
| Francesca Vitali | University of Arizona, USA |
| Dimitrios Vogiatzis | ACG Deree, NCSR "Demokritos", Greece |
| Juexin Wang | Indiana University Indianapolis, USA |
| Junbai Wang | Radium Hospital, Norway |

| | |
|---|---|
| Jens Weber | University of Victoria, Canada |
| Chunhua Weng | Columbia University, USA |
| Szymon Wilk | Poznań University of Technology, Poland |
| Huanmei Wu | Temple University, USA |
| Sejung Yang | Yonsei University, South Korea |
| Ye Ye | University of Pittsburgh, USA |
| Rui Zhang | University of Minnesota, USA |
| W. Jim Zheng | U Texas Health Science Houston, USA |
| Pierre Zweigenbaum | Université Paris-Saclay, CNRS, LISN, France |
| Paweł Śniatała | Poznań University of Technology, Poland |
| Martin Špendl | University of Ljubljana, Slovenia |

## Sponsors

We would like to thank the following organizations for sponsoring the conference:

**Platinum Sponsors**

Institut du Savoir Montfort (ISM)

Ottawa Academic Health Network (OAHN)

Telfer School of Management

Faculty of Medicine

**Keynote Sponsor**

CarMa Global Enterprise

**Silver Sponsors**

The University of Ottawa Heart Institute

**Other Sponsors and Partners**

Springer

Artificial Intelligence journal

uOttawa INNOVA

# Contents

# 1 Introduction

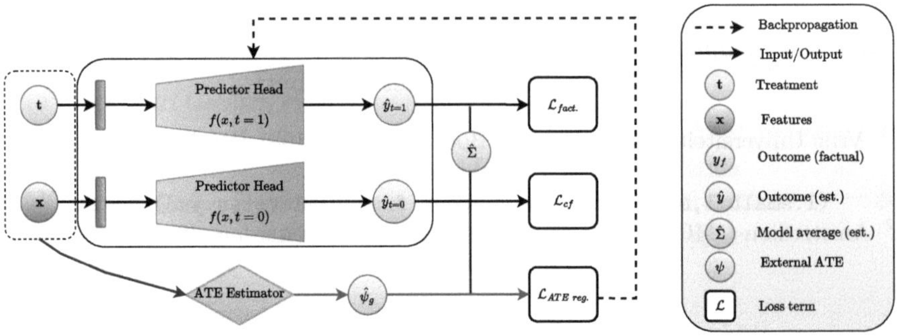


**Fig. 1.** Overview of the AnchorNet framework, illustrating external clinical verification of the population-level ATE and its use as a training-time constraint to anchor individualized treatment-effect predictions.

Clinical decisions increasingly rely on models that estimate how individual patients will respond to treatment. Causal machine learning (ML), a set of methods aimed at producing individual treatment effect estimations from observational data, has therefore attracted significant interest in personalized medicine [2,13]. Despite its potential, many practitioners remain hesitant to deploy state-of-the-art causal models in clinical settings due to concerns about validation, plausibility of the results and trustworthiness [3,10,16].

Assessing the plausibility of the estimates made by a causal model is limited by the fact that for a given individual, treated and untreated outcomes cannot both be observed [6]. As a result, individualized treatment effect (ITE) predictions generated by causal ML models cannot be directly verified, making them inherently difficult to trust in clinical practice. Previous work has sought to address this limitation by deriving bounds on counterfactual error [20], offering theoretical guarantees on estimation accuracy. However, such guarantees are largely driven by abstract theoretical assumptions rather than grounding in variables that correspond to measurable clinical quantities, and therefore leave a gap between abstract causal modeling guarantees and clinically measurable quantities needed to support trustworthy clinical decision-making.

Addressing the disconnect between theory and practice requires a certain level of grounding with respect to externally verifiable quantities such as the odds ratio or average treatment effect. Such quantifies can be observed (or inferred) in the real world could therefore provide a "linkage" between the unverifiable individual model estimates and group level estimates. In particular, introducing group-level grounding offers two key benefits: (1) the model's global behavior can be validated and compared against established clinical knowledge, improving clinical assurance; and (2) population-level quantities align naturally with how clinical evidence is generated and summarized, enabling direct comparison with evidence from clinical trials and guidelines.

We operationalize this group-level anchoring in a causal learning method called AnchorNet (Fig. 1). AnchorNet uses population-level treatment effects as clinically meaningful references to guide individualized predictions, while enforcing bounded and clinically plausible heterogeneity. Among such population-level quantities, we focus on the average treatment effect (ATE) as a canonical and practically estimable reference. The use of an *externally* estimated ATE is motivated by the following considerations: the ATE can generally be estimated consistently under standard causal inference assumptions [1,4,7,18]. In contrast, averaging conditional or individualized treatment effect predictions produced by a causal ML model does not, in general, yield a reliable estimate of the ATE. The quantity produced is a model-internal quantity rather than an externally estimable reference, and therefore cannot serve as an independent check on model behavior [9,19].

In summary, our contributions are threefold: (1) we propose a clinically informed causal ML anchoring approach that constrains individualized treatment effect estimation using population-level causal quantities; (2) we provide a theoretical analysis, including a generalization bound, that characterizes error control under bounded heterogeneity; and (3) we empirically validate our framework on real-world pediatric and geriatric medical use cases, demonstrating clinically coherent treatment policies without sacrificing predictive performance. We also release the accompanying codebase.[1]

## 2 Related Work

Existing approaches to individualized treatment effect (ITE) estimation include meta-learners such as the X-learner [12] and counterfactual regression (CFR) methods that balance treated and control representations using integral probability metrics (IPM) [20]. Despite strong predictive performance, predictions made by the current generation of off-the-shelf models often remains difficult to validate and assess in practice. Our work builds on these approaches by explicitly addressing the challenge of clinical grounding.

Recent studies show that averaging conditional average treatment effect predictions produced by individual-effect models is not a reliable way to recover the average treatment effect (ATE) [19]. A key insight is that estimating the ATE amounts to recovering a single scalar quantity, whereas estimating the conditional average treatment effect (CATE) requires learning an entire function of the covariates [9], making CATE estimation statistically more challenging and typically incurs substantially larger estimation error for a given sample size. These observations motivate a two-tiered approach: we first estimate the ATE, and then use this validated quantity to guide personalized prediction models.

Foundational work by Pearl [15] established that the average treatment effect (ATE) can be consistently estimated from observational data under standard

[1] https://github.com/ljsmalbil/AnchorNet.

causal assumptions. Subsequent advances include doubly robust and debiased estimation methods [4], as well as tree-based approaches for treatment effect estimation [1]. In contrast to approaches that recover the ATE by aggregating individualized predictions, our work leverages this line of research by independently estimating the ATE and incorporating it as a population-level constraint.

## 3 Methodology

**Notations and Definitions.** We formalize our approach using the Neyman–Rubin potential outcomes framework [8]. Each individual $i$ has covariates $x^i$, binary treatment $t^i \in \{0,1\}$, potential outcomes $Y_0^i, Y_1^i$, and observed outcome $y^i = t^i Y_1^i + (1-t^i) Y_0^i$. Let $\mathbb{I}[\cdot]$ denote the indicator function and $\bar{Y}_t$ the mean of a treatment group. We define the conditional outcome functions $m_t(x) = \mathbb{E}[Y_t \mid x]$, the individual (conditional average) treatment effect $\tau(x) = m_1(x) - m_0(x)$, and the population average treatment effect (ATE) $\psi = \mathbb{E}_x[\tau(x)]$. Estimates of the ATE are denoted $\hat{\psi}_g$, where $g$ indexes the estimator (we use $\hat{\psi}_f$ to denote the estimate made by the model $f$). We model both potential outcomes using a single predictor $f : \mathcal{X} \times 0,1 \to \mathbb{R}$ with $f(x,t) \approx m_t(x)$. We use $f$ to denote the neural network used for modelling. For analysis, we define the maximum deviation of the CATE from the ATE, $\sup_x |\tau(x) - \psi|$, assumed finite. This quantity is essentially measure of the maximum spread of the treatment distribution. The factual and counterfactual squared errors $\epsilon_F$ and $\epsilon_{CF}$; the estimated CATE $\hat{\tau}_f(x) = f(x,1) - f(x,0)$; and the PEHE $\epsilon_{\text{PEHE}}(f) = \mathbb{E}_x[(\hat{\tau}_f(x) - \tau(x))^2]$, which measures the error in the estimated treatment effect and real treatment effect.
**Assumptions.** We assume strong ignorability, $(Y_0, Y_1) \perp t \mid x$, implying that after adjusting for clinical covariates (e.g., demographics, comorbidities, prior utilization), treatment assignment is unbiased. We also assume overlap (positivity), $0 < p(t = 1 \mid x) < 1$, meaning that similar patients can plausibly receive either treatment in practice. Together, these assumptions identify the average treatment effect (ATE) and allow consistent estimation using standard causal methods, including doubly robust estimators [4,5]. We use these to anchor the externally estimated ATE $\hat{\psi}_g$ to the model-predicted ATE $\hat{\psi}_f$.

### 3.1 Estimation Generalization Bound

A key advantage of existing causal inference approaches is the theoretical control they provide over the estimation error [20]. Our approach builds on this principle by transferring such guarantees from the population-level estimand to individualized predictions. Proposition 1 formalizes this connection and shows how anchoring to a reliable average treatment effect induces control over individual-level errors.

**Proposition 1 (PEHE Bound).** *Let* $m_t(x) = \mathbb{E}[Y_t \mid x]$, $\tau(x) = \mathbb{E}[Y_1 \mid x] - \mathbb{E}[Y_0 \mid x]$, $\hat{\tau}_f(x) = f(x,1) - f(x,0)$, $u = \Pr(T = 1)$, $\bar{Y}_t$ *the mean outcome in* *group $t$, and $\psi$ the population average treatment effect. Define the heterogeneity modulus $H = \sup_x |\tau(x) - \psi|$. Under unconfoundedness and positivity,*

$$\epsilon_{\text{PEHE}}(f) \leq 2\Big[(1-u)\big(\mathbb{E}_x[(f(x,1) - (\bar{Y}_0 + \psi))^2] + \mathbb{E}_x[(f(x,0) - m_0(x))^2]\big) + u\big(\mathbb{E}_x[(f(x,1) - m_1(x))^2] + \mathbb{E}_x[(f(x,0) - (\bar{Y}_1 - \psi))^2]\big)\Big] + 2H.$$

*Proof.* By $(a-b)^2 \leq 2(a^2+b^2)$, we have $\epsilon_{\text{PEHE}}(f) \leq 2\mathbb{E}_x[(f_1 - m_1)^2] + 2\mathbb{E}_x[(f_0 - m_0)^2]$. Decomposing $\mathbb{E}_x$ into factual and counterfactual terms weighted by $u$ yields factual errors on $\mathbb{E}_{x|T=t}$. For counterfactuals, we substitute $m_1(x) = m_0(x) + \tau(x)$ and anchor the unobserved $\tau(x)$ to the population ATE $\psi$. Applying the quadratic inequality to the surrogates $\bar{Y}_0 + \psi$ and $\bar{Y}_1 - \psi$ introduces the heterogeneity modulus $H = \sup_x |\tau(x) - \psi|$. Collecting terms yields the result.

Proposition 1 shows that the error in estimating individualized treatment effects is bounded by the factual prediction error, a counterfactual surrogate error term, and an irreducible term capturing deviation from the population average treatment effect. From a clinical perspective this implies that anchoring to a reliable population-level estimate stabilizes patient-level treatment-effect predictions by constraining individualized estimates to remain coherent with the estimate based on the data, thereby enforcing global behavior consistent with validated population-level effects. Furthermore, the proposed bound can be readily incorporated into existing error bounds (e.g., [20]), preserving theoretical guarantees on estimation accuracy while additionally enforcing a clinically meaningful plausibility constraint.

The heterogeneity modulus $H$ appearing in Proposition 1 reflects intrinsic biological variation in treatment response. As such, the bound tightens when treatment effects are more homogeneous across the population. In this sense, anchoring individualized predictions to the ATE induces a form of clinically grounded regularization: when plausible treatment-effect ranges are narrow, deviations from the population estimate are necessarily limited. Corollary 1 formalizes this intuition by showing that ATE-guided anchoring yields a PEHE guarantee expressed directly in terms of clinically meaningful effect ranges, without relying on uninterpretable representation-balancing constraints.

**Corollary 1 (Clinically bounded heterogeneity).** *If treatment effects satisfy $\tau(x) \in [\tau_{\min}, \tau_{\max}]$ for all $x$, then $\psi \in [\tau_{\min}, \tau_{\max}]$ and the heterogeneity modulus in Proposition 1 obeys $H = \sup_x |\tau(x) - \psi| \leq (\tau_{\max} - \tau_{\min})/2$.*

### 3.2 Algorithmic and Architectural Details

Algorithmically, we instantiate a predictor $f(x, t; \theta)$ and train it using a combination of factual loss, ATE-guided counterfactual loss, and an ATE-matching regularizer. Architecturally, our approach lies between classical meta-learners [12] and treatment-agnostic representation network (TARNet)–type models [20]. Following a two-tiered approach, we first estimate the population ATE $\psi$ using estimators $g$, for which we can use methods such as double/debiased estimation [4]. Second, we then proceed with the following training objective:

**Algorithm 1** AnchorNet Training

**Input:** Data $\{(x^i, t^i, y^i)\}_{i=1}^n$, loss $\mathcal{L}$, estimator $g$, model $f$, step size $\gamma$, regularization $\lambda$, treatment prevalence $u = \Pr(T = 1)$, $\hat{Y}_t = \frac{1}{n}\sum_{i=1}^n Y_t \approx \bar{Y}_t$. **Output:** $\hat{y}_0^i = f(x^i, 0; \theta)$, $\hat{y}_1^i = f(x^i, 1; \theta)$.

1: Estimate $\hat{\psi}_g$ using $g$
2: **for** each training iteration **do**
3: $\mathcal{L}_{\text{fact}} = (1-u)\mathcal{L}(f(x^i, 0; \theta), y^i)\mathbb{I}[t^i = 0] + u\mathcal{L}(f(x^i, 1; \theta), y^i)\mathbb{I}[t^i = 1]$
4: $\mathcal{L}_{\text{cf}} = (1-u)\mathcal{L}(f(x^i, 1; \theta), \hat{Y}_0 + \hat{\psi}_g)\mathbb{I}[t^i = 0] + u\mathcal{L}(f(x^i, 0; \theta), \hat{Y}_1 - \hat{\psi}_g)\mathbb{I}[t^i = 1]$
5: $\mathcal{R} = \left(\frac{1}{n}\sum_i (f(x^i, 1; \theta) - f(x^i, 0; \theta))) - \hat{\psi}_g\right)^2$
6: $\theta \leftarrow \theta - \gamma\nabla_\theta(\mathcal{L}_{\text{fact}} + \mathcal{L}_{\text{cf}} + \lambda\mathcal{R})$
7: **end for**

$$\min_\theta \ \mathcal{L}_{\text{fact}} + \mathcal{L}_{\text{cf}} + \lambda\mathcal{R},$$

where $\mathcal{L}_{\text{fact}}$ penalizes prediction error on observed outcomes, $\mathcal{L}_{\text{cf}}$ enforces coherence with the ATE-induced counterfactual surrogates $\hat{Y}_0 + \hat{\psi}_g$ and $\hat{Y}_1 - \hat{\psi}_g$, and $\mathcal{R}$ aligns the average predicted treatment effect with $\hat{\psi}_g$, thereby serving as a complementary interpretability constraint. Algorithm 1 summarizes the resulting AnchorNet training procedure.

# 4 Experiments

We conduct two sets of experiments. First, we provide an empirical evaluation on two real-world medical use cases. Second, we include two ablation studies. In the first ablation study, we examine the effect of the ATE-matching regularizer's weight, and in the second one, we conduct a synthetic analysis assessing the model's robustness to biased ATE estimates while comparing it to previously proposed bounds [20].

We present two versions of AnchorNet: (1) **AnchorNet** and (2) **AnchorNet$_{\text{NDT}}$**, a neural decision tree–based (NDT) model inspired by Kontschieder et al. (2015) [11], included to demonstrate that our approach can be seamlessly integrated with other model classes. The default model **AnchorNet** is a neural network, following the TARNet architecture [20]. We include the following baselines: a classical tree-based approach called Causal Forest [1]. We also include two counterfactual regression methods: CFR with Wasserstein distance (CFR$_{\text{Wass}}$) [20], an improved version of CFR$_{\text{Wass}}$ called Similarity SITE-CFR (Preserved Individual Treatment Effect) [21]. Lastly, we include an autoencoder-based approach called TEDVAE (Treatment Effect with Disentangled Autoencoder) [22], a state-of-the art method. We use a double/debiased estimator $g_{\text{DR}}$ proposed by Chernozhukov et al. (2018) [4] as $\hat{\psi}_g$.

## 4.1 Evaluation on Medical Use-Cases

**(1) IBenC (Identifying Best Practices for Care-Dependent Elderly).** This dataset consists of longitudinal records for $n = 1594$ older adults receiving community care across Europe [17]. Our outcome is binarized functional independence (decline or improvement), measured using the short-form activities of daily living (ADL) scale [14]. Our treatment is physiotherapy (PT), measured in minutes in the past week. The goal is therefore to predict the to extent to which PT has a positive effect on ADL. Following [20], performance is evaluated using policy risk,$R_{\text{pol}}(\pi_f) = 1 - \mathbb{E}\left[Y_{\pi_f(X)} \mid T = \pi_f(X)\right], \pi_f(x) = \mathbb{1}\{f(x,1) > f(x,0)\}$. It measures how well the model-guided PT decisions improve functional independence, and can be estimated by averaging outcomes of patients whose received PT matches the model's recommendation, without requiring access to true counterfactuals. We further report (average treatment effect of the treated) ATT error, defined as $\epsilon_{\text{ATT}} = \left|\text{ATT} - \frac{1}{n}\sum_{i=1}^{n} \Delta_f(x_1^i)\right|, \quad \Delta_f(x) = f(x,1) - f(x,0)$ with a ground-truth sample ATT of $-0.25$.

**(2) IHDP (Infant Health and Development Program).** IHDP is a semi-simulated pediatric benchmark [20], where the treatment is assignment to the early childhood social support intervention program, and the outcome is the child's cognitive development score measured by the Bayley Scales. The dataset includes 747 subjects with 25 covariates. We use the standard benchmark version with $n = 1000$ replications and report the $\sqrt{\text{PEHE}}$. A low $\sqrt{\text{PEHE}}$ indicates accurate estimation of individual treatment effects, whereas a high value reflects poor recovery of heterogeneous effects.

**Table 1.** Performance comparison of causal inference methods on the IHDP and IBenC datasets across PEHE, policy risk, and ATT metrics (lower values is better). Best performers (paired t-test, $p < 0.05$) are bold faced.

| | IHDP | | IBenC | | |
|---|---|---|---|---|---|
| Method | $\sqrt{\epsilon_{pehe}}^{\text{in-s}}$ | $\sqrt{\epsilon_{pehe}}^{\text{oos}}$ | $R_{pol}^{\text{in-s}}$ | $R_{pol}^{\text{oos}}$ | $\epsilon_{\text{ATT}}$ |
| CausalForest | 3.80 (0.20) | 3.80 (0.20) | 0.84 (0.00) | 0.90 (0.03) | 0.46 (0.02) |
| TEDVAE | 1.30 (1.00) | 1.36 (1.24) | 0.81 (0.03) | 0.85 (0.04) | 0.23 (0.06) |
| $\text{CFR}_{\text{Wass}}$ | 0.93 (0.10) | 0.84 (0.05) | 0.62 (0.23) | 0.66 (0.42) | 0.21 (0.12) |
| SITE-CFR | **0.65** (0.07) | **0.73** (0.28) | 0.51 (0.24) | 0.53 (0.14) | **0.21** (0.03) |
| $\text{AnchorNet}_{\text{NDT}}$ | 2.28 (0.07) | 2.45 (0.41) | **0.45** (0.06) | **0.45** (0.10) | **0.20** (0.01) |
| AnchorNet | **0.63** (0.04) | **0.71** (0.18) | 0.65 (0.04) | 0.66 (0.05) | **0.18** (0.07) |

**Results.** Table 1 summarizes performance on the IHDP and IBenC datasets. On IBenC, AnchorNet variants achieve strong performance on clinically relevant decision metrics: $\text{AnchorNet}_{\text{NDT}}$ attains the lowest policy risk ($0.45 \pm 0.06$ in-sample; $0.45 \pm 0.10$ out-of-sample), while also achieving competitive policy risk and low ATT error ($0.18 \pm 0.07$). Anchoring maintains predictive accuracy while ensuring the resulting treatment policies remain coherent with the externally estimated population-level evidence. On IHDP, AnchorNet's performance is tied with the state-of-the art SITE-CFR model $\sqrt{\text{PEHE}}$ ($0.63 \pm 0.04$ in-sample; $0.71 \pm 0.18$ out-of-sample), demonstrating accurate individualized effect estimation while maintaining global coherence. Additional results in Table 2 show that

**Table 2.** Out-of-sample PEHE for different ATE estimators used as plug-in anchors for **AnchorNet**. The third column reports absolute deviation from the true ATE.

| Estimator | $\sqrt{\epsilon_{pehe}}^{oos}$ | $\sum\lvert\hat{\psi}_g - \psi\rvert$ |
|---|---|---|
| Double/debiased | 0.71 (0.18) | 0.03 |
| InversePropensity | 0.84 (0.29) | 0.34 |
| CausalForest | 0.74 (0.21) | 0.17 |
| Mean | 0.76 (0.32) | 0.19 |

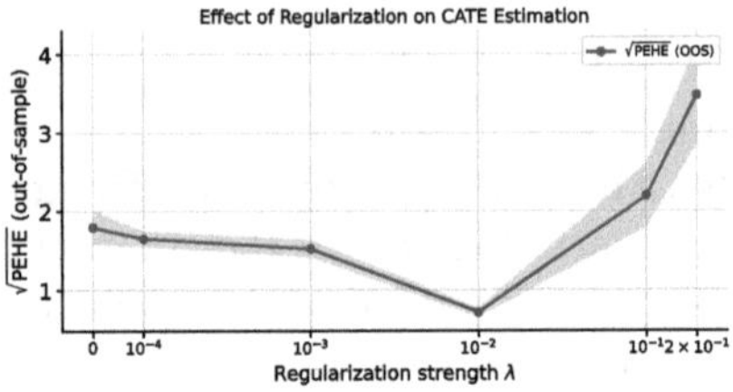


**Fig. 2.** Out-of-sample $\sqrt{\text{PEHE}}$ of **AnchorNet** as a function of the regularization strength $\lambda$ on IHDP.

our approach is also robust to the choice of ATE estimator: estimates closer to the true ATE yield lower $\sqrt{\text{PEHE}}$ and more interpretable anchoring, whereas poorly aligned estimates degrade performance (albeit not too much).

### 4.2 Additional Experiments and Ablation Studies

**Hyperparameter Sensitivity.** ATE regularization impacts performance. In particular, weight values that are too low weaken grounding, while values that are too large cause individual predictions to cluster around the average. Figure 2 shows the effect of the ATE-matching regularization strength $\lambda$ on out-of-sample performance on the IHDP dataset. $\sqrt{\text{PEHE}}$ decreases as $\lambda$ increases up to an intermediate optimum (approximately $10^{-2}$), after which stronger regularization degrades accuracy. Clinically, this reflects a trade-off: insufficient regularization weakens anchoring to population-level evidence, while excessive regularization overly constrains the model and suppresses patient-level heterogeneity.

**Bias–Variance Trade-off.** We investigate the limits of grounding-based approaches by asking: *under what conditions does a method that explicitly models variability outperform anchoring?* To answer this question, we compare the AnchorNet bound with the IPM-based bound of Shalit et al. (2017) [20] under synthetic settings with correlated covariates, nonlinear treatment assignment, and heterogeneous treatment effects. We vary treatment-effect heterogeneity ($\sigma_\tau$) and introduce controlled ATE misspecification to model clinically plausible bias–variance trade-offs. As shown in Fig. 3, our bound is tighter for small to moderate heterogeneity, while the alternative bound becomes competitive only under substantial heterogeneity, indicating that anchoring is most effective when patient

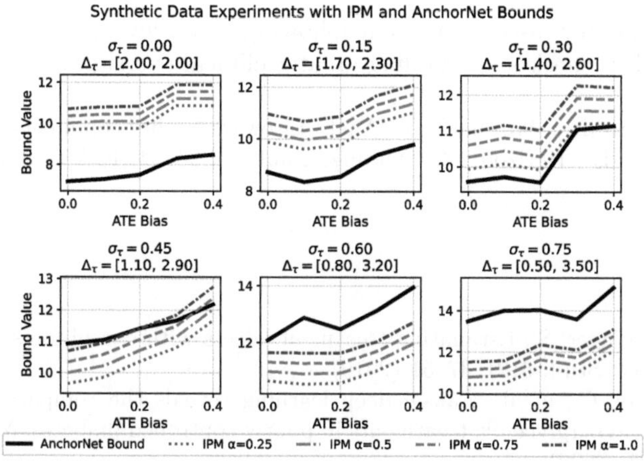


**Fig. 3.** AnchorNet and IPM-based error bounds under increasing treatment-effect heterogeneity $\sigma_\mathcal{T}$. $\alpha$ denotes an imbalance penalty. $\Delta_\mathcal{T}$ denotes treatment range.

responses vary within biologically plausible ranges. Interestingly, the impact of bias appears to be roughly the same across approaches.

# 5 Discussion and Conclusion

We introduced AnchorNet, a clinically grounded approach to conditional average treatment-effect estimation that incorporates an external population-level treatment effect as an interpretability constraint. We showed that AnchorNet achieves performance that is on par with or better than existing methods, suggesting that anchoring individualized predictions to clinically meaningful group-level quantities may improve model plausibility assessment without sacrificing accuracy. Our theoretical analysis clarifies when anchoring is most effective: while representation-balancing methods may be preferable under extreme treatment-effect heterogeneity, AnchorNet performs particularly well when heterogeneity is present but clinically bounded, a common scenario in practice.

A theoretical limitation of AnchorNet is the assumption that the ATE quantity is unbiased. While our experiments indicate that AnchorNet is relatively robust to moderate bias in the anchor, formally characterizing this robustness remains an important direction for future work. Further, if clinical consensus aligns with an incorrect population-level estimate or if the ATE is estimated from the same observational data used to train the outcome model and unmeasured confounding persists, AnchorNet enforces consistency with a biased reference, a challenge shared by causal machine learning methods more broadly. Beyond the ATE, an interesting extension would be to anchor predictions to other group-level quantities commonly reported in clinical research, such as odds ratios or hazard ratios. Finally, the two-tiered structure of AnchorNet naturally admits an additional doctor-in-the-loop stage following group-level prediction, providing an extra validity check and enabling greater clinical oversight.

**Acknowledgements.** We thank Dr. Aneta Lisowska for her comments and feedback. We acknowledge EU Horizon 2020 funding, grant No. 96534 (ICARE4OLD).

## References

1. Athey, S., Wager, S.: Estimating treatment effects with causal forests: an application. Observ. Stud. **5**(2), 37–51 (2019)
2. Belthangady, C., et al.: Causal deep learning reveals the comparative effectiveness of antihyperglycemic treatments in poorly controlled diabetes. Nat. Commun. **13**(1), 6921 (2022)
3. Caruana, R., Lou, Y., Gehrke, J., Koch, P., Sturm, M., Elhadad, N.: Intelligible models for healthcare: Predicting pneumonia risk and hospital 30-day readmission. In: Proceedings of the 21st ACM SIGKDD International Conference on Knowledge Discovery and Data Mining, pp. 1721–1730 (2015)
4. Chernozhukov, V., Chetverikov, D., Demirer, M., Duflo, E., Hansen, C., Newey, W., Robins, J.: Double/Debiased Machine Learning for Treatment and Structural Parameters. Oxford University Press, Oxford (2018)
5. Funk, M.J., Westreich, D., Wiesen, C., Stürmer, T., Brookhart, M.A., Davidian, M.: Doubly robust estimation of causal effects. Am. J. Epidemiol. **173**(7), 761–767 (2011)
6. Holland, P.W.: Statistics and causal inference. J. Am. Stat. Assoc. **81**(396), 945–960 (1986)
7. Imbens, G.W.: Nonparametric estimation of average treatment effects under exogeneity: a review. Rev. Econ. Stat. **86**(1), 4–29 (2004)
8. Imbens, G.W., Rubin, D.B.: Causal Inference in Statistics, Social, and Biomedical Sciences. Cambridge University Press (2015)
9. Kennedy, E.H., Balakrishnan, S., Robins, J.M., Wasserman, L.: Minimax rates for heterogeneous causal effect estimation. Ann. Stat. **52**(2), 793 (2024)
10. Kleinberg, S., Hripcsak, G.: A review of causal inference for biomedical informatics. J. Biomed. Inform. **44**(6), 1102–1112 (2011)
11. Kontschieder, P., Fiterau, M., Criminisi, A., Bulo, S.R.: Deep neural decision forests. In: Proceedings of the IEEE International Conference on Computer Vision, pp. 1467–1475 (2015)
12. Künzel, S.R., Sekhon, J.S., Bickel, P.J., Yu, B.: Metalearners for estimating heterogeneous treatment effects using machine learning. Proc. Natl. Acad. Sci. **116**(10), 4156–4165 (2019)
13. Msaouel, P., Lee, J., Karam, J.A., Thall, P.F.: A causal framework for making individualized treatment decisions in oncology. Cancers **14**(16), 3923 (2022)
14. interRAI Organization: interRAI activities of daily living (ADL) short form scale (2021). https://interrai.org/applications/status-and-outcome-scales/. Accessed 12 Mar 2025
15. Pearl, J.: Causality. Cambridge University Press (2009)
16. Petersson, L., et al.: Challenges to implementing artificial intelligence in healthcare: a qualitative interview study with healthcare leaders in Sweden. BMC Health Serv. Res. **22**(1), 850 (2022)

17. van der Roest, H.G., van Eenoo, L., van Lier, L.I., Onder, G., Garms-Homolová, V., Smit, J.H., Finne-Soveri, H., Jónsson, P.V., Draisma, S., Declercq, A., et al.: Development of a novel benchmark method to identify and characterize best practices in home care across six European countries: design, baseline, and rationale of the IBENC project. BMC Health Serv. Res. **19**, 1–11 (2019)
18. Rubin, D.B.: Causal inference using potential outcomes: design, modeling, decisions. J. Am. Stat. Assoc. **100**(469), 322–331 (2005)
19. Salditt, M., Eckes, T., Nestler, S.: A tutorial introduction to heterogeneous treatment effect estimation with meta-learners. Admin. Policy Mental Health Mental Health Serv. Res. **51**(5), 650–673 (2024)
20. Shalit, U., Johansson, F.D., Sontag, D.: Estimating individual treatment effect: generalization bounds and algorithms. In: International Conference on Machine Learning, pp. 3076–3085. PMLR (2017)
21. Yao, L., Li, S., Li, Y., Huai, M., Gao, J., Zhang, A.: Representation learning for treatment effect estimation from observational data. In: Advances in Neural Information Processing Systems, vol. 31 (2018)
22. Zhang, W., Liu, L., Li, J.: Treatment effect estimation with disentangled latent factors. In: Proceedings of the AAAI Conference on Artificial Intelligence, vol. 35, pp. 10923–10930 (2021)

# Learning to Segment Using Summary Statistics and Weak Supervision

Omkar Kulkarni[1(✉)], Edward Raff[2], and Tim Oates[1]

[1] University of Maryland, Baltimore County, Baltimore, MD, USA
{omkar.kulkarni,oates}@umbc.edu
[2] Crowdstrike, Austin, TX, USA
edward.raff@crowdstrike.com

**Abstract.** Medical experts often manually segment images to obtain diagnostic statistics and discard the resulting annotations. We aim to train segmentation models to alleviate this burden, but constrained to the retained summary statistics (e.g., the area of the annotated region). Empirical results suggest that statistics alone are insufficient for this task, but adding weak information in the form of a few pixels within the area of interest significantly improves performance. We use a novel loss function that combines terms for image reconstruction quality, matching to summary statistics, and overlap between the predicted foreground and the weak supervisory signal. Experiments on standard image, ultrasound (breast cancer), and Computed Tomography (CT) scan (kidney tumors) data demonstrate the utility and potential of the approach.

**Keywords:** Weak Supervision · Image Segmentation · Medical Images · Limited Labels

## 1 Introduction

Our work is motivated by an attempted collaboration with physicians at the University of Maryland School of Medicine. Multiple research projects, such as [6,7,9], involved months of manual effort by physicians and physician trainees to label images pixel-by-pixel and categorize cell types. The ultimate goal of this activity was to produce a clinically relevant ratio for the subject under study. Our interest in helping these physicians accelerate their work by using AI to segment the images was thwarted by the discovery that the original segmentation masks, the ground truth labels we would train and evaluate on, were routinely discarded as "not relevant" to the clinical question. *Only the ratio was saved.* The effort to relabel even a few hundred images was measured in half-year increments, depending on the project and the required details. This problem motivates our work to develop a new approach to semi-supervised segmentation that directly addresses this common clinical scenario. Despite the difficulty of learning under these constraints, our results can be surprisingly useful—as demonstrated in Fig. 1.

© The Author(s), under exclusive license to Springer Nature Switzerland AG 2027
P. Andreev et al. (Eds.): AIME 2026, LNAI 16748, pp. 12–16, 2027.
https://doi.org/10.1007/978-3-032-30710-1_2

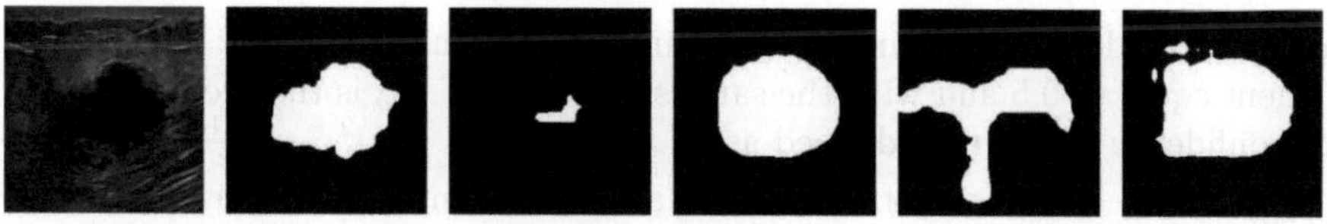

(a) Input Image (b) Ground truth (c) Weak mask (d) Our Method (e) Only weak mask (f) Only statistics

**Fig. 1.** Example images from the BUSI dataset, showing that we can obtain reasonably accurate segmentations even under highly restrictive and minimal learning signals from the physician.

Numerous prior works have investigated medical image segmentation as summarized in [8], however, these are all fully supervised methods. Recent approaches toward weakly/semi supervised segmentation use skeletonization methods to encode domain knowledge, regularization algorithms, or incomplete labels (most similar to our work) [3]. To wit, none have dealt with the kind of label scarcity or interdisciplinary hurdles to leveraging historical data. In tackling this problem, we find that a combination of self-supervised and weak signals can deliver practical and reasonable results.

## 2 Methods and Architecture

We use a **percentage of ROI (Region of Interest)** as a summary statistic that represents the ROI's size relative to the image's size. Physicians conducting research often record this information for analysis, e.g., the percentage of fat cells vs. regular cells in [9]. Physicians calculate this by labeling the image, and then the labeled image is discarded for perceived uselessness, recording only the summary statistic for posterity. It is simply the fraction of pixels in the ROI to the total number of pixels in the image. Mathematically, this is defined as $\bar{M} = \frac{1}{I \times J} \sum_{i=1}^{I} \sum_{j=1}^{J} M_{i,j}$. As noted, our experiments use a ratio equal to the ground-truth fraction of pixels in the segmentable class. A degenerate solution we encountered is that the sigmoid prediction mask would learn to produce a constant value near the target ratio. While this got the correct "summary statistic", it failed to meaningfully segment any of the image content.

To tackle this, we came up with a **'weak mask'** that contains information about the location and shape of the ROI. Let $X$ be the medical image, $M$ be its corresponding ground truth mask, and $M_w$ be the weak mask. It is easier to obtain a coarse localization of the ROI, typically at its center, than to accurately hand-annotate and obtain $M$. Thus for a given $X$, it is easier to obtain $M_w$ than to obtain $M$, i.e., $M_w \subset M$. Since $M$ already exists for the datasets used in this research, we obtain $M_w$ from $M$ by eroding $M$ to mimic how a radiology technician would obtain $M_w$ from $X$ - annotate only some pixels of the ROI, primarily the ones at the center.

We also want to ensure that the predictions are highly confident, so we avoid output values close to 0.5 or any other constant ratio. To achieve this, we implement a "confidence" loss function. We initialize a constant matrix $I_c$ with each element equal to 0.5 and with the same size as $M_p$. If $M_p$ is the predicted mask, the confidence loss here is defined as $L_c = \frac{1}{\text{size}(I_c)} \sum_{i,j} (I_c)^2_{i,j} - \frac{1}{\text{size}(I_c)} \sum_{i,j} (I_c - M_p)^2_{i,j}$. Thus, each element that is 0.5 accrues the maximum penalty possible of 0.25. This encourages the model to output near-0 or near-1 values across the matrix and avoids degenerate solutions. The second form of self-supervision is a **reconstruction loss**, $L_r(I, Y) = \|I - Y\|_1$, as in an autoencoder. If the network can use the intermediate representation to reconstruct the input, it has likely learned to encode structural patterns in the input image that can improve segmentation. Since the loss $L_r$ and the preceding confidence loss $L_c$ are used in all experiments, they will not be stated explicitly when their inclusion would clutter the page or diagram. We now describe the **weak supervision loss** ($L_{ws}$) between the predicted mask and the weak mask as follows: Let $M_p$ be the predicted mask, $M$ be the ground truth mask, and $M_w$ be the weak mask. We only have the weak mask and assume no knowledge of the remaining pixels. Hence, we consider only the pixels for which we know information when computing a loss. We do an element-wise multiplication of the weak mask with the predicted mask, thus zeroing out all other pixels. The loss is then $L_{ws}(M_w, M_p) = -[M_w \odot \log(M_w \odot M_p) + (1 - M_w) \log(1 - M_w \odot M_p)]$, where '$\odot$' denotes element-wise multiplication. By enforcing that the weak mask is sufficiently small for a domain expert to quickly mark the unambiguous portion of an image (i.e., 'center mass' avoiding the edges), we replicate and evaluate how much expert physician relabeling may be needed in future studies. The **statistics loss** ($L_s$) we use is simply the L1 loss between the percentage of ROI in the predicted mask and the actual mask, $L_s(M, M_p) = \|\bar{M} - \bar{M}_p\|_1$.

## 3 Results

We demonstrate our method on two datasets. The Breast Ultrasound Tumor (BUSI) dataset [1] and the KiTS23 dataset [5]. Volumetric data are treated as 2D in our tests by selecting the volume slice with the largest ROI. We use the DeepLabV3 [2] architecture with a ResNet-50 [4] backbone across all our experiments. In addition to the primary predictions from segmentation maps, we use the auxiliary output as an autoencoder, forcing it to reconstruct the input image. This helps preserve the image's 2D structure, which is useful for segmentation under weak supervision. We use IoU (Intersection over Union) as our standard evaluation metric. For both medical imagery datasets, the best performance is seen in the setting where both losses, $L_s$ and $L_{ws}$, are used. The summary statistics loss ($L_s$) appears to be more significant than the weak supervision loss ($L_{ws}$). Table 1 summarizes our results from each dataset in all the settings tested.

An example image from the KiTS dataset is shown in Fig. 2, which illustrates the benefits and risks of our strategy. The top row shows the ground-truth and weak ground-truth used in training. The bottom row shows the kidney and tumor predictions for the three combinations of $L_s$ and $L_{ws}$. Notice that the kidney

**Table 1.** IoU achieved with three weak mask sizes ([4–12%]), ablating where either one of the losses is disabled, as well as with a fully supervised scenario. The table shows that we can achieve results that are not far from those of fully supervised learning by combining the $L_s$ and $L_{ws}$ loss functions. Also to be noted is that both loss functions are necessary to achieve this result.

| Dataset | $L_s$ only | 4% | 8% | 12% | $L_{ws}$ only | Fully Supervised |
|---|---|---|---|---|---|---|
| BUSI | 36.95 | 45.70 | **48.13** | 45.29 | 26.33 | 63.15 |
| KiTS23 | 12.65 | 29.22 | **37.23** | 28.43 | 8.75 | 59.85 |

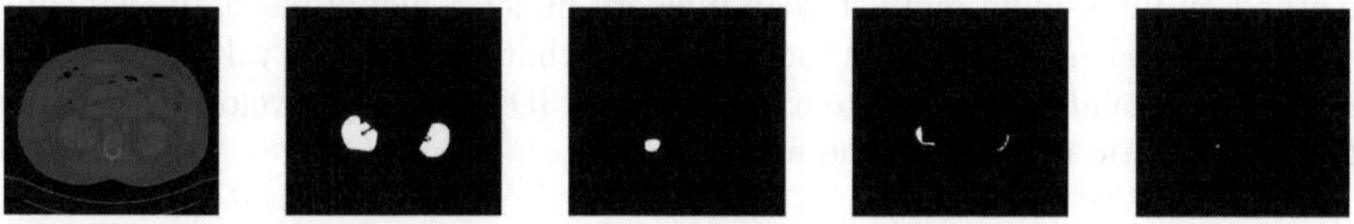

(a) Input CT scan (b) Kidney mask (c) Tumor mask (d) Weak kidney mask (e) Weak tumor mask

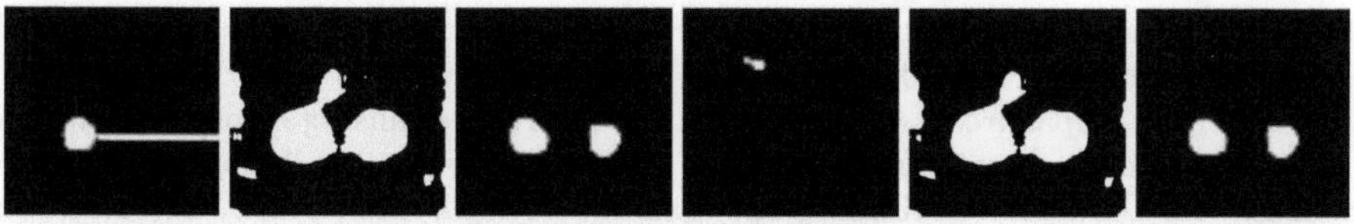

(f) Kidney: $L_s$ (g) Kidney: $L_{ws}$ (h) Kidney: $L_s, L_{ws}$ (i) Tumor: $L_s$ (j) Tumor: $L_{ws}$ (k) Tumor: $L_s, L_{ws}$

**Fig. 2.** A sample from the KiTS dataset, showing reasonably accurate segmentation masks even under highly restrictive and minimal learning signals. While the tumor prediction is less accurate, the kidney prediction is very close to the ground truth mask.

mask is produced with high accuracy despite the limited labeling, whereas the tumor prediction has devolved to predicting the kidneys, resulting in a much lower 7% IoU compared to 66% for the kidney.

At the macro scale, the image poses the problem that the mask is small over a non-visually distinct portion of the image for the tumor, which has a similar scale ratio of mask foreground to background pixels. This makes it difficult for the model to determine which actual content is intended to be segmented, especially since there is no negative signal in invalid regions to select (i.e., the weak segmentation loss $L_{ws}$ has only positive signals, with no negative signals). When combined with the reconstruction loss, this means the model can misattribute a segmentation signal to a different, more visually distinct, but similarly sized organ (in this case, the kidneys).

This result indicates that, in our current results, medical tasks with more visually distinct content will be better application areas. This is still a large time savings, as informed by our physician counterparts, especially when considering irregular cell structures that may have highly irregular borders but be visually distinct from the surrounding tissue.

## 4 Conclusion

Our results show that it is possible to obtain reasonably accurate segmentations with weak supervision without high-quality ground truth for medical image data. Our method performs best when the content of interest is visually distinct from the surrounding tissue in medical images. We successfully demonstrate our method on ultrasound and CT scan imagery under a highly restrictive labeling scenario prevalent in hospitals today, proving that there is still value in the limited labels available. We plan to expand this to 3D data, and develop this further for probabilistic masking in the future.

## References

1. Al-Dhabyani, W., Gomaa, M., Khaled, H., Fahmy, A.: Dataset of breast ultrasound images. Data Brief **28**, 104863 (2020)
2. Chen, L.C., Papandreou, G., Schroff, F., Adam, H.: Rethinking atrous convolution for semantic image segmentation (2017). https://arxiv.org/abs/1706.05587
3. Das, A., Gorade, V., Kumar, K., Chakraborty, S., Mahapatra, D., Roy, S.: Confidence-guided semi-supervised learning for generalized lesion localization in XRAY images. In: MICCAI, pp. 242–252 (2024)
4. He, K., Zhang, X., Ren, S., Sun, J.: Deep residual learning for image recognition. In: CVPR, pp. 770–778 (2016). https://doi.org/10.1109/CVPR.2016.90
5. Heller, N., et al.: The kits21 challenge: automatic segmentation of kidneys, renal tumors, and renal cysts in corticomedullary-phase CT (2023)
6. Klein, A., Jauregui, J.J., Raff, E., Henn, R.F., Hasan, S.A., Gilotra, M.: Early outcomes and complications of obese patients undergoing shoulder arthroplasty: a meta-analysis. J. Clin. Orthopaedics Trauma (2019)
7. Kolakowski, L., et al.: NEER award 2018: benzoyl peroxide effectively decreases preoperative cutibacterium acnes shoulder burden: a prospective randomized controlled trial. J. Shoulder Elbow Surgery **27**(9) (2018)
8. Rayed, M.E., Islam, S.S., Niha, S.I., Jim, J.R., Kabir, M.M., Mridha, M.: Deep learning for medical image segmentation: state-of-the-art advancements and challenges. Inf. Med. Unlocked **47**, 101504 (2024)
9. Valencia, A.P., et al.: Fatty infiltration is a prognostic marker of muscle function after rotator cuff tear. Am. J. Sports Med. **46**(9) (2018)

# SemAS - Semantic Alignment Score for XAI Applications in Clinical Decision Support

Laura Bergomi[1(✉)], Martin Michalowski[2], Szymon Wilk[3], Marc Carrier[4], Grégoire Le Gal[4], Tzu-Fei Wang[4], and Wojtek Michalowski[5]

[1] University of Pavia, Pavia, Italy
laura.bergomi01@universitadipavia.it
[2] University of Minnesota, Minneapolis, MN, USA
[3] Poznan University of Technology, Poznan, Poland
[4] The Ottawa Hospital, Ottawa, ON, Canada
[5] University of Ottawa, Ottawa, ON, Canada

**Abstract.** This paper introduces SemAS, a novel tool designed to assess the semantic alignment between clinical encounter data and textual explanations of decision support outputs, with the goal of evaluating their actual clinical usefulness for patient management. It extracts meaningful information (i.e., relations between medical concepts) and applies semantic search to relation embeddings to compute an alignment score using a cosine-similarity-based ranking scheme. We compare the performance of SemAS with that of the LLM-as-a-judge (LaaJ) paradigm and show that SemAS provides a more fine-grained, nuanced assessment of alignment, whereas LaaJ can only distinguish extreme cases of alignment, missing intermediate levels. A clinician evaluation of sample explanations largely agrees with the SemAS results, but reveals inconsistencies in identifying alignment in more nuanced cases. Overall, the preliminary analysis highlights the strength of SemAS as a dedicated, traceable scoring approach that leverages meaningful clinical information to deliver a finer-grained assessment of explanation than LaaJ, representing a significant advancement for XAI evaluation in clinical decision support.

**Keywords:** Explainable AI · Clinical Decision Support · Clinical Usefulness · Semantic Alignment Score · LLM-as-a-judge

## 1 Introduction

Clinical decision support systems (CDSS) increasingly incorporate opaque, difficult-to-interpret artificial intelligence (AI) models. Thus, the explainability of a model's output has become an important function of CDSS, as the ability to interpret these outputs can directly impact patient safety and outcomes. However, the quality of explanations is context-dependent [1], indicating that if explanations are misaligned with the underlying clinical encounter data (hereafter referred to as 'encounter data'), they may obscure rather than assist in patient management.

© The Author(s), under exclusive license to Springer Nature Switzerland AG 2027
P. Andreev et al. (Eds.): AIME 2026, LNAI 16748, pp. 17–27, 2027.
https://doi.org/10.1007/978-3-032-30710-1_3

In our earlier work [9], we introduced the concept of clinical usefulness of an explanation as "the ability of the explanation to aid subsequent decision-making of the user in a clinical setting." Building on this work, we present an advanced measure – *Semantic Alignment Score* (SemAS) – that assesses the alignment of an explanation with encounter data. We posit that for an explanation to support patient management, it must be contextualized by encounter data, as observed in [4]. Thus, SemAS plays an important role in evaluating the clinical usefulness of explanations generated by a CDSS.

Systematic reviews [15] have shown that evaluation practices of explanations remain inconsistent and rarely employ standardized, objective metrics. Many studies rely on subjective human ratings or qualitative clinician feedback, which, while valuable, are resource-intensive and difficult to scale. This gap has prompted the exploration of automated evaluation strategies, including using large language models (LLMs) as automated judges of explanation quality, known as the *LLM-as-a-judge* (LaaJ) paradigm.

In this paper, we begin by presenting a structured format for explanations based on Toulmin's argument structure. Then, we describe a dedicated computational pipeline that implements SemAS. This is followed by an evaluation study focused on assessing the alignment of explanations with encounter data. As part of this study, first, we established a reference alignment provided by physicians. Second, we used LaaJ, in which an LLM is prompted to rate the alignment of explanations with the encounter data. Third, we used SemAS to automatically quantify alignment. We discuss the evaluation study design and present its results. We conclude by outlining study limitations and highlighting the novel contributions of our work.

## 2 Related Work

One challenge in evaluating a textual explanation associated with CDSS outputs is determining its clinical usefulness using a proxy measure of its alignment with the encounter data. Comparing explanations with encounter data is not a simple n-gram (i.e., sequence of words) comparison, as the explanations are generated based on encounter data but often include additional information, such as evidence-based motivations [6]. LLMs have increasingly been employed for context-sensitive scoring and ranking beyond strict lexical matching [8]. This has led to the emergence of the LaaJ paradigm, which combines the scalability of automated evaluation with the potential for approximating expert judgment [6, 12]. LaaJ has been applied to evaluate LLM-generated text across various tasks. While offering a convenient approach for evaluating explanations, it is limited in its reproducibility, reliability, and bias [6].

Recent benchmarks utilize LLMs and a human-centered perspective to assess the clinical usefulness of textual responses. Notable examples include HealthBench [2] and MedHELM [3]. HealthBench is designed to evaluate the quality of the explanations generated by LLMs by grading open-ended responses against physician-written, conversation-specific rubrics. One of the evaluation axes is context awareness, which measures whether the model effectively incorporates contextual cues. MedHELM is a taxonomy-guided benchmark suite to assess LLM performance on medical tasks. Free-text generations are evaluated by a three-member LLM-jury ensemble against gold-standard responses in terms of accuracy, completeness, and clarity, demonstrating strong agreement with clinician ratings. However, these two benchmarks focus on alignment with end-user perceptions rather than with encounter data.

Building on our earlier work [9], this paper introduces SemAS as a dedicated, encounter-centered automated evaluation tool agnostic to medical specialty that measures the alignment of textual explanations with encounter data, enabling a more precise and traceable assessment of their clinical usefulness.

## 3 Methods

The key methodological components of our proposed method for computing SemAS are structured explanations, as described in Sect. 3.1, and the scoring algorithm, presented in Sect. 3.2.

### 3.1 Toulmin's Argument Structure

The topic of how evidence should be presented to physicians is a recurring theme in several publications on evidence-based medicine. Structured formats, such as Toulmin's argumentation framework [13], have been shown to clarify the role of evidence in clinical reasoning [14] and have been applied in decision support systems (e.g., the WOZ explanation framework embedded in the ATHENA system [10]). As part of the research described here, we presented three physicians with sample explanations in both free-text and Toulmin's structured formats, and they unanimously preferred the structured format, confirming that it is sufficiently clear and descriptive for readability and comprehension. Therefore, we adopted Toulmin's structure (hereafter referred to as the 'structured format') to organize explanations systematically, enabling physicians to quickly locate relevant clinical information rather than searching through free text. We use Toulmin's core elements – *data*, *claim*, and *warrant* – where *data* summarizes selected data items that characterize the clinical encounter, *claim* includes the recommended clinical action, and *warrant* provides a summary of the clinical knowledge that supports deriving the recommendation from the available data. Importantly, this structure is applied post-hoc: any free-text explanation, regardless of style, is mapped automatically onto Toulmin's elements.

### 3.2 Semantic Alignment Score (SemAS)

The calculation of the semantic alignment score relies on identifying meaningful information in encounter data and explanations, which are captured as relations between medical concepts. The pseudo-code for SemAS is given in Fig. 1 and the corresponding source code is publicly available on GitHub[1]. SemAS takes as input the encounter data and the explanation for a specific action from the management plan, and returns a numerical score in the range $[0, 1]$.

```
1  function semas(enc, expl):
       input  : enc: encounter data, expl: explanation
       output: score: alignment score for enc and expl
       /* Step 1: Extract relations                                    */
2      enc_relations:= extract_relations(enc)
3      expl_relations:= extract_relations(expl)
       /* Step 2: Generate embeddings for relations                    */
4      enc_rel_embeddings:= generate_embeddings(enc_relations)
5      expl_rel_embeddings:= generate_embeddings(expl_relations)
       /* Step 3: Calculate the alignment score                        */
6      search_scores:= []
7      for qry ∈ expl_rel_embeddings do
8          similarity_scores:= max(0, cosine_similarity(qry,
             enc_rel_embeddings))
9          append(search_scores, percentile(similarity_scores, 90))
10     score:= mean(search_scores)
11     return score
```

**Fig. 1.** Pseudo-code for SemAS.

The computational pipeline is composed of three main steps:

1. *Relation extraction from the encounter data and explanation* (lines 2–3). For the encounter data, relations are extracted from the entire textual content and from the data core element of the explanation. Specifically, an LLM is prompted to extract all possible relations between medical concepts, constrained by the predefined set of relation types coming from [7]: *improves, worsens, causes, is administered for, is not administered because of, reveals, is conducted to investigate*, and *indicates*. These relations capture the semantic meaning of text for the encounter data and the explanation.
2. *Generation of embeddings for extracted relations* (lines 4–5). We use the PubMedBERT base model fine-tuned with Sentence-Transformers[2], applied to each of the extracted relations.
3. *Computation of the alignment score* (lines 6–10). We adopt a semantic search approach in which the cosine similarity between the explanation's relation embeddings and the embeddings of all relations in the encounter data is computed. Then, the 90th percentile of the resulting similarity distribution is identified as the *semantic search score* and stored. Through experimentation,

[1] https://github.com/laurabergomi/SemAS.
[2] https://huggingface.co/NeuML/pubmedbert-base-embeddings.

we found that using the 90th percentile yielded more robust results than using the maximum, mean, or median. Finally, the semantic alignment score is calculated by averaging the semantic search scores for specific relations obtained from the explanation.

# 4 Evaluation

Here, we describe the evaluation study that uses structured explanations and compares two evaluation methods: LaaJ and SemAS, with reference alignment provided by physicians. We describe the experimental design in Sect. 4.1 and the clinical encounters developed for the evaluation study in Sect. 4.2. Finally, we present the study's results in Sect. 4.3.

## 4.1 Experimental Design

We followed a three-step experimental design. In each experiment, we used all clinical encounters described in Sect. 4.2. First, we established a reference alignment provided directly by physicians. Three physicians assessed the alignment between structured explanations and the corresponding encounter data using a 5-point Likert scale, ranging from 1 (no alignment) to 5 (very good alignment). The assessments were further grouped into 3 alignment classes by collapsing responses of 2, 3, and 4 (weak, moderate, and good alignment) into a single 'moderate' category. The extreme assessments (low alignment and high alignment) were preserved. Those classes were used in the subsequent analysis. Second, within the LaaJ paradigm, the OpenAI o3 model[3] was selected as the judge, chosen for its top performance on the HealthBench benchmark. The model was prompted to act as a clinical evaluator and assess how well the given explanation aligned with the encounter data, returning a numerical score directly comparable with SemAS. Third, SemAS was used to automatically quantify alignment. In the SemAS pipeline, we used GPT-4o mini[4] for relation extraction, as this task is structured rather than requiring complex interpretive reasoning. By contrast, for the LaaJ evaluation, we employed the o3 reasoning model, which is better suited for nuanced, justification-driven assessments.

We conducted statistical analyses in two stages. First, to characterize the physicians' evaluation, inter-physician agreement was quantified using pairwise Cohen's kappa, and the relationship between physicians' assessments and the results of SemAS and LaaJ was evaluated using Pearson correlations. Second, to compare evaluation methods (i.e., LaaJ vs SemAS), differences in median alignment scores across clinical encounters within the same experiment were assessed using the Friedman test, followed, when significant effects were detected, by Dunn's post-hoc test with false discovery rate correction (Benjamini-Hochberg) to identify specific pairwise differences. All analyses were conducted at a significance level of $\alpha = 0.05$. Given the limited sample size and consequently low

[3] Snapshot: o3-2025-04-16.

[4] Snapshot: gpt-4o-mini-2024-07-18.

statistical power to validate significance, we complemented these inferential tests with a descriptive statistical analysis to better characterize patterns in the data. Finally, to deepen our understanding of the results, we leveraged the intrinsic traceability of the SemAS computational pipeline to examine how individual relations aligned between the explanations and the encounter data.

### 4.2 Data

Four clinical encounters were used to evaluate the SemAS tool and the LaaJ responses. These encounters represent realistic patient cases observed by physicians in clinical practice, but use simulated data. To represent and report encounter data, we adopted the general format of a structured clinical note [5]. General descriptions of the encounters, along with their a priori expected level of alignment with the explanations, are provided in Table 1.

The encounters were chosen to elicit different levels of alignment (i.e., high, moderate, low), with considered explanations. Those explanations describe actions from the treatment plan developed for Encounter 1 – prescribing apixaban, nitrostat, and pantoprazole, scheduling a follow-up visit, and encouraging physical activity – and refer to Encounter 1 data.

**Table 1.** Clinical encounters and their a priori expected level of alignment with the explanations: *High* – explanation pertains to encounter data; *Moderate* – explanation partially overlaps with encounter data; *Low* – explanation is completely misaligned with encounter data.

| Encounter type | Description | Expected alignment |
|---|---|---|
| Encounter 1 (CAD/DVT/GIB) | A 68-year-old male patient with stable coronary artery disease (CAD), deep vein thrombosis (DVT), and upper gastrointestinal bleeding (GIB). | *High* |
| Encounter 2 (SD/CAD/DVT) | An 85-year-old male patient with seizure disorder (SD), stable coronary artery disease (CAD), and deep vein thrombosis (DVT). | *Moderate* |
| Encounter 3 (Afib/CKD/HTN) | A 70-year-old male patient with persistent, highly symptomatic atrial fibrillation (AFib), chronic kidney disease (CKD), and hypertension (HTN). | *Moderate* |
| Encounter 4 (AE) | An 8-year-old female patient with acute asthma exacerbation (AE). | *Low* |

### 4.3 Results

Physicians' evaluation of explanation alignment with the encounter data is reported in Fig. 2. To enable easier comparison with SemAS and LaaJ results, their ratings were rescaled to [0, 1] range. For all physicians, Encounter 1 received the highest alignment ratings, except for nitrostat and physical activity for participant 2. In contrast, Encounter 4 was consistently rated the lowest in alignment across all explanations. Encounters 2 and 3 received intermediate to low ratings, with some variability across explanations and participants.

Overall agreement among physicians was variable, as indicated by pairwise Cohen's kappa: participants 1–2 = 0.595 (weak agreement), 2–3 = 0.345 (minimal agreement), and 1–3 = 0.704 (moderate agreement). Nevertheless, all physicians consistently agreed on cases with expected high alignment (Encounter 1) and on cases with no alignment (Encounter 4).

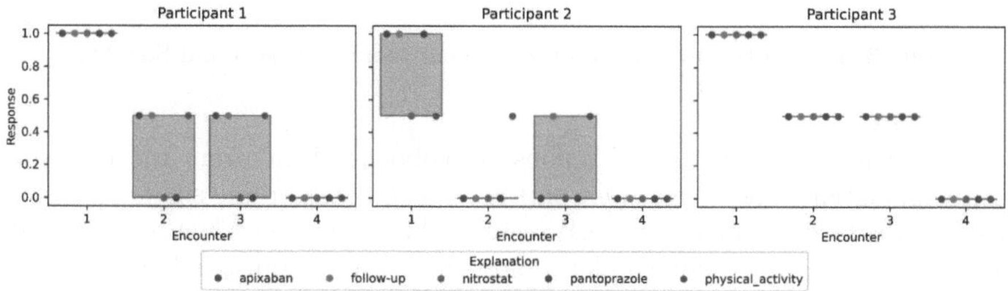


**Fig. 2.** Physicians' responses to explanation alignment with each encounter.

Figure 3 illustrates the distribution of alignment scores generated by LaaJ and SemAS via box plots and rescaled to [0, 1]. This distribution reveals outliers in most encounters, which are primarily related to physical activity and nitrostat explanations. Across all experiments, Encounter 1 showed the highest semantic alignment, Encounters 2 and 3 had lower but similar mean scores, and Encounter 4 had the lowest score, consistent with the experimental setup. Specifically, LaaJ distinguished only between high and low alignment, failing to recognize the moderate alignment level. In contrast, SemAS successfully identified three levels of alignment. Furthermore, physicians' evaluations were more consistent with SemAS than with LaaJ results, except for participant 2. Pearson correlation coefficients between physicians' ratings and LaaJ and SemAS, respectively, were 0.827 and 0.837 for participant 1, 0.847 and 0.833 for participant 2, and 0.794 and 0.864 for participant 3, with all $p$-values $< 0.0001$.

According to the Friedman test, LaaJ and SemAS evaluations yielded $p$-values $< 0.05$. Dunn's post-hoc test confirmed a significant difference in alignment between Encounter 1 and 4, as these encounters represent opposite ends of the alignment spectrum. For LaaJ, Encounter 1 also differed significantly from both Encounters 2 and 3. For SemAS, no other pairwise comparisons were significant because the limited sample size did not allow detection of small differences. Nevertheless, the significant difference in alignment between Encounters 1 and 4 demonstrates that SemAS reliably distinguishes strong from no alignment.

A key advantage of SemAS is the score's intrinsic traceability. Specifically, for each relation from the explanation, the similarity with all encounter relations can be examined. An illustrative example is shown in Fig. 4, which specifically presents this for the relation "long-term warfarin use → is administered

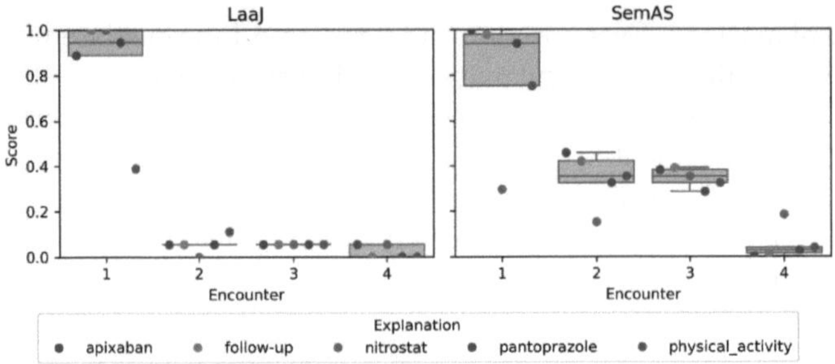


**Fig. 3.** Box plots for explanation alignment scores for LaaJ and SemAS.

for → secondary prevention of venous thromboembolism" from the follow-up visit explanation. The scatter plot on the left shows the cosine similarity scores between the target explanation relation and all relations in each encounter. Blue dots indicate the maximum similarity scores, with the corresponding encounter relation shown on the right, while red dots represent the 90th percentile, used as a representative measure for each explanation relation. Although Encounters 2 and 3, respectively, include "thromboprophylaxis" and "prevention of thromboembolism" – both semantically close to Encounter 1's "prevention of recurrent venous thromboembolism" – their 90th percentiles (0.57 and 0.44, respectively) reveal weaker overall similarity to the target follow-up visit relation compared to Encounter 1 (0.74). This is because the remaining relations in those encounters are less similar, reducing the overall alignment. Finally, Encounter 4 shows very low similarity across all relations, resulting in markedly poor alignment (0.13).

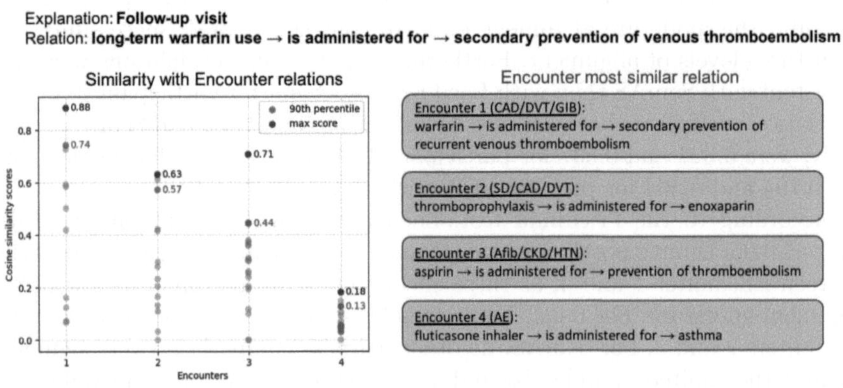


**Fig. 4.** Inspection of the SemAS computation, highlighting the similarity between individual encounter relations and a given explanation relation. The 90th percentile of the similarity distribution (red dots) is the representative score of the explanation relation. The most similar relation for each encounter (blue dots) is shown on the right. (Color figure online)

This relation-level inspection provides local traceability by directly linking each component of the SemAS score to specific semantic matches and by identifying which explanation relations drive higher or lower alignment.

# 5 Discussion and Future Work

The alignment of explanations with encounter data is a crucial proxy for assessing their clinical usefulness in patient management. In this paper, we propose SemAS to automatically evaluate the degree to which explanations align with encounter data. We demonstrate the advantage of a dedicated score to assessing this alignment over existing approaches, such as LaaJ. While we use an LLM to extract relations, it is tasked with obtaining very specific information and is better focused than when used as a judge to evaluate alignment.

A key strength of SemAS lies in its use of meaningful (i.e., knowledge-driven) information, combined with a well-defined computational pipeline, which provides intrinsic traceability. Specifically, for each relation in the explanation, the corresponding cosine similarity with the encounter relations can be inspected. Qualitative inspection of these similarities shows that encounters associated with similar presentations may still exhibit varying degrees of alignment, depending on the presence of supporting, semantically related relations in the explanation. As we also observed in the physicians' evaluation, identifying explanation–encounter data pairs with strong or no alignment is straightforward, and SemAS performs this task effectively. For more nuanced situations (i.e., Encounters 2 and 3), the inconsistencies in physicians' evaluations highlighted the need for careful attention. SemAS can identify this "grey area alignment", directing the physician's attention to it, and supporting a subsequent assessment of partial or ambiguous alignment between an explanation and encounter data.

While the experimental results are very encouraging, this study has several limitations. First, the evaluation considered a limited number of clinical encounters and explanations, which restricts the generalizability of the results. While the encounters covered a wide range of patient cases and possible alignments, increasing the sample size would enable a more thorough assessment. Furthermore, only a single LLM (o3) was used in the LaaJ paradigm, as this study is intended as a proof-of-concept for SemAS; an ensemble of models might improve LaaJ's performance. Additionally, SemAS produces raw scores, while categorical values might be easier for physicians to interpret. Finally, evaluating only a single structured format prevented us from assessing how other formats might affect SemAS.

This work makes an important contribution to research on assessing the quality of explanations in terms of their alignment with encounter data, an important dimension for quantifying explanations' clinical usefulness. Currently, we are working with our clinical partners to establish thresholds for categorizing SemAS values and to increase the number of encounters and explanations, with external validation by a broader panel of physicians. We are studying alternatives to Toulmin's structure, such as those based on HL7 FHIR [11], to assess SemAS's sensitivity to changes in structured formats. We are continuously evaluating the ability of new LLM models to extract relations from text and integrating the best-performing ones into the pipeline.

**Acknowledgments.** The first author acknowledges funding support provided by the Italian project PRIN PNRR 2022 InXAID - Interaction with eXplainable Artificial Intelligence in (medical) Decision-making, CUP: H53D23008090001, funded by the European Union - Next Generation EU.

**Disclosure of Interests.** The authors have no competing interests to declare that are relevant to the content of this article.

## References

1. Amann, J., Vetter, D., Blomberg, S.N., et al.: To explain or not to explain?-Artificial intelligence explainability in clinical decision support systems. PLOS Digit. Health **1**(2) (2022). https://doi.org/10.1371/journal.pdig.0000016
2. Arora, R.K., Wei, J., Hicks, R.S., et al.: HealthBench: evaluating large language models towards improved human health (2025). https://doi.org/10.48550/arXiv.2505.08775, http://arxiv.org/abs/2505.08775
3. Bedi, S., Cui, H., Fuentes, M., et al.: MedHELM: holistic evaluation of large language models for medical tasks (2025). https://doi.org/10.48550/arXiv.2505.23802
4. Bruckert, S., Finzel, B., Schmid, U.: The next generation of medical decision support: a roadmap toward transparent expert companions. Front. Artif. Intell. **3**, 507973 (2020). https://doi.org/10.3389/frai.2020.507973
5. Ebbers, T., Kool, R.B., Smeele, L.E., et al.: The impact of structured and standardized documentation on documentation quality; a multicenter, retrospective study. J. Med. Syst. **46**(3), 46 (2022)
6. Gu, J., Jiang, X., Shi, Z., et al.: A survey on LLM-as-a-judge (2025). https://doi.org/10.48550/arXiv.2411.15594, http://arxiv.org/abs/2411.15594
7. Islamaj Doğan, R., Névéol, A., Lu, Z.: A context-blocks model for identifying clinical relationships in patient records. BMC Bioinformat. **12**, S3 (2011). https://doi.org/10.1186/1471-2105-12-S3-S3, https://www.ncbi.nlm.nih.gov/pmc/articles/PMC3111589/
8. Li, D., Jiang, B., Huang, L., et al.: From generation to judgment: opportunities and challenges of LLM-as-a-judge (2025). https://doi.org/10.48550/arXiv.2411.16594, http://arxiv.org/abs/2411.16594
9. Michalowski, M., Wilk, S., Bauer, J.M., et al.: CUE-x: A framework for the automatic evaluation of clinical usefulness of explanations for the multimorbidity problem. In: Bellazzi, R., Juarez Herrero, J.M., Sacchi, L., Zupan, B. (eds.) Artificial Intelligence in Medicine, pp. 293–303. Springer Nature Switzerland (2025). https://doi.org/10.1007/978-3-031-95838-0-29
10. Shankar, R.D., Tu, S.W., Musen, M.A.: Medical arguments in an automated health care system. In: Argumentation for Consumers of Healthcare, AAAI Spring Symposium Series. pp. 96–104. AAAI Press, Stanford, CA (2006)
11. Strasberg, H.R., Rhodes, B., Fiol, G.D., et al.: Contemporary clinical decision support standards using health level seven international fast healthcare interoperability resources. J. Am. Med. Inform. Assoc. **28**(8), 1796–1806 (2021). https://doi.org/10.1093/jamia/ocab070

12. Thakur, A.S., Choudhary, K., Ramayapally, V.S., et al.: Judging the judges: evaluating alignment and vulnerabilities in LLMs-as-judges (2025). https://doi.org/10.48550/arXiv.2406.12624, http://arxiv.org/abs/2406.12624
13. Toulmin, S.E.: The Uses of Argument, 2nd edn. Cambridge University Press (2003)
14. Upshur, R.E.G., Colak, E.: Argumentation and evidence. Theor. Med. Bioeth. **24**(4), 283–299 (2003). https://doi.org/10.1023/a:1026006801902
15. Xu, Q., Xie, W., Liao, B., et al.: Interpretability of clinical decision support systems based on artificial intelligence from technological and medical perspective: a systematic review. J. Healthc. Eng. **2023**, 9919269 (2023). https://doi.org/10.1155/2023/9919269

# Addressing Incomplete Data in Survival and Quality of Life Prediction: A Pancreatic Cancer Case Study

Aneta Lisowska[1,2(✉)], Floris den Hengst[1], Syed Ihtesham Hussain Shah[1], Annette ten Teije[1], Omar Bohoudi[3], Pauline Vissers[4,5], Mahsoem Ali[2], Laura Leeuwenburgh[2,4], Martijn Stommel[5], Amber Lamoré[2,6], Inez Verpalen[2,6], Marjolein Homs[7], Bas Groot Koerkamp[7], Judith De Vos-Geelen[8], Sven Mieog[9], Jeanin E. Van Hooft[9], Lois Daamen[10], Vincent E. De Meijer[11], Hanneke Wilmink[2,12], Hanneke van Laarhoven[2,12], Marc Besselink[2,13], Geert Kazemier[2,14], and for the Dutch Pancreatic Cancer Group

[1] Vrije Universiteit, Department Computer Science, Amsterdam, The Netherlands
[2] Cancer Center Amsterdam, Amsterdam, The Netherlands
a.j.lisowska@vu.nl
[3] Amsterdam UMC, loc. VU, Department Radiotherapy, Amsterdam, The Netherlands
[4] IKNL, Department Research and Development, Utrecht, The Netherlands
[5] Radboud UMC, Department Surgery, Nijmegen, Netherlands
[6] Amsterdam UMC, loc. UvA, Department Radiology, Amsterdam, The Netherlands
[7] Erasmus MC, Rotterdam, The Netherlands
[8] Maastricht UMC, Maastricht UMC, Department Internal Medicine, GROW Research Institute for Oncology and Reproduction, Maastricht, The Netherlands
[9] Leiden UMC, Department Gastroenterology and Hepatology, Leiden, The Netherlands
[10] Utrecht UMC, Division of Imaging and Oncology, Utrecht, The Netherlands
[11] University of Groningen and UMC, Department Surgery, Groningen, The Netherlands
[12] Amsterdam UMC, loc. UvA, Department Medical Oncology, Amsterdam, The Netherlands
[13] Amsterdam UMC, loc. UvA, Department Surgery, Amsterdam, The Netherlands
[14] Amsterdam UMC, loc. VU, Department Surgery, Amsterdam, The Netherlands

**Abstract.** Models that predict the survival and quality of life (QoL) in patients with malignancies can support prognostic counselling and patient-centered evaluation of disease trajectories.

Challenges in the development of such models include incomplete data in real-world registries, including missing baseline measurements and irregular, sparse availability of longitudinal QoL outcomes during treatment. These limitations complicate the incorporation of QoL into survival prediction and the reliable modeling of QoL over time.

We address these limitations with a novel framework to predict survival and quality of life in the face of sparse data. The framework consists of a regularized missingness-avoiding random survival forest (MA-RSF)

© The Author(s), under exclusive license to Springer Nature Switzerland AG 2027
P. Andreev et al. (Eds.): AIME 2026, LNAI 16748, pp. 28–37, 2027.
https://doi.org/10.1007/978-3-032-30710-1_4

for survival prediction, and a conditional diffusion-based approach to predict QoL at various follow-up intervals.

We apply the approach to a pancreatic cancer use-case, and evaluate it on a nationwide Dutch cohort.

We find that our approach maintains high predictive accuracy (C-index 0.77) for survival prediction and minimizes reliance on sparse pre-treatment data, including QoL PROMs. In addition, we demonstrate that the QoL prediction expressed as the Static-Dynamic diffusion architecture reduces trajectory prediction error (RMSE) at key follow-up intervals compared to standard conditional generation (e.g. 12.9 vs 14.0 RMSE at 7 months).

The proposed framework facilitates the prediction of survival and QoL outcomes in settings characterized by incomplete data and could enhance prognostic counseling in patients with malignancies, including pancreatic cancer.

**Keywords:** Quality of Life · Survival Analysis · Generative Diffusion Models · Missing Data/Missingness-Avoidance · Pancreatic Cancer

## 1 Introduction

Shared decision-making for patients with poor prognosis involves a consideration of both therapeutic goals such as extending survival and palliative goals such as preserving quality of life (QoL). For example, the median overall survival duration for patients diagnosed with pancreatic ductal adenocarcinoma (PDAC) is 4 months and 5-year survival is as low as 4%, and QoL is an important factor in shared decision-making [5]. Additionally, QoL has been established as an independent predictor of overall survival [6]. QoL and its relation with survival are therefore becoming increasingly important in shared decision-making.

Treatment planning in settings with a poor survival outlook is characterized by weighing potential survival benefits of interventions against their associated impact on QoL [9]. Prognostic survival models have been developed to assist with patient counselling with time-to-event analysis at Concordance Index (C-index) values in the range of 0.70–0.73 for overall survival [2,4], and have demonstrated improved accuracy over traditional staging systems. However, these models often do not incorporate QoL in their predictions, limiting their usefulness for holistic shared decision-making.

QoL is typically quantified using patient-reported outcome measures (PROMs) that are obtained directly from patients via questionnaires. Gold standards for QoL PROMs have long been established for a multitude of conditions [1]. However, as these instruments rely on active patient participation, they suffer from limited longitudinal availability. Specifically, patients can be enrolled at various phases of their care journey which results in missing pre-treatment QoL measures, and measures at irregular intervals during treatment.

These characteristics are illustrated by the Dutch Pancreatic Cancer Project (PACAP), which collects clinical data and patient-reported outcome measures

(PROMs) from a multicenter cohort of patients with PDAC [7]. The resulting sparsity at both the onset of and during treatment provides technical challenges for standard prognostic modeling techniques.

In this paper, we propose a joint modeling framework to predict survival and QoL in the face of incomplete data. The framework integrates two components:

**Missingness-Aware Random Survival Forest (MA-RSF)** which employs RSF-specific regularization during node splitting to minimize reliance on features with high missingness. [1]

**Static-Dynamic Architecture** a ConDOR [3] adaptation that explicitly disentangles conditioning factors, restricting the Regional Diffusion Model (RDM) to time-invariant patient covariates and the Temporal Diffusion Model (TDM) to dynamic treatment impulses, to better capture treatment-associated temporal patterns in the QoL progression.

We validate our framework through a clinical case study. Results demonstrate that MA-RSF maintains high survival prediction accuracy with lower reliance on sparse pre-treatment data. Furthermore, the Static-Dynamic diffusion architecture significantly reduces QoL trajectory prediction error (RMSE) at key follow-up intervals compared to static conditional generation.

## 2 Methodology

This section details our contributions to the challenge of predicting survival and QoL outcomes in the face of data incompleteness. First, we address missing explanatory variables prior to treatment with a random forest robust to missing data, including QoL, clinical, and demographics data. Second, we address missing QoL data during the treatment with a generative conditional diffusion model.

### 2.1 Missingness Avoidance Random Survival Forest

We address missing pretreatment explanatory variables for survival prediction by extending random survival forests (RSF) with techniques from the missingness-avoidance (MA) paradigm, motivated by Stempfle et al. who argued that existing approaches, such as mean imputation or missingness indicators, often introduce bias or obscure model interpretability [8]. We first provide a high-level overview of RSF and then describe the extension to the MA framework.

The RSF algorithm constructs an ensemble of de-correlated decision trees, where each tree is grown through a recursive process of node splitting. At every node, the algorithm evaluates a subset of candidate features to find the optimal data partition that maximizes the survival difference between the resulting child nodes. In traditional RSF, this is achieved via a log-rank split criterion $L_{\mathrm{LR}}(j, \tau)$ for feature $j$ and split thresholds $\tau$, which calculates a test statistic to identify the feature and threshold that best separate distinct survival distributions for the data subset associated with the current node.

[1] We release the open-source Python package https://pypi.org/project/masurvival/.

We adopt the MA paradigm to survival analysis by extending its log-rank split criterion with an additional term to minimize reliance on sparse pretreatment variables. Our approach penalizes the use of missing data in its splitting criterion by using what we refer to as the missingness-aware log-rank criterion:

$$L_{\mathrm{MALR}}(j, \tau) := L_{\mathrm{LR}}(j, \tau) - \alpha N_{\mathrm{missing},j} \tag{1}$$

where $j$ and $\tau$ are as before, and $N_{\mathrm{missing},j}$ the number of samples in the current node with a missing value for feature $j$, and $\alpha \geq 0$ a regularization hyperparameter to control the penalty strength. The algorithm identifies a model within the Rashomon set that optimizes predictive accuracy while minimizing reliance on sparse variables. While this missingness-avoiding regularization mitigates instability from Missing At Random patterns, and $\alpha$ ensures that informative Missing Not At Random predictors are retained if their utility outweighs the risk to model reliability.

## 2.2 Longitudinal QoL Prediction with Conditional Diffusion

Longitudinal QoL prediction is complicated by non-linear dynamics arising from the stochastic interplay between disease progression and interventions. Conventional imputation, such as linear interpolation, fails to characterize these fluctuations, while standard forecasting architectures like RNNs and Transformers are typically optimized for discrete, equidistant sequences. In clinical settings, assessments often occur at irregular intervals. To address the resulting temporal sparsity, we utilize ConDOR (Conditional Diffusion with Ordinal Regression) [3].

Our framework instantiates ConDOR as a two-stage conditional diffusion model and introduces a static–dynamic decomposition. A first denoising network (RDM) estimates the pretreatment QoL state $x_0$ at $t = 0$:, $x_0 = g_\phi(s)$, based on static covariates $s$ (e.g., demographics and pretreatment laboratory measurements), providing a patient-specific initialization. A second denoising network (TDM) models longitudinal state updates from $t$ to $t+1$: $x_{t+1} = x_t + f_\theta(x_t, t, s, u_t)$, where $u_t$ represents time-varying treatment factors at time $t$, including intervention type (e.g., surgery/systemic therapy), treatment initiation indicators, and elapsed time since treatment start. Therefore, Stage 2 learns how treatment exposure modifies the QoL trajectory over time, conditional on the patient baseline context $s$. The two-stage design separates (i) baseline heterogeneity across patients (captured by $g_\phi(s)$) from (ii) treatment-driven temporal evolution (captured by $f_\theta(x_t, t, s, u_t)$), enabling generation of individualized QoL trajectories under different intervention schedules.

Unlike the original ConDOR model, we drop the cohort-level priors and rely solely on individual trajectories to prevent sparse-data averages from smoothing over acute changes stemming from interventions.

## 3 Experimental Setup

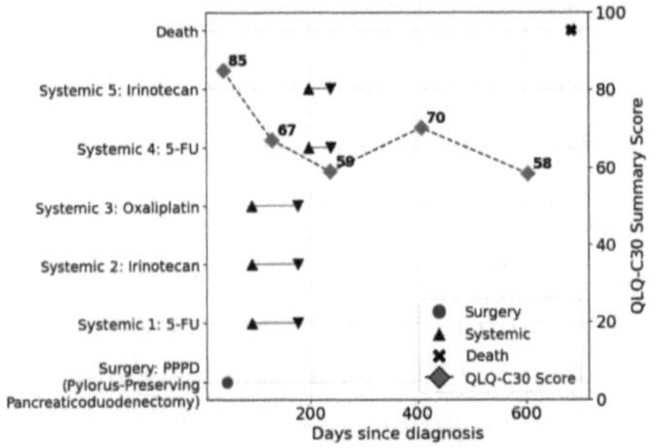


(a) **Example patient records.** The gray squares represent time points at which the QoL PROM was completed by the patient (from PACAP). Treatment time points, here surgery and systemic therapy, are taken from the NCR registry.

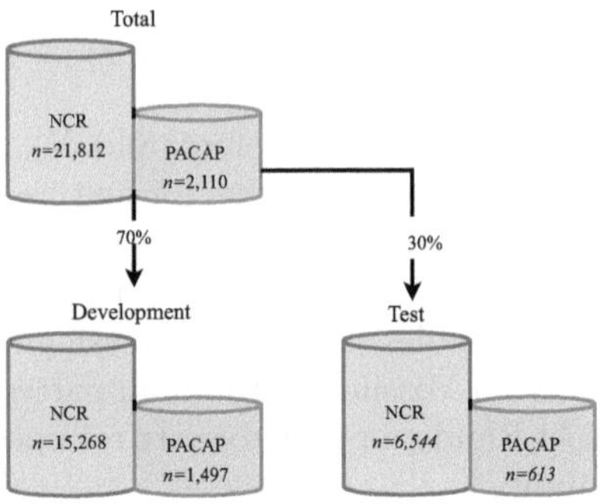


(b) **Development and test splits.** PACAP is a subset of NCR, $n$ the number of patients.

**Fig. 1.** Visualisation of NCR registry joined with PACAP self-reported QoL data.

A retrospective cohort study is used with data from two merged national Dutch sources. The study period includes patients diagnosed between January 1, 2015, and December 31, 2024. Clinical, demographic, and tumor-related data are extracted from the Netherlands Cancer Registry (NCR), a comprehensive, nationwide population-based registry. Longitudinal QoL PROMs are obtained from PACAP [10] using the EORTC QLQ-C30 questionnaire [1].

The PACAP cohort represents a 9.8% subset of the full NCR registry (See Fig. 1b). Merging these datasets enables the integration of static pretreatment clinical variables with dynamic longitudinal QoL trajectories as depicted in Fig. 1a. The 2,110 patients in the PACAP development set provide a total of 5,441 PROMs throughout their care trajectory, with a mean of 3.6 responses per patient (median 3, max 15). Both selection bias (due to informed consent for PACAP-PROMS) and response bias make it unlikely that the PACAP-PROMS cohort is representative of the entire NCR cohort. The study uses two outcomes defined as follows:

**Overall Survival (OS)**: the time from diagnosis to death from any cause,
**Quality of Life (QoL)**: the EORTC QLQ-C30 Summary Score [1], calculated following EORTC guidelines as the mean of 13 component scales, with symptom scales reversed so that higher scores indicate better QoL consistently.

Models were trained to predict these outcomes using 5-fold cross-validation on the development set. For MA-RSF, we additionally performed a 10-fold parameter search, identifying $\alpha = 0.1$ as the optimal regularization value. Performance was evaluated via the C-index and RMSE on held-out test sets stratified by cohort (PACAP vs. Full NCR) to assess generalization to broader populations.

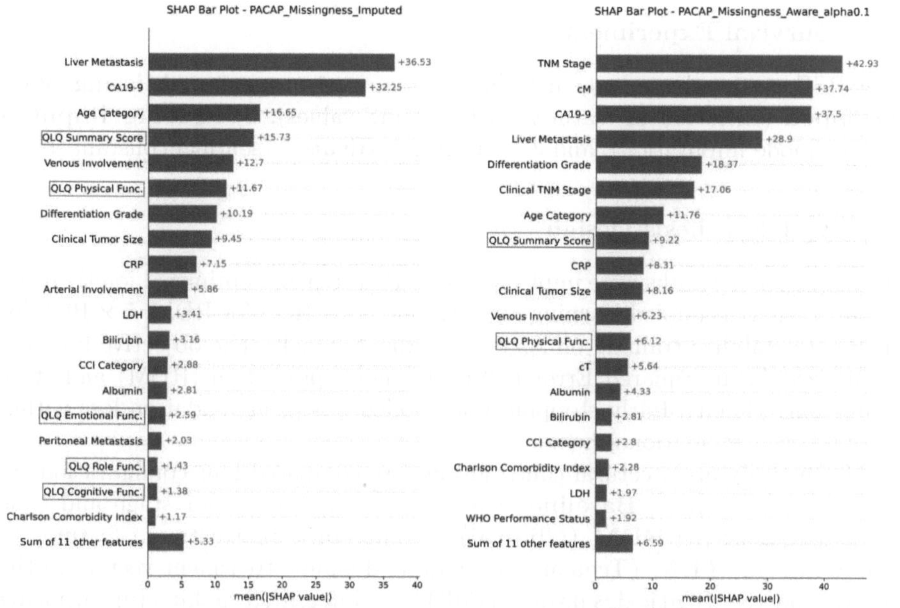


(a) RSF (Missing Imputed), $\alpha = 0.0$ (b) MA-RSF, $\alpha = 0.1$

**Fig. 2.** Feature importance (SHAP) comparison between standard imputation and missingness-avoiding regularization ($\alpha = 0.1$) on the PACAP test set.

### 3.1 Data Pre-processing and Feature Representation

For the MA-RSF survival prediction model, static pretreatment variables captured at diagnosis were included, including demographics (age, sex), WHO performance status, comorbidities (Charlson Comorbidity Index), laboratory values (e.g., CA19-9, Albumin, CRP), and tumor characteristics (e.g. metastasis status, vasculature involvement). The functioning and summary scores of the QLQ-C30 were included where available. In the PACAP development cohort, 9% lacked valid PROMs. Baseline PROMs were defined as the first valid PROM prior to treatment initiation, or the first valid PROM overall for untreated patients. Baseline PROMs were available for 47% of patients and occurred on average 20 d after diagnosis. Features were organized for the static-dynamic ConDOR model for QoL trajectory prediction as follows. Both models were conditioned on time since diagnosis (continuous) and clinical tumor stage (ordinal). For the *static* diffusion model that predicts pretreatment baselines, time-invariant features including age, sex, season of diagnosis, CCI, and pretreatment laboratory values were used. For the *dynamic* model a time-dependent vector capturing treatment events was used. Both surgery and systemic therapy were encoded using: 1) a binary feature indicating treatment occurrence; 2) a *cumulative status* (post-event binary flag); and 3) a *time-since-event* counter to model non-linear recovery.

### 3.2 Survival Experiment Design

MA-RSF was evaluated against three common strategies: 1) **Missing Vars Dropped** (exclusion of features with missing values); 2) **Missing Imputed** (mean/mode imputation); and 3) **Missing Indicated** (sentinel constant -999).

### 3.3 QoL Synthesis Design

The diffusion networks were implemented in PyTorch and optimized jointly using Adam with a decoupled learning rate strategy ($1 \times 10^{-3}$ for RDM; $5 \times 10^{-4}$ for TDM) to stabilize training on sparse treatment signals. The objective function minimized Mean Squared Error (MSE) for noise prediction (RDM) and state transitions (TDM). Early stopping was applied based on validation loss within a 5-fold cross-validation scheme.[2]

To quantify architectural contributions, we compared four configurations in an *ablation study*: (i) **Baseline**, conditioned solely on tumor stage and time since diagnosis; (ii) **RDM (Clinical)**, adding static pretreatment features to the RDM; (iii) **TDM (Treatment)**, adding dynamic treatment vectors to the TDM; and (iv) **Static-Dynamic (Full)**, the integrated architecture utilizing demographic/clinical static features and dynamic treatment impulses.

**Table 1.** Survival Prediction Performance on the test set (C-index ↑ [std]). The best and second-best performance within each training–test set block are highlighted.

| Training set | Missingness handling strategy | PACAP | NCR |
|---|---|---|---|
| PACAP | Missing Vars Dropped | 0.691 [0.002] | 0.664 [0.003] |
| | Missing Imputed | 0.705 [0.002] | 0.696 [0.005] |
| | Missing Indicated | 0.704 [0.002] | 0.693 [0.005] |
| | Missing Avoiding | 0.706 [0.002] | 0.701 [0.003] |
| | Missing Vars Dropped + Treatment | 0.760 [0.002] | 0.731 [0.002] |
| | Missing Imputed + Treatment | 0.760 [0.002] | 0.749 [0.006] |
| | Missing Indicated + Treatment | 0.760 [0.002] | 0.740 [0.009] |
| | Missing Avoiding + Treatment | 0.761 [0.002] | 0.748 [0.005] |
| NCR | Missing Vars Dropped | 0.701 [0.003] | 0.683 [0.001] |
| | Missing Imputed | 0.729 [0.002] | 0.744 [0.000] |
| | Missing Indicated | 0.727 [0.002] | 0.743 [0.001] |
| | Missing Avoiding | 0.731 [0.002] | 0.744 [0.001] |
| | Missing Vars Dropped + Treatment | 0.769 [0.001] | 0.730 [0.001] |
| | Missing Imputed + Treatment | 0.775 [0.002] | 0.772 [0.001] |
| | Missing Indicated + Treatment | 0.774 [0.001] | 0.770 [0.001] |
| | Missing Avoiding + Treatment | 0.775 [0.001] | 0.770 [0.001] |

[2] https://github.com/anli66/panc-surv-qol.

# 4 Results

## 4.1 Overall Survival

We validated the effectiveness of the MA penalty by analyzing feature importance (SHAP) distributions (Fig. 2). In the unregularized model ($\alpha = 0.0$), the QLQ Summary Score ranked as the fourth most important predictor. Conversely, the MA-RSF ($\alpha = 0.1$) successfully deprioritized this frequently missing variable, dropping it to eighth place while maintaining predictive performance. Notably, the importance of variables with low missingness (e.g., arterial involvement, 3.5% missing) was also reduced, indicating the regularization successfully isolates the most robust core predictors.

Table 1 reports predictive performance. As anticipated, dropping incomplete variables significantly degraded performance (paired Student's $t$-test on aligned fold-specific C-index $p < 0.01$). While standard imputation performed comparably to the missingness-aware (MA) approach within the training distribution (PACAP), the MA-RSF showed more robust generalization to the broader NCR cohort, achieving competitive accuracy while reducing reliance on sparsely observed inputs. However, this advantage diminishes when treatment variables are introduced or when the model is trained on the full NCR registry. The differences between MA-RSF and Imputation are not significant.

## 4.2 Longitudinal QoL

Ablation results (Table 2) confirm the efficacy of the Static-Dynamic architecture. While paired Student's t-tests showed no significant differences in baseline ($T_0$) prediction errors, the S-D configuration (RDM Clinical + TDM Treatment) achieved the lowest overall trajectory error. This full model significantly outperformed the RDM (Clin.) ($p = 0.03$) and demonstrated a borderline-significant improvement over the baseline ($p = 0.05$).

For the PACAP study, questionnaires are sent every three months; our analysis focused on months in the test set where at least 100 patients responded. Monthly RMSEs were obtained from 5-fold CV on the Black Envelope set, and

**Table 2.** QoL Synthesis Ablation (RMSE).

| **Config.** | $T_0$ | **Full** |
|---|---|---|
| Baseline | 25.60 | 12.85 |
| RDM (Clin.) | 25.10 | 13.50 |
| TDM (Treat.) | 26.37 | 12.58 |
| Full Model (S-D) | 26.26 | 12.20 |

**Table 3.** Monthly RMSE: Baseline vs. S-D

| Month | Base. | S-D | $p$-val |
|---|---|---|---|
| 1 | 25.99 | 24.53 | 0.149 |
| 3 | 14.07 | 13.97 | 0.711 |
| 4 | 13.41 | 12.90 | 0.005** |
| 6 | 14.18 | 13.80 | 0.014* |
| 7 | 14.01 | 12.92 | 0.006** |
| 10 | 13.15 | 11.89 | 0.052 |
| 13 | 11.93 | 10.83 | 0.031* |

Baseline vs. Static–Dynamic (S-D) differences were assessed with paired two-sided $t$-tests on fold-matched RMSEs ($n$=5 folds), since errors are not independent across models. Table 3 shows significant improvements ($p < 0.05$) at 4, 6, 7, and 13 months. Across-month $p$-values are correlated and should be interpreted as exploratory.

## 5 Discussion and Conclusion

This study addresses the challenges of baseline feature missingness and longitudinal sparsity in oncological survival and QoL modeling. Our results demonstrate that incorporating missingness-avoidance regularization into survival forests (MA-RSF) effectively shifts model reliance away from sparse baseline variables toward robust clinical variables. Unlike standard imputation, which risks introducing bias when data are structurally missing (e.g., patients referred late in the care pathway), the MA approach learns a valid decision policy within the Rashomon set that prioritizes observable features. Consequently, the model maintains generalization performance across the broader NCR population where pretreatment QoL is frequently unavailable.

For longitudinal prediction, the proposed Static-Dynamic adaptation of ConDOR offers a methodological advancement over static conditional diffusion. By architecturally disentangling static patient phenotypes from dynamic treatment impulses, the model is constrained to learn state transitions as responses to interventions rather than demographic correlations. This yielded improvements in RMSE at 4, 7, and 10 months—critical windows for evaluating treatment efficacy. However, the absolute RMSE values remain relatively high, reflecting the inherent stochasticity of self-reported well-being and the complexity of unmeasured confounders in registry data.

*Limitations:* Our validation is restricted to a Dutch cohort, which may limit generalizability to healthcare systems with different care pathways. In addition, the PACAP-PROMS cohort is subject to both selection bias and response bias, which together reduce the representativeness of the QoL trajectory relative to the full population of patients. Our current framework also relies on pretreatment clinical variables that are updated only by treatment events for the primary tumor and does not incorporate time-varying clinical biomarkers (e.g., longitudinal CA19-9 or albumin), which could provide important physiological context to further refine trajectory predictions.

*Conclusion:* We present a robust pipeline for PDAC prognosis that navigates the irregularities of real-world clinical data. By harmonizing missingness-avoidant survival analysis with conditional QoL trajectory generation, this framework moves closer to enabling personalized, holistic risk assessment in oncology.

**Declaration of AI Assistance Technologies During Manuscript Preparation.** The authors used Google Gemini for AI Activity Class 1 and Cursor for AI Activity Classes 6 and 7. The authors reviewed the results and take full responsibility for the contents of the manuscript.

**Acknowledgments.** This work has been partly supported by the PersOn project (P21-03) and the Hybrid Intelligence center (grant no. 024.004.022), both funded by Nederlandse Organisatie voor Wetenschappelijk Onderzoek (NWO).

## References

1. Aaronson, N.K., et al.: The European organization for research and treatment of cancer QLQ-C30: a quality-of-life instrument for use in international clinical trials in oncology. JNCI: J. Nat. Cancer Inst. **85**(5), 365–376 (1993)
2. van den Boorn, H.G., et al.: Source-PANC: a prediction model for patients with metastatic pancreatic ductal adenocarcinoma based on nationwide population-based data. J. Natl. Compr. Canc. Netw. **19**(9), 1045–1053 (2021)
3. Cho, H., Wei, Z., Lee, S., Dan, T., Wu, G., Kim, W.H.: Conditional diffusion with ordinal regression: longitudinal data generation for neurodegenerative disease studies. In: The Thirteenth International Conference on Learning Representations (2025)
4. Deng, Q.L., et al.: Development and validation of a nomogram for predicting survival in patients with advanced pancreatic ductal adenocarcinoma. Sci. Rep. **7**(1), 11524 (2017)
5. Latenstein, A.E., et al.: Nationwide trends in incidence, treatment and survival of pancreatic ductal adenocarcinoma. Eur. J. Cancer **125**, 83–93 (2020)
6. Mackay, T.M., et al.: Relationship between quality of life and survival in patients with pancreatic and periampullary cancer: a multicenter cohort analysis. J. Nat. Comprehensive Cancer Netw. **18**(10), 1354–1363 (2020)
7. Seelen, L.W., et al.: Quality of life among patients with locally advanced pancreatic cancer: a prospective nationwide multicenter study. J. Natl. Compr. Canc. Netw. **23**(3), 97–104 (2025)
8. Stempfle, L., Matsson, A., Mwai, N., Johansson, F.D.: Prediction models that learn to avoid missing values. In: Forty-second International Conference on Machine Learning (2025)
9. Valverde, C.P.T., et al.: Impact of short-course palliative radiation therapy on pancreatic cancer-related pain: prospective phase 2 nonrandomized PAINPANC trial. Int. J. Radiation Oncol. Biol. Phys. **118**(2), 352–361 (2024)
10. Van Den Braak, R.C., et al.: Nationwide comprehensive gastro-intestinal cancer cohorts: the 3P initiative. Acta Oncol. **57**(2), 195–202 (2018)

# From Many to Meaningful: Feature-Guided Zero-Shot Chronic Kidney Disease Screening Using Large Language Models

Muhammad Ashad Kabir[1(✉)] and Sirajam Munira[2]

[1] School of Computing, Mathematics and Engineering, Charles Sturt University, Bathurst, NSW, Australia
akabir@csu.edu.au

[2] Department of Computer Science, Rensselaer Polytechnic Institute, Troy, NY, USA
munirs@rpi.edu

**Abstract.** Early screening of chronic kidney disease (CKD) is essential for preventing irreversible progression; however, many machine learning (ML)-based screening methods remain difficult to deploy in community and resource-limited screening settings due to their reliance on large labeled datasets, resource-intensive pathology tests, or high-dimensional clinical features, and limited robustness to population and distributional shifts. This study examines the feasibility of using large language models (LLMs) for early-stage CKD screening in a zero-shot setting, without dataset-specific training. We propose a feature-guided zero-shot framework that evaluates LLM performance using a selected set of clinically meaningful, readily available community-based features, rather than exhaustive clinical inputs. Feature selection was guided by ML-based analysis to identify a compact, clinically relevant subset of variables. Tabular patient records were subsequently serialized into text using standardized prompt templates to enable zero-shot inference. The zero-shot performance of four LLMs (LLaMA-3, Qwen-3, Mistral, and GPT-4o-mini) was evaluated using both the full feature set and the selected subset. Generalizability was assessed across three heterogeneous CKD datasets spanning three countries. Across models and datasets, the selected feature set yielded consistent and statistically significant improvements in balanced accuracy and probability estimates, achieving performance levels suitable for screening purposes. These findings suggest that LLMs can support clinically meaningful, training-free CKD screening using minimal community-accessible patient features, offering a practical complement to conventional ML methods in real-world screening contexts.

**Keywords:** Chronic Kidney Disease · Large Language Model · Zero-shot · Tabular data · Classification · Feature guided

© The Author(s), under exclusive license to Springer Nature Switzerland AG 2027
P. Andreev et al. (Eds.): AIME 2026, LNAI 16748, pp. 38–48, 2027.
https://doi.org/10.1007/978-3-032-30710-1_5

## 1 Introduction

Chronic kidney disease (CKD) is a progressive condition characterized by sustained loss of kidney function or persistent kidney damage. If undetected, it can lead to end-stage renal disease requiring costly and lifelong treatment [9]. Globally, CKD affects approximately 850 million individuals, with a disproportionate burden in low- and middle-income countries, where access to early diagnosis and preventive care remains limited [13]. In South Asia, particularly in Bangladesh, community-based studies report high CKD prevalence and low awareness in rural and peri-urban populations [2,12]. Early-stage CKD (stages 1–3) is often asymptomatic, yet timely detection can significantly slow disease progression [9].

Standard CKD screening relies on laboratory markers such as serum creatinine, estimated glomerular filtration rate (eGFR), and urine albumin-to-creatinine ratio, which require well-equipped facilities and trained personnel [9]. In many parts of South Asia, particularly rural and peri-urban areas, limited diagnostic infrastructure and financial constraints restrict access to these tests [13]. While conventional machine learning (ML) models have shown promising performance for CKD detection, they depend on large labeled datasets, predefined feature spaces, and retraining for new populations [11]. Such requirements reduce adaptability in heterogeneous, real-world screening contexts.

Recent advances in large language models (LLMs) have shown strong zero-shot generalization across diverse classification and reasoning tasks [3]. In nephrology, LLMs have been explored for various applications [6], including patient education and personalized dietary advice [8], diagnostic support [14], and medication management [11]. However, their use for systematic CKD screening – particularly in zero-shot settings and based on non-diagnostic or readily accessible community-level features – remains largely unexplored.

Motivated by this gap, we investigate whether LLMs can achieve clinically meaningful zero-shot CKD detection without any dataset-specific training or finetuning. This study makes three primary contributions: (i) we evaluate the zero-shot screening performance of four state-of-the-art LLMs (LLaMA-3, Qwen-3, Mistral, and GPT-4o-mini); (ii) we systematically compare the use of comprehensive feature sets with a compact subset of clinically meaningful variables, examining whether feature reduction improves or maintains screening performance; (iii) we assess generalizability by evaluating the approach on a community-based population and validating it on two additional datasets from different countries. Although the datasets do not share identical feature spaces, a harmonized subset of selected features was available across datasets. Across models and datasets, the selected feature subset achieved comparable or improved performance relative to using all available features. These findings suggest that meaningful feature selection can enhance zero-shot LLM-based CKD screening, which is critical for resource-constrained settings, and demonstrate cross-population robustness.

## 2 Methods

Figure 1 provides an overview of the proposed zero-shot LLM framework for CKD screening. The workflow consists of three main steps: (i) feature harmonization and selection, (ii) prompt construction, and (iii) inference using large language models.

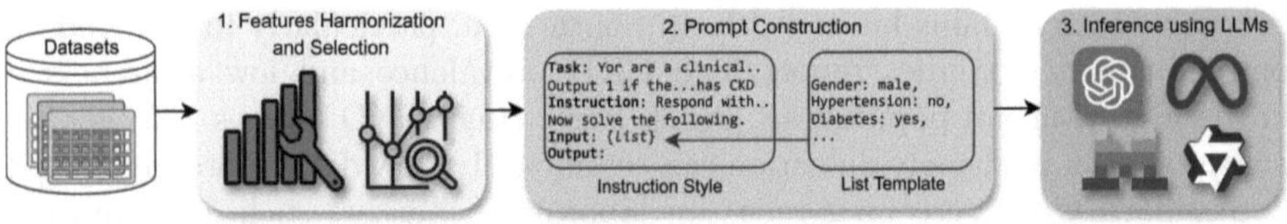


**Fig. 1.** Schematic overview of the zero-shot LLM pipeline for CKD detection.

### 2.1 Datasets

We evaluated the proposed zero-shot LLM framework using three heterogeneous CKD datasets, summarized in Table 1, representing both community-based (Dataset-1) and hospital-based populations (Dataset-2 and Dataset-3) across three countries: Bangladesh, India, and the UAE. To align with our research objective, gold-standard pathology tests used for direct CKD diagnosis, such as serum creatinine, urinary albumin, urinary creatinine, eGFR, and uACR, were excluded from all datasets. These markers are direct clinical identifiers of CKD. Therefore, including them would trivialize the prediction task. Moreover, such pathology tests are costly and not always accessible in low-resource or community settings. By excluding these features, we assess whether LLMs can detect CKD using more accessible and non-gold-standard clinical information.

**Table 1.** Summary of CKD datasets used in this study

| Dataset | Country | Sample size | | | CKD Stage | Considered Features | | | | | |
|---|---|---|---|---|---|---|---|---|---|---|---|
| | | CKD | Non-CKD | Total | | SD | LH | MH | CE | Path* | Total |
| Dataset-1 [12] | Bangladesh | 112 | 172 | 284 | 1–3 | 5 | 3 | 7 | 4 | 5 | 24 |
| Dataset-2 [10] | India | 250 | 150 | 400 | – | 1 | 1 | 3 | 5 | 13 | 23 |
| Dataset-3 [1] | UAE | 56 | – | 56 | 3–5 | 2 | 1 | 8 | 1 | 2 | 14 |

*Excluding gold-standard pathology tests for CKD diagnosis, such as serum creatinine, urinary albumin, urinary creatinine, eGFR, and uACR

Dataset-1 [12] is a community-based CKD survey conducted in the Mirzapur, sub-district of Tangail, Bangladesh. This dataset was collected through age-stratified random sampling of adults aged 18 years and above under the Mirzapur demographic surveillance system. CKD was diagnosed based on reduced kidney function (eGFR) and/or elevated urine albumin-to-creatinine ratio (uACR) according to standard clinical guidelines. After removing incomplete records, the final dataset included 284 participants, consisting of 112 early-stage CKD cases (stages 1–3) and 172 non-CKD individuals. The dataset contains 24 variables covering socio-demographic (SD), lifestyle habits (LH), medical history (MH), clinical examination (CE), and pathology test (Path) features.

Dataset-2 [10] is the UCI 2015 CKD dataset, collected from a hospital in India and widely used as a benchmark for CKD detection research. It contains clinical records from 400 patients admitted over two months, including 250 CKD cases and 150 non-CKD controls. Following the removal of gold-standard pathology markers, 23 variables were retained across socio-demographic, lifestyle, medical history, clinical examination, and non-gold-standard pathology features. CKD stages were not reported in this dataset.

Dataset-3 [1] is the UAE CKD dataset derived from hospital records at Tawam Hospital in Al-Ain City, Abu Dhabi, UAE. It includes 56 patients diagnosed with moderate-to-advanced CKD (stages 3–5). CKD, with stages 1–2, was not clearly separated from healthy individuals in the original data; therefore, only confirmed CKD cases were used in our analysis. After excluding gold-standard tests and redundant features, 14 features were retained across demographic, lifestyle, medical history, clinical, and pathology.

**Table 2.** All features and selected features (underlined) retained after harmonization for each dataset.

| Dataset | Considered features |
|---|---|
| Dataset-1 | <u>Age</u>, <u>Gender</u>, Illiterate, Occupation, Marital status, <u>Sleeping duration</u>, Tobacco smoker, Smokeless tobacco, <u>History of hypertension</u>, <u>History of diabetes</u>, Heart disease, Stroke, Family history of diabetes, <u>Family history of hypertension</u>, Family history of CKD, <u>Body mass index</u>, Abdominal obesity, Undernutrition, <u>Anemia</u>, <u>Presence of red blood cells in urine</u>, Serum albumin, Hyper-cholesterolemia, HDL cholesterol, Hypertriglyceridemia |
| Dataset-2 | Age, Blood pressure, Specific gravity, Albumin, Sugar, <u>Presence of red blood cells in urine</u>, Pus cell, Pus cell clumps, Bacteria, Blood glucose random, Blood urea, Sodium, Potassium, Hemoglobin, Packed cell volume, White blood cell count, Red blood cell count, <u>History of hypertension</u>, <u>History of Diabetes</u>, Coronary artery disease, Appetite condition, Pedal edema, <u>Anemia</u> |
| Dataset-3 | <u>Age</u>, <u>Gender</u>, History of heart disease, Vascular disease, History of dyslipidemia, <u>History of hypertension</u>, <u>History of diabetes</u>, Tobacco smoker, <u>Body mass index</u>, Hyper-cholesterolemia, Consuming dyslipidemia medication, Consuming diabetes medication, Consuming hypertension medication, HbA1C |

### 2.2 Features Harmonization and Selection

To ensure consistency across datasets, we performed systematic feature harmonization before model evaluation. Variables representing the same clinical concepts were harmonized across three datasets by standardizing both feature names and value encodings into a unified, semantically interpretable format to facilitate zero-shot LLM inference. This harmonization enabled consistent prompt construction and comparable evaluation across datasets. The complete list of harmonized features considered in this study is presented in Table 2.

Feature selection was informed by our prior machine learning analysis on the community-based Dataset-1 [7], which includes diverse and accessible variables spanning socio-demographic characteristics, lifestyle factors, medical history, clinical examination findings, and selected pathology measures. In [7], ten complementary feature selection methods (including recursive feature elimination with multiple ML estimators) were applied to identify a compact subset of clinically meaningful and readily obtainable variables most predictive of early-stage CKD. The selected features are underlined in Table 2. The selected features from Dataset-1 were subsequently mapped to Dataset-2 and Dataset-3 by identifying variables with equivalent clinical interpretation. As the datasets did not share identical feature spaces, only variables matching the selected features in Dataset-1 were retained as selected features in Datasets 2 and 3.

### 2.3 Prompt Construction

We represent each patient record (tabular instance) by serializing feature-value pairs into a structured list format (Appendix A). This design follows prior findings demonstrating that list-based serialization preserves feature boundaries, reduces ambiguity, and performs comparably to free-text or sentence-style representations when applying LLMs to tabular inference [5]. The serialized representation enables the model to reason over individual attributes while preserving the original tabular semantics.

We adopt an instruction-style, role-conditioned prompting strategy (chat-style for GPT-4o-mini) in which each serialized record is embedded within a structured instruction–input–output format [15]. The prompt (Appendix A) explicitly specifies the task objective, assigns the model a functional role, defines the expected binary output space, and presents the serialized input record. This design is consistent with instruction-tuning paradigms used in modern LLM training, which have been shown to enhance zero-shot generalization [16]. Unlike native chat-style templates, instruction-style prompts avoid reliance on model-specific control tokens, improving robustness and cross-model generalizability. Furthermore, explicit output constraints reduce generation variability and support more deterministic predictions, which is advantageous for zero-shot binary classification of structured clinical data.

The prompt text was formulated by adapting instruction templates aligned with model instruction-tuning paradigms and iteratively refined through empirical validation, consistent with prior work on instruction-based prompt optimization in in-context learning settings [4].

### 2.4 Inference Using LLMs

We evaluated four large language models, LLaMA-3 8B, Qwen-3 8B, Mistral 7B, and GPT-4o-mini, selected to represent architectural diversity, variation in parameter scale, and differences in training paradigms (open-weight vs. proprietary). These models have been pretrained on large-scale, heterogeneous corpora that include biomedical and clinical knowledge, making them suitable for zero-shot reasoning in healthcare-related tasks such as CKD screening. Additionally, all selected models expose token-level log-probabilities, enabling probabilistic classification based on likelihood comparisons over predefined label tokens—an important capability not consistently available in many LLMs.

Inference was conducted in a zero-shot setting without task-specific training or parameter updates. For each patient record, the constructed instruction-style prompt was provided to the model, and binary predictions (CKD vs. non-CKD) were derived using log-probability scores over the constrained output space. Deterministic decoding was applied where supported to ensure reproducibility. Each record was processed independently, and no in-context examples were provided.

## 3 Results

Figure 2 compares the use of all available features versus the selected feature subset across LLMs and datasets using balanced accuracy, with statistical signif-

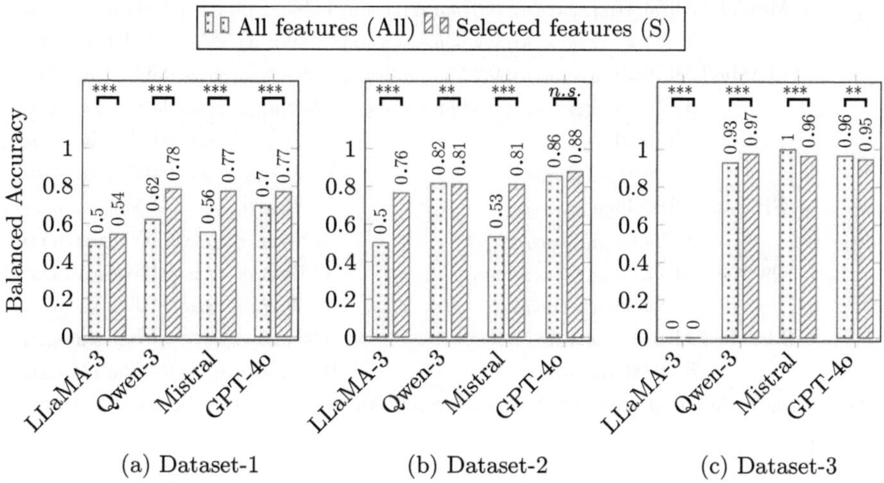


**Fig. 2.** Comparison of *all* versus *selected* features and the performance of different LLMs. Bars report balanced accuracy, while statistical significance between all- and selected-feature settings is assessed using a paired permutation test on per-sample Brier loss, with pairing over shared test samples. Significance levels are indicated by asterisks: $^{*}p < 0.05$, $^{**}p < 0.01$ and $^{***}p < 0.001$.

icance assessed using a paired permutation test on per-sample Brier loss to provide a distribution-free, paired comparison of probabilistic predictions. Table 3 reports the detailed zero-shot performance metrics, including balanced accuracy, macro AUROC, macro F1-score, and Brier score, along with 95% confidence intervals estimated using nonparametric bootstrap resampling at the sample level using percentile intervals to quantify metric uncertainty.

**Table 3.** Zero-shot performance of LLMs using all features and selected features, reported as balanced accuracy, macro AUROC, macro F1-score, and Brier loss with 95% confidence intervals computed using nonparametric bootstrap.

| Dataset | Model | FS | B. Accuracy (%) | Macro AUROC | Macro F1 (%) | Brier loss (↓) |
|---|---|---|---|---|---|---|
| Dataset-1 | Qwen-3 | All | $62.04_{(57.14-66.79)}$ | $0.735_{(0.676-0.794)}$ | $55.90_{(50.17-61.67)}$ | $0.253_{(0.227-0.280)}$ |
| | | S | $78.32_{(73.43-83.42)}$ | $0.836_{(0.786-0.884)}$ | $78.63_{(73.71-83.62)}$ | $0.161_{(0.131-0.192)}$ |
| | LLaMa-3 | All | $50.00_{(50.00-50.00)}$ | $0.749_{(0.689-0.804)}$ | $37.69_{(35.31-39.83)}$ | $0.264_{(0.232-0.297)}$ |
| | | S | $54.26_{(51.30-57.31)}$ | $0.816_{(0.766-0.865)}$ | $47.58_{(42.32-53.17)}$ | $0.207_{(0.181-0.235)}$ |
| | GPT-4o | All | $69.69_{(65.19-73.94)}$ | $0.803_{(0.751-0.855)}$ | $64.21_{(58.60-69.39)}$ | $0.330_{(0.280-0.382)}$ |
| | | S | $77.11_{(72.48-81.79)}$ | $0.851_{(0.808-0.892)}$ | $75.77_{(70.93-80.51)}$ | $0.212_{(0.170-0.256)}$ |
| | Mistral | All | $55.53_{(53.23-58.08)}$ | $0.794_{(0.739-0.848)}$ | $39.61_{(34.33-45.18)}$ | $0.505_{(0.448-0.558)}$ |
| | | S | $77.27_{(72.38-82.16)}$ | $0.838_{(0.791-0.883)}$ | $76.51_{(71.66-81.34)}$ | $0.212_{(0.169-0.255)}$ |
| Dataset-2 | GPT-4o | All | $85.57_{(81.85-89.25)}$ | $0.925_{(0.896-0.950)}$ | $85.40_{(81.73-89.01)}$ | $0.131_{(0.098-0.165)}$ |
| | | S | $88.00_{(85.34-90.54)}$ | $0.943_{(0.921-0.964)}$ | $84.82_{(81.30-88.12)}$ | $0.145_{(0.114-0.178)}$ |
| | Qwen-3 | All | $81.61_{(78.60-84.49)}$ | $0.901_{(0.866-0.934)}$ | $76.95_{(72.69-80.98)}$ | $0.170_{(0.150-0.191)}$ |
| | | S | $81.24_{(78.14-84.29)}$ | $0.843_{(0.796-0.885)}$ | $76.50_{(72.43-80.67)}$ | $0.207_{(0.171-0.244)}$ |
| | Mistral | All | $53.47_{(51.13-56.05)}$ | $0.822_{(0.779-0.860)}$ | $46.92_{(42.48-51.45)}$ | $0.341_{(0.297-0.388)}$ |
| | | S | $85.22_{(82.35-88.04)}$ | $0.932_{(0.908-0.956)}$ | $81.40_{(77.46-85.16)}$ | $0.179_{(0.143-0.216)}$ |
| | LLaMa-3 | All | $50.20_{(50.00-50.62)}$ | $0.923_{(0.895-0.948)}$ | $27.68_{(25.09-30.32)}$ | $0.326_{(0.304-0.348)}$ |
| | | S | $76.45_{(73.22-79.67)}$ | $0.849_{(0.810-0.887)}$ | $70.46_{(65.92-74.99)}$ | $0.212_{(0.186-0.239)}$ |
| Dataset-3 | Mistral | All | $100.0_{(100.0-100.0)}$ | – | $100.0_{(100.0-100.0)}$ | $0.003_{(0.000-0.010)}$ |
| | | S | $96.48_{(91.07-100.0)}$ | – | $56.40_{(47.66-100.0)}$ | $0.035_{(0.000-0.088)}$ |
| | GPT-4o | All | $96.48_{(91.07-100.0)}$ | – | $56.40_{(47.66-100.0)}$ | $0.035_{(0.000-0.088)}$ |
| | | S | $94.65_{(87.50-100.0)}$ | – | $50.84_{(46.67-100.0)}$ | $0.054_{(0.002-0.122)}$ |
| | Qwen-3 | All | $92.89_{(85.71-98.21)}$ | – | $49.19_{(46.15-49.55)}$ | $0.084_{(0.031-0.152)}$ |
| | | S | $96.48_{(91.07-100.0)}$ | – | $56.40_{(47.66-100.0)}$ | $0.036_{(0.001-0.089)}$ |
| | LLaMa-3 | All | $0.00_{(0.00-0.00)}$ | – | $0.00_{(0.00-0.00)}$ | $0.670_{(0.663-0.678)}$ |
| | | S | $0.00_{(0.00-0.00)}$ | – | $0.00_{(0.00-0.00)}$ | $0.489_{(0.468-0.514)}$ |

B. Accuracy: Balanced accuracy, FS: Feature set, All: All features, S: Selected features

For Dataset-1, the selected feature set consistently yields higher balanced accuracy across all models, with statistically significant improvements ($p < 0.001$). The largest gains are observed for Qwen-3 and Mistral, where balanced accuracy increases from 0.62 to 0.78 and from 0.56 to 0.77, respectively. GPT-4o-mini improves from 0.70 to 0.77, while LLaMA-3 shows a modest but significant increase from 0.50 to 0.54. These improvements are accompanied by higher macro AUROC and macro F1-scores and lower Brier loss, indicating enhanced discrimination and calibration. For example, Qwen-3's AUROC increases from 0.735 to 0.836, macro F1-score from 55.90% to 78.63%, and Brier loss decreases from 0.253 to 0.161. The bootstrap-derived 95% confidence intervals remain well separated in settings with large performance gains, reinforcing the statistical stability of the observed improvements. Similar patterns are observed across the other models, suggesting that restricting inputs to clinically selected features improves both predictive performance and probabilistic reliability.

For Dataset-2, selected features again yield improved or comparable balanced accuracy across all models, with statistically significant gains observed in several cases. The most substantial improvement is seen for Mistral, where balanced accuracy increases from 0.53 to 0.81 ($p < 0.001$). LLaMA-3 also demonstrates a marked improvement from 0.50 to 0.76. Qwen-3 maintains strong performance under both feature configurations, indicating robustness to feature redundancy. While GPT-4o-mini shows a slight increase, that difference is not statistically significant. These performance patterns are consistent with changes in AUROC, F1-score, and Brier loss. For example, Mistral's AUROC increases from 0.822 to 0.932, and its Brier loss decreases from 0.341 to 0.179, indicating improved discrimination and probabilistic calibration when using selected features.

For Dataset-3, a different pattern is observed, likely reflecting its focus on moderate-to-advanced CKD cases. LLaMA-3 yields a balanced accuracy of 0 under both feature configurations, indicating an inability to identify CKD cases, although the difference between all and selected features remains statistically significant in terms of Brier loss. The most notable improvement is observed for Qwen-3, where balanced accuracy increases from 0.93 to 0.97 with statistical significance ($p < 0.001$). In contrast, Mistral and GPT-4o-mini show slight decreases when using selected features, from 1.00 to 0.96 and from 0.96 to 0.95, respectively; however, overall performance remains high. These patterns are also reflected in AUROC and Brier scores. For example, Qwen-3's Brier loss decreases from 0.084 to 0.036, indicating improved probabilistic calibration in selected features, while Mistral and GPT-4o-mini maintain strong discrimination despite marginal reductions in balanced accuracy.

Overall, the results consistently indicate that the selected feature set improves or maintains balanced accuracy, AUROC, F1-score, and probabilistic calibration across datasets, despite differences in feature space composition. This consistency across heterogeneous cohorts supports the robustness of the approach and suggests that zero-shot LLM-based CKD screening can generalize across populations using a compact, clinically harmonized set of features.

## 4 Discussions

The most pronounced gains were observed in early-stage community screening (Dataset-1), where reducing redundant or less informative inputs substantially improved predictive stability and calibration. This finding suggests that in settings where disease signals are subtle, compact, and clinically meaningful features may enhance zero-shot reasoning by reducing noise and guiding the model toward salient risk factors. In hospital-based cohorts (Dataset-2), feature selection yielded particularly great improvements for smaller or open-weight models, whereas higher-capacity models such as GPT-4o-mini demonstrated relative robustness to feature redundancy. In the advanced-stage CKD cohort (Dataset-3), performance remained high under both feature configurations, indicating that feature reduction does not compromise discrimination when disease signals are more pronounced.

Our previous supervised ML study using the same selected feature subset reported a best balanced accuracy of 90.4% on Dataset-1 using 10-fold cross-validation and 79.33% when trained on Dataset-1 and externally tested on Dataset-2 [7]. In comparison, the zero-shot LLM approach achieved up to 78.32% on Dataset-1 (Qwen-3) and 88% on Dataset-2 (GPT-4o-mini) without any dataset-specific training, demonstrating competitive performance with strong practical applicability.

Collectively, these results suggest that feature-guided prompting enhances the reliability and stability of zero-shot LLM-based screening, particularly in early-stage and resource-constrained settings. While larger models appear less sensitive to redundant inputs, a compact and clinically grounded feature set provides clearer and more consistent performance gains across diverse model architectures without sacrificing predictive quality.

Several limitations should be acknowledged. First, the datasets are moderate in size and limited to three geographic regions, which may restrict generalizability. Second, zero-shot prompting relies on prompt design and instruction tuning characteristics, which may vary across future model releases. Third, Dataset-3 contains only CKD-positive cases, limiting full binary evaluation in that context.

## 5 Conclusions and Future Work

This study demonstrates that LLMs can support clinically meaningful zero-shot CKD screening using a compact, harmonized feature set without dataset-specific training or retraining. Across heterogeneous community- and hospital-based cohorts, restricting inputs to clinically selected features consistently improved or preserved accuracy, discrimination, and probabilistic calibration.

Future work should evaluate larger and more diverse cohorts, explore structured uncertainty estimation for screening thresholds, and investigate few-shot or retrieval-augmented extensions to further enhance robustness. Integration into community screening workflows and prospective validation in real-world settings will be critical to assess clinical impact.

**Acknowledgments.** Authors thank Dr. Mohammad Habibur Rehman Sarker (ICDDRB) for sharing Dataset-1.

# A Zero-Shot Prompt Template

**Table A1.** Example of the instruction-style prompt used for zero-shot inference.

```
Task: You are a clinical classification model. Classify whether a patient has chronic kidney
disease (CKD) based on the patient input features. 1 indicates CKD and 0 indicates non-
CKD.
Output 1 if the patient has CKD. Output 0 if the patient does not have CKD.
Instruction: Respond with exactly one token: 0 or 1.
Now solve the following.
Input:
Patient features:
History of diabetes: Yes,
History of hypertension: No,
...
Output:
```

## References


1. Al-Shamsi, S., Regmi, D., Govender, R.D.: Chronic kidney disease in patients at high risk of cardiovascular disease in the United Arab Emirates: a population-based study. PLOS ONE **13**(6) (2018)
2. Banik, S., Ghosh, A.: Prevalence of chronic kidney disease in Bangladesh: a systematic review and meta-analysis. Int. Urol. Nephrol. **53**(4), 713–718 (2021)
3. Brown, T.B., et al.: Language models are few-shot learners. In: Advances in Neural Information Processing Systems, vol. 33 (2020)
4. Cui, W., et al.: SEE: Strategic exploration and exploitation for cohesive in-context prompt optimization. In: Proceedings of the 63rd Annual Meeting of the Association for Computational Linguistics, pp. 29575–29627 (2025)
5. Hegselmann, S., Buendia, A., Lang, H., Agrawal, M., Jiang, X., Sontag, D.: TabLLM: few-shot classification of tabular data with large language models. In: International Conference on Artificial Intelligence and Statistics, pp. 5549–5581 (2023)
6. Hu, Y., Liu, J., Jiang, W.: Large language models in nephrology: applications and challenges in chronic kidney disease management. Renal Failure **47**(1) (2025)
7. Kabir, M.A., Munira, S., Azad, D.T., Ikram, S.M., Sarker, M.H.R., Hanifi, S.M.A.: Community-based early-stage chronic kidney disease screening using explainable machine learning for low-resource settings. Int. J. Med. Informat. **214** (2026)
8. Kairat, M., Adilmetova, G., Ibraimova, I., Gaipov, A., Varol, H.A., Chan, M.Y.: Benchmarking ChatGPT and other large language models for personalized stage-specific dietary recommendations in chronic kidney disease. J. Clin. Med. **14**(22) (2025)
9. Levey, A.S., Coresh, J.: Chronic kidney disease. The Lancet **399**(10391) (2022)
10. Rubini, L., Soundarapandian, P., Eswaran, P.: Chronic kidney disease. UCI Mach. Learn. Reposit. (2015). https://doi.org/10.24432/C5G020
11. Sabanayagam, C., et al.: Artificial intelligence in chronic kidney disease management: a scoping review. Theranostics **15**(10), 4566–4578 (2025)
12. Sarker, M.H.R., et al.: Community-based screening to determine the prevalence, health and nutritional status of patients with CKD in rural and peri-urban Bangladesh. Therapeutic Adv. Chronic Dis. **12** (2021)

13. Stanifer, J.W., Muiru, A., Jafar, T.H., Patel, U.D.: Chronic kidney disease in low- and middle-income countries. Nephrol. Dial. Transplant. **31**(6), 868–874 (2016)
14. Syeda, M.Z., Bukhari, S.U.K., Hussain, M., Khan, W.A., Shah, S.S.H.: LLM-based kidney disease diagnostic framework for pathologists. In: 46th Annual International Conference of the IEEE Engineering in Medicine and Biology Society. IEEE (2024)
15. Wang, Y., et al.: Self-instruct: aligning language models with self-generated instructions. In: Proceedings of the 61st Annual Meeting of the Association for Computational Linguistics, pp. 13484–13508 (2023)
16. Wei, J., et al.: Finetuned language models are zero-shot learners. In: International Conference on Learning Representations (2022)

# Making Conformal Predictors Robust in Healthcare Settings: a Case Study on EEG Classification

Arjun Chatterjee[1,2(✉)], Sayeed Sajjad Razin[2,3], John Wu[1,2(✉)], Siddhartha Laghuvarapu[1,2], Jathurshan Pradeepkumar[1,2], and Jimeng Sun[1]

[1] University of Illinois Urbana-Champaign, Urbana, IL 61801, USA
{arjunc4,johnwu3}@illinois.edu
[2] PyHealth, Urbana, IL 61801, USA
[3] Bangladesh University of Engineering and Technology, Dhaka, Bangladesh

**Abstract.** Quantifying uncertainty in clinical predictions is critical for high-stakes diagnosis tasks. Conformal prediction offers a principled approach by providing prediction sets with theoretical coverage guarantees. However, in practice, patient distribution shifts violate the i.i.d. assumptions underlying standard conformal methods, leading to poor coverage in healthcare settings. In this work, we evaluate several conformal prediction approaches on EEG seizure classification, a task with known distribution shift challenges and label uncertainty. We demonstrate that personalized calibration strategies can improve coverage by over 20% points while maintaining comparable prediction set sizes. Our implementation is available via PyHealth, an open-source healthcare AI framework: https://github.com/sunlabuiuc/PyHealth.

**Keywords:** Conformal Prediction · Distribution Shift · EEG Signal Classification · Uncertainty Quantification · Robustness

## 1 Introduction

For many healthcare tasks, uncertainty is intrinsic to the problem itself. This is exemplified by EEG classification, where labels are derived from group voting among expert neurologists [2,7]. Whether due to measurement noise or patient-to-patient variance, expert disagreements on waveform readings are not uncommon [2,10], as illustrated in Fig. 1. Single-class predictions can therefore be overconfident or misleading.

Conformal prediction [8] directly addresses this by producing prediction sets rather than point predictions for uncertain samples. However, it assumes i.i.d. calibration and test distributions, a condition that EEG classification routinely violates due to patient differences and recording conditions [13]. We demonstrate that under patient-level distribution shift, conventional conformal prediction techniques fail to provide adequate coverage.

© The Author(s), under exclusive license to Springer Nature Switzerland AG 2027
P. Andreev et al. (Eds.): AIME 2026, LNAI 16748, pp. 49–53, 2027.
https://doi.org/10.1007/978-3-032-30710-1_6

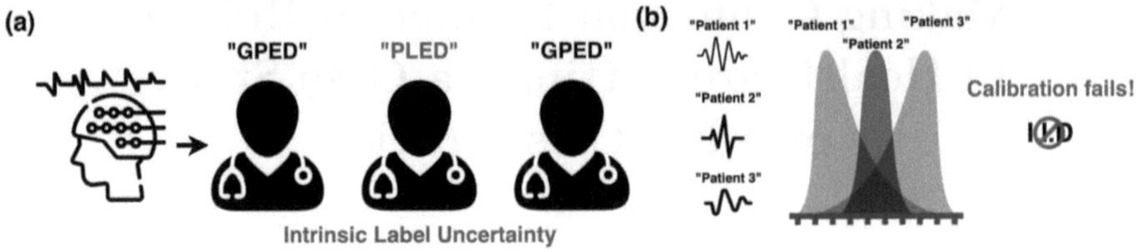


**Fig. 1.** EEG Classification Challenges. EEG tasks often violate key aspects of a typical machine learning pipeline. (a) Their annotation process consistently leaves room for uncertainty, which is then passed onto the models. (b) Training, validation, and test distributions are not i.i.d. due to patient distribution shift [13]. Both issues make EEG classification a very challenging machine learning problem.

We explore conformal prediction approaches robust to such shifts using ContraWR [14] on TUAB [6] and TUEV [4], evaluated under both random and patient-level splits. **Our contributions are: (1) a neighborhood conformal prediction (NCP) approach that improves coverage by up to 20% over baselines; (2) theoretical results showing NCP yields provably better coverage under covariate shift; (3) prediction set sizes that remain relatively stable; and (4) a modular PyHealth integration enabling easy replication in other clinical settings.**

## 2 Experiments and Results

**Datasets.** We evaluate on two benchmark tasks under two splitting regimes from the TUH EEG Corpus [7]: **TUEV** [4], a six-class EEG event classification task (SPSW, GPED, PLED, EYEM, ARTF, BCKG), and **TUAB** [6], a binary normal/abnormal detection task. In the **random split** setting, all samples are pooled and divided globally at 60%, 10%, 15%, and 15% for the training, validation, calibration, and test sets, respectively. In the **patient split** setting, patients are partitioned first, with the train partition further split at 60%, 20%, and 20% for train, validation, and calibration sets respectively, and held-out patients forming the test set, introducing realistic cross-patient distribution shift.

**Models and Conformal Approaches.** We train **ContraWR** [14], a ResNet-based 2D CNN over multi-channel spectrograms, from scratch across five random seeds. We compare four conformal prediction (CP) approaches: **Naive CP** [8] (standard split conformal prediction assuming i.i.d. calibration and test), **Covariate CP** [11] (likelihood-ratio reweighting via KDE [5]), **K-means CP** (threshold derived from the nearest cluster's calibration samples), and **NCP** [3] (sample-specific calibration via k-nearest neighbors with relevance weighting). The first two are non-personalized; the latter two are personalized. More theoretical results are provided in [1] (Fig. 4).

**Covariate CP does not improve coverage over Naive CP.** As seen in Fig. 2, the two methods track similarly across all $\alpha$ values and both datasets,

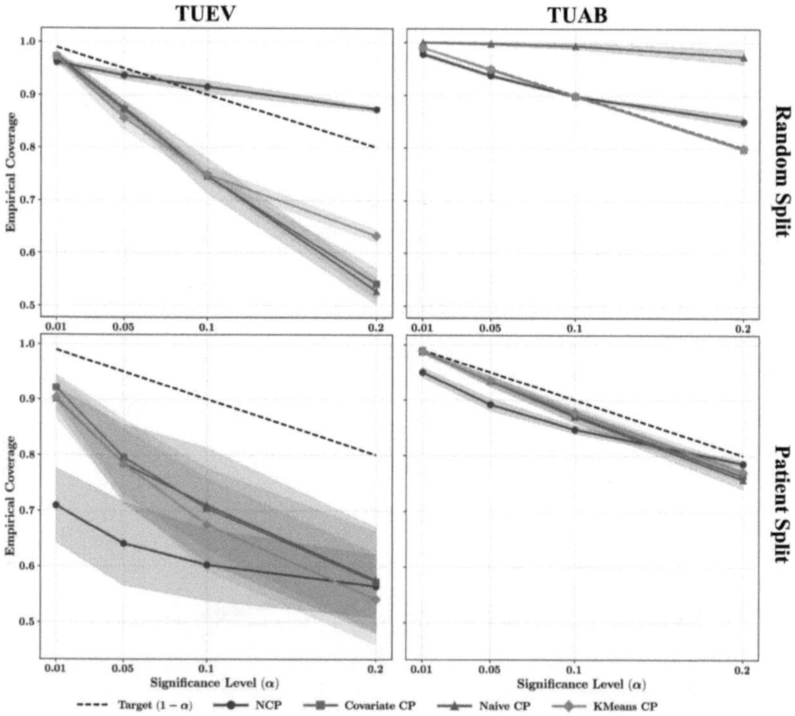


**Fig. 2.** Empirical coverage under random (top) and patient (bottom) splits. The dotted line is target coverage $1 - \alpha$. Under the random split, NCP substantially outperforms non-personalized baselines on TUEV. Under the patient split, all methods fall short of target coverage, reflecting the difficulty of cross-patient distribution shift.

as likelihood-ratio estimation via KDE is unreliable in high-dimensional EEG feature spaces [5].

**NCP substantially improves coverage on the random split.** On TUEV under the random split, NCP achieves around **34% greater coverage** than Naive CP at $\alpha = 0.2$ (0.87 vs. 0.53), with a modest increase in average prediction set size (1.22 vs. 0.90) (Fig. 3). On TUAB, where Naive CP already satisfies coverage due to the easier binary task, the personalization benefit is less pronounced but NCP still produces notably more compact prediction sets.

**Patient-level splits reveal the limits of all approaches.** Ensuring calibration and test patients are disjoint causes all methods to fall well short of target coverage on TUEV, with high variance across seeds, and a smaller but still present gap on TUAB. NCP's smaller set sizes under this split suggest its personalization yields overly tight prediction sets under strong distribution shift.

**Empirical coverage remains imperfect.** No method consistently achieves $1-\alpha$ coverage across all settings, and cross-patient distribution shift remains an open challenge for conformal prediction in EEG classification.

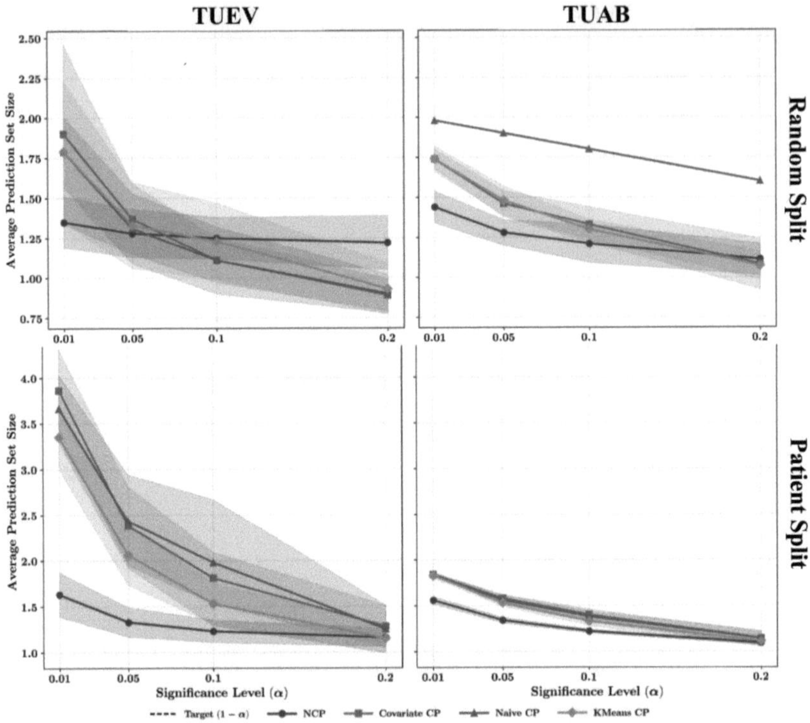


**Fig. 3.** Average prediction set sizes under random (top) and patient (bottom) splits. NCP consistently maintains smaller prediction sets than non-personalized methods despite achieving competitive or higher coverage.

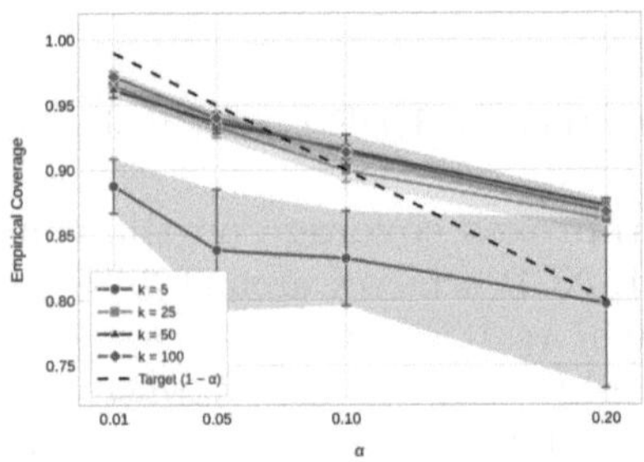


**Fig. 4.** Empirical coverage vs. $\alpha$ for NCP using varying calibration set sizes $k$. Shaded regions denote $\pm 1$ std. The dashed line is target coverage $1-\alpha$.

# 3 Discussion

**Future Directions.** Our EEG case study highlights distribution shift challenges common across healthcare [12,13]. Applying personalized conformal predictors more broadly could reveal which shift types these methods handle well. NCP's coverage could also improve with stronger EEG foundation model embeddings, such as TFM-Tokenizer [9], which better characterizes signal structure. Finally, all implementations are available via `pip install pyhealth` to lower barriers and encourage adoption of conformal prediction in safety-critical healthcare AI.

**Disclosure of Interests.** There are no competing interests.

## References


1. Chatterjee, A., Razin, S.S., Wu, J., Laghuvarapu, S., Pradeepkumar, J., Sun, J.: Making conformal predictors robust in healthcare settings: a case study on EEG classification (2026). https://arxiv.org/abs/2602.19483v1
2. Ge, W., et al.: Deep active learning for interictal ictal injury continuum EEG patterns. J. Neurosci. Methods **351**, 108966 (2021)
3. Ghosh, S., Belkhouja, T., Yan, Y., Doppa, J.R.: Improving uncertainty quantification of deep classifiers via neighborhood conformal prediction: novel algorithm and theoretical analysis. Proc. AAAI Conf. Artif. Intell. **37**(6), 7722–7730 (2023)
4. Harati, A., Golmohammadi, M., Lopez, S., Obeid, I., Picone, J.: Improved EEG event classification using differential energy. IEEE Signal Processing in Medicine and Biology Symposium (2015)
5. Laghuvarapu, S., Lin, Z., Sun, J.: CoDrug: conformal drug property prediction with density estimation under covariate shift. Adv. Neural. Inf. Process. Syst. **36**, 37728–37747 (2023)
6. Lopez, S., Suarez, G., Jungreis, D., Obeid, I., Picone, J.: Automated identification of abnormal adult EEGs. IEEE Signal Processing in Medicine and Biology Symposium (2015)
7. Obeid, I., Picone, J.: The temple university hospital EEG data corpus. Front. Neurosci. **10**, 196 (2016)
8. Papadopoulos, H., Vovk, V., Gammerman, A.: Conformal prediction with neural networks. In: 19th IEEE International Conference on Tools with Artificial Intelligence (ICTAI 2007), vol. 2, pp. 388–395. IEEE (2007)
9. Pradeepkumar, J., Piao, X., Chen, Z., Sun, J.: Tokenizing single-channel EEG with time-frequency motif learning (2026). https://arxiv.org/abs/2502.16060
10. Shah, V., J.: The temple university hospital seizure detection corpus. Front. Neuroinformatics **12** (2018)
11. Tibshirani, R.J., Foygel Barber, R., Candes, E., Ramdas, A.: Conformal prediction under covariate shift. In: Advances in Neural Information Processing Systems, vol. 32 (2019)
12. Wu, Z., Yao, H., Liebovitz, D., Sun, J.: An iterative self-learning framework for medical domain generalization. In: Advances in Neural Information Processing Systems, vol. 36, pp. 54833–54854 (2023)
13. Yang, C., Westover, M.B., Sun, J.: ManyDG: Many-domain generalization for healthcare applications. In: The 11th International Conference on Learning Representations, ICLR 2023 (2023)
14. Yang, C., Xiao, D., Westover, M.B., Sun, J.: Self-supervised EEG representation learning for automatic sleep staging. JMIR AI (2023)

# Beyond Performance Metrics: Nurses' Concerns and Comfort with Clinical AI Use in Canada

Amanda Kutenski, Tarek Khalil, and Mirou Jaana(✉)

Telfer School of Management, University of Ottawa, Ottawa, ON, Canada
jaana@telfer.uottawa.ca

**Abstract.** Nurses represent frontline users of Artificial Intelligence (AI) enabled decision support, monitoring, and workflow systems, but their perspectives remain underrepresented in AI implementation research. This study examines the nature and level of concerns affecting nurses' comfort with AI use in Canada. Secondary data from the 2023 Canada Health Infoway nurses' survey (N = 1,907) were analyzed to examine the association between self-reported comfort (dependent variable) and concerns with AI use (independent variables). Multivariate ordinal logistic regression analyses assessed the relationship between *comfort with AI use* and *nine concern items* (4-point Likert Scale, 1 = very uncomfortable or concerning to 4 = very comfortable or not at all concerning) covering three concern areas (i.e. ethical/legal; human-relationship; workforce), while controlling for age and gender. Most respondents were female (91.5%) and [35–54] years old (53.7%). Median concern levels ranged from 1 to 2, with highest concerns related to data privacy and reduced human interaction (median = 1, respectively). Comfort with AI use was moderate (median = 2). Lower comfort was significantly associated with older age ($\tau = -0.066$) and female gender ($\chi^2$ (2) = 6.18). Multivariate analyses showed that greater concerns with medical liability ($\beta = 0.363$), negative patient-provider relationship impact ($\beta = 0.409$), and mistrust in AI ($\beta = 0.498$) are significantly associated with lower comfort. Nurses' comfort with AI use is associated with AI trust and accountability concerns. Future research should build on these findings and investigate how AI knowledge may affect this relationship. Designing AI tools requires in addition to algorithmic transparency and performance validation, liability frameworks, explainability, and clinician-centered interaction models that alleviate users' concerns.

**Keywords:** Artificial Intelligence · Concerns · Adoption · Comfort · Nursing

## 1 Introduction

Artificial intelligence (AI) enabled digital health technologies are increasingly deployed in healthcare systems to address rising costs and improve system efficiency. Emerging AI technologies include predictive analytics, smart home support, virtual health care assistants and robotic systems [1]. Within clinical environments, nurses represent one of the largest groups of end-users of digital health technologies. However, nurses still report persistent ambivalence toward adopting AI-enabled technologies. Accordingly,

© The Author(s), under exclusive license to Springer Nature Switzerland AG 2027
P. Andreev et al. (Eds.): AIME 2026, LNAI 16748, pp. 54–58, 2027.
https://doi.org/10.1007/978-3-032-30710-1_7

nurses have raised concerns regarding the ethical implications of AI integration in care delivery [2]. Such concerns act as barriers to adoption and may undermine the realization of the potential AI benefits, including early detection of patient deterioration, workload management, documentation automation and medication safety [3]. These tools are not intended to replace nurse judgement and work, and successful implementation not only depends on algorithmic performance, but also on nurses' knowledge, attitudes, and readiness to engage with these tools [1].

Classical technology acceptance frameworks (i.e., Technology Acceptance Model, Unified Theory of Acceptance and Use, and extensions) emphasize perceived usefulness, effort expectancy, social influence and facilitating conditions as predictors of adoption, with age/gender/experience as moderators [4]. Although these models help explain intention to use conventional systems, they may be insufficient for AI-enabled technologies, which can disrupt established workflow and raise concerns about effects on workforce and care practices [5]. Furthermore, prior work suggests that knowledge of AI mechanisms alone does not fully explain nurses' comfort with AI technologies [6]. AI-enabled technology considerations may involve simultaneous recognition of potential benefits and perceived risks [6]. *Thus, understanding how specific risk perceptions affect comfort is critical for human-centered AI design and adoption.*

This study investigates the relationship between specific AI-related concerns and Canadian nurses' comfort with AI use in healthcare, taking into consideration sociodemographic factors (i.e. age and gender). By identifying the domains of concern most strongly associated with comfort, the findings can inform human-centered AI design and implementation strategies in Canadian healthcare settings.

## 2 Methods

### 2.1 Data Source

We used secondary data from the 2023 Canada Health Infoway national survey of nurses (N = 1,907). The survey assessed nurses' experiences and readiness across six domains: digital nursing practice, clinical interoperability, electronic prescriptions, use of AI-enabled technologies, barriers to adoption of digital technologies, and demographic characteristics [7]. For this study, we focus on the questions related to AI concerns and comfort with AI use.

### 2.2 Measures

The primary outcome is nurses' self-reported comfort with AI use in healthcare (4-point Likert Scale, 1 = very uncomfortable to 4 = very comfortable). Nine items assessed perceived concerns regarding AI use (4-point Likert Scale, 1 = very concerning to 4 = not at all concerning), across three domains: ethical and legal issues; human relationship issues; and workforce implications (Fig. 1). To improve distributional balance [8], response categories were collapsed into three ordinal levels. Comfort categories "Very" and "moderately uncomfortable", and concern categories "not very concerning" and "not at all concerning" were merged, respectively. Age was recoded into three categories ($\leq$34; 35–54; $\geq$55).

### 2.3 Statistical Analysis

All analyses were conducted using IBM SPSS V.30. Descriptive statistics (i.e., frequencies, medians) were computed. Bivariate associations were examined using nonparametric tests. Kruskal–Wallis H assessed differences in AI comfort across gender categories. Kendall's tau-b correlation coefficient was used to assess associations between comfort and age, and between comfort and concerns. Ordinal logistic regression was conducted including concern variables, and age and gender as covariates (Fig. 1).

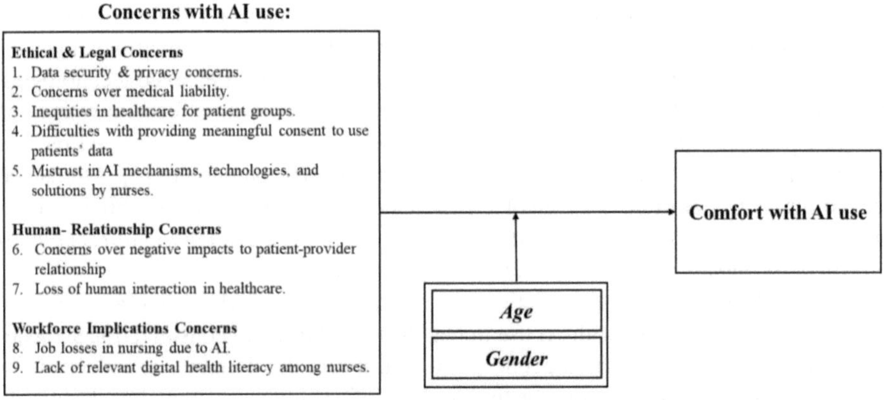


**Fig. 1.** Conceptual framework guiding multivariable ordinal logistic regression.

## 3 Results

### 3.1 Descriptive Results

Survey respondents were predominantly female (91.5%) and 35–54 years old (53.7%). More than half of the respondents (55.3%) indicated being uncomfortable with AI use; 27.5% were moderately comfortable and only 6.3% reported being comfortable. Overall, respondents expressed considerable concerns regarding AI use (median = 1–2) The highest level of concerns (median = 1) were associated with potential loss of human interaction in healthcare (56%) and data security and privacy risks (47.7%). Respondents were somewhat concerned across all other domains (median = 2, 29.5–42%), whereas 7.1–16.6% of respondents reported uncertainty regarding specific concerns.

### 3.2 Bivariate Analyses

**Age/Gender and Comfort.** Higher age categories were significantly associated with lower comfort levels ($\tau = -0.066$, $p = .017$). Comfort levels differed across gender categories ($\chi2(2) = 6.18$, $p = .045$), with men reporting higher mean rank comfort scores.

**Concerns and Comfort.** Higher levels of concern were significantly associated with lower comfort across all items ($p < .001$). The strongest associations were observed for concerns related to the potential negative impacts of AI on the patient–provider relationship ($\tau = 0.310$), mistrust in AI mechanisms and technologies ($\tau = 0.294$), and the loss of human interaction in healthcare ($\tau = 0.284$).

### 3.3 Multivariate Analysis

Lower levels of concerns related to medical liability ($\beta = 0.363$, $p = .005$), negative impacts on the patient–provider relationship ($\beta = 0.409$, $p = .005$), and mistrust in AI mechanisms and technologies ($\beta = 0.498$, $p < .001$) were significantly associated with greater comfort with AI use. Age and gender were not significant in the model, indicating that demographic characteristics did not explain variability in comfort levels once perceptions of AI-related risks were considered.

## 4 Discussion and Conclusions

This study examined how specific AI-related concerns are related to nurses' comfort with AI use in healthcare. Although all concerns were significantly associated with comfort with AI use in the bivariate analyses, only three remained significant in the adjusted model: *mistrust in AI mechanisms*, *perceived negative impact on the patient-provider relationship*, and *concerns about medical liability*. Age and gender did not affect these relationships, underscoring that perceived concerns/risks primarily drive variability in comfort with AI use. These findings suggest that comfort with AI is linked to perceptions of relational integrity, system trustworthiness and professional accountability rather than by broader workforce concerns (i.e., job losses and digital health literacy), in line with previous studies assessing determinants of nurses' comfort with AI [3, 9]. Thus, AI integration strategies should emphasize transparent risk communication, articulation of systems capabilities, and clear governance mechanisms. Reported uncertainty by up to 17% of nurses regarding concerns highlights an opportunity for proactive engagement through education, and co-design activities targeting modifiable beliefs about AI.

Prior human-centered interaction principles emphasize that trust calibration, explainability and participatory design are central to successful human-AI collaborations in healthcare [10]. By empirically distinguishing which concern domains are most strongly associated with comfort, we propose priority targets for human-centered AI interventions. Designing AI tools for clinical environments should therefore enable transparency of algorithmic reasoning; ensure that systems support a clear delineation of accountability and liability on the provider; and embed elements to preserve clinical-patient relational presence. Addressing these dimensions through participatory and human-centered AI design approaches may reduce nurses' dissonance and improve readiness/willingness for AI adoption.

The robust associations from the large sample size provide useful avenues for practical and further theoretical examination. We are further expanding our analysis to investigate how AI knowledge moderates the relationship between concerns and comfort.

Extending this framework to physicians and other healthcare professionals may further inform interdisciplinary AI design strategies.

**Disclosure of Interests.** The authors have no competing interests to declare that are relevant to the content of this paper.

## References

1. Wei, Q., Pan, S., Liu, X., Hong, M., Nong, C., Zhang, W.: The integration of AI in nursing: addressing current applications, challenges, and future directions. Front Med (Lausanne). **12**, 1545420 (2025). https://doi.org/10.3389/fmed.2025.1545420
2. Rony, M.K.K., Numan, S.M., Akter, K., Tushar, H., Debnath, M., Johra, F., et al.: Nurses' perspectives on privacy and ethical concerns regarding artificial intelligence adoption in healthcare. Heliyon. **10**, e36702 (2024). https://doi.org/10.1016/j.heliyon.2024.e36702
3. Ruksakulpiwat, S., Phianhasin, L., Benjasirisan, C., Su, T., Riangkam, C., Thorngthip, S., et al.: Artificial intelligence in nursing research: a systematic review of applications, benefits, and challenges. Int. Nurs. Rev. **72**, e70080 (2025)
4. Ammenwerth Elske: Technology acceptance models in health informatics: TAM and UTAUT. In: Studies in Health Technology and Informatics. IOS Press (2019). https://doi.org/10.3233/SHTI190111
5. Abdelwanis, M., Simsekler, M.C.E., Gabor, A.F., Sleptchenko, A., Omar, M.: Artificial intelligence adoption challenges from healthcare providers' perspectives: a comprehensive review and future directions. Saf. Sci. **193**, 107028 (2026). https://doi.org/10.1016/j.ssci.2025.107028
6. Li, A.K.C., Rauf, I.A., Keshavjee, K.: Knowledge is not all you need for comfort in use of AI in healthcare. Public Health. **238**, 254–259 (2025). https://doi.org/10.1016/j.puhe.2024.11.019
7. Canada Health Infoway: Infoway Insights: 2023 Canadian Survey of Nurses. https://insights.infoway-inforoute.ca/2023-nursing-survey
8. Koo, M., Yang, S.-W.: Likert-type scale. Encyclopedia. **5**, 18 (2025). https://doi.org/10.3390/encyclopedia5010018
9. Pare, G., Raymond, L., Etindele Sosso, F.A.: Nurses' intention to integrate AI into their practice: survey study in Canada. JMIR Nurs. **8**, e76795–e76795 (2025). https://doi.org/10.2196/76795
10. Majumder, N.N., Adebiyi, B.O.: Human-centered AI in healthcare. In: Handbook of Human-Centered Artificial Intelligence, pp. 1–55. Springer, Singapore (2026). https://doi.org/10.1007/978-981-97-8440-0_112-1

# Privacy-Preserving Generation of Synthetic Pathology Reports for Information Extraction

Alejandra Lorenzo[1,3(✉)], Adrien Coulet[2], and Claire Gardent[3]

[1] U2R, Unité de Radiothérapie République, Clermont-Ferrand, France
[2] Inria, Inserm, Université Paris Cité, HeKA UMR1346, Paris, France
Adrien.Coulet@inria.fr
[3] CNRS, Université de Lorraine, Loria UMR7503, Nancy, France
{alejandra.abdelnur,Claire.Gardent}@loria.fr

**Abstract.** A long-standing goal in clinical NLP is extracting key variables from clinical text, but progress is hindered by domain shift, limited annotated data, and privacy constraints. In this paper, we propose a novel privacy-preserving method to generate synthetic report/data pairs that support information extraction by associating LLM-generated pathology reports with thirteen variables commonly found in real reports for breast cancer patients. We first generate synthetic tabular data for these variables and their possible values, comparing several tabular synthesizers and selecting PATE-CTGAN for its strong statistical fidelity and differential privacy guarantees. We then generate pathology reports using three LLMs to maximize linguistic diversity and conditioning generation on synthetic variable–value sets.

We show that a model fine-tuned on the resulting synthetic data substantially outperforms the same model without fine-tuning and improves performance over a 3-shot baseline using synthetic in-context examples, achieving 0.79 accuracy compared to 0.38 and 0.64, respectively. These results show that high-quality synthetic data can effectively compensate for limited annotated clinical data while enabling accurate and privacy-preserving clinical information extraction. The code is available at https://gitlab.inria.fr/aabdelnu/syntheticpreports.

**Keywords:** Clinical text · Information Extraction · Synthetic data · Differential privacy

## 1 Introduction

Cancer diagnosis and treatment rely on the accurate interpretation of pathology reports, which contain essential information about tumor location, grade, morphology, and classification. Extracting this information to populate structured diagnosis forms is critical for clinical decision-making, yet manual extraction is time-consuming and error-prone. Large language models (LLMs) offer a promising avenue for automating this process, but their effectiveness depends on access

© The Author(s), under exclusive license to Springer Nature Switzerland AG 2027
P. Andreev et al. (Eds.): AIME 2026, LNAI 16748, pp. 59–69, 2027.
https://doi.org/10.1007/978-3-032-30710-1_8

to substantial annotated data and the use of real clinical text is constrained by patient privacy regulations, leading to a scarcity of training data—an issue that is particularly acute for languages with fewer resources than English [13]. Synthetic data generation provides a potential solution by enabling the creation of datasets that retain the statistical properties of real data while reducing privacy risks. Thus [12] generate table/text pairs by first, generating tabular data using a Bayesian network whose dependencies are defined by domain-experts and second, using this data as input to an LLM to generate clinical texts. Similarly, [15] automatically extracts table/text pairs from pdf files and uses these to train a table-to-text summarisation system.

In this work, we propose a novel privacy-preserving method to generate synthetic data for information extraction. This method consists in first creating realistic clinical tabular data and second, converting it into matching French reports using LLMs. We show that fine-tuning an LLM on these pairs significantly outperforms both zero- and few-shot baselines.

## 2 Generating Synthetic Tabular Data

Based on 3,880 breast cancer patient records, we derive synthetic data for thirteen clinically relevant variables (e.g., diagnosis, size and position of the tumor, Estrogen Receptor Status) in three main steps: discretization, comparison of four existing synthesizers and application of the selected synthesizer to the cancer data. Patient data were extracted from four French clinics belonging to the U2R group. Patient information and data pseudonymisation were performed in accordance with French regulation and the GDPR.

### 2.1 Discretization

First, we discretize variable values in order to aggregate fine-grained variables into clinically meaningful and broader categories. Categorical variables are consolidated into broader classes (e.g., *tumorectomie avec curage axillaire* → *tumorectomie*), while numerical variables are discretized into clinically meaningful ranges (e.g., tumor size (mm) → 0, 1–5, 6–10, 11–20, 21–50, 50+ mm). Discretization helps strengthen privacy protection as exact numerical values can make individuals more easily identifiable, especially for rare or extreme measurements. By grouping values into intervals, we reduce data granularity, which lowers the risk of linkage attacks based on unique numerical patterns, and we increase the size of equivalence classes (more patients share the same combination of variables) again reducing re-identification probability. Discretization was also shown to facilitate and stabilise synthetic data generation. In particular, differentially private tabular synthesizers, like MST or PATE-CTGAN, were shown to handle categorical distributions more effectively than continuous variables with wide or heavy-tailed ranges and [5] showed that optimizing the discretizer and number of bins improves utility.

### 2.2 Comparing Synthesizers

We compare four existing synthesizers from two libraries, Synthetic Data Vault (SDV) [11] and SmartNoise [8]: a probabilistic model based on copulas (Gaussian Copulas from SDV), a generative adversarial network adapted to tabular data (CTGAN from SDV), and two variants that incorporate differential privacy guarantees (PATE-CTGAN, MST, from SmartNoise). The *Gaussian Copula Synthesizer* [11] learns marginal distributions, transforms them to a normal scale, estimates the covariance matrix, and samples synthetic rows from the resulting multivariate Gaussian before mapping them back to the original domain. *CTGAN* [16] is a conditional generative adversarial network designed specifically for tabular data, which extends the standard GAN framework with three innovations: a conditional generator to better model rare categorical values, Mode-Specific Normalization using Gaussian Mixture Models for continuous data, and conditional sampling to balance discrete categories. *PATE-CTGAN* [6] takes the state-of-the-art CTGAN tabular data synthesizer and applies PATE (Private Aggregation of Teacher Ensemble), to ensure Differential Privacy. Finally, *Maximum Spanning Tree (MST)* [10] is a simple probabilistic tabular data synthesizer that models dependencies between variables using a maximum spanning tree. While the Gaussian Copula preserves correlations and CTGAN captures complex non-linear relationships, both can still reproduce rare combinations, posing re-identification risks. Because of these risks, stronger guarantees are needed. Differential Privacy (DP) [4] provides a rigorous, mathematically provable standard for privacy protection. Under DP, the risk of any individual being identified is nearly the same whether or not their data is included in the dataset, making it resistant to membership inference and reconstruction attacks. This is particularly important when dealing with high-dimensional tabular data, where correlations and rare variable combinations can inadvertently expose individuals.

*Evaluation Metrics.* To determine which synthesizer best captures data distribution while preserving privacy, we evaluate the synthesized data along three main dimensions: fidelity, similarity and novelty.

Fidelity assesses the synthetic data's ability to reproduce the statistical distributions observed in the real data, both at the marginal level for individual variables and at the level of inter-variable relationships. We evaluate fidelity using *Accuracy* [14], the agreement between real and synthetic data, measured across univariate (single column), bivariate (column pairs), and trivariate (column triplets) distributions via averaged L1 distance.

Similarity [14] assesses whether the synthetic data preserves the overall structure of the real data within a learned representation space, without aiming for a one-to-one correspondence at the individual record level. First, the synthetic and training instances are represented as vectors in an embedding space, then the cosine distance between the centroid of each dataset is computed.

Finally, novelty focuses on privacy preservation. Here, the goal is to detect whether certain synthetic records are excessively close to real individuals. We use four metrics for novelty: *the proportion of identical matches between synthetic and training data*, NNDR (Nearest Neighbor Distance Ratio), DCR share (Distance to Closest Record share) [14] and DCR Overfitting Score [3]. *NNDR* compares how close a synthetic record is to its nearest training *vs.* holdout record, where values near 1 mean balanced, below 1 suggest overfitting, and above 1 indicate high novelty. *DCR share* shows the proportion of synthetic records that are closer to some training record than to any holdout record. If this share is too large, it suggests overfitting/memorization. Ideally the synthetic data should behave similarly to holdout data in this respect. Lastly, *DCR Overfitting Score* evaluates whether synthetic samples are excessively close to the real (training) data compared to unseen holdout data. It computes a normalized ratio between 0 and 1, where lower scores (close to 0) indicates that a large fraction of synthetic samples are closer to real training data, suggesting possible overfitting or memorization, whereas higher scores (approaching 1) reflect greater novelty and privacy preservation.

*Hyper-Parameters.* We apply our synthesizers to 3,880 sets of variable-values pairs associated with anatomical pathology reports written by physicians for breast cancer patients. For the novelty metrics, this data was split 50/50 into training and holdout sets. For each synthesizer, ten independent synthetic datasets were generated and the resulting datasets evaluated, giving ten measurements per synthesizer. We then average the ten results to get the final score. The privacy budget $\epsilon$ was empirically evaluated across multiple values (from 2 to 5), and $\epsilon$=3 was selected as it provides the best balance between data utility and privacy risk, consistent with findings in [1].

**Table 1.** Comparing the four Synthesisers.

| Metric \ Synthesizer | Gaussian Copula | CTGAN | PATE-GAN | MST |
|---|---|---|---|---|
| **Fidelity** | | | | |
| Overall Accuracy | 86.59% | 74.57% | 82.56% | **92.22%** |
| Accuracy - Univariate | 96.57% | 86.68% | 93.46% | **98.36%** |
| Accuracy - Bivariate | 86.46% | 74.17% | 82.34% | **92.22%** |
| Accuracy - Trivariate | 76.72% | 62.86% | 71.87% | **86.07%** |
| **Similarity** | | | | |
| Cosine Similarity | 0.984 | 0.886 | 0.973 | **0.999** |
| **Novelty** | | | | |
| ↓ % Identical Matches | 5.85% | **1.76%** | 3.68% | 17.62% |
| ↑ NNDR | 0.961 | 0.560 | **1.080** | 1.189 |
| ↓ DCR – Share | 55.10% | 56.47% | 54.90% | **52.36%** |
| DCR Overfitting Score | **1.0** | **1.0** | **1.0** | **1.0** |

*Results and Synthesizer Selection.* Following [7], who emphasize that the optimal synthetic data generator is not necessarily the one with the highest raw accuracy, but rather the one that achieves the best trade-off between fidelity and privacy protection, we aim to strike a balance between realism and privacy: generating synthetic data that is sufficiently faithful to support the training of performant models, while remaining sufficiently distinct from the original data to ensure patient protection.

Table 1 reports the results for the four synthesizers. They show that CTGAN has the lowest and MST the highest fidelity. However, MST also produces the largest number of identical matches, indicating a higher risk of memorization and lower novelty. Gaussian Copula and PATE-CTGAN exhibit comparable fidelity, but PATE-CTGAN yields fewer identical matches. Balancing fidelity, and novelty, we therefore select PATE-CTGAN for synthetic medical data generation.

### 2.3 Generating Synthetic Sets of Variable-Value Pairs

Using the PATE-CTGAN synthesizer, we generate 4,000 synthetic data instances (sets of 13 variable-value pairs) and select a representative subset of 1,000 instances to compare the outputs of three different LLMs while maintaining textual diversity and reducing generation and evaluation costs. To obtain this representative sample, we performed a stratified, frequency-weighted subsampling. First, we quantified data completeness by counting non-missing (non-"unknown") variables per instance and used this measure to define quartiles. Within each quartile, we examined the joint distribution of two clinically relevant variables namely, MORPHOLOGY and NUMBER OF LYMPH NODES REMOVED. For each quartile, we sampled 60 examples from the two most frequent variable combinations, 30 examples from the next two most frequent combinations, and 70 examples from all remaining combinations. This yielded 250 samples per quartile, totaling 1,000 records that preserve both category structure and completeness heterogeneity.

## 3 Generating Synthetic Pathology Reports

This second step uses LLMs to generate synthetic textual pathology reports conditioned on the previously generated variable-value pairs.

*Data Preprocessing and Input Structuring.* The tabular data is first transformed into a format suitable for prompting an LLM. This preprocessing is particularly important for variable values previously discretized as numerical ranges. To ensure clinical plausibility while allowing narrative flexibility, these ranges are converted into descriptive expressions within the prompt. For instance, the tabular entry *lymph nodes examined: 6–12*, is transformed into the French version of *Number of lymph nodes examined: to be selected within the range of 6 to 12, depending on clinical consistency.* In this way, the LLM is informed of the possible values but is left free to choose within the given range.

Although the "diagnostic test" variable is mandatory in pathology reports, we observed cases in both real and synthetic data where it was missing. To address this issue, we apply the following expert rule: if the test is not specified but the instance includes a tumor size value, the "diagnostic test" is set to "breast lumpectomy" (the most frequent diagnostic test with "tumor size" variable); otherwise, it is set to "biopsy" (the most frequent diagnostic test when no tumor size is indicated). We also observed that "hormonal receptors" values were systematically generated as either negative or positive whereas pathology reports also report a percentage of positivity when this variable is positive. To reproduce similar values, we provide the LLM with a random value drawn from a range of valid positivity percentages.

*Models.* We select three LLMs for text generation based on their various expected strengths: Mixtral-8×7B for strong French generation, MedGemma-27B for medical-domain specialization, and Qwen3-30B-A3B as a large, instruction-tuned generalist model. For all three models, inference is performed using deterministic greedy decoding with temperature 0.

*Evaluation.* As reference texts are unavailable, standard reference-based metrics such as BLEU or ROUGE cannot be used. Hence we adopt an LLM-as-Judge evaluation protocol using two LLMs (GPT-5.1 and Gemini-2.5-Pro) to assess both the faithfulness between texts and variable-value pairs and the global consistency of the document. For faithfulness, the LLM judge outputs, for each input variable-value pair, a JSON object with two fields: the field 'correct (yes/no)', indicates whether the text correctly mentions the input variable–value; the field 'reference', provides the supporting text span when applicable. For consistency, we prompt the LLMs to detect explicit contradictions for key clinical variables (e.g., tumor size, receptor status, grade, margins, lymph nodes) and assign each text a single consistency label out of the three possible ones {PASS, FAIL, or UNKNOWN}.

We assess the reliability of the LLM judges by comparing their predictions against human judgments. Two clinical experts were asked to manually annotate 50 synthetic pathology reports with their matching attribute-value pairs. The Kappa [2] value between the two human annotators reaches 0.90 for faithfulness (almost perfect) and 0.67 for consistency. For Humans–LLM agreement, we use Krippendorff's $\alpha$ [9], which is suitable for multiple annotators ($n = 3$ in our case). For both LLMs, the results show high consistency with human annotators for faithfulness $\alpha$ scores of 0.90 for GPT 5.1 and 0.82 for Gemini-2.5-Pro. Results are lower for consistency: 0.53 and 0.59, respectively. Based on these results, we used GPT 5.1 for faithfulness evaluation and Gemini-2.5-Pro for consistency.

We also assess the distribution gap between synthetic and real reports using lexical richness, repetition, entropy, compression, and structural-formatting metrics.

*Results.* Table 2 presents the faithfulness and consistency evaluations for the three LLMs. For each clinical variable, the table reports the per variable accuracy, defined as the proportion of variable-value pairs correctly mentioned in the generated report relative to the input data. The table also reports the overall accuracy, computed as the average across all variables, and the consistency score, defined as the proportion of reports assigned a"PASS" value by the consistency evaluation. The overall accuracy across all variables is relatively high, with faithfulness ranging from 0.747 to 0.888 and consistency ranging from 0.792 to 0.929. The medical LLM MedGemma performs well in terms of both faithfulness (0.878) and consistency (0.929). For Qwen3, the lower accuracy on the *diagnostic_test* variable can be explained by the frequent use of generic report titles that do not clearly specify the procedure type and may be incompatible with biopsy reports.

Table 3 shows the distribution of document-level accuracy for each LLM. For each document, accuracy is defined as the proportion of clinical variables that exactly match the reference. Documents are then grouped into bins according to this proportion, and the table reports the percentage of documents falling into each bin. MedGemma and Mixtral achieve moderate to high document level accuracy for 92.9% of the documents.

Finally, the distribution gap analysis shows that real reports are longer, more lexically diverse, and more structurally segmented, whereas synthetic reports are shorter, more repetitive, more predictable, and less faithful to clinical formatting conventions. Details are provided in the code repository.

**Table 2.** Accuracy and Consistency of Synthetic Reports

| Variable | Qwen3 | MedGemma | Mixtral |
|---|---|---|---|
| diagnostic_test | 0.125 | 1.000 | 0.994 |
| number_lymph_nodes_removed | 0.840 | 0.872 | 0.851 |
| number_lymph_nodes_affected | 0.519 | 0.871 | 0.728 |
| extracapsular_tumor_spread | 0.848 | 0.884 | 0.925 |
| tumor_size | 0.483 | 0.709 | 0.840 |
| estrogen_receptor_status | 0.961 | 0.974 | 0.957 |
| progesterone_receptor_status | 0.960 | 0.995 | 0.977 |
| lymphovascular_invasion | 0.405 | 0.712 | 0.605 |
| her2_status | 0.903 | 0.991 | 0.992 |
| clear_margins | 0.943 | 0.552 | 0.731 |
| Ki67_percentage | 0.923 | 0.996 | 0.983 |
| morphology | 0.992 | 0.948 | 0.974 |
| sbr_grade | 0.815 | 0.917 | 0.987 |
| **Overall** | 0.747 | 0.878 | 0.888 |
| consistency | 0.885 | 0.929 | 0.792 |

## 4 Information Extraction

To evaluate whether the synthetic training data improves IE in real world scenarios, we use it to fine-tune Mistral-7B-Instruct and compare the resulting model (Mistral-FT) with the same model in a 0- (Mistral-0S) and a 3-shot (Mistral-3S) setting. The fine-tuning data is composed of report/variable-value pairs, where each variable-value pair corresponds to those correctly generated within the report by any of the three LLMs. This yielded 33,277 training examples, i.e., about 2,500 reports for each of the thirteen variables. For each training instance, the input consists of a prompt including a pathology report, the variable to be extracted, its possible values or range and the required JSON output schema ({"value": ..., "reference": ...}. The output is the expected variable value. We fine-tuned using LoRA adaptation.

**Table 3.** Document-level accuracy of Synthetic Reports (percentage of documents that achieved a given proportion of correctly generated clinical variables, N = 1000)

| Accuracy Bucket - % of Correct Vars. | Qwen3 | MedGemma | Mixtral |
|---|---|---|---|
| Perfect - 100% | 0.3% | 20.8% | 27.2% |
| High - 85–99% | 7.7% | 30.8% | 30.3% |
| Moderate - 70–84% | 50.8% | 41.3% | 35.4% |
| Low - 50–69% | 40.0% | 7.1% | 6.6% |
| Very Low - < 50% | 1.2% | 0.0% | 0.5% |

We evaluated the IE performance of the three models on a test set of 377 real breast cancer pathology reports manually annotated with gold standard labels for all target variables by experts.

*Results.* Table 4 shows the results.

Adding synthetic examples as in-context demonstrations significantly improves performance over zero-shot prompting, showing their value even without fine-tuning. However, the fine-tuned model performs best overall, surpassing the 3-shot baseline, particularly on variables requiring numerical extraction or specific mention detection (e.g., Ki-67, tumor size, lymph nodes, extracapsular spread).

For some variables, the 3-shot baseline is competitive or slightly better. These correspond to attributes with a small, well defined set of possible values (e.g., positive/negative/unknown) and standardized phrasing in the reports, such as estrogen and progesterone receptor status, clear margins and diagnostic type. In such settings, a small number of in-context examples is often sufficient for the model to generalize.

Morphology is the hardest variable across settings, likely because the prompt uses an ICD-O classification name instead of a fixed label set, forcing the model to generate or extract free text instead of choosing from a limited set of labels.

**Table 4.** IE Accuracy and F1 Scores for Fine-Tuned, 0- and 3-Shot Models.

| Variable | Acc-0S | Acc-3S | Acc-FT | F1-0S | F1-3S | F1-FT |
|---|---|---|---|---|---|---|
| morphology | 0.07 | 0.15 | **0.44** | 0.05 | 0.07 | **0.47** |
| diagnostic_type | 0.48 | **0.73** | 0.71 | 0.52 | **0.76** | 0.75 |
| lymphovascular_invasion | 0.55 | 0.63 | **0.79** | 0.69 | 0.68 | **0.72** |
| sbr_grade | 0.46 | 0.84 | **0.90** | 0.55 | 0.83 | **0.90** |
| her2_status | 0.47 | 0.71 | **0.82** | 0.55 | 0.79 | **0.82** |
| Ki67_percentage | 0.39 | 0.69 | **0.89** | 0.23 | 0.64 | **0.87** |
| clear_margins | 0.28 | 0.67 | **0.77** | 0.41 | **0.53** | 0.50 |
| number_lymph_nodes_affected | 0.24 | 0.66 | **0.84** | 0.24 | 0.36 | **0.71** |
| number_lymph_nodes_removed | 0.22 | 0.57 | **0.81** | 0.14 | 0.32 | **0.69** |
| estrogen_receptor_status | 0.71 | **0.83** | 0.80 | 0.79 | **0.88** | 0.83 |
| progesterone_receptor_status | 0.66 | **0.88** | 0.85 | 0.71 | **0.89** | 0.85 |
| extracapsular_tumor_spread | 0.15 | 0.37 | **0.98** | 0.14 | 0.13 | **0.62** |
| tumor_size | 0.24 | 0.53 | **0.77** | 0.15 | 0.27 | **0.63** |
| **Overall** | 0.38 | 0.64 | **0.79** | 0.41 | 0.58 | **0.74** |

## 5 Conclusion and Discussion

We propose a novel privacy-preserving approach for generating synthetic pathology reports from structured data. Applied to real-world breast cancer variables, the resulting synthetic report/data pairs remain faithful to real world distribution while avoiding the exposure of protected health information, thereby creating novel opportunities for the development of robust information extraction systems. We show that a model fine-tuned on this synthetic data achieves strong and consistent improvements in extraction performance across nearly all variables compared to the base model, while also improving overall performance over a 3-shot baseline that uses the generated synthetic pathology reports as in-context examples.

A limitation of this evaluation is that the extraction task targets the same variables used to generate the synthetic reports, so it does not assess generalization beyond the predefined schema. However, the approach can be extended to any new set of clinical variables. As it does not require annotated data, our approach can be applied to other types of clinical texts, provided the corresponding structured data are available. An important direction for future work would be to extend it to additional clinical domains and to other languages.

**Acknowledgments.** The authors thank SELARL U2R for providing the data and supporting this research. This work received government funding managed by the French National Research Agency under France 2030, reference number "ANR-23-IACL-0004." (AI Chair Gardent: "Semantically Consistent LLM Based Text Generation"). It was also granted access to the HPC resources of IDRIS under the allocation AD011016561 made by GENCI.

**Ethics Statement.** The study received approval from the institution's internal bodies. The mandatory declaration was completed with the French regulatory authority in accordance with Reference Methodology MR-004 (ref. MR-004, no. 28088412).

**Disclosure of Interests.** Alejandra Lorenzo is affiliated with the organization that provided the data used in this study. The authors declare that this affiliation did not influence the design, analysis, or reporting of the results.

## References


1. Appenzeller, A., Leitner, M., Philipp, P., Krempel, E., Beyerer, J.: Privacy and utility of private synthetic data for medical data analyses. Appl. Sci. **12**(23), 12320 (2022)
2. Cohen, J.: A coefficient of agreement for nominal scales. Educ. Psychol. Measur. **20**(1), 37–46 (1960). https://doi.org/10.1177/001316446002000104
3. DataCebo, Inc.: Synthetic Data Metrics (2023). https://docs.sdv.dev/sdmetrics/, version 0.12.0
4. Li, N., Lyu, M., Su, D., Yang, W.: Differential Privacy. In: International Colloquium on Automata, Languages, and Programming, pp. 1–12. Springer, Cham (2006). https://doi.org/10.1007/978-3-031-02350-7
5. Ganev, G., Annamalai, M.S.M.S., Mahiou, S., De Cristofaro, E.: The importance of being discrete: measuring the impact of discretization in end-to-end differentially private synthetic data, (2025). arXiv preprint arXiv:2504.06923
6. Jordon, J., Yoon, J., Van Der Schaar, M.: PATE-GAN: generating synthetic data with differential privacy guarantees. In: International Conference on Learning Representations (2018)
7. Kiran, A., Kumar, S.S.: A methodology and an empirical analysis to determine the most suitable synthetic data generator. IEEE Access **12**, 12209–12228 (2024)
8. Kopp, A.: Microsoft smart noise differential privacy machine learning case studies. Microsoft Azure White Papers 14 (2021)
9. Krippendorff, K.: Computing Krippendorff's alpha-reliability. Annenberg School for Communication. University of Pennsylvania, Tech. rep. (2011)
10. McKenna, R., Miklau, G., Sheldon, D.: Winning the NIST contest: a scalable and general approach to differentially private synthetic data. arXiv preprint arXiv:2108.04978 (2021)
11. Patki, N., Wedge, R., Veeramachaneni, K.: The synthetic data vault. In: IEEE International Conference on Data Science and Advanced Analytics (DSAA), pp. 399–410 (2016). https://doi.org/10.1109/DSAA.2016.49
12. Rabaey, P., Heytens, S., Demeester, T.: Simsum-simulated benchmark with structured and unstructured medical records. J. Biomed. Semantics **16**(1), 20 (2025)
13. Richter-Pechanski, P., et al.: Clinical information extraction for lower-resource languages and domains with few-shot learning using pretrained language models and prompting. Nat. Lang. Process. **31**(5), 1210–1233 (2025). https://doi.org/10.1017/nlp.2024.52
14. Sidorenko, A., Platzer, M., Scriminaci, M., Tiwald, P.: Benchmarking synthetic tabular data: a multi-dimensional evaluation framework (2025). arXiv preprint arXiv:2504.01908

15. Wu, H.Y., Zhang, J., Ive, J., Li, T., Gupta, V., Chen, B., Guo, Y.: Medical scientific table-to-text generation with synthetic data under data sparsity constraint. In: NeurIPS 2022 Workshop on Synthetic Data for Empowering ML Research (2023)
16. Xu, L., Skoularidou, M., Cuesta-Infante, A., Veeramachaneni, K.: Modeling tabular data using conditional GAN. In: Advances in Neural Information Processing Systems, vol. 32 (2019)

# Evaluating SSL Representations, Temporal Modeling, and Fine-Tuning Strategies for Low-Resource Speech-Based TBI Detection


Adebanji Adeleye[1], Olayinka Adeleye[2(✉)], and Victor Mayowa[3]

[1] Department of Computer Science, Auckland University of Technology, Auckland, New Zealand
adebanji.adeleye@aut.ac.nz

[2] Department of Information Technology, Otago Polytechnic, Dunedin, New Zealand
ola.adeleye@op.ac.nz

[3] Department of Engineering and Computing, University of East London, London, UK
u2680504@uel.ac.uk



**Abstract.** Traumatic Brain Injury (TBI) is a major public health concern for which early detection is critical. Speech-based TBI detection offers a scalable, non-invasive alternative to conventional clinical assessment, yet progress is hindered by extreme data scarcity, conditions under which deep models often overfit and generalize poorly. While self-supervised learning (SSL) models can be leveraged to address data scarcity within a transfer learning pipeline, the relative contributions of representation quality, temporal modeling, and fine-tuning strategies remain poorly understood under such constraints. We conduct a systematic evaluation of wav2vec 2.0, HuBERT, and WavLM across frozen feature extraction, partial fine-tuning, and end-to-end adaptation, combined with both traditional classifiers and temporal neural architectures. A layer-wise analysis identifies the most TBI-discriminative SSL representations. Subject-independent evaluation shows that frozen intermediate SSL features paired with lightweight classifiers achieve the highest performance (95.2% accuracy), demonstrating strong robustness under severe data scarcity. Temporal modeling provides significant gains over static aggregation when model complexity is controlled (90.5% vs. 76.2%), but deeper end-to-end architectures overfit and generalize poorly. Critically, any fine-tuning of the SSL encoder, whether partial (76.5%) or end-to-end (51.8%), degrades performance, as the limited data cannot support effective adaptation without destabilizing pretrained representations. These results establish practical guidelines for deploying SSL-based speech biomarkers in low-resource clinical settings, emphasizing the importance of preserving frozen pretrained features.



**Keywords:** Traumatic Brain Injury · Self-Supervised Learning · Transfer Learning · Speech Analysis · Temporal Modeling · Data Scarcity



© The Author(s), under exclusive license to Springer Nature Switzerland AG 2027


P. Andreev et al. (Eds.): AIME 2026, LNAI 16748, pp. 70–80, 2027.
https://doi.org/10.1007/978-3-032-30710-1_9

## 1 Introduction

Traumatic brain injury (TBI) is a neurological disorder caused by external mechanical forces that disrupt normal brain function, impairing cognition, communication, and speech production [6]. It is a major cause of long-term neurological disability, affecting over 55 million individuals worldwide, approximately 0.7% of the global population [4]. In the United States alone, more than 1.4 million new cases occur annually [6]. Beyond acute injury, TBI often leads to persistent cognitive, emotional, and motor impairments across all severity levels, increasing the risks of complications and re-hospitalization [5]. Continuous monitoring is therefore essential for tracking recovery and enabling timely intervention.

Conventional TBI assessment relies on neuropsychological testing and neuroimaging, which are costly, time-consuming, and require specialized clinical infrastructure. These limitations restrict accessibility, particularly for routine monitoring of mild-to-moderate cases and in low-resource settings. Consequently, scalable non-invasive approaches based on behavioral biomarkers, including gait and speech analysis, have attracted growing interest [15]. Speech-based assessment is especially promising, since TBI disrupts the articulatory, phonatory, and prosodic subsystems of speech production [13,14]. These disruptions manifest as measurable changes in speech rate, voice quality, and articulation that evolve throughout recovery, making speech well suited for continuous monitoring. These impairments have been examined in clinical speech pathology [8] and more recently leveraged for automated TBI detection using vocal biomarkers [7,13].

Despite its potential, progress in speech-based TBI detection remains constrained by severe data scarcity. Ethical, logistical, and financial challenges limit the collection of annotated clinical speech corpora, resulting in small and homogeneous datasets typically containing fewer than 150 subjects. This extreme low-resource regime renders deep learning approaches prone to overfitting and poor generalization. Even the largest publicly available corpus contains recordings from only slightly over one hundred participants [3].

Recent advances in self-supervised learning (SSL) for speech have demonstrated that pretrained models can provide rich transferable representations that improve performance in low-resource clinical tasks [10,17,18]. However, their application to speech-based TBI detection remains largely unexplored. Existing studies rely primarily on handcrafted features or shallow neural networks [7,12,13,15,16], failing to exploit modern pretrained representations. Moreover, under severe data constraints, the relative contributions of representation depth, temporal modeling, and fine-tuning strategies remain unclear. In this work, we present a controlled investigation, isolating the roles of SSL representation quality, transfer strategy, and temporal modeling in low-resource speech-based TBI detection. We systematically evaluate wav2vec 2.0, HuBERT, and WavLM across frozen, partially adapted, and fully fine-tuned configurations, complemented by a layer-wise analysis and a strict subject-independent train–test split for performance evaluation, with additional analysis highlighting variability under different data partitions. Our contributions are summarized as follows, we present:

- A unified evaluation framework isolating the effects of representation quality, temporal modeling, and fine-tuning in low-resource TBI detection.
- A systematic benchmark quantifying performance and generalization stability under realistic clinical data constraints.

## 2 Related Work

Early speech-based TBI detection employed traditional machine learning with handcrafted acoustic features (MFCCs, fundamental frequency, jitter, shimmer, prosodic measures) [7,8,13,14]. While demonstrating feasibility, these approaches were limited by manual feature engineering and restricted representational capacity. Recent work has shifted toward deep learning that learns hierarchical representations from spectrograms or minimally processed speech [6,12,16]. Wall et al. [16] applied attention-based BiLSTM to athlete speech, achieving high sensitivity despite small cohorts. Helfer et al. [8] analyzed formant coordination, reporting AUROC 0.94–0.97. Talkar et al. [15] fused speech and gait features, achieving 98% AUROC versus 89% for speech-only CNNs. Rojas et al. [12] employed ResNet-based classification with Grad-CAM interpretability but highlighted instability under small samples. Ditthapron et al. [6] proposed cascading GRU with parametrized sinc filters, achieving 83.9% accuracy on the Coelho corpus. Despite advances, end-to-end deep models remain constrained by labeled data scarcity (often <120 subjects), raising overfitting concerns. Ditthapron et al. [5] investigated transfer learning through cross-task, multi-task, and meta-learning frameworks. While improving performance, these entangle representation quality, temporal modeling, and adaptation mechanisms. In related clinical domains, particularly mental health [10,17,18], SSL models pretrained on large-scale unlabeled corpora consistently demonstrate robustness in low-resource settings by capturing transferable acoustic-temporal structures. However, their application to TBI detection remains unexplored, with studies continuing to rely on handcrafted features or auxiliary labeled supervision. This work leverages SSL encoders pretrained on large-scale unlabeled speech as foundational backbones for TBI detection, systematically evaluating frozen extraction and selective fine-tuning under extreme data scarcity while disentangling contributions of representation quality, temporal modeling architecture, and layer depth.

## 3 Material and Methods

### 3.1 Problem Formulation

Given a speech recording $x_i \in \mathbb{R}^{T_i}$ from participant $i$ with variable duration $T_i$ and binary label $y_i \in \{0,1\}$ (0: healthy, 1: TBI), we learn a classifier $f : \mathbb{R}^{T_i} \to \{0,1\}$ predicting TBI status from raw speech. The dataset

$\mathcal{D} = \{(\mathbf{x}_i, y_i)\}_{i=1}^{N}$ contains $N = 107$ subjects ($N_{\text{TBI}} = 55$, $N_{\text{control}} = 52$), representing a severe low-resource regime where conventional deep learning overfits. Rather than training from scratch, we leverage pretrained SSL models as feature extractors: $\mathbf{h}_i = g_\theta(\mathbf{x}_i) \in \mathbb{R}^d$, where $g_\theta$ denotes an SSL encoder (HuBERT, Wav2Vec2, or WavLM) with parameters $\theta$, producing $d$-dimensional ($d = 768$) contextual representations. Each model comprises a 7-layer convolutional encoder and 12-layer Transformer (768 dimensions, 12 attention heads).

For input $\mathbf{x}_i$, the encoder produces layer-wise hidden states $\{\mathbf{H}_i^{(\ell)}\}_{\ell=0}^{12}$, where $\mathbf{H}_i^{(\ell)} \in \mathbb{R}^{T' \times d}$ denotes layer $\ell$ output with $T'$ frames. We aggregate via mean pooling: $\mathbf{h}_i^{(\ell)} = \frac{1}{T'} \sum_{t=1}^{T'} \mathbf{H}_i^{(\ell)}[t,:] \in \mathbb{R}^d$. Classification then reduces to learning lightweight classifier $f_\phi$ on layer $\ell$ representations: $\hat{y}_i = f_\phi(\mathbf{h}_i^{(\ell)})$, where $\phi$ denotes trainable parameters. Figure 1 illustrates the self-supervised learning (SSL) representation and transfer learning evaluation pipeline for speech-based traumatic brain injury (TBI) detection.

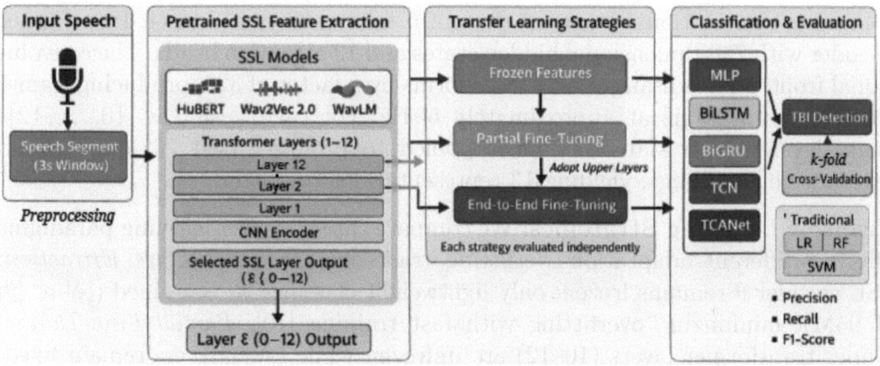


**Fig. 1.** Systematic SSL Representation and Transfer Learning Evaluation Pipeline for Speech-Based TBI Detection, comprising: (1) Preprocessing, (2) SSL Feature Extraction, (3) TBI Classification.

**Table 1.** Demographic and Clinical Summary of the Coelho TBI Speech Corpus

| Characteristic | TBI Group | Control Group |
|---|---|---|
| Sample size (n) | 55 | 52 |
| Age (years), mean (range) | 28.6 (16–69) | 31.9 (16–63) |
| Education (years), mean (range) | 13.0 (9–21) | 14.2 (11–22) |
| Sex (M:F) | 45:10 | 41:11 |
| Injury severity | Moderate to severe | – |
| Primary task | Story retelling, conversation | |

### 3.2 Data Preprocessing and SSL Feature Extraction

We use the Coelho TBI corpus [3] comprising story retelling and conversational speech from 55 TBI patients and 52 controls. Participant-only segments were extracted using transcript timestamps, resampled to 16 kHz, normalized, and segmented into 3-second overlapping windows (50% overlap). Table 1 summarizes demographics. For evaluation, we employ stratified 5-fold subject-independent cross-validation to ensure robust performance estimation and prevent data leakage. The dataset is partitioned at the subject level, preserving class balance, with performance reported as the mean across folds. Subject independence is strictly enforced by assigning all segments from each subject to a single fold.

**SSL Feature Extraction:** We extract layer-wise representations from three state-of-the-art SSL models pretrained on large-scale unlabeled corpora: *wav2vec 2.0* [1] (960h LibriSpeech, contrastive masked prediction); *HuBERT* [9] (iterative masked prediction with unsupervised clusters); *WavLM* [2] (94,000h speech, unified contrastive objectives with gated relative position bias). Each model comprises convolutional frontend (layer 0), followed by a 12-layer Transformer encoder with 768-dimensional hidden states and 12 attention heads. The convolutional frontend downsamples raw waveforms by a factor of 320, producing frame-level representations at approximately 50 Hz. For each layer $\ell \in \{0, \ldots, 12\}$, frame-level hidden states are mean-pooled to produce fixed 768-dimensional utterance embeddings, yielding 13 representations per utterance.

**Transfer Learning Strategies.** We compare three transfer learning paradigms offering different adaptation-overfitting trade-offs: *Frozen Feature Extraction:* SSL encoder $\theta$ remains frozen; only lightweight classifier $f_\phi$ is trained ($|\phi| \ll |\theta|$ of 95M), minimizing overfitting with fast training [10]. *Partial Fine-Tuning:* Upper transformer layers (10–12) are unfrozen while lower layers remain fixed, yielding 2.1M trainable parameters (2.2% of total). Low learning rates prevent catastrophic forgetting. *End-to-End Fine-Tuning:* All SSL encoder and classifier parameters are jointly optimized ( 95M parameters). Very low learning rate ($5\times10^{-6}$), dropout (0.3), weight decay, and early stopping mitigate overfitting.

### 3.3 Classifiers

**Traditional Machine Learning:** Segment-level embeddings are temporally averaged per participant and $z$-score normalized before training. We evaluate four conventional classifiers: Support Vector Machine (SVM) with linear and RBF (Radial Basis Function) kernels, Random Forest (100 trees, max depth 10), and Logistic Regression. These baselines assess the linear and nonlinear discriminability of SSL representations independently of any temporal modeling.

**Deep Learning Architectures:** All deep learning models operate on sequences of segment-level embeddings $\{\mathbf{h}_t\}_{t=1}^{T}$, where $\mathbf{h}_t \in \mathbb{R}^{768}$. Sequences are padded to a fixed maximum length, with binary masks used to ignore non-speech timesteps. A shallow MLP (one hidden layer, 8 units, dropout 0.4) serves as a non-temporal baseline, operating on the temporally averaged representation $\bar{\mathbf{h}} = \frac{1}{T}\sum_{t=1}^{T}\mathbf{h}_t$, isolating nonlinear discrimination from sequential modeling. We evaluate four compact temporal classifier heads to model sequential dependencies in SSL representations, each using a hidden dimension of 8 per direction with dropout set to 0.3 to mitigate overfitting in the low-resource regime. These include a Bidirectional GRU for parameter-efficient recurrent modeling, a Bidirectional LSTM with explicit memory cells for longer-range temporal dependencies, a Temporal Convolutional Network (TCN) employing stacked dilated causal convolutions to achieve large receptive fields with parallel computation [11], and an Attention-enhanced BiLSTM that weights diagnostically salient speech segments via additive attention.

## 4 Experiments and Results

*Experimental Setup:* We investigate three aspects of SSL-based TBI detection: (i) which SSL model and encoder layer provide the most discriminative and stable representations; (ii) whether temporal modeling improves performance beyond static feature aggregation without sacrificing generalization; and (iii) which transfer learning paradigm offers the optimal balance between accuracy, overfitting resistance, and computational efficiency for robust clinical deployment under low-resource conditions. All experiments are conducted on a single NVIDIA GeForce RTX 4080 SUPER GPU with 16 GB memory. Frozen-feature models are trained using Adam (lr $= 3 \times 10^{-3}$, batch $= 16$), partial fine-tuning with lr $= 1 \times 10^{-5}$ and batch $= 4$, and end-to-end fine-tuning with lr $= 5 \times 10^{-6}$ and batch $= 4$. All models employ weight decay ($10^{-4}$), gradient clipping (5.0), learning-rate scheduling, and early stopping. Performance is evaluated in terms of accuracy, weighted F1-score, and AUC.

**Impact of Temporal Modeling on Generalization Performance:** Figures 2a and 2b reveal a clear sample-efficiency trade-off between static aggregation and temporal modeling. Static classifiers consistently achieve superior performance, with SVC-Linear and Logistic Regression reaching 95.24% accuracy compared to 90.48% for the best temporal model (LSTM+Attention), reflecting their lower complexity and robustness under extreme data scarcity. In contrast, temporal architectures (BiGRU, BiLSTM, TCN) require substantially more data to generalize reliably and are more susceptible to overfitting. When model capacity is comparable, however, explicit temporal modeling provides clear benefits: LSTM+Attention significantly outperforms the Static-MLP (90.48% vs. 76.19%), indicating that sequence-aware architectures capture clinically relevant speech dynamics more effectively. The weak performance of simpler temporal models (BiGRU at 61.90%, BiLSTM at 76.19%) reflects training instability rather than limitations of temporal structure. Training curves in Fig. 3b confirm that temporal models fail primarily due to data scarcity rather than architectural inadequacy. While Static-MLP converges stably with minimal overfitting (0.61% gap), BiGRU and LSTM+Attention achieve high training accuracy (85–90%) but exhibit large generalization gaps (15.67% and 21.89%),

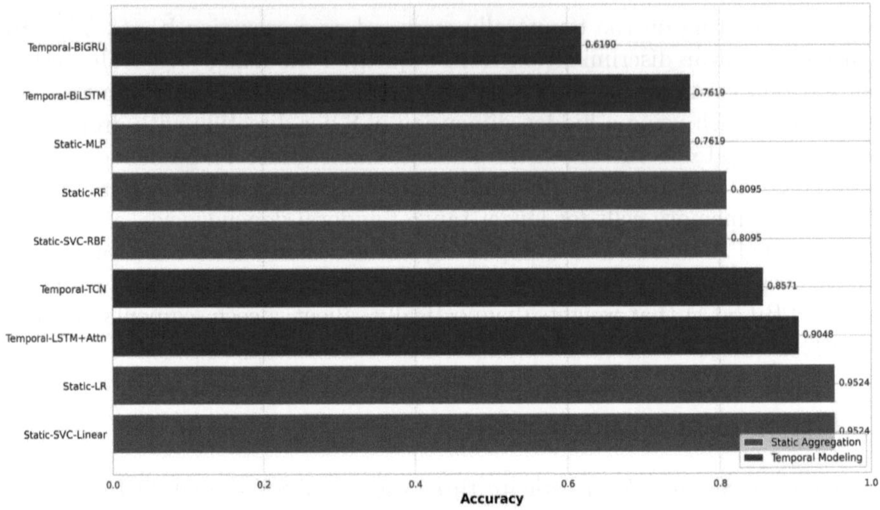


(a) Models Performance Comparison

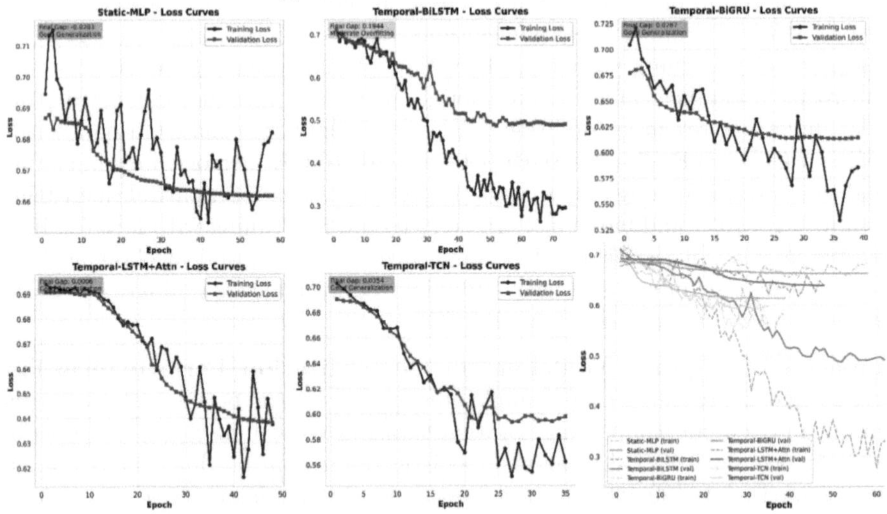


(b) Training and validation losses for Temporal Models

**Fig. 2.** (a) Comparison of model performance. (b) Training and validation loss curves for the temporal models.

demonstrating strong representational capacity that does not transfer under limited samples. TCN partially mitigates this through inductive bias, showing a negative generalization gap (-9.98%). Consistently, static models exhibit tightly clustered performance (median AUC $\approx$ 0.93), whereas temporal methods show greater variance and lower medians (accuracy and F1 $\approx$ 0.81).

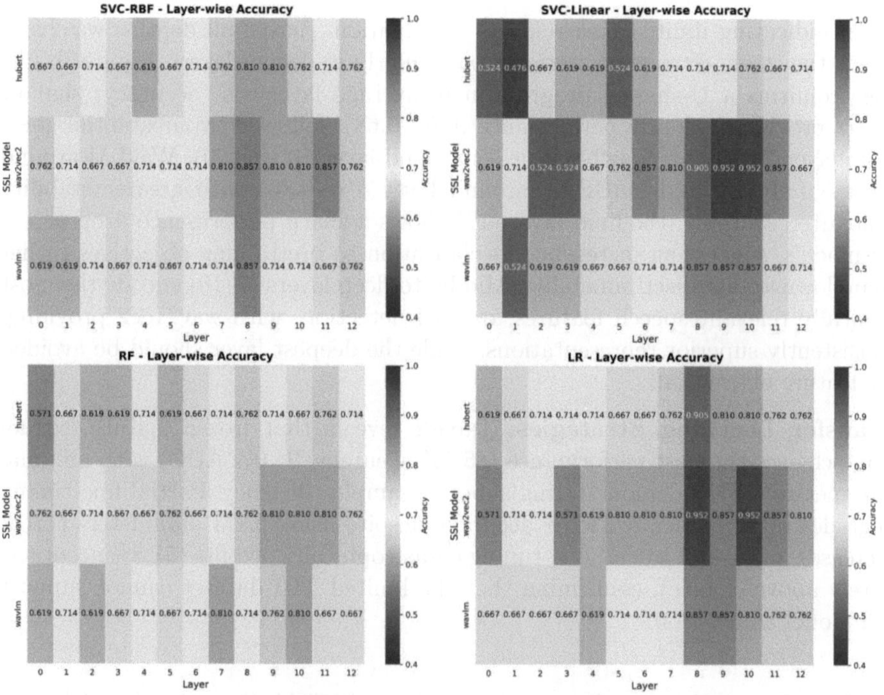


(a) Layer-wise accuracy heatmap across classifiers and SSL models.

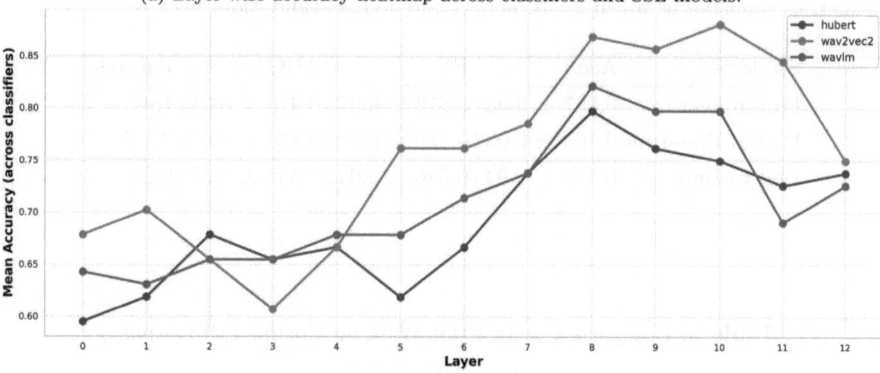


(b) Average discriminability across SSL layers.

**Fig. 3.** Layer-wise analysis of SSL representations for TBI detection.

**SSL Representation Quality and Layer-wise Discriminability:** Figure 3a shows clear depth-dependent performance trends across classifiers and SSL models. Linear classifiers (SVC-Linear, Logistic Regression) achieve peak accuracy in middle-to-deep layers (8–11), exceeding 0.90 and reaching above 0.95 with wav2vec2, whereas non-linear models (SVC-RBF, Random Forest) exhibit flatter profiles with lower peaks (0.81–0.86). Early layers (0–4) consistently underperform, indicating limited task-relevant information. Across all depths, wav2vec2 yields the strongest representations, particularly in deeper layers. Figure 3b further confirms a U-shaped progression in average layer-wise accuracy: shallow layers provide moderate performance (0.60–0.68), followed by substantial gains from layer 7 onward. Wav2vec2 peaks around layer 10 ($\sim$0.90), WavLM around layer 8 ($\sim$0.82), and HuBERT around layer 8 ($\sim$0.80) with greater stability thereafter. Notably, the final layer (12) shows a sharp performance drop across all models, suggesting increasing specialization to pretraining objectives rather than downstream discriminability. Middle-to-deep layers (7–10) encode the most clinically relevant speech features for TBI detection, with wav2vec2 providing consistently superior representations, while the deepest layer should be avoided for feature extraction.

**Transfer Learning Strategies:** Table 2 reveals that frozen feature extraction achieves the best performance (85.7% accuracy, 94.0% AUC) with minimal parameters (18K), demonstrating superior sample efficiency. Partial fine-tuning degrades performance to 76.5% accuracy despite using 2.1M parameters (116$\times$ increase), while end-to-end fine-tuning catastrophically overfits (51.8% accuracy, barely above chance), confirming that the limited TBI dataset cannot support full model adaptation.

**Table 2.** Transfer Learning Strategy Comparison (BiLSTM+Attention, Wav2Vec2.0). All metrics reported as mean ± std across 5-fold cross-validation.

| Strategy | Acc. | F1 | AUC | Params |
|---|---|---|---|---|
| Frozen Features | 0.857 ± 0.024 | 0.870 ± 0.021 | 0.940 ± 0.012 | 18K |
| Partial Fine-tune | 0.765 ± 0.032 | 0.780 ± 0.028 | 0.835 ± 0.025 | 2.1M |
| End-to-End | 0.518 ± 0.045 | 0.540 ± 0.042 | 0.535 ± 0.051 | 95M |

**Table 3.** Comparison with Prior Work on Coelho TBI Corpus

| Study | Features | Classifier | Accuracy |
|---|---|---|---|
| Ditthapron et al. (2022) | Sinc filters | Cascading GRU | 83.9% |
| This work (Frozen) | wav2vec 2.0 | SVC-Linear | **95.2%** |
| This work (Frozen) | wav2vec 2.0 | LSTM+Attn | 90.5% |

Intermediate SSL representations captured from frozen encoders best preserve the prosodic and organizational speech features disrupted by TBI, while avoiding overfitting. Attempting to fine-tune the pretrained encoder, whether partially or fully, destabilizes the robust representations learned during large-scale pretraining, leading to performance degradation as the limited TBI data cannot support effective adaptation without overfitting. Table 3 contextualizes our results within existing literature on the Coelho corpus. Our frozen SSL approach (95.2% accuracy with SVC-Linear) outperforms the current state-of-the-art (Ditthapron et al. 2022: 83.9%) by 11.3% points while using substantially simpler classifiers (linear SVM vs. cascading GRU).

## 5 Conclusion and Future Directions

This study demonstrates that robust speech-based TBI detection in low-resource clinical settings is best achieved using frozen intermediate SSL representations with lightweight classifiers. Traditional classifiers on frozen features excel due to sample efficiency, achieving 95.2% accuracy, while temporal architectures with attention outperform static neural baselines(90.5% vs. 76.2%) when model complexity is controlled, demonstrating that sequential modeling captures clinically relevant speech dynamics. Transfer learning experiments confirm that frozen feature extraction outperforms both partial (76.5%) and end-to-end (51.8%) fine-tuning, as the limited TBI data cannot support effective encoder adaptation without catastrophic overfitting. For limitations, all experiments were conducted on the Coelho TBI corpus, the largest publicly available dataset for this task. While this is the established benchmark, external validation on independent cohorts is essential to confirm generalizability across different clinical populations, recording conditions, and speech tasks. Our findings should be interpreted as establishing proof-of-concept and methodological best practices, with external validation as a critical next step. These findings provide practical guidelines for deploying SSL-based diagnostic systems in real-world healthcare contexts, highlighting the critical importance of preserving pretrained representations under severe data constraints. Future directions include: (i) interpretability analysis through attention visualization and feature attribution to identify clinically relevant acoustic biomarkers, and (ii) data augmentation strategies to improve temporal model generalization under severe data constraints.

## References


1. Baevski, A., Zhou, Y., Mohamed, A., Auli, M.: wav2vec 2.0: a framework for self-supervised learning of speech representations. Adv. Neural. Inf. Process. Syst. **33**, 12449–12460 (2020)
2. Chen, S., et al.: WavLM: large-scale self-supervised pre-training for full stack speech processing. IEEE J. Sel. Top. Signal Process. **16**(6), 1505–1518 (2022)
3. Coelho, C.A., Youse, K.M., Le, K.N.: Conversational discourse in closed-head-injured and non-brain-injured adults. Aphasiology **16**(4–6), 659–672 (2002)
4. Dewan, M.C., et al.: Estimating the global incidence of traumatic brain injury. J. Neurosurg. **130**(4), 1080–1097 (2018)
5. Ditthapron, A., Agu, E.O., Lammert, A.C.: Learning from limited data for speech-based traumatic brain injury detection. In: 2021 20th IEEE International Conference on Machine Learning and Applications (ICMLA), pp. 1482–1486. IEEE (2021)

6. Ditthapron, A., Lammert, A.C., Agu, E.O.: Continuous TBI monitoring from spontaneous speech using parametrized sinc filters and a cascading GRU. IEEE J. Biomed. Health Inform. **26**(7), 3517–3528 (2022)
7. Falcone, M., Yadav, N., Poellabauer, C., Flynn, P.: Using isolated vowel sounds for classification of mild traumatic brain injury. In: 2013 IEEE International Conference on Acoustics, Speech and Signal Processing, pp. 7577–7581. IEEE (2013)
8. Helfer, B.S., et al.: Articulatory dynamics and coordination in classifying cognitive change with preclinical mTBI. In: Fifteenth Annual Conference of the International Speech Communication Association (2014)
9. Hsu, W.N., Bolte, B., Tsai, Y.H.H., Lakhotia, K., Salakhutdinov, R., Mohamed, A.: Hubert: self-supervised speech representation learning by masked prediction of hidden units. IEEE/ACM Trans. Audio, Speech Lang. Process. **29**, 3451–3460 (2021)
10. Huang, X., et al.: Depression recognition using voice-based pre-training model. Sci. Rep. **14**(1) (2024)
11. Lea, C., Vidal, R., Reiter, A., Hager, G.D.: Temporal convolutional networks: a unified approach to action segmentation. In: Hua, G., Jégou, H. (eds) European Conference on Computer Vision, pp. 47–54. Springer, Cham (2016). https://doi.org/10.1007/978-3-319-49409-8_7
12. Rojas, F., Madanian, S., Templeton, J.M., Poellabauer, C., Schneider, S.L.: Exploring deep learning and grad-cam for speech-based detection of mild traumatic brain injury. In: 2024 IEEE International Conference on Big Data (BigData), pp. 6108–6116. IEEE (2024)
13. Rubaiat, R., Templeton, J.M., Schneider, S.L., De Silva, U., Madanian, S., Poellabauer, C., et al.: Exploring speech biosignatures for traumatic brain injury and neurodegeneration. JMIR Neurotechnol. **4**(1), e64624 (2025)
14. Talkar, T., et al.: Acoustic indicators of speech motor coordination in adults with and without traumatic brain injury. Interspeech, 21–25 (2021)
15. Talkar, T., et al.: Detection of subclinical mild traumatic brain injury (mTBI) through speech and gait. In: INTERSPEECH, pp. 135–139 (2020)
16. Wall, C., et al.: A deep learning-based approach to diagnose mild traumatic brain injury using audio classification. PLoS ONE **17**(9), e0274395 (2022)
17. Wu, W., Zhang, C., Woodland, P.C.: Self-supervised representations in speech-based depression detection. In: ICASSP 2023-2023 IEEE International Conference on Acoustics, Speech and Signal Processing (ICASSP), pp. 1–5. IEEE (2023)
18. Zhang, X., Zhang, X., Chen, W., Li, C., Yu, C.: Improving speech depression detection using transfer learning with wav2vec 2.0 in low-resource environments. Sci. Rep. **14**(1), 9543 (2024)

# FC-CL: Contrastive Learning-Based Sleep Stage Classification Considering Surrounding Epochs in EEG Signals

Zhengting Wang[1,2], Vijdan Khalique[1,3(✉)], Kazumasa Horie[1,3], Fusae Kawana[4], Toshio Kokubo[1], Masashi Yanagisawa[1,5], and Hiroyuki Kitagawa[1]

[1] International Institute for Integrative Sleep Medicine (WPI-IIIS), TIAR, University of Tsukuba, Tsukuba, Japan
wangzhengting@kde.cs.tsukuba.ac.jp,
{khalique.vijdan.gt,toshio.kokubo.fp,yanagisawa.masa.fu}@u.tsukuba.ac.jp,
{horie,kitagawa}@cs.tsukuba.ac.jp

[2] Graduate School of Science and Technology, University of Tsukuba, Tsukuba, Japan

[3] Center for Computational Sciences (CCS), University of Tsukuba, Tsukuba, Japan

[4] Graduate School of Medicine, Juntendo University, Tokyo, Japan
nadeshiko.kawana@gmail.com

[5] Department of Molecular Genetics, University of Texas Southwestern Medical Center, Dallas, TX, USA

**Abstract.** Supervised learning-based automatic sleep stage classification methods rely on the availability of a large amount of labeled sleep data. On the other hand, in-home EEG devices are emerging as an alternative to polysomnography (PSG). A recent work employed contrastive learning - a self-supervised learning method - for label-efficient sleep stage classification on an in-home EEG dataset. However, this method classified each sleep epoch independently without considering the short-range temporal context. This work proposes *FC-CL*, a simple two-step framework that integrates temporal context at the feature level for contrastively pretrained sleep stage classification. *Step 1* (*CL*) performs contrastive pretraining on unlabeled multi-channel in-home EEG, followed by supervised fine-tuning to obtain a baseline 5-stage classifier. *Step 2* (*FC*) concatenates the per-epoch feature of a target epoch with those of its temporally surrounding epochs, and trains a classifier while keeping the pretrained encoder fixed. Thus, our method accounts for the transitional properties of the sleep stages without introducing complex sequential models. In the experiments, we demonstrate the effectiveness of *FC-CL* compared to other methods.

**Keywords:** Sleep stage classification · In-home EEG · Contrastive learning · Temporal context · Feature concatenation

© The Author(s), under exclusive license to Springer Nature Switzerland AG 2027
P. Andreev et al. (Eds.): AIME 2026, LNAI 16748, pp. 81–91, 2027.
https://doi.org/10.1007/978-3-032-30710-1_10

# 1 Introduction

Sleep is essential for human health, and insufficient or disrupted sleep has been associated with several health risks, such as depression and cardiovascular diseases. To analyze human sleep, polysomnography (PSG) is used by sleep experts, which records electroencephalogram (EEG), electromyogram (EMG), and electrooculogram (EOG) signals. The 30-second epochs are analyzed and scored into five sleep stages, i.e., wake (W), rapid eye movement (R), and three non-rapid eye movement (N1-3) stages. However, PSG has its limitations as it can be performed in the sleep clinics by the experts, hindering scalable sleep monitoring. Recently, in-home EEG devices have been developed to address these drawbacks.

Automatic sleep stage classification has been extensively studied with supervised deep learning approaches being commonly used. However, the performance of these approaches heavily relies on the availability of large amounts of labeled sleep data.

Self-supervised learning (SSL) provides an effective alternative by learning representations from unlabeled EEG data. In particular, contrastive learning has demonstrated strong label efficiency for sleep stage classification by enforcing augmentation-invariant yet stage-discriminative representations [7,8]. The key idea of contrastive learning is to increase the agreement between pairs of augmentations derived from the same signal while decreasing the agreement between the augmentations from different signals. Recently, [9] applied contrastive pretraining to a three-channel in-home EEG device, followed by supervised fine-tuning with limited labeled data. Despite improved overall performance, the method does not capture the transitional properties of the sleep epochs and classifies each epoch independently.

Sleep stages exhibit strong short-term temporal continuity, suggesting that contextual information from neighboring epochs can aid stage disambiguation. Inspired by the practice of human sleep annotators, who routinely consider surrounding epochs when labeling a target epoch, we propose to explicitly integrate such temporal context at the feature level.

In this work, we introduce Feature Concatenated Contrastive Learning, referred to as *FC-CL*, which uses a contrastively pretrained sleep stage classifier by concatenating feature representations of a target epoch with those of its temporal neighbors. Using multi-channel in-home EEG data collected by a portable device (*Insomnograf*) developed by S'UIMIN [4], our pipeline consists of two steps: (1) contrastive pretraining on unlabeled EEG followed by supervised fine-tuning to obtain a baseline classifier (*CL*), and (2) a lightweight context integration step that concatenates neighboring-epoch features for supervised training. Experimental results show that *FC-CL* consistently improves sleep stage classification performance under label-efficient settings without modifying the feature encoder or introducing complex sequential models.

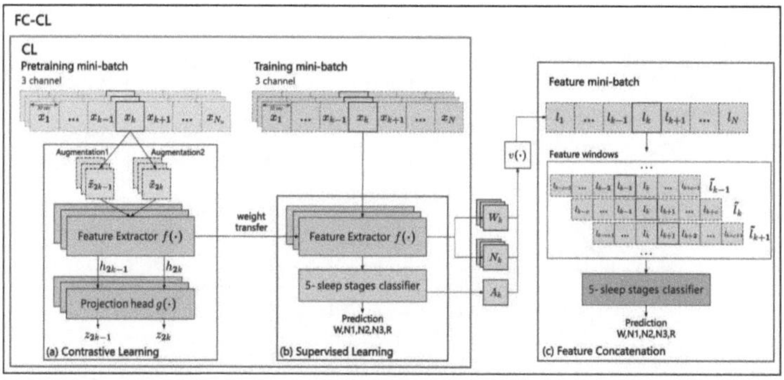


**Fig. 1.** Overview of *FC-CL*.

## 2 Related Work

Supervised deep learning approaches employing convolutional and sequence-based models have been widely used for automated sleep stage classification on PSG data [5,6]. Some works have shown improved prediction accuracy and interpretability by leveraging multi-view modeling and transformer-based learning [10,11]. For in-home EEG, supervised methods have been adapted to address device-specific challenges such as signal variability and electrode contact instability [2,3]. Overall, these methods are dependent on a large amount of labeled sleep data, and label-efficient approaches are needed.

Recently, contrastive learning - a self-supervised learning approach - has been effective for label-efficient sleep stage classification for PSG data [7,8]. Approaches incorporating temporal or contextual contrasting further emphasize the importance of local temporal structure in EEG signals [12]. Another work applied contrastive pretraining to multi-channel in-home EEG, followed by supervised fine-tuning with limited labeled data, achieving strong overall performance [9]. Nevertheless, ambiguous transitional stages such as N1 remain difficult to classify, as epochs are treated independently during finetuning. Hence, mechanisms are required to incorporate short-range temporal context for more accurate sleep stage classification.

## 3 Method

### 3.1 Overview

Figure 1 presents an overview of the proposed Feature Concatenated Contrastive Learning (*FC-CL*) framework. The method follows a two-stage training pipeline with a lightweight context integration step. First, a feature extractor is pretrained on unlabeled in-home EEG using contrastive learning to obtain robust representations (Fig. 1 (a)). We adopt two augmentation methods (permutation and crop & resize) as [9] with parameter values 10 and 20%, respectively. Permutation divides an epoch into 10 equal segments and shuffles them randomly,

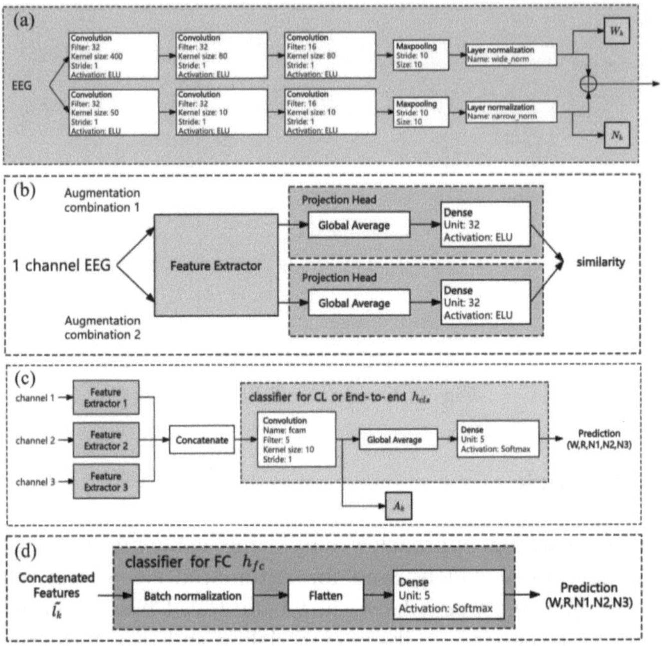


**Fig. 2.** Architectures of (a) feature extractor, (b) *CL* model, (c) 5-sleep stages classification model, and (d) feature concatenation model.

and crop & resize randomly samples 20% of an epoch and scales it. The pretrained weights are then transferred to a sleep stage classifier, and subsequently fine-tuned using a limited amount of labeled data in supervised learning settings (Fig. 1 (b)). Thus, it forms the baseline contrastive learning model (*CL*).

To incorporate short-range temporal context, *FC-CL* operates on the intermediate features extracted by the pretrained feature extractor. For each target epoch, its per-epoch feature representation is concatenated with features of its temporally surrounding epochs within a sliding window (Fig. 1(c)). The resulting feature window is used as input to a new 5-sleep-stage classifier, which is trained in a supervised manner using the label of the target epoch. During this stage, the parameters of the feature extractor and the supervised classifier remain fixed, and only the context-aware classifier is trained. By integrating contextual information at the feature level, *FC-CL* improves sleep stage classification accuracy without modifying the encoder architecture or introducing complex sequential models.

### 3.2 *FC-CL*

We adopt narrow and wide filters, as in [13], to capture features at fine and coarse granularities, respectively. Since our target data is three-channel EEG signal, the input to the feature extractor is a per-channel EEG signal represented

**Algorithm 1.** *FC-CL*: Two-Step Training

**Input:** Unlabeled data $\mathcal{D}^U$, labeled data $\mathcal{D}^L$; record length $N$; context size $c$
**Given**: Encoder $f$, projection head $g$, *CL* classifier $h_{\text{cls}}$, *FC* classifier $h_{\text{fc}}$.
**Step 1:** ***CL***
Initialize $f$ and $g$.
Pretrain the model $g \cdot f$ in Fig 2 (b) via contrastive learning using $D^U$ as [9].
Perform supervised finetuning of $h_{\text{cls}} \cdot f$.
**Step 2:** ***FC***
Freeze $f$; initialize $h_{\text{fc}}$.
**for** each labeled recording $x=\{x_1, \ldots, x_N\} \in \mathcal{D}^L$ **do**
    Extract per-epoch features $\ell_k$.
    **for** $k = c+1$ to $N - c$ **do**
        $\hat{y}_k \leftarrow h_{\text{fc}}([\ell_{k-c}, \ldots, \ell_k, \ldots, \ell_{k+c}])$
        Update only $h_{\text{fc}}$ with cross-entropy loss$(\hat{y}_k, y_k)$.
    **end for**
**end for**

as ${x_k}^{(C)} \in \mathbb{R}^L$, where $L$ is the temporal length of one epoch EEG signal, and channel $C \in \{1, 2, 3\}$. Figure 2 (a) illustrates the architecture of the feature extractor. The branch outputs $W_k$ from the narrow and $N_k$ from the wide filters used later in computing the mapping $v(\cdot)$.

The contrastive learning model inputs augmented pairs of the original signal, as shown in Fig. 2 (b). The contrastive pretraining procedure and the loss function follow the paper [9]. After contrastive pretraining, the feature extractor is transferred and fine-tuned for the sleep stage classification task.

As shown in Fig. 2 (c), each EEG channel is processed by an independent feature extractor; with three-channel input, the three outputs are concatenated and fed to a common classifier. In this work, we adopt the contrastive-learning-based training scheme (*CL*): the feature extractor is first pretrained via contrastive learning on unlabeled sleep records and then fine-tuned on a limited amount of labeled data to obtain a sleep stage classifier. Moreover, the output (denotes as $A_k$) of the convolutional layer in the classifier (*fcam* shown in Fig. 2 (c)) is used later by the *FC* classifier (Fig. 2 (d)) for constructing the feature mapping with $v(\cdot)$.

To further leverage intermediate representations learned during *CL*, we extract per-epoch features from the trained model and then concatenate short-range temporal context, as depicted in Fig. 2 (d). After *CL* is completed, for each epoch $x_k^{(C)}$ where $C \in \{1, 2, 3\}$, the contrastively pretrained feature extractor outputs wide ($W_k$) and narrow ($N_k$) features at the final normalization layers (Fig. 2 (a)). Temporal mean and max pooling are applied to each branch, and the resulting summaries are concatenated to form a per-channel representation $\boldsymbol{\phi}_k^{(C)} \in \mathbb{R}^{64}$. Concatenating the three channels yields the wide-narrow feature vector $\boldsymbol{\phi}_k = [\boldsymbol{\phi}_k^{(1)}, \boldsymbol{\phi}_k^{(2)}, \boldsymbol{\phi}_k^{(3)}] \in \mathbb{R}^{192}$. In addition, we extract $A_k$, a cross-channel representation from the convolutional activation map of the *CL* classifier head (Fig. 2 (c)). After temporal mean and max pooling, this yields

$\psi_k \in \mathbb{R}^{10}$. Finally, the per-epoch feature $([\phi_k, \psi_k] \in \mathbb{R}^{202})$ used for epoch concatenation is obtained as $\ell_k = v(W_k, N_k, A_k)$. For each target epoch $k$ with sufficient neighbors, we concatenate context features within a symmetric window $\tilde{\ell}_k$ of size $2c+1$ as $\tilde{\ell}_k = [\ell_{k-c}, \ldots, \ell_{k-1}, \ell_k, \ell_{k+1}, \ldots, \ell_{k+c}]$, $\tilde{\ell}_k \in \mathbb{R}^{(2c+1)\times 202}$, where $k = c{+}1, \ldots, N{-}c$ and $N$ is the record length.

As shown in Fig. 2 (d), given a feature window $\tilde{\ell}_k$ of the target epoch $k$ and its label, the *FC* classifier is trained in supervised learning settings, where the weights of the feature extractor and the supervised classifier are not updated. Hence, the *FC* classifier is trained to predict the correct label given the features of the target and its neighboring epochs.

In summary, we present *FC-CL* as a two-step pipeline: *Step 1 (CL)* performs contrastive pretraining on unlabeled in-home EEG and then fine-tunes the encoder with limited labeled data to obtain a strong baseline; *Step 2 (FC)* freezes the encoder, concatenates neighboring epoch features to inject short-range temporal context, and trains a lightweight classifier on the concatenated features using the same limited amount of labeled data. The complete workflow is summarized in Algorithm 1.

# 4 Experiments and Results

## 4.1 Dataset

S'UIMIN [4] provided the in-home EEG device (called *Insomnograf)* dataset, consisting of 1,053 recordings from 256 subjects. The device has 4-electrodes: Fp1, Fp2, M1 and M2. Three montages - $Fp1 - Ma$, $Fp2 - Ma$ and $Fp1 - Fp2$, where $Ma = (M1 - M2)/2$ - were used as input to all models. The sampling frequency is 200 Hz, with each 30-second sleep epoch annotated by human experts under AASM guidelines [1]. The sleep records were pre-processed using the bandpass filtering and per-channel normalization following [9]. Moreover, we partitioned the data into a non-overlapping pool of 891 records for contrastive pretraining and a labeled pool of 162 records for downstream evaluation. In contrastive learning, we used 90% for training and 10% for validation. We applied subject-wise 5-fold cross-validation for the supervised fine-tuning and training.

## 4.2 Experimental Settings

We compared *FC-CL* with other configurations, briefly described as follows:

1. ***CL***: The model using only the features of the target epochs without considering the surrounding epochs. The feature extractor are pretrained using contrastive learning.
2. ***End-to-end***: Supervised end-to-end training of the model in Fig. 2 (c) where feature extractors are randomly initialized.
3. ***FC-end-to-end***: This model has the same architecture as *FC-CL*, but builds the feature concatenation mechanism (Fig. 1 (c)) and its sleep stage classifier (Fig 2 (d)) on top of *End-to-end* model.

For reference, we also evaluated the performance of these models under a 1-channel ($Fp1 - Ma$) setting. For contrastive pretraining, we used a batch size of 512, $1 \times 10^{-4}$ learning rate, and temperature $\tau = 0.5$. For supervised model training, a batch size of 32 and $1 \times 10^{-5}$ learning rate was used. All models were trained for 100 epochs, and the best model was used. These hyperparameter settings were found optimal in [9]. $c = 3$ was used for *FC-CL* as it showed the best performance. Furthermore, to analyze how performance changes with label availability, we vary the volume of labeled data used in supervised training from 10% to 100% and report the corresponding test performance.

### 4.3 Results and Discussion

***Performance Overview.*** Figure 3 compares the 4 models across accuracy, macro F1-score, and Cohen's kappa under different labeled-data proportions, under both the 3-channel ($Fp1 - Ma$, $Fp2 - Ma$ and $Fp1 - Fp2$) and 1-channel ($Fp1 - Ma$) settings. All models improve monotonically as more labeled data is available.

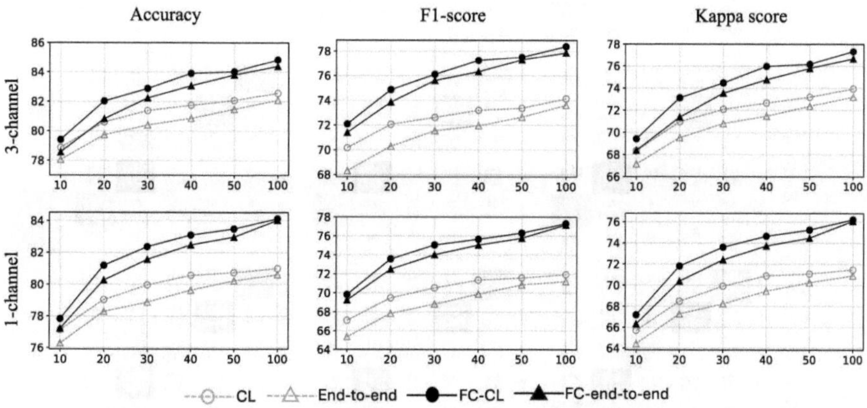


**Fig. 3.** Comparison of all methods across labeled data proportions (x-axis).

Across all metrics and label budgets, *FC-CL* consistently achieves the best performance. While feature concatenation also improves the supervised backbone (*FC-end-to-end*), its gains remain smaller than those of *FC-CL*, indicating that contrastively pretrained representations provide a more effective basis for exploiting short-range temporal context. This advantage is particularly evident under low-label regimes.

As the proportion of labeled data increases, the performance gap between *FC-CL* and *FC-end-to-end* narrows, especially under the 1-channel setting, where both models approach similar accuracies under full supervision. Nevertheless, *FC-CL* maintains a slight advantage in the 3-channel case and attains the highest overall accuracies (84.83% for 3- and 84.12% for 1-channel), suggesting that it approaches the dataset's performance ceiling.

Overall, these results demonstrate that contrastive pretraining substantially enhances the effectiveness of feature concatenation for sleep stage classification, particularly when labeled data are limited.

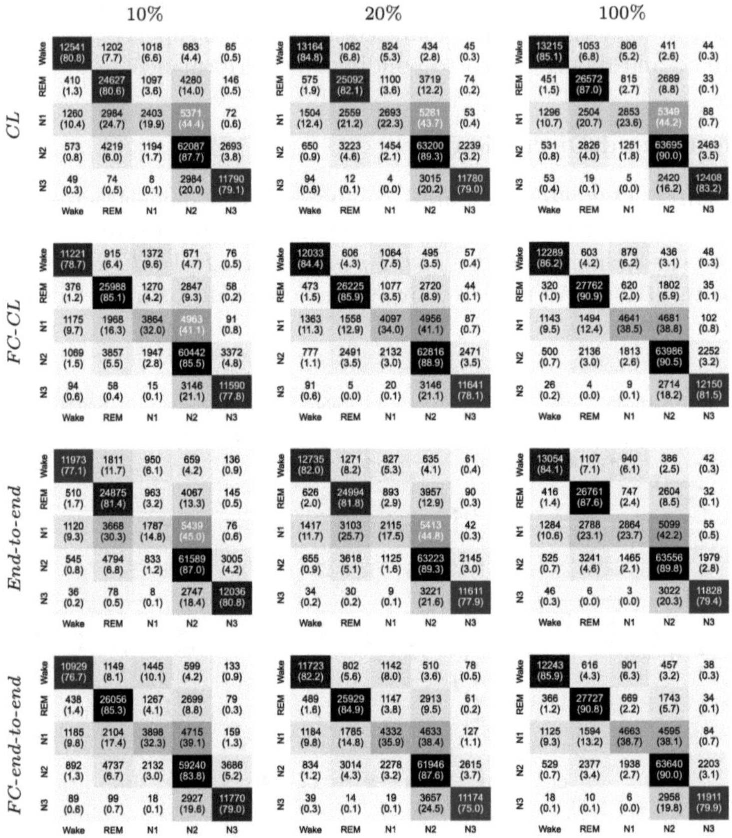


**Fig. 4.** Confusion matrices showing the number of epochs and % in brackets.

***Stage-wise Analysis.*** To complement the overall results, we examine per-stage behavior using the confusion matrices in Fig. 4. At label budgets of 10%, 20%, and 100%, both *FC-CL* and *FC-end-to-end* show clear improvements on the more ambiguous stages—especially N1—where confusions with W and N2 are most common. Across budgets, adding temporal context increases N1 recall for both supervised backbones, and similar but smaller gains can be observed for stage R, while stable stages such as N3 remain largely unchanged.

Although *FC-end-to-end* shows larger relative gains than *FC-CL*, this mainly reflects differences in backbone strength: the weaker *End-to-end* benefits more from added context, while the contrastively pretrained encoder leaves less room for relative improvement. In absolute terms, *FC-CL* still provides the strongest and most balanced stage-wise performance.

Overall, these results indicate that temporal context is particularly useful for improving recognition of transitional stages such as N1, and that contrastive representations enable the *FC-CL* variant to make more effective absolute use of this context, even when *FC-end-to-end* shows larger relative improvements due to its weaker baseline.

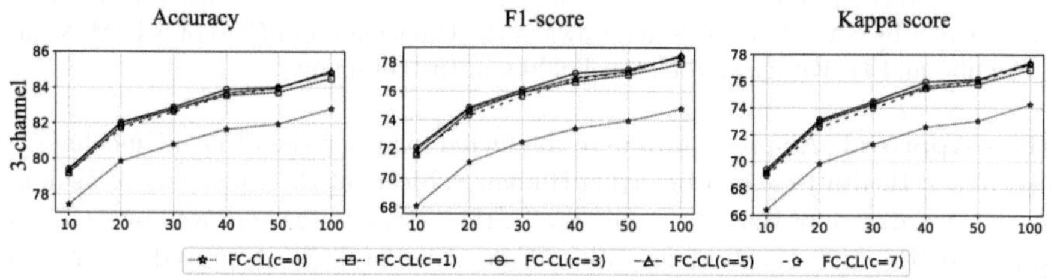


**Fig. 5.** Performance of *FC-CL* with different context sizes $c \in \{0, 1, 3, 5, 7\}$.

***Effect of Context Size.*** To assess how the amount of temporal context influences the effectiveness of feature concatenation, we vary the context size $c \in \{0, 1, 3, 5, 7\}$, corresponding to window lengths of 1, 3, 7, 11, and 15 epochs, respectively. The special case $c$=0 represents a degenerated configuration in which the classifier receives only the target epoch's feature without any neighboring information.

Figure 5 shows that incorporating even minimal context ($c$=1) leads to a clear improvement over the $c$=0 variant across all label budgets and evaluation metrics. Across $c \in \{1, 3, 5, 7\}$, performance curves remain close, indicating that *FC* is robust to the precise choice of window length. Nevertheless, a mild inverted-U trend is observable: increasing $c$ from 1 to 3 consistently improves accuracy, macro F1-score, and Cohen's kappa, suggesting that additional nearby context provides useful complementary information. For $c \geq 5$, a slight decline was observed, implying that more distant epochs may contribute diminishing or even noisy contextual cues. Empirically, $c$=3 yields the strongest and most stable performance across metrics and label proportions.

## 5 Conclusion

In conclusion, this work presented *FC-CL*, a two-step pipeline for label-efficient sleep staging on 3-channel in-home EEG: (i) contrastive pretraining followed by supervised fine-tuning (*CL*), and (ii) a lightweight feature concatenation head (*FC*) that injects short-range temporal context at the representation level. Across different label budgets and training strategies, *FC-CL* outperformed supervised and self-supervised vanilla contrastive learning baselines. Overall, *FC-CL* is a simple and effective way of using unlabeled sleep data for self-supervised pretraining and improving label-efficient downstream sleep staging. It will be interesting to compare our approach with the state-of-the-art methods using open datasets.

**Acknowledgments.** This work was supported by JSPS KAKENHI (JP23K28089, JP23K16988, JP24H00894, JP25K22810, JP26K15054), JSPS RECONNECT (JP22K21351), MEXT WPI, AMED (JP21zf0127005, PreF), F-MIRAI Collaboration Research, and collaboration research with S'UIMIN [4]. The dataset used in this study was provided by S'UIMIN. M. Yanagisawa is the Chairman and CSO of S'UIMIN, and T. Kokubo and H. Kitagawa are stakeholders in the company.

**Ethics Approval.** All procedures were conducted following the Ethical Guidelines for Medical and Health Research Involving Human Subjects at the University of Tsukuba and the Declaration of Helsinki. Additionally, this research was approved by TCReDO (Approved ID# H29-177) and the Ethics Committee of CCS (Approved ID#25-001) at the University of Tsukuba.

## References

1. Berry, R.B.: The AASM manual for the scoring of sleep and associated events: rules, terminology and technical specifications. Version 2 (2012)
2. Almanza, J.C.N., Ota, L., Horie, K., Kawana, F., Kokubo, T., Yanagisawa, M., Kitagawa, H.: Sleep and arousal scoring for in-home EEG signals: a multitask learning approach. In: The 12th IEEE International Conference on Healthcare Informatics 2024, pp. 147–156 (2024)
3. Horie, K., et al.: An ensemble method for improving robustness against the electrode contact problems in automated sleep stage scoring. Sci. Rep. **14**(1), 21894 (2024)
4. S'UIMIN Inc., Official website of S'UIMIN Co., Ltd., https://www.suimin.co.jp/. Accessed 2025
5. Supratak, A., Dong, H., Wu, C., Guo, Y.: DeepSleepNet: a model for automatic sleep stage scoring based on raw single-channel EEG. IEEE Trans. Neural Syst. Rehabil. Eng. **25**(11), 1998–2008 (2017)
6. Perslev, M., Jensen, M., Darkner, S., Jennum, P.J., Igel, C.: U-Time: a fully convolutional network for time series segmentation applied to sleep staging. In: Advances in Neural Information Processing Systems, vol. 32 (2019)
7. Eldele, E., Ragab, M., Chen, Z., Wu, M., Kwoh, C.K., Li, X.: Self-supervised learning for label-efficient sleep stage classification: a comprehensive evaluation. IEEE Trans. Neural Syst. Rehabil. Eng. **31**, 1333–1342 (2023)
8. Jiang, X., Zhao, J., Du, B., Yuan, Z.: Self-supervised contrastive learning for EEG-based sleep staging. In: International Joint Conference on Neural Networks, pp. 1–8 (2021)
9. Khalique, V., Wang, Z., Horie, K., Kawana, F., Kukobo, T., Yanagisawa, M., Kitagawa, H.: Label-efficient self-supervised learning for sleep stage classification using multi-channel in-home EEG data. In: The 13th IEEE International Conference on Healthcare Informatics, pp. 174–183 (2025)

10. Phan, H., Chen, O.Y., Tran, M.C., Koch, P., Mertins, A., Vos, D., M.: XSleepNet: multi-view sequential model for automatic sleep staging. IEEE Trans. Pattern Anal. Mach. Intell. **44**(9), 5903–5915 (2022)
11. Phan, H., Mikkelsen, K., Chen, O.Y., Koch, P., Mertins, A., Vos, D., M.: SleepTransformer: automatic sleep staging with interpretability and uncertainty quantification. IEEE Trans. Biomed. Eng. **69**(8) (2022)
12. Eldele, E., Ragab, M., Chen, Z., Wu, M., Kwoh, C.-K., Li, X., Guan, C.: Timeseries representation learning via temporal and contextual contrasting. In: 30th International Joint Conference on Artificial Intelligence, pp. 2352–2359 (2021)
13. Suzuki, Y., et al.: Accurate in-home sleep assessment by combining a userfriendly electroencephalography device and automated sleep-stage scoring. Submitted (2025)

# How Explanation Framing Shapes Reliance on AI in Clinical Decision Support

Federico Cabitza[1,2], Alessia Papale[1(✉)], Lucía Vicente[3], and Rossella Tomaiuolo[4]

[1] Università degli Studi di Milano-Bicocca, Milano, Italy
{federico.cabitza,alessia.papale}@unimib.it
[2] Digital Health and Wellbeing, Fondazione Bruno Kessler (FBK), Trento, Italy
fcabitza@fbk.eu
[3] Universidad de La Rioja, La Rioja, Spain
lucia.vicente@unirioja.es
[4] Università Vita-Salute San Raffaele, Milano, Italy
tomaiuolo.rossella@hsr.it

**Abstract.** The integration of AI-based decision-support systems in clinical settings has raised concerns about how professionals interpret and rely on algorithmic recommendations. In particular, explainable AI (XAI) systems are not only technical tools but communicative artifacts that can shape user behavior. Within this context, the persuasive impact of linguistic framing in AI-generated explanations remains underexplored. This study addresses this gap by reporting findings from a controlled experiment in which 52 training nurses completed obstetric decision-making tasks with AI support, examining how neutral, cost-oriented, and gain-oriented explanation framings affect performance, confidence, and reliance behavior among clinical professionals. Results show that while both cost- and gain-oriented framings improved diagnostic accuracy over neutral explanations, cost-oriented framing uniquely increased appropriate reliance, deference, and automation bias. Conversely, self-anchoring bias was lowest under cost-oriented framing. These findings suggest that framing not only affects performance but can increase susceptibility to flawed AI suggestions, calling for design strategies that balance rhetorical effectiveness with professional autonomy in safety-critical environments.

**Keywords:** Human-AI Interaction · Explainable AI · framing effect · reliance · decision support systems

## 1 Introduction

Across a wide range of domains, decision-making is susceptible to how information is framed. Decades of classic research in prospect theory and cognitive psychology have shown that even objectively equivalent descriptions–whether emphasizing gains (e.g., "lives saved") or losses (e.g., "lives lost")–can

© The Author(s), under exclusive license to Springer Nature Switzerland AG 2027
P. Andreev et al. (Eds.): AIME 2026, LNAI 16748, pp. 92–102, 2027.
https://doi.org/10.1007/978-3-032-30710-1_11

systematically influence judgment and behavior [21]. In healthcare, subtle differences in how treatment outcomes are presented–e.g., "90% survival" versus "10% mortality"–can significantly shape clinicians' choices and perceptions [18]. Consistently, individuals become more risk-seeking when attention is drawn to avoiding losses and more risk-averse when it is directed toward achieving gains [11,18,21].

As Artificial Intelligence (AI) becomes increasingly embedded in high-stakes environments, recent advances in eXplainable AI (XAI) emphasize that AI-generated explanations are not merely vehicles of technical transparency, but communicative artifacts situated in social contexts that shape trust, comprehension, and behavioral responses [16].

Prior research in human–AI interaction has examined how framing information about an AI system's attributes, such as its accuracy, reliability, or intended role, affects users' trust and willingness to rely on the system [15,19]. A well-documented example shows how describing an AI as "80% accurate" or reporting a "20% error rate", although informationally equivalent, produces different levels of trust and reliance [12,13], consistent with classical effects of highlighting success or failure rates [14]. As AI systems gain increasingly sophisticated natural language capabilities, how they frame their own recommendations and explanations becomes especially consequential. Prior research shows that linguistic framing in explanations can amplify or mitigate cognitive biases, shape perceptions of system competence, and influence human judgment and reliance on AI [2,3]. For example, Balog and colleagues [2] found that positively or negatively biased AI-generated movie recommendations led users to make suboptimal choices, demonstrating that bias embedded in natural language outputs directly affects decision-making. The existence of framing effects has been widely documented also in medical decision-making [14]. For instance, physicians are more likely to choose a surgical procedure when outcomes are framed positively in terms of survival rates rather than negatively in terms of mortality rates [17,18].

These findings resonate with a growing shift in XAI research that is increasingly moving from explaining *how* an AI system operates, merely functioning as technical accounts of model logic, to explaining *why* its recommendations deserve consideration or use [16]. Thus, domain expertise fundamentally shapes what counts as a meaningful explanation [7]. For instance, explanations aligned with goal-oriented framing can emphasize why a recommended action is beneficial or harmful rather than how the underlying model works. Such explanations provide domain-relevant, actionable guidance that may be particularly valuable in high-stakes contexts like healthcare [16].

In this light, how an AI-based CDSS frames its explanations should be carefully considered by designers, as it can significantly influence how decision-makers perceive risk, make decisions, or interpret the consequences of their choices. Whether AI explanations should emphasize potential benefits of compliance (gain-oriented) or costs of non-compliance (cost-oriented) remains an unresolved design dilemma. Even within medical decision research, evidence is mixed, indicating that there are probably moderating factors such as task demands, context, and domain [1,10]. Although some work suggests that users may be more receptive to AI advice when risks are emphasized [8], it remains unclear whether gain- or cost-oriented framing better supports appropriate reliance, or whether framing meaningfully affects user behavior at all. Within the clinical domain, where the consequences of diagnostic errors are severe, the trade-off between persuasive influence and user autonomy becomes particularly salient. Understanding the influence of such framings is essential to ensure that AI augments, rather than undermines, critical clinical judgment.

To address this gap, we conducted a controlled experiment simulating human–AI collaboration in obstetric decision-making. Fifty-two nurses specializing in obstetrics evaluated 15 clinical scenarios supported by an AI-based Clinical Decision Support System (CDSS) that provided identical diagnostic recommendations, each accompanied by one of three explanation framings–gain-oriented, cost-oriented, or neutral. Our study was designed and conducted to address the following research question: (**RQ1**) how does explanation framing influence human accuracy, self-reported confidence, and reliance behavior–operationalized via metrics such as Appropriate Reliance, Deference, Automation Bias, and Self-Anchoring Bias–in AI-assisted clinical decision-making?

This study advances the understanding of how AI-based explanations can steer expert behavior in high-stakes domains, offering actionable insights for the design of XAI systems.

## 2 Methods

Adopting a within-subjects design, our study investigates how different linguistic framings of AI-generated explanations–namely, gain-oriented, cost-oriented, and neutral–affect nurses' accuracy, self-assessed confidence, and reliance behavior when interacting with a simulated CDSS in decision-making tasks.

The methodological approach was quantitative, using experimental manipulation embedded in a simulated decision-making task to avoid any real-world clinical risks, to ensure consistency across participants, and to retain control over the independent variable (i.e., explanation framing). The CDSS used in the study was a mock-up, specifically created for the purpose of experimental control; its behavior was fully predetermined and integrated via a custom-built interface on the LimeSurvey platform.

Participants were 52 nurses enrolled in an obstetrics specialization program at Università Vita-Salute San Raffaele in Milan, Italy. Each nurse completed the study individually in a supervised session of approximately one hour, accessing the experiment through a web-based interface on their own device, within the university facilities. Data were collected across two waves in March and June 2025, allowing for participation from two distinct course cohorts.

Each participant completed 15 obstetric clinical cases presented in randomized order and developed in collaboration with a professor of Clinical Pathology and Clinical Biochemistry, who also taught the participants' course. The cases focused on type and screen procedures, relevant to transfusion safety and prenatal diagnosis, and were intentionally designed to be moderately complex but solvable using curricular knowledge, independent of participants' clinical work experience. This ensured a consistent baseline of domain knowledge across the sample, thereby isolating the effect of the manipulated AI explanations.

For each case, participants first reviewed a brief clinical scenario (e.g., "Anna, 35 years old, at 32 weeks of gestation, presents with hypertension and proteinuria. The type and screen result is negative.") and selected one of two diagnostic or treatment options (e.g., "What is the most likely diagnosis? A. Preeclampsia B. Maternal-fetal incompatibility"), forming their First Human Decision (HD1). They then rated their confidence in this initial choice (C1) on a 4-point Likert scale, ranging from 1 (*Not at all confident*) to 4 (*Completely confident*). Confidence scores were subsequently normalized to the [0, 1] range for analysis. Following the initial decision, the same scenario was shown again, now accompanied by the AI system's advice and explanation, whose framing varied across cases. Each participant received five cases in each of the three framing conditions: gain-oriented emphasizes benefits of agreement (e.g., "Detecting preeclampsia in time is essential to protect mother and fetus."), cost-oriented highlights risks of non-compliance (e.g., "Neglecting the possibility of preeclampsia could expose mother and fetus to serious risks."), and neutral offers factual, guideline-based justification ("Signs of hypertension and proteinuria suggest preeclampsia. Maternal–fetal incompatibility is ruled out by the negative Type and Screen."). Framing assignment was counterbalanced across cases to control for order and content effects. To reflect realistic AI performance, the mock system was accurate in 80% of cases–slightly exceeding baseline human accuracy–and deliberately wrong in 20% of cases, with one incorrect advice per framing type. These incorrect cases were crafted to appear plausible, simulating the ambiguity common in real-world clinical decisions. After reviewing the AI's advice and explanation, participants were asked to make a Final Human Decision (FHD) between the same two options and rate their confidence in this last choice (FC) again on the same scale subsequently normalized to the [0, 1] range for analysis. This human-first paradigm enabled the measurement of reliance patterns, including whether and when participants updated their decisions in response to AI advice.

The study focused on three outcomes: decision accuracy, self-assessed confidence, and reliance behavior. Accuracy was measured at both pre-AI (HD1) and post-AI (FHD) stages, with a difference score ($\Delta$ accuracy) reflecting the extent to which AI support altered performance. Confidence was likewise measured before and after AI exposure, with a difference score ($\Delta$ confidence) capturing any increase or decrease related to AI support. Reliance behavior was operationalized using a triplet coding scheme based on whether the initial human decision, the AI advice, and the final human decision were correct (1) or incorrect (0) (e.g., 011 indicates a shift from incorrect to correct under AI guidance). Following the metric framework introduced by Campagner and colleagues [5], four derived indices were calculated: Appropriate Reliance (AR), Deference (D), Automation Bias (AB), and Self-Anchoring Bias (SAB). AR captured the ability to accept correct AI advices and reject incorrect ones, incorporating directional changes in confidence (see Eq. 1). D represented the extent to which participants changed their initial decisions to align with the AI's advice (see Eq. 2). AB indicated the susceptibility to being misled by incorrect AI advices and was calculated as the log-odds of following incorrect AI advice relative to rejecting it (see Eq. 3). SAB measured the tendency to ignore correct AI advice due to overconfidence in one's initial judgment, also via log-odds (see Eq. 4).

$$\text{Appropriate Reliance} = \frac{N_{011} + N_{101} + N_{001} + N_{111}\uparrow + N_{000}\downarrow}{N} \tag{1}$$

$$\text{Deference} = \frac{N_{011} + N_{100}}{N_{011} + N_{100} + N_{010} + N_{101}} \tag{2}$$

$$\text{Automation Bias} = \log\left(\frac{N_{100}\,/\,(N - N_{100})}{(N - N_{101})\,/\,N_{101}}\right) \tag{3}$$

$$\text{Self-Anchoring Bias} = \log\left(\frac{N_{010}\,/\,(N - N_{010})}{(N - N_{011})\,/\,N_{011}}\right) \tag{4}$$

To ensure that task difficulty was evenly distributed across conditions, baseline accuracy rates from unaided decisions were compared using paired McNemar tests. No significant differences were found between framing conditions, confirming the internal validity of the experimental design. Behavioral outcome measures were then analyzed using condition-specific point estimates and confidence intervals, both at 83% and 95% confidence intervals. For proportions such as accuracy and AR, Wilson score intervals were used. For difference scores, we employed the Newcombe–Wilson hybrid method. Log odds ratios for AB and SAB were accompanied by confidence intervals computed using the standard asymptotic method, where standard errors were estimated from reciprocal cell frequencies [4]. To facilitate visual inference, we reported 83% confidence intervals. Under standard assumptions of independence and approximate normality, non-overlap of 83% confidence intervals between two estimates is approximately equivalent to rejecting a two-sided null hypothesis at the 5% significance level (i.e., $p < 0.05$), corresponding to statistical significance at the 95% confidence level [9]. Overall, analyses were conducted comparing all valenced conditions (gain- and cost-oriented) against the neutral framing, and then directly comparing all three framings to isolate any framing-specific effects.

All procedures adhered to ethical guidelines for research involving human participants. No real clinical decisions were involved and no identifiable personal data were collected. Participation was voluntary and informed consent was obtained prior to the study.

## 3 Results

Point estimates and confidence intervals for all outcome variables are reported in Table 1.

With respect to accuracy, decision-makers' performance in the final decision was higher when explanations were framed with risk valence than when

**Table 1.** Point estimates and 83% Confidence Intervals (CIs) by dimension and experimental condition. Blue labels indicate non-overlapping CIs for the comparison between *valenced* and *neutral* conditions, while red labels indicate non-overlapping CIs for the comparison between *cost-oriented*, *gain-oriented*, and *neutral* conditions.

| Dimension | Condition | Value [CI] |
|---|---|---|
| Accuracy | *Valenced* | 0.77 [0.74, 0.80] |
| | Gain-Oriented | 0.77 [0.74, 0.81] |
| | Cost-Oriented | 0.77 [0.73, 0.80] |
| | *Neutral* | 0.70 [0.66, 0.73] |
| Confidence | Valenced | 0.80 [0.78, 0.82] |
| | Gain-Oriented | 0.81 [0.77, 0.84] |
| | Cost-Oriented | 0.80 [0.76, 0.83] |
| | Neutral | 0.75 [0.72, 0.79] |
| $\Delta$ Accuracy | *Valenced* | 0.06 [0.03, 0.10] |
| | Gain-Oriented | 0.07 [0.01, 0.12] |
| | Cost-Oriented | 0.06 [0.01, 0.11] |
| | *Neutral* | -0.04 [-0.09, 0.02] |
| $\Delta$ Confidence | Valenced | 0.18 [0.14, 0.21] |
| | Gain-Oriented | 0.16 [0.11, 0.22] |
| | Cost-Oriented | 0.19 [0.13, 0.24] |
| | Neutral | 0.14 [0.08, 0.19] |
| Appropriate Reliance | Valenced | 0.52 [0.49, 0.55] |
| | *Gain-Oriented* | 0.47 [0.43, 0.52] |
| | *Cost-Oriented* | 0.57 [0.53, 0.61] |
| | Neutral | 0.51 [0.47, 0.55] |
| Deference | *Valenced* | 0.66 [0.64, 0.69] |
| | *Gain-Oriented* | 0.54 [0.50, 0.58] |
| | *Cost-Oriented* | 0.79 [0.75, 0.82] |
| | *Neutral* | 0.55 [0.51, 0.59] |
| Automation Bias | Valenced | 0.59 [0.20, 0.98] |
| | *Gain-Oriented* | -0.24 [-0.78, 0.31] |
| | *Cost-Oriented* | 1.60 [0.91, 2.29] |
| | *Neutral* | -0.03 [-0.36, 0.30] |
| Self-Anchoring Bias | Valenced | -0.83 [-1.13, -0.53] |
| | *Gain-Oriented* | -0.40 [-0.81, 0.02] |
| | *Cost-Oriented* | -1.32 [-1.79, -0.85] |
| | Neutral | -0.66 [-1.09, -0.23] |

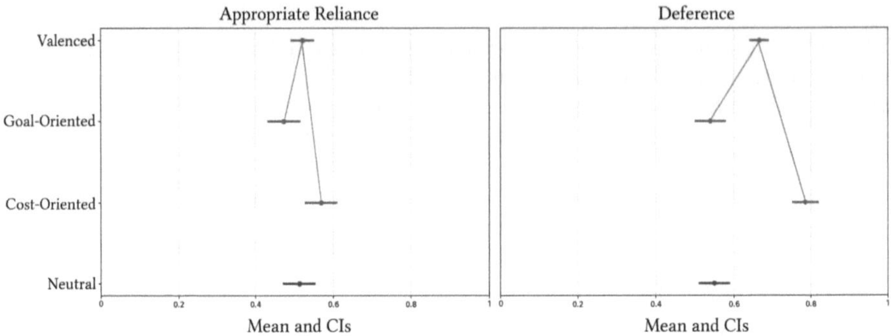


**Fig. 1.** Means and CIs for appropriate reliance and deference (range 0–1) by condition.

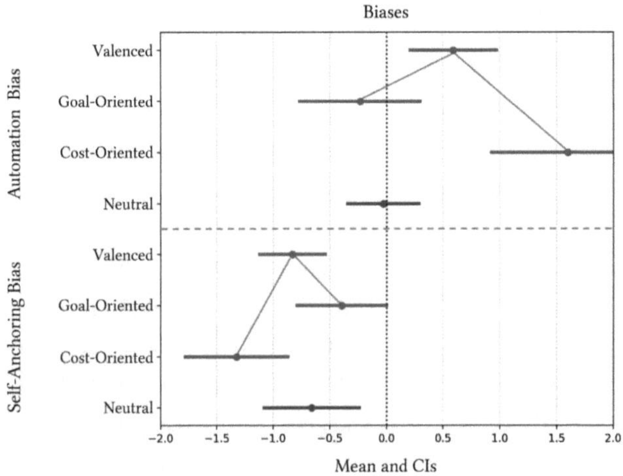


**Fig. 2.** Means and CIs for automation bias and self-anchoring bias (log OR), stratified by condition.

they were framed neutrally. Specifically, final accuracy was higher overall in the valenced framing condition (0.77, 83% CI [0.74, 0.80]) compared to the neutral framing condition (0.70, 83% CI [0.66, 0.73]). A similar pattern emerges considering change scores, as accuracy changed in opposite directions across the two main framings. In the aggregated valenced condition, accuracy increased after exposure to AI advice ($\Delta = 0.06$, CI [0.03, 0.10]), whereas in the neutral condition it slightly decreased ($\Delta = -0.04$, CI [−0.09, 0.02]). The corresponding CIs do not overlap, indicating a clear divergence. By contrast, although confidence increased after AI advice in all conditions, there is no visually compelling evidence of framing-related differences in confidence change.

A different pattern emerges for reliance-related outcomes (see Fig. 1 and Fig. 2). Cost-oriented explanations were associated with higher appropriate reliance (0.57, CI [0.53, 0.61]) than gain-oriented explanations (0.47, CI [0.43,

0.52]) and higher deference (0.79, CI [0.75, 0.82]) than both gain-oriented explanations (0.54, CI [0.50, 0.58]) and neutral ones (0.55, CI [0.51, 0.59]), always with non-overlapping CIs. Finally, bias-related measures show pronounced separation between cost- and gain-oriented framings. Automation bias was substantially higher under cost-oriented framing (log OR = 1.60, CI [0.91, 2.29]) than under gain-oriented (log OR = −0.24, CI [−0.78, 0.31]) and neutral framing (log OR = −0.03, CI [−0.38, 0.30]). Self-anchoring bias was also lower under cost-oriented framing (log OR = −1.32, CI [−1.79, −0.85]) than under gain-oriented framing (log OR = −0.40, CI [−0.81, 0.02]), again with non-overlapping CIs.

## 4 Discussion

This study examined how linguistic framing in AI-based explanations influences clinical decision accuracy, confidence, and reliance behavior among professionals. Specifically, we assessed the effects of cost-oriented, gain-oriented, and neutral explanation framings on nurses' interactions with an AI-based CDSS across 15 obstetric scenarios.

The most significant result concerned the persuasive impact of cost-oriented explanations. Compared with both gain-oriented and neutral framings, cost-oriented explanations elicited the highest levels of appropriate reliance and deference toward the system's recommendations but also the highest levels of automation bias and the lowest levels of self-anchoring bias. In practical terms, this indicates that while participants were generally more likely to rely correctly on the system's suggestions and less likely to ignore correct AI advice due to overconfidence in their initial judgment, they were also more prone to revising their initial decisions, also in favor of incorrect recommendations. Persuasive explanations may thus enhance performance when the AI is right but erode critical oversight when it is wrong, an effect especially problematic in safety-critical contexts where unchecked overreliance can compromise care quality [6,20]. These effects were not attributable to baseline differences in task difficulty or accuracy across conditions, confirming the robustness of the framing manipulation. While valenced framings improved overall accuracy relative to neutral framing, only cost-oriented explanations substantially shifted participants' decision patterns and susceptibility to flawed AI suggestions.

This strong influence of cost-oriented framing aligns with prior research on prospect theory [11,21] and framing in medical decision-making [10,17,18], which shows that risk-oriented advices tends to heighten compliance and bias, even among professionals, due to stronger affective responses or risk aversion. Our findings extend this literature to human–AI interaction in healthcare, demonstrating that AI-based explanations do not merely inform but can strategically steer users' behavior. Cost-oriented language appears to act as a rhetorical cue, increasing the perceived urgency or consequences of non-compliance and thereby nudging users toward AI alignment regardless of advice accuracy.

Overall, these findings underscore the role of linguistic framing in shaping user behavior within AI-supported clinical workflows. Thus, choices about how to present explanations are not neutral or merely stylistic. The main implication for XAI design is that, when the goal is to improve human accuracy, explanations should be treated as valenced rather than neutral, and framed in terms of costs rather than gains, because this latter framing yields significantly higher levels of appropriate reliance on the DSS. Importantly, this effect appears contingent on the AI being more accurate than the average human decision-maker. By contrast, if the AI were less accurate, the substantially higher automation bias typically observed under such cost-oriented condition would likely offset–or reverse–any positive effects of employing a persuasive decision aid.

This study's controlled simulation environment ensured high internal validity but limits the generalizability of the findings, also due to the small sample size, making it an exploratory study. The experiment was conducted with nurses from a single institution within a specific obstetric type-and-screen decision context and relied on static mock CDSS scenarios. Thus, the findings should be interpreted within clearly defined boundary conditions and their generalization to other specialties or real-world workflows characterized by dynamic interactions, time pressure, and competing cognitive demands requires further validation. Future research should therefore replicate and extend these results across multiple professional roles (e.g., experienced physicians) and clinical domains, as well as in real-time decision-support environments embedded in routine workflows. Additionally, future studies should investigate how framing effects vary across different decision contexts, such as simpler versus more complex cases, and across users with different levels of expertise. More broadly, there is a need for adaptive explanation systems capable of tailoring their rhetorical style to user characteristics and task demands, with the goal of maximizing decision support while preserving professional autonomy. Understanding how framing effects interact with trust, interpretability, and accountability remains a key frontier for human-centered AI design in healthcare.

## 5 Conclusion

This study explored how linguistic framing in AI-generated explanations affects diagnostic decision-making and reliance behavior among clinical professionals. Specifically, we examined whether gain-oriented, cost-oriented, or neutral explanation framings would differentially influence the diagnostic accuracy, confidence, and reliance patterns of nurses making high-stakes obstetric decisions.

Our findings reveal that while both gain- and cost-oriented framings improve diagnostic accuracy relative to neutral framing, cost-oriented explanations exert a uniquely strong influence on behavior. They significantly increase appropriate reliance and deference on AI recommendations but also elevate automation bias, indicating a greater tendency to accept incorrect AI advice. Overall, explanation strategies that maximize AI influence can enhance performance under favorable conditions, yet also increase vulnerability to overreliance. This underscores the need for explanation designs that balance decisional impact with safeguards against automation bias, especially in safety-critical domains.

**Acknowledgments.** The authors acknowledge funding support provided by the Italian projects AMAR (CUP: D53C22002380006) and InXAID (CUP: H53D23008090001), both funded by the European Union (Next Generation EU).

**Disclosure of Interests.** The authors have no competing interests to declare that are relevant to the content of this article.

## References

1. Ainiwaer, A., Zhang, S., Ainiwaer, X., Ma, F.: Effects of message framing on cancer prevention and detection behaviors, intentions, and attitudes: Systematic review and meta-analysis. J. Med. Internet Res. **23**(9), e27634 (2021)
2. Balog, K., Radlinski, F., Petrov, A.: Measuring the impact of explanation bias: a study of natural language justifications for recommender systems. CHI EA ' 23, (2023) ACM
3. Bertrand, A., Belloum, R., Eagan, J.R., Maxwell, W.: How cognitive biases affect XAI-assisted decision-making: a systematic review. In: AAAI/ACM AIES '22, pp. 78–91. ACM (2022)
4. Bland, J.M., Altman, D.G.: The odds ratio. BMJ **320**(7247), 1468 (2000)
5. Campagner, A., Fregosi, C., Natali, C., Cabitza, F.: Under what influence: measuring AI influence to fit user profiles in decision-making. Int. J. Hum Comput Stud. **210**(103763) (2026)
6. Dratsch, T., et al.: Automation bias in mammography: the impact of artificial intelligence bi-rads suggestions on reader performance. Radiology **307**, e222176 (2023)
7. Ehsan, U., et al.: The who in XAI: how AI background shapes perceptions of AI explanations. In: CHI '24, pp. 1–32. ACM (2024)
8. Fahnenstich, H., Rieger, T., Roesler, E.: Trusting under risk-comparing human to AI decision support agents. Comput. Hum. Behav. **153**, 108107 (2024)
9. Goldstein, H., Healy, M.J.: The graphical presentation of a collection of means. J. R. Stat. Soc. A. Stat. Soc. **158**(1), 175–177 (1995)
10. Gong, J., et al.: The framing effect in medical decision-making: a review of the literature. Psychol. Health Med. **18**(6), 645–653 (2013)
11. Kahneman, D.: A perspective on judgment and choice: mapping bounded rationality. Am. Psychol. **58**(9), 697–720 (2003)
12. Kim, T., Song, H.: Communicating the limitations of AI: the effect of message framing and ownership on trust in artificial intelligence. Int. J. Hum.-Comput. Int. **39**(4), 790–800 (2023)
13. Kunar, M.A., Watson, D.G.: Framing the fallibility of computer-aided detection aids cancer detection. Cogn. Res. **8**(1), 30 (2023). https://doi.org/10.1186/s41235-023-00485-y
14. Levin, I.P., Schneider, S.L., Gaeth, G.J.: All frames are not created equal: a typology and critical analysis of framing effects. Organ. Behav. Hum. Decis. Process. **76**(2), 149–188 (1998)
15. Liao, M., Sundar, S.S.: How should AI systems talk to users when collecting their personal information? Effects of role framing and self-referencing on human-AI interaction. In: CHI '21, ACM (2021)
16. Liu, H., Su, Y., Lease, M.: Rhetorical XAI: explaining AI's benefits as well as its use via rhetorical design (2025). https://arxiv.org/abs/2505.09862

17. Marteau, T.M.: Framing of information: its influence upon decisions of doctors and patients. Br. J. Soc. Psychol. **28**(1), 89–94 (1989)
18. McNeil, B.J., Pauker, S.G., Sox, H.C., Tversky, A.: On the elicitation of preferences for alternative therapies. N. Engl. J. Med. **306**(21), 1259–1262 (1982)
19. Pataranutaporn, P., Liu, R., Finn, E., Maes, P.: Influencing human–AI interaction by priming beliefs about ai can increase perceived trustworthiness, empathy and effectiveness. Nat. Mach. Intell. **5**, 1076–1086 (2023)
20. Schemmer, M., Kuehl, N., Benz, C., Bartos, A., Satzger, G.: Appropriate reliance on AI advice: conceptualization and the effect of explanations. In: IUI '23, pp. 410–422 (2023)
21. Tversky, A., Kahneman, D.: The framing of decisions and the psychology of choice. Science **211**(4481), 453–458 (1981)

# FedVendorBC: Accurate Multi-vendor Federated Learning for Privacy-Preserving and Generalizable Breast Cancer Diagnosis Using Ultrasound Images

Faisal Ahmed[1,2(✉)], David Sánchez[1], Zouhair Haddi[2], and Josep Domingo-Ferrer[1]

[1] Department of Computer Engineering and Mathematics, ComSCIAM-Center for Computational Science and Applied Mathematics, CYBERCAT-Center for Cybersecurity Research of Catalonia, Universitat Rovira i Virgili, Tarragona, Catalonia

[2] NVISION Systems and Technologies SL, Barcelona, Catalonia

faisal.ahmed@nvision.es

**Abstract.** Manual ultrasound-based breast cancer diagnosis is labor-intensive, time-consuming, and prone to errors, a burden that AI-assisted diagnostic systems can help alleviate. However, developing accurate and generalizable diagnostic models requires large-scale multi-vendor data collected across multiple hospitals, which are difficult to obtain due to privacy concerns, data ownership restrictions, and regulatory constraints. Federated learning (FL) enables privacy-preserving and regulation-compliant collaborative training. Nevertheless, conventional FL often underperforms in multi-vendor breast ultrasound settings due to substantial data heterogeneity across vendors. To tackle this issue, we propose FedVendorBC, an FL framework tailored for accurate, privacy-preserving training of breast cancer diagnostic models across multi-vendor ultrasound imaging settings. Experiments show that FedVendorBC achieves relative improvements in diagnostic performance of 7.85% in recall, 5.55% in F1-score, 2.51% in auROC, and 12.72% in sensitivity at a 5% false-positive rate over standard baselines.

**Keywords:** Breast cancer diagnosis · Data privacy · Data heterogeneity · Federated learning · Multi-vendor generalization

## 1 Introduction

Breast cancer is a leading cause of cancer-related mortality among women, where early diagnosis significantly improves outcomes. Ultrasound (US) imaging is widely used for detection due to its cost-effectiveness and real-time capability, but manual interpretation is time-consuming and expertise-dependent. Accurate AI-assisted diagnosis from US images is thus essential to reduce this burden.

© The Author(s), under exclusive license to Springer Nature Switzerland AG 2027
P. Andreev et al. (Eds.): AIME 2026, LNAI 16748, pp. 103–108, 2027.
https://doi.org/10.1007/978-3-032-30710-1_12

However, developing accurate and generalizable deep learning models requires large-scale, multi-institutional datasets covering diverse populations and clinical settings. Such data collection is challenging due to privacy constraints, data ownership, and regulatory restrictions.

Federated learning (FL) [1] has emerged as a promising paradigm for collaborative training of AI models across multiple institutions that does not require them to share their (sensitive) data. However, FL on multi-vendor datasets remains challenging because US images originating from different vendors are inherently heterogeneous. This heterogeneity arises from variations in image-acquisition hardware and reconstruction pipelines and is further amplified by differences in imaging protocols and diverse demographics of patients. These compound distribution shifts can significantly degrade the convergence and generalization of the model if not explicitly addressed. To tackle this issue, we propose FedVendorBC, a federated learning framework for training AI models for breast cancer diagnosis using multi-vendor US images. Empirical results conducted in a realistic multi-vendor clinical setting show that FedVendorBC offers superior performance than three baseline FL methods.

## 2 FedVendorBC

FedVendorBC incorporates two innovative strategies along with the vanilla FL workflow: i) it employs a gradient correction mechanism to align all parameters of local models in the same direction before aggregating them at the server, in order to overcome the gradient conflict that arises from training each local model on images of a different vendor; and ii) it regulates local training on the vendor-specific data at the client side using an early-stopping strategy guided by clinically meaningful evaluation criteria.

**Local Training Regularization at the Client Level.** In clinical breast ultrasound practice, benign lesions substantially outnumber malignant cases, resulting in a class imbalance. This can bias learning toward the majority (benign) class and may degrade diagnostic reliability, leading to excessive false-positive predictions that result in unnecessary biopsies, increased healthcare costs, and additional patient burden. To ensure training is performed under clinically realistic operating conditions and to promote clinically meaningful performance while mitigating overfitting, FedVendorBC regulates local training by using an early-stopping strategy based on sensitivity measured at a fixed 5% false-positive rate (FPR) on the local validation set. This low-FPR operating point aligns with practical clinical requirements, where the false-positive rate must remain limited while maintaining a high sensitivity to cancer detection.

More specifically, after each local training epoch, FedVendorBC evaluates the current model on the client's vendor-specific validation set and terminates the training if the sensitivity at 5% FPR does not improve for a predefined patience period. The model achieving the highest validation sensitivity at this operating point is retained as the final local model and is sent to the server.

**Gradient Correction at the Server.** Due to non-IID data distributions across clients –arising from US images acquired with devices from different vendors– the locally learned model parameters can diverge and conflict with one another, degrading the quality of the global model. To tackle this problem, FedVendorBC employs a gradient correction mechanism inspired by the *projecting conflicting gradients (PCGrad)* strategy [8]. FedVendorBC treats each vendor's local model as a separate task and projects a vendor's gradient onto the normal plane of the gradient of other vendors with conflicting gradients before local parameter aggregation. Specifically, in round $t$, FedVendorBC computes the local gradient $g_t^k$ for each client $k$ by determining the difference between the locally updated model parameters $\theta_t^k$ and the previous global model parameters $\theta_{t-1}$. Then it flattens these gradient vectors into a vector form to enable pairwise gradient correction and projection. The gradient of client $k$ is formally defined as $g_t^k = \text{vec}\big(\theta_t^k - \theta_{t-1}\big)$, where $\text{vec}(\cdot)$ denotes the vectorization (flattening) operator. Subsequently, for each client $k$, FedVendorBC randomly selects another client $j \neq k$ from the remaining $K-1$ clients and computes the inner product $\langle g_t^k, g_t^j \rangle$ between their respective gradient vectors. If the inner product is negative, that is, $\langle g_t^k, g_t^j \rangle < 0$, the two gradients are interpreted as being in conflict, indicating that they point in opposite directions. In this scenario, $g_t^k$ is projected onto the normal plane of $g_t^j$ to eliminate the conflicting component. The gradient is corrected as follows:

$$\bar{g}_t^k = \begin{cases} g_t^k - \dfrac{\langle g_t^k, g_t^j \rangle}{\|g_t^j\|_2^2}\, g_t^j, & \text{if } \langle g_t^k, g_t^j \rangle < 0, \\ g_t^k, & \text{otherwise.} \end{cases} \tag{1}$$

The gradient $\bar{g}_t^k$ is then reshaped back to match the parameter $\theta_t^k$ tensor structure of the target model and used to obtain the corrected local model parameter $\bar{\theta}_t^k$, as $\bar{\theta}_t^k = \theta_{t-1} + \text{unvec}(\bar{g}_t^k)$, where $\text{unvec}(\cdot)$ denotes the inverse vectorization operator that reshapes a vector back into the original parameter tensor structure. The server finally aggregates these corrected parameters to compute the global model update for the next training round $t+1$ using the Federated Averaging (FedAvg) [5] algorithm.

## 3 Experiments

**Datasets and Model.** We curated five datasets from public sources: *BUS-BRA* [4], *BUSI* [2], *QAMEBI* [3], *BUS-UCLM* [6] and *UDIAT* [7]. The BUS-BRA dataset contains images acquired using ultrasound systems from *GE Healthcare* and *Toshiba Medical Systems* (now Canon Medical Systems). Images in the BUSI dataset were also acquired using ultrasound systems from *GE Healthcare*. BUS-UCLM and UDIAT both include images acquired using ultrasound machines from *Siemens Healthineers*. The QAMEBI dataset comprises images captured using ultrasound system from *Supersonic Imagine*. Based on the manufacturer specifications, we organized the data into four vendor-specific datasets. We preprocessed all images using a standard transformation pipeline used in

[1]. We retrained ResNet-18 as the prediction model, modifying its input layer to accept two channels: a grayscale US image and its corresponding mask. We also replaced its final layer with a single output neuron for binary classification between benign and malignant.

**Results and Discussion.** We conducted leave-one-vendor-out validation to evaluate the effectiveness of FedVendorBC and compared it against three standard FL baselines (FedAvg, FedProx, and SCAFFOLD) using the following evaluation metrics: accuracy, precision, recall, sensitivity at 5% false-positive rate (S-5-F), F1-score, and area under the receiver operating characteristic curve (auROC). The results for four unseen external vendors across all metrics, as well as the average results across the vendors, are presented in Table 1.

**Table 1.** Performance of FedVendorBC and baselines on external vendor datasets. Averages are computed over per-vendor point estimates; best result per metric in bold.

| Vendor | Method | Accuracy | Precision | Sensitivity | Specificity | S-5-F | F1-score | auROC |
|---|---|---|---|---|---|---|---|---|
| GE | FedVendorBC | **87.16** | **76.53** | **85.31** | **88.00** | **72.63** | **0.807** | **0.929** |
| | FedAvg | 84.77 | 72.18 | 83.85 | 85.19 | 62.62 | 0.776 | 0.915 |
| | FedProx | 84.73 | 73.62 | 80.11 | 86.84 | 60.61 | 0.767 | 0.909 |
| | SCAFFOLD | 84.47 | 70.62 | 86.65 | 83.48 | 61.95 | 0.778 | 0.912 |
| Siemens | FedVendorBC | **78.59** | 64.96 | **86.36** | 74.29 | **37.50** | **0.742** | **0.852** |
| | FedAvg | 73.33 | 58.94 | 82.39 | 68.34 | 31.25 | 0.687 | 0.817 |
| | FedProx | 77.17 | 66.15 | 73.30 | 79.31 | 37.50 | 0.695 | 0.832 |
| | SCAFFOLD | 78.59 | **69.23** | 71.59 | **82.45** | 33.52 | 0.704 | 0.816 |
| Supersonic | FedVendorBC | **81.90** | 80.92 | **86.18** | 77.06 | **51.22** | **0.835** | **0.872** |
| | FedAvg | 78.88 | 83.64 | 74.80 | **83.49** | 42.28 | 0.790 | 0.866 |
| | FedProx | 79.74 | **83.93** | 76.42 | **83.49** | **51.22** | 0.800 | 0.868 |
| | SCAFFOLD | 79.74 | 83.33 | 77.24 | 82.57 | 41.46 | 0.802 | 0.839 |
| Toshiba | FedVendorBC | **89.21** | 90.77 | 86.76 | 91.55 | **75.00** | **0.887** | **0.944** |
| | FedAvg | 84.89 | **94.34** | 73.53 | **95.77** | 73.53 | 0.826 | 0.903 |
| | FedProx | 82.01 | 77.22 | **89.71** | 74.65 | 57.35 | 0.830 | 0.899 |
| | SCAFFOLD | 82.01 | 82.09 | 80.88 | 83.10 | 33.82 | 0.815 | 0.836 |
| Avg±SD | FedVendorBC | **84.22 ± 4.85** | **78.30 ± 10.70** | **86.15 ± 0.61** | 82.72 ± 8.35 | **59.09 ± 17.93** | **0.818 ± 0.060** | **0.899 ± 0.044** |
| | FedAvg | 80.47 ± 5.52 | 77.28 ± 15.21 | 78.64 ± 5.23 | **83.20 ± 11.30** | 52.42 ± 19.15 | 0.770 ± 0.059 | 0.875 ± 0.044 |
| | FedProx | 80.91 ± 3.22 | 75.23 ± 7.43 | 79.88 ± 7.10 | 81.07 ± 5.22 | 51.67 ± 10.10 | 0.773 ± 0.058 | 0.877 ± 0.034 |
| | SCAFFOLD | 81.20 ± 2.67 | 76.32 ± 7.43 | 79.09 ± 6.25 | 82.90 ± 0.47 | 42.69 ± 13.47 | 0.775 ± 0.049 | 0.851 ± 0.042 |

FedVendorBC shows a substantial generalization improvement over FedAvg across all evaluation metrics except specificity, without incurring additional costs in terms of communication efficiency and bandwidth usage. Performance improvements are more substantial for sensitivity, F1-score, auROC and sensitivity at a fixed 5% false-positive rate, which are clinically significant metrics for breast cancer diagnosis. Compared to standard baselines, FedVendorBC achieves relative performance gains of 7.85% in recall, 5.55% in F1-score, 2.51% in auROC, and 12.72% in sensitivity at a 5% false-positive rate. These gains indicate improved cancer-detection performance under clinically realistic low-false-positive operating conditions. A vendor-specific analysis shows that GE HealthCare and Siemens Healthineers, whose datasets exhibit a more realistic ratio of malignant to benign samples, demonstrate consistently superior diagnostic performance across all evaluation metrics compared to FedAvg. The data distributions for these two vendors closely reflect real-world clinical practice, where benign lesions substantially outnumber malignant cases, further highlighting the practical relevance of FedVendorBC. In contrast, for SuperSonic Imagine and Toshiba Medical Systems, FedVendorBC shows a relatively lower specificity, as also reflected in the overall average specificity score. This reduced specificity can be attributed to the atypical class distributions in these datasets, where the balance between malignant and benign samples deviates from realistic clinical prevalence.

## 4 Conclusions

FedVendorBC addresses the data heterogeneity that arises in collaborative trained AI models using multi-vendor US imaging systems for breast cancer diagnosis. By explicitly accounting for inter-vendor heterogeneity, FedVendorBC enables robust and stable learning across hospitals operating scanners from different manufacturers. Future work will extend FedVendorBC to additional imaging modalities and cancer types, and include an ablation study to identify which component drives the performance gains.

**Acknowledgments.** This work is funded by the European Commission (GA 101073222), the Government of Catalonia (ICREA Acadèmia Prizes to J. Domingo-Ferrer and D. Sánchez), and MCIN/AEI grant PID2024-157271NB-I00 "CLEARING-IT".

**Disclosure of Interests.** The authors have no competing interests to declare.

## References

1. Ahmed, F., Sánchez, D., Domingo-Ferrer, J., Haddi, Z.: FedBC: privacy-preserving breast cancer diagnosis from ultrasound images using federated learning. In: Deep Breast Workshop on AI and Imaging for Diagnostic and Treatment Challenges in Breast Care, pp. 31–40. Springer (2025)
2. Al-Dhabyani, W., Gomaa, M., Khaled, H., Fahmy, A.: Dataset of breast ultrasound images. Data Brief **28**, 104863 (2020)
3. Ardakani, A.A., Mohammadi, A., Mirza-Aghazadeh-Attari, M., Acharya, U.R.: An open-access breast lesion ultrasound image database: applicable in artificial intelligence studies. Comput. Biol. Med. **152**, 106438 (2023)
4. Gómez-Flores, W., Gregorio-Calas, M.J., Coelho de Albuquerque Pereira, W.: BUS-BRA: a breast ultrasound dataset for assessing computer-aided diagnosis systems. Med. Phys. **51**(4), 3110–3123 (2024)
5. McMahan, B., Moore, E., Ramage, D., Hampson, S., y Arcas, B.A.: Communication-efficient learning of deep networks from decentralized data. In: Artificial Intelligence and Statistics, pp. 1273–1282. PMLR (2017)
6. Vallez, N., Bueno, G., Deniz, O., et al.: BUS-UCLM: breast ultrasound lesion segmentation dataset. Sci. Data **12**, 242 (2025)

7. Yap, M.H., et al.: Automated breast ultrasound lesions detection using convolutional neural networks. IEEE J. Biomed. Health Inform. **22**(4), 1218–1226 (2017)
8. Yu, T., Kumar, S., Gupta, A., Levine, S., Hausman, K., Finn, C.: Gradient surgery for multi-task learning. Adv. Neural. Inf. Process. Syst. **33**, 5824–5836 (2020)

# Regression vs. Medical LLMs: A Comprehensive Study for CVD and Mortality Risk Prediction

Samuel Desire Kom Sande[1(✉)], Maciej Skorski[1], Martin Theobald[1], Jochen Schneider[2], and Winfried März[3]

[1] Department of Computer Science, University of Luxembourg, Esch-sur-Alzette, Luxembourg
{samuel.kom,maciej.skorski,martin.theobald}@uni.lu

[2] Luxembourg Center for Systems Biomedicine, University of Luxembourg, Esch-sur-Alzette, Luxembourg
jochen.schneider@uni.lu

[3] University Hospital Heidelberg and SYNLAB Academy, Augsburg, Germany
winfried.maerz@synlab.com

**Abstract.** Cardiovascular Diseases (CVDs) remain a leading cause of mortality worldwide, driving the demand for predictive tools that enable early detection and preventive intervention. Machine Learning (ML) models—such as linear and logistic regression, support vector machines (SVMs), and tree ensembles—have long underpinned CVD and mortality risk estimation. Recent advances in Generative Artificial Intelligence (GenAI) and Large Language Models (LLMs) are however increasingly shifting this paradigm. This paper demonstrates that the gap between LLMs and leading ML techniques diminishes and can be bridged with appropriate biomarker selection and prompt engineering—with LLMs achieving up to 85% AUROC in 1-year all-cause mortality prediction on the Ludwigshafen Risk and Cardiovascular Health Study (LURIC), proving them competitive to recent boosting-based ML algorithms and established clinical scores (CoroPredict, SMART, SCORE2).

**Keywords:** Cardiovascular Diseases & Mortality Risk Prediction · Medical Large Language Models · Regression & Boosting · Calibration & Stratification

## 1 Introduction

GenAI rapidly transforms various domains, including the Life Sciences and Healthcare. Its recent advances have sparked a growing interest in leveraging LLMs for mortality prediction in patients diagnosed with CVD [4], which remains a leading cause of mortality worldwide, with an estimated annual cost of over $400B in the US and €282B in the EU. ML models, such as SVMs, tree ensembles and Artificial Neural Networks (ANNs), traditionally dominate CVD mortality prediction [7,9,10] and remain the standard choice in top medical publications [3]. Previous LLM studies, on the other hand, fall short in three key aspects:

© The Author(s), under exclusive license to Springer Nature Switzerland AG 2027
P. Andreev et al. (Eds.): AIME 2026, LNAI 16748, pp. 109–114, 2027.
https://doi.org/10.1007/978-3-032-30710-1_13

(i) **limited domain-specific tuning**—as they mostly apply commercial LLMs in zero-shot settings [4,11,13]; (ii) **performance gap of open LLMs**—openly available models lag behind commercial ones [8]; and (iii) **predominant focus on textual input**—finetuning approaches mostly rely on clinical notes and discharge summaries [1,2], both of which are often only inconsistently available across domains and expensive to produce.

**Contributions and Outline.** Motivated by these limitations, we explore routinely collected lab markers and comorbidity profiles as a cost-effective and widely available alternative to clinical notes. Our contributions include:

- a comprehensive study of **leading regression techniques** (SVMs, LinearBoost, XGBoost, CatBoost, RealMLP) in comparison to both **open Medical LLMs** (MedGemma, Med42, MMed, Meditron, OpenBioLLM) and **general-purpose commercial models** (ChatGPT, Gemini, Claude);
- a wide range of **curated biomarkers**, covering routine and specialized tests, assembled via expert knowledge, literature mining, and algorithmic selection;
- a universal **tabular-to-clinical-note** prompting scheme that converts structured lab and biomarker records into natural-language prompts, proven effective across open and commercial models for both **inference** and **finetuning**;
- **established tuning techniques** via few-shot prompting to enable in-context learning, supervised finetuning, and post-hoc calibration.

## 2 Cohort Selection and Methodology

**Cohorts.** We focus on the LURIC study [12], a large prospective investigation of 3,316 patients enrolled between 1997 and 2000. It is one of the most comprehensive CVD cohorts available, with a high prevalence of CAD (79%) and other cardio-metabolic conditions (62% dyslipidemia, 58% hypertension), a broad array of biomarkers (inflammatory, coagulation, lipid, endothelial) derived from over 115 ml of fasting blood, and more than 25 years of follow-up on all-cause and cardiovascular mortality. Among all patients, 2,600 (78.4%) were diagnosed with CVD, enabling comparisons against established clinical scores such as CoroPredict [6]. We therefore derived two cohorts, to assess generalizability on the full population and enable comparison against clinical baselines:

- the **full-cohort** of LURIC consisting of 3,316 patients; and
- the **sub-cohort** of LURIC consisting of 2,112 CVD patients.

**Outcomes.** 1-year all-cause mortality (**1YM**), a standard prognostic endpoint for CVD risk, is defined as "death within 12 months of follow-up". This occurred for 139 (4.2%) patients in the full-cohort and for 86 (4.1%) in the sub-cohort.

**Biomarkers and Comorbidity Profiles.** We curated five biomarker sets as input for our ML and GenAI analyses on LURIC, comprehensively representing a clinical baseline from RiskyCAD (**Risk-12**), routine low-cost tests (**Core-20**), literature-mined markers at two scales (**Lit-21** & **Ext-64**), as well as a comprehensive compilation of all prior sets (**Comp-94**); we refer to [5] for details.

**ML Models.** We evaluate SVMs as a classic baseline, gradient-boosting ensembles including competition-winning CatBoost and XGBoost (proven effective for medical prediction [3]) as well as LinearBoost, and a state-of-the-art Tabular Foundation Model RealMLP—pre-tuned to bridge deep learning and gradient boosting on tabular data (so far unexploited in the medical literature). Hyper-parameters were tuned via Bayesian optimization using `Optuna` with 200 trials per cohort and biomarker selection; also here we refer to [5] for details.

**LLM Prompting.** We convert tabular biomarker records into structured clinical-note-like prompts (see Fig. 1) under the following two schemes:

- **zero-shot prompts** for direct mortality risk assessment; and
- **few-shot prompts** which prepend the zero-shot prompt by three fixed synthetic patient records with given risk scores.

Open LLMs were deployed on two GPUs via `vLLM` for efficient inference, while commercial models were queried via their APIs—both using identical prompts.

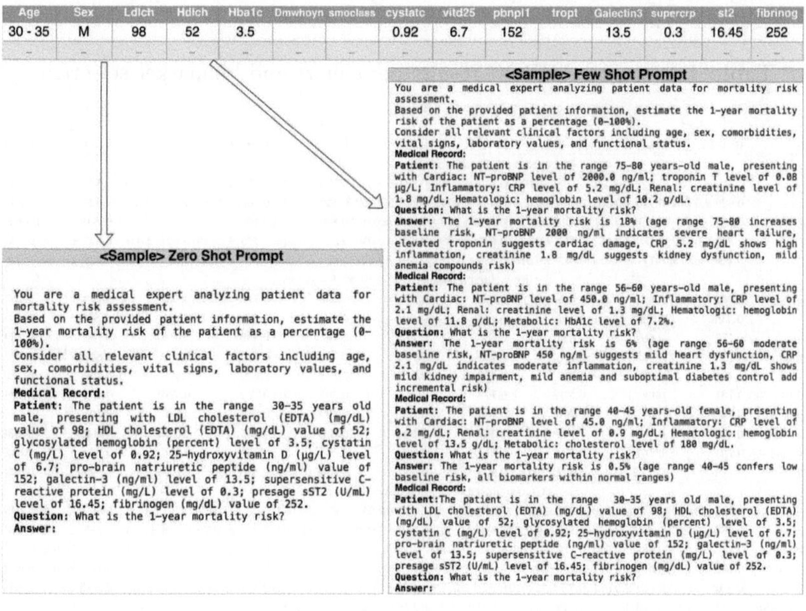


**Fig. 1.** Prompting for the **Risk-12** biomarkers (anonymized patient data).

Model outputs were carefully parsed to extract risk scores; libraries such as `Instructor` can further unify querying and simplify parsing effort.

**Supervised Finetuning.** We finetuned the open LLMs directly on the zero-shot prompts by using the 1YM labels as targets, allowing them to learn clinical patterns while preserving natural-language inference. Due to computational costs, finetuning was limited to the 4B version of MEDGEMMA and the 8B variants of the other (Llama-based) models, using LoRA adapters and accelerated distributed training with `DeepSpeed` (8 epochs, batch size 16, learning rate 1e-4, cosine scheduling) on an Nvidia H100 NVLink dual-GPU platform.

## 3 Evaluation

**Methodology.** For a robust assessment given the cohort size and class imbalance, we used stratified cross-validations (CVs) with 10 and 5 splits for the classical and finetuned models, respectively. Prompting-based experiments used direct 3-shot in-context learning without CVs. Missing values were imputed with per-attribute medians for classical models only, while they were skipped for the prompting schemes. AUROC was used to assess the discriminative performance of risk scores, as is customary for risk prediction.

**Results.** Table 1 reports detailed AUROC results for both LURIC cohorts, and under all combinations of biomarker sets and models. Top selections of the corresponding ROC plots are depicted in Fig. 2 for the sub-cohort of LURIC. We

**Table 1.** Detailed AUROC results per cohort and biomarker selection.

| Model | Full-Cohort | | | | | Sub-Cohort | | | | |
|---|---|---|---|---|---|---|---|---|---|---|
| | Risk-12 | Base-20 | Lit-21 | Ext-64 | Comp-94 | Risk-12 | Base-20 | Lit-21 | Ext-64 | Comp-94 |
| | | | | | REGRESSION: BOOSTING & TABULAR FOUNDATION MODELS | | | | | |
| SVM | 0.817 ±0.059 | 0.722 ±0.047 | 0.765 ±0.044 | 0.819 ±0.062 | 0.823 ±0.058 | 0.829 ±0.032 | 0.778 ±0.065 | 0.741 ±0.055 | 0.827 ±0.037 | 0.805 ±0.063 |
| LinearBoost | 0.826 ±0.051 | 0.776 ±0.050 | 0.795 ±0.057 | 0.826 ±0.042 | 0.826 ±0.052 | 0.836 ±0.047 | **0.802** ±0.047 | 0.772 ±0.070 | 0.827 ±0.052 | 0.834 ±0.037 |
| CatBoost | 0.829 ±0.052 | **0.792** ±0.049 | **0.816** ±0.047 | **0.839** ±0.051 | **0.841** ±0.053 | **0.838** ±0.048 | 0.796 ±0.055 | 0.814 ±0.049 | **0.849** ±0.039 | **0.846** ±0.041 |
| XGBoost | 0.829 ±0.052 | 0.780 ±0.057 | 0.810 ±0.044 | 0.825 ±0.055 | 0.828 ±0.050 | 0.825 ±0.043 | 0.775 ±0.049 | **0.815** ±0.047 | 0.825 ±0.046 | 0.825 ±0.044 |
| RealMLP | **0.830** ±0.017 | 0.777 ±0.024 | 0.813 ±0.013 | 0.836 ±0.023 | 0.839 ±0.021 | 0.824 ±0.021 | 0.775 ±0.029 | 0.799 ±0.021 | 0.826 ±0.015 | 0.825 ±0.019 |
| | | | | | FEW-SHOT PROMPTING (3-SHOT PROMPTS) | | | | | |
| MedGemma-27B | 0.762 | 0.698 | 0.698 | 0.762 | 0.749 | 0.767 | 0.719 | 0.728 | 0.784 | 0.765 |
| Med42-70B | **0.796** | **0.727** | 0.649 | **0.815** | **0.786** | **0.810** | **0.739** | 0.644 | **0.818** | **0.814** |
| MMed-70B | 0.770 | 0.609 | 0.624 | 0.806 | 0.714 | 0.780 | 0.635 | 0.619 | 0.787 | 0.729 |
| JSL-MedLlama-8B | 0.726 | 0.652 | 0.715 | 0.785 | 0.754 | 0.755 | 0.675 | 0.683 | 0.810 | 0.753 |
| meditron-70b | 0.728 | 0.632 | 0.687 | 0.779 | 0.716 | 0.727 | 0.635 | 0.698 | 0.752 | 0.747 |
| OpenBioLLM-70B | 0.731 | 0.698 | **0.722** | 0.777 | 0.743 | 0.765 | 0.722 | **0.739** | 0.801 | 0.696 |
| Llama-3.1-70B | 0.741 | 0.641 | 0.707 | 0.765 | 0.723 | 0.739 | 0.685 | 0.670 | 0.791 | 0.713 |
| Gemini-3-Flash | **0.804** | 0.766 | 0.744 | **0.820** | **0.812** | **0.837** | 0.791 | **0.753** | **0.849** | **0.838** |
| Claude-Sonnet-4.5 | 0.795 | 0.767 | **0.749** | 0.815 | 0.810 | 0.828 | 0.783 | 0.743 | 0.832 | 0.812 |
| ChatGPT-5.2 | 0.710 | **0.772** | 0.672 | 0.808 | 0.800 | 0.786 | **0.807** | 0.712 | 0.829 | 0.820 |
| | | | | | CLASSIFICATION FINETUNING (0-SHOT PROMPTS) | | | | | |
| MedGemma-4B | 0.740 ±0.020 | 0.654 ±0.059 | 0.772 ±0.027 | 0.814 ±0.021 | 0.750 ±0.056 | 0.659 ±0.067 | 0.628 ±0.087 | 0.761 ±0.074 | 0.809 ±0.025 | 0.665 ±0.088 |
| Med42-8B | 0.783 ±0.040 | **0.697** ±0.050 | 0.718 ±0.034 | 0.816 ±0.031 | 0.743 ±0.052 | 0.777 ±0.074 | 0.712 ±0.070 | 0.718 ±0.047 | 0.785 ±0.018 | 0.716 ±0.135 |
| MMed-8B | 0.780 ±0.040 | 0.668 ±0.031 | 0.771 ±0.048 | 0.815 ±0.018 | 0.805 ±0.050 | 0.783 ±0.037 | 0.672 ±0.099 | 0.730 ±0.046 | 0.813 ±0.032 | 0.741 ±0.067 |
| JSL-MedLlama-8B | 0.782 ±0.041 | 0.682 ±0.077 | 0.766 ±0.022 | 0.808 ±0.033 | 0.726 ±0.080 | 0.754 ±0.077 | **0.729** ±0.069 | 0.713 ±0.073 | 0.792 ±0.045 | 0.699 ±0.104 |
| Meditron3-8B | **0.813** ±0.045 | 0.684 ±0.087 | **0.784** ±0.019 | **0.826** ±0.025 | **0.809** ±0.028 | **0.806** ±0.033 | 0.732 ±0.084 | **0.745** ±0.055 | **0.815** ±0.025 | **0.811** ±0.032 |
| OpenBioLLM-8B | 0.784 ±0.052 | 0.686 ±0.028 | 0.749 ±0.041 | 0.810 ±0.027 | 0.773 ±0.035 | 0.789 ±0.033 | 0.688 ±0.054 | 0.723 ±0.050 | 0.791 ±0.025 | 0.714 ±0.099 |
| Llama-3.1-8B | 0.778 ±0.048 | 0.658 ±0.063 | 0.706 ±0.071 | 0.824 ±0.026 | 0.753 ±0.059 | 0.790 ±0.034 | 0.688 ±0.064 | 0.719 ±0.041 | 0.798 ±0.024 | 0.694 ±0.145 |

remark that the provided **CoroPredict** [6] scores over this sub-cohort yield an AUROC of **0.841**, while SMART and SCORE2 yield 0.729 and 0.668, respectively (available however only for different LURIC cohorts).

**Model Stratification and Calibration.** LLMs tend to over-predict mortality when prompted for risk scores, which can be improved via calibration techniques such as Platt scaling. The effect is depicted in Fig. 3, which shows that the Expected Calibration Error (ECE) can be reduced by up to 60–90%.

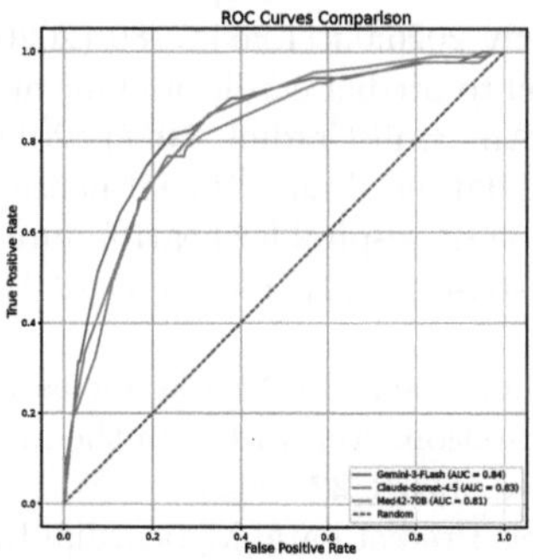


**Fig. 2.** Selected ROC plots.

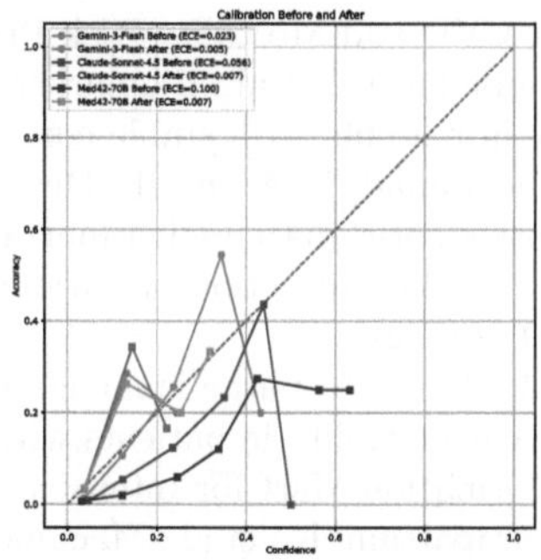


**Fig. 3.** Selected calibration plots.

## 4 Conclusions

Our study demonstrates the strong potential of both open and commercial LLMs for predicting 1-year all-cause mortality in CVD patients under routinely collected biomarkers. Our key findings include: (a) large open LLMs (70B) achieve up to 82% AUROC with few-shot prompting, competitive with CoroPredict (84% AUROC on the LURIC sub-cohort); (b) smaller finetuned LLMs (8B) match or surpass larger and commercial models (ChatGPT-5.2, Claude-Sonnet-4.5), exceeding 82% AUROC; (c) LLMs exhibit a systematic mortality over-prediction (ECE: 0.05–0.10), while Platt scaling reduces miscalibration by 60–90%. Overall, our study reveals large gains of recent LLMs for CVD mortality prediction compared to earlier results [1,2,7,8], where LLMs still lagged behind ML methods and CoroPredict. Most remarkably, Gemini-3-Flash matches the best ML models and CoroPredict via few-shot prompting alone—without any domain-specific tuning, a significant gain over prior prompting results [4,13].

## References

1. Anisuzzaman, D., et al.: Fine-tuning large language models for specialized use cases. Mayo Clinic Proc. Digital Health **3**(1) (2025)
2. Ben Shoham, O., Rappoport, N.: CPLLM: clinical prediction with large language models. PLOS Digital Health **3**(12) (2024)
3. Bibi, I., et al.: Cardiovascular risk assessment enhanced by automated machine learning in a multi-phase study. Nat. Sci. Rep. **15**(1) (2025)
4. Han, C., et al.: Evaluation of GPT-4 for 10-year cardiovascular risk prediction: insights from the UK Biobank and KoGES data. iScience **27**(2) (2024)
5. Kom Sande, S.D., et al.: Regression vs. Medical LLMs: A Comprehensive Study for CVD and Mortality Risk Prediction. medRxiv 2026.03.11.26347789 (2026)
6. Lindholm, D., et al.: Biomarker-based risk model to predict cardiovascular mortality in patients with stable coronary disease. J. Am. Coll Cardiol. **70**(7) (2017)
7. Mohammad, M.A., et al.: Development and validation of an artificial neural network algorithm to predict mortality and admission to hospital for heart failure after myocardial infarction: a nationwide population-based study. Lancet Digit Health **4**(1) (2022)
8. Shi, B., et al.: Large language models and artificial neural networks for assessing 1-year mortality in patients with myocardial infarction: Analysis from the Medical Information Mart for Intensive Care IV database. JMIR **27** (2025)
9. Tsarapatsani, K., et al.: Machine Learning Models Predict Fatal Myocardial Infarction Within 10-Years Follow-Up Utilizing Explainable AI. In: BIBE (2023)
10. Tsarapatsani, K., et al.: Machine learning models to predict myocardial infarction within 10-years follow-up of cardiovascular disease progression. In: EMBS (2022)
11. Wang, X., Wang, H., Fu, R.: Boosting cardiovascular disease prediction accuracy: a hybrid AI strategy integrating LLM-generated risk scores. In: HIDA (2025)
12. Winkelmann, B.R., et al.: Rationale and design of the LURIC study—a resource for functional genomics, pharmacogenomics and long-term prognosis of cardiovascular disease. Pharmacogenomics **2**(1) (2001)
13. Zanab, T., et al.: Advancing cardiovascular disease prediction using LLMs. In: ICMLAS (2025)

# Epistemologically Guided LLM Reasoning for Differential Diagnosis

Simone Rancati(✉), Laura Bergomi, Enea Parimbelli, Giovanna Nicora, and Riccardo Bellazzi

BMI lab "Mario Stefanelli", Department of Electric, Computer and Biomedical Engineering, University of Pavia, Pavia, Italy
{simone.rancati01,laura.bergomi01}@universitadipavia.it

**Abstract.** Large language models (LLMs) have been widely tested on their ability to perform "clinical reasoning" especially since the emergence of Large Reasoning Models (LRM). Yet much of the available evidence derives from medical question–answering benchmarks, which oversimplify the reality of real-world clinical practice scenarios. Performance measures reported in such benchmarks often highlight the correctness of final answers alone, offering limited insights into how the LLM reached the correct conclusion. In this study, we propose a novel way of guiding LLM clinical reasoning, grounded on an epistemological model described in the 90 s for knowledge-based Clinical Decision Support Systems (CDSS) by Ramoni et al. We validate our approach on a diagnosis task using ten real-world annotated case records from the Massachusetts General Hospital. Our method constrains LLM inference to follow the epistemological framework's reasoning phases of abstraction, abduction, hypothesis generation, deduction, and induction. We compare our proposed approach against a range of out-of-the-box open-weights LLMs, including reasoning models. Performance is assessed over repeated runs reporting ranking-oriented metrics and diagnostic accuracy at Top-1 and Top-10. Across most cases and metrics, the implemented epistemologically guided reasoning performs comparably to, or better than, baselines, while exhibiting higher consistency and stability across repeated runs. Beyond accuracy, a key contribution is the improved interpretability: the explicit hypothesis generation and testing steps provide a structured reasoning trace that supports clinician review. Overall, these findings reinforce the need for evaluation protocols that transcends aggregate performance scores, and motivate future work on reliability-aware, epistemology grounded clinical AI systems.

**Keywords:** Clinical Reasoning · Decision Support · Diagnosis · Generative AI · Interpretability

## 1 Introduction

Large language models (LLMs) are increasingly reported to demonstrate "clinical reasoning" across diagnostic and decision-support tasks. Much of the evidence, however, still comes from medical question–answering (QA) benchmarks that only weakly

Authors Simone Rancati and Laura Bergomi have equally contributed to this chapter.
Enea Parimbelli, Giovanna Nicora, Riccardo Bellazzi are co-senior authors.

© The Author(s), under exclusive license to Springer Nature Switzerland AG 2027
P. Andreev et al. (Eds.): AIME 2026, LNAI 16748, pp. 115–124, 2027.
https://doi.org/10.1007/978-3-032-30710-1_14

approximate real clinical practice, where information is incomplete, temporally distributed, and frequently clarified through iterative questioning [1]. This mismatch has motivated a shift toward more challenging evaluation settings that better reflect clinical workflows and safety requirements. Recent work has systematically characterized limitations of LLMs in clinical decision-making and explored mitigation strategies, highlighting the gap between benchmark performance and deployable behavior in practice [2]. Similarly, studies using complex diagnostic challenges show that apparent diagnostic competence can be brittle when cases demand multi-step inference and robust integration of heterogeneous findings [3]. Importantly, when tasks are reframed into more realistic interaction conditions—such as transforming clinical vignettes into clinician–patient dialogues—performance can drop substantially, underscoring how sensitive LLM behavior is to presentation, context, and information acquisition dynamics [4]. Together, these findings reinforce the need for evaluation protocols that go beyond a single "final answer" and instead test the process by which a diagnosis is reached.

A second, closely related barrier to the clinical adoption of LLMs is interpretability. QA evaluations typically score only the final diagnosis, providing limited insight into why a model is correct—or incorrect—on a given case. This is crucial for clinical validation, auditing, and accountable deployment, because clinicians and institutions need to understand the motivations of a recommendation, identify potential errors, and ensure that the system's reasoning aligns with medical knowledge and practice standards [2, 4]. Moreover, this is an explicit requirement of AI regulation in Europe.

Medical AI has a long tradition of knowledge representation and explicit reasoning models. Classic knowledge-based systems, such as MYCIN, showed that diagnostic support can be built around transparent rule-based inference and domain knowledge, enabling inspection and critique of intermediate steps [5]. More broadly, the AI in MEdicine (AIME) community[1] has developed formal models of diagnostic reasoning and architectures for consultation systems grounded in epistemology and cognitive structure rather than purely data-driven mappings [6–8]. Specifically, Ramoni et al. [6] proposed an epistemological model, called Select-And-Test Model (ST-Model), that breaks medical reasoning into well-defined phases, which are interpretable by construction. Recent comparative evidence also suggests that dedicated expert systems can remain competitive against generative LLM-based approaches for clinical diagnosis, emphasizing the enduring value of explicit structure in the development of AI applications in healthcare [9].

Indeed, while a new wave of LLM-based diagnostic agents has emerged, incorporating iterative information gathering [10–13], the "reasoning model" remains often implicit—encoded within the LLM and its prompting strategy—rather than expressed as an explicit and controllable system. This can make it difficult to separate clinical knowledge, inference strategy, and language generation, and to provide clinicians with a transparent reasoning trace that supports validation.

In this work, we aim to combine the flexibility and generative power of LLMs with the transparency and rigor of classic knowledge-based medical reasoning. We implemented and evaluated an LLM-based clinical reasoning framework grounded in the ST-Model. The framework constrains and organizes LLM inference into structured phases, so that

[1] https://aimedicine.info/aime/

intermediate outputs form a coherent trace that can be inspected, compared across runs, and reviewed by clinicians. We evaluate this approach on differential diagnosis cases provided and annotated by Massachusetts General Hospital [14], reporting ranking-oriented metrics aggregated over repeated runs.

Overall, the contribution of this paper is twofold: (i) the integration of an epistemologically grounded reasoning model with LLM-based diagnostic inference, and (ii) the evaluation of our framework against a range of out-of-the-box open-weights LLMs, including reasoning models.

# 2 Methods

## 2.1 Reasoning on the Basis of an Epistemological Model

We adopt an epistemological model of medical diagnostic reasoning originally applied in the context of knowledge-based consultation systems by Ramoni et al. [6]. It follows the Generate-and-Test paradigm, in which an initial hypothesis selection phase uses the available information to generate a set of candidate hypotheses, followed by a hypothesis testing phase, where the selected hypotheses are used to predict expected consequences that are then compared with available or newly acquired information to confirm or refute them. This approach can be described as a process of abduction, understood as inference to the best explanation. This type of inference is defeasible and therefore non-monotonic, since its conclusions may be overturned by additional evidence. It is at the basis of scientific discovery, theory revision, and both selective and creative reasoning. The ST (Select and Test) model was proposed by Ramoni et al. [6] as a general framework for automated medical reasoning that formalizes inference to the best explanation as an iterative sequence of elementary inferential steps.

Reasoning by the ST-model is articulated as an iterative cycle of hypothesis selection and testing. It begins with *abstraction*, where the clinical narrative and observations are transformed into a compact representation of salient, higher-level features. On the basis of this representation, the reasoning proceeds through two abductive stages: *unfocused abduction* opens a broad hypothesis space (e.g., syndromes or diagnostic families), and *focused abduction* refines it into more specific competing or complementary hypotheses grounded in the available evidence. Candidate hypotheses are then subjected to an explicit *ranking* phase driven by clinically meaningful preference criteria (i.e., parsimony, danger, cost, and curability), which prioritizes what should be tested first. From the first ranked hypothesis, *deduction* determines which findings have to be expected if the hypothesis is true, assuming everything else stays the same; these expectations may motivate requests for additional clinical or laboratory examinations when relevant consequences are not yet observed. *Induction* then matches expected against observed findings to corroborate, revise, or reject hypotheses, and also supports the termination decision (i.e., whether a satisfactory explanation has been achieved or further testing is warranted). The cyclic structure of the model stresses the nonmonotonic character of medical reasoning: previously entertained hypotheses can be withdrawn whenever new information becomes available. A schematic mapping between the epistemological phases and their computational instantiation in our study is provided in Fig. 1A.

## 2.2 Epistemologically Guided Implementation

The ST-model has been implemented in Python as a directed state graph using LangGraph, where each reasoning phase is implemented in a node that stores intermediate artifacts in a shared state. To enforce structured and replicable intermediate representations, each node is constrained by Pydantic schemas to return a JSON output. The graph uses the same phases described in Sect. 2.1. The abstraction node extracts and organizes features into clinically meaningful categories (i.e., medical history, physical examination, investigations, medications, allergies, and social determinants–related elements). The abductive node, implementing both *unfocused* and *focused abduction*, returns the hypotheses' list in which each hypothesis includes a concise diagnostic label, a rationale, and explicit links to supporting abstracted features. The *ranking* node orders the list of hypotheses generated in the previous node, together with criterion-specific justifications aligned with the preference criteria of the original epistemological model (i.e., parsimony, danger, cost, and curability). In our framework, parsimony favors hypotheses that require the least therapeutic intervention while achieving equivalent outcomes; danger prioritizes hypotheses for which delayed diagnosis or treatment would pose greater risk to the patient; cost favors hypotheses whose confirmation and management require fewer resources (e.g., money, time, labor); and curability favors hypotheses for which effective cure or healing is possible.

For testing each hypothesis, the *deduction* node outputs a compact set of expected consequences annotated by type (e.g., manifestation, test result, clinical course) and priority, while the *induction* node evaluates these predicted consequences against the observed case evidence, labeling them as confirmed, not observed, or contradicted, and producing an overall plausible/refuted judgment together with a termination recommendation. All intermediate outputs are persistently recorded in a structured log file (per case and run), enabling retrospective inspection of the complete reasoning trace and supporting auditability and qualitative analysis.

The entire clinical reasoning is guided: at each node, the LLM generates the phase-specific structured output under schema constraints, while LangGraph orchestrates control flow and state propagation across phases. To assess how the epistemological pipeline behaves across models with different capacity, we tested our approach using four widely used open-weights LLMs spanning a range of parameter scales and families—gpt-oss-120B, gpt-oss-20B, llama-3.3-70b-instruct, and qwen3-14B—keeping prompts, schemas, and graph logic fixed so that differences can be attributed to the underlying LLM. In the original ST-model, an explicit information-seeking phase can be added to resolve uncertainty by requesting additional observations or tests and iterating until sufficient evidence discriminates among hypotheses (Fig. 1B). When the clinical presentation is provided upfront as a fixed narrative, with no interactive channel to obtain new data (such as in retrospective evaluation), we perform a single pass of hypothesis generation and testing on the given text; after *induction*, we invoke the *ranking* node again using the induction-annotated hypotheses (including tested expectations and their evaluation) to produce the final ordered list of differential diagnoses. This substitutes the "ask-for-more-information" iteration with a post-testing prioritization step, yielding an auditable trace that links extracted evidence, hypotheses and expectations against the case narrative, consistent with the epistemological foundations of the framework. The code of the framework is available at https://github.com/bmi-labmedinfo/Epistemological_framework.

### 2.3 Case Reports Benchmark

We evaluate our approach using CPC-Bench[2], a benchmark designed to assess the clinical reasoning capabilities of AI models using expert-curated Clinicopathological Conference (CPC) cases from the Massachusetts General Hospital licensed from The New England Journal of Medicine [14]. CPC-Bench defines 10 distinct tasks spanning multiple facets of clinical reasoning—ranging from differential diagnosis generation to multimodal tasks such as medical image interpretation—thereby enabling evaluation beyond single-answer QA settings. In this study, we focus specifically on the Differential Diagnosis task, which assesses a model's ability to generate a comprehensive, ranked list of plausible diagnoses from the clinical presentation of the cases. Concretely, we use a subset of 10 published cases of CPC-Bench. For each case, we use: (i) the full clinical narrative and (ii) the reference final diagnosis provided by the benchmark.

### 2.4 Evaluation

As a baseline, we implement a zero-shot differential diagnosis setting in which the LLM is directly prompted to output the top-10 most likely diagnoses given the full case narrative, without any explicit intermediate reasoning phases. This produces a ranked list that is directly comparable to the hypotheses returned by the final step of our approach and aligns with the evaluation setup commonly adopted in CPC-oriented benchmarking [14].

For each case and run, we evaluate performance using both accuracy and ranking-based measures. Specifically, we compute accuracy at Top-1—whether the reference diagnosis is ranked first—and accuracy at Top-10—whether the reference diagnosis appears anywhere among the top 10 predicted diagnoses. In addition, we compute the rank, defined as the position of the reference diagnosis in the model's ranked list (with a penalty rank of 11 when the correct diagnosis is not present in the top 10), and we summarize this as the mean rank across runs to quantify how the correct diagnosis is prioritized even when it is not top-1.

To reduce spurious mismatches due to synonyms, lexical variation, or differing diagnostic specificity, we map both the reference diagnosis and each predicted diagnosis to ICD-10-CM standardized clinical codes using a MetaMap-based concept mapping procedure: we count a prediction as correct when the predicted and reference code sets coincide [15]. When code mapping is unavailable or inconclusive, we apply a conservative fallback based on diagnosis-string matching (exact match or substring match). All metrics are computed per run and then aggregated across repeated runs for each LLM. To compare our approach against the zero-shot baseline under repeated runs, we perform paired statistical analyses. Differences in diagnostic prioritization are tested using the Wilcoxon signed-rank test on the rank's results, while paired differences in accuracy at

[2] https://cpcbench.com/

Top-1 and Top-10 are assessed using an exact McNemar test implemented via a binomial test on discordant pairs. We report both raw p-values and multiple-testing–corrected results using Benjamini–Hochberg False Discovery Rate (FDR) and Holm corrections.

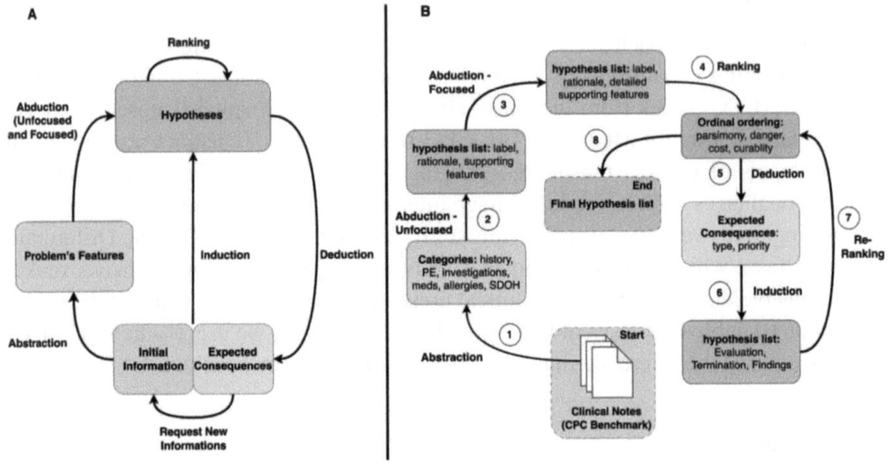


**Fig. 1.** **A)** The ST-model [6]. **B)** LLM based on ST-model implementation. Our approach processes a raw clinical case through reasoning nodes. Evidence is abstracted into clinically meaningful features, which support unfocused and focused abduction to generate diagnostic hypotheses. Hypotheses are then ranked with criterion-specific justifications, tested through the deduction of expected consequences and against observed evidence via induction. The final inducted hypothesis list is eventually ranked and the reasoning terminates.

## 3 Results

### 3.1 Intrinsic Interpretability

Our approach provides intrinsic interpretability by producing an explicit, machine-readable reasoning trace (Fig. 2). For every run, all intermediate artifacts are persistently saved in a structured log, enabling retrospective inspection of how hypotheses were generated, prioritized, and tested. Concretely, the logs record the abstracted clinical findings, the evolving hypothesis sets with links to supporting evidence, an explicit ranking justified by clinically meaningful preference criteria, and a deduction–induction comparison of predicted versus observed findings that marks hypotheses as corroborated, contradicted, or unsupported. This produces an auditable trace that can be reviewed to understand why a diagnosis was prioritized and which evidence supported or challenged each alternative. In contrast, the zero-shot baseline returns only the final ranked differential diagnosis (optionally accompanied by free text justifications), making the reasoning process substantially harder to audit.

---- Abstraction Phase ----
ABSTRACTION – The features abstracted by the text are:
* [1] The category is "Social & Community Context" for the finding "Age" .....
* [2] The category is "Current Medications" for the finding "Vitamin B12 supplement".....
* [3] The category is "Family History" for the finding "Brother"....
---- Abduction Phase (Unfocused) ----
ABDUCTION (UNFOCUSED) – Diagnostic hypotheses generated:
1. Endogenous hyperinsulinemic hypoglycemia (e.g., insulinoma)
Why: Recurrent fasting hypoglycemia.....
Supporting features:
- Fingerstick glucose at EMS – 39 mg/dL (2.2 mmol/L)
- Fingerstick glucose on ED arrival – 36 mg/dL (2.0 mmol/L)
---- Abduction Phase (Focused) ----
ABDUCTION (FOCUSED) – Diagnostic hypotheses generated:
1. Insulinoma (pancreatic neuroendocrine tumor)
Why: Focal endogenous hyperinsulinemic hypoglycemia...
Supporting features:
- Fingerstick glucose at EMS – 39 mg/dL (2.2 mmol/L)
- Fingerstick glucose on ED arrival – 36 mg/dL (2.0 mmol/L)
---- Ranking Phase ----
RANKING – Hypotheses ordered by plausibility:
#1 – Insulinoma (pancreatic neuroendocrine tumor)
Parsimony: Single neoplastic lesion...
Danger: Unrecognized insulinoma can cause...
Cost: Initial biochemical work-up....
Curability: Surgical resection is curative in >90 % of cases....
---- Deduction Phase ----
DEDUCTION – Expected consequences per hypothesis:
• Insulinoma (pancreatic neuroendocrine tumor)
- [HIGH | clinical_course] fasting glucose <55 mg/dL with Whipple's triad....
- [HIGH | clinical_course] inappropriately high serum insulin (>3 μIU/mL) during hypoglycemia....
---- Induction Phase ----
INDUCTION – Matching expected vs observed:
• Insulinoma (pancreatic neuroendocrine tumor)
Evaluation: plausible
Termination: continue_testing
Why: continue_testing
Findings summary: ✓ 2 | ? 6 | ✗ 0
Findings:
- ✓ E1: fasting glucose <55 mg/dL with Whipple's triad...
- ? E2: inappropriately high serum insulin (≥3 μIU/mL) during hypoglycemia
---- Ranking Phase ----
RANKING – Hypotheses ordered by plausibility:
#1 – Insulinoma (pancreatic neuroendocrine tumor)
Parsimony: Requires a single pathological entity (a tumor) to explain Whipple's triad; no additional physiologic abnormalities needed.
Danger: Recurrent, severe hypoglycemia can be life-threatening if not identified and resected.
Cost: Initial biochemical work-up (insulin, C-peptide, sulfonylurea screen) is low-cost; imaging is moderate but essential only after biochemical confirmation.
Curability: Surgical removal is curative in >90% of cases.

**Fig. 2.** Example of reasoning trace for one CPC case (abstraction → abduction → ranking → deduction → induction, with post-induction re-ranking), enabling transparent and auditable diagnostic prioritization. The full example is reported on the GitHub repository.

## 3.2 Metrics Performance

Using the case-level distribution across the 10 CPC cases (metrics averaged across runs per case, then summarized across cases with median and IQR), our approach is overall competitive with zero-shot baseline and shows a clear pattern of greater stability across cases (tighter IQRs), even when Top-1 accuracy remains challenging in this benchmark. In terms of prioritization quality (i.e., rank; lower is better), our approach performs better than baseline for the two larger gpt-oss models (gpt-oss-120B and gpt-oss-20B), while it is essentially comparable for llama-3.3-70B-instruct. Notably, for gpt-oss-120B, the improvement over the baseline is statistically significant according to the Wilcoxon signed-rank test ($p < 0.05$). The main exception is qwen3-14B, where our approach yields a worse median rank ($p < 0.05$). A similar picture emerges for Top-10 accuracy:

our approach improves median Top-10 inclusion for gpt-oss-120B and gpt-oss-20B, remains close to the baseline for llama-3.3-70B-instruct, and is worse ($p < 0.05$) for qwen3-14B. Overall, the consistently smaller IQRs under our approach (Table 1) indicate more stable case-to-case behavior, particularly for larger models, while benefits may diminish (or reverse) for smaller models.

**Table 1. Case-level performance across CPC cases (median and IQR).** The table reports, for each LLM, the distribution across the 10 cases of (i) the rank (lower is better), (ii) **Top-1 accuracy** (higher is better), and (iii) **Top-10 accuracy** (higher is better), comparing the **epistemological pipeline (EP)** against the **zero-shot baseline (ZS)**. For each case, metrics are first averaged across repeated runs and then summarized across cases as **median (IQR)**.

| Models | Rank-EP | Rank-ZS | Top-1-EP | Top-1-ZS | Top-10-EP | Top-10-ZS |
|---|---|---|---|---|---|---|
| gpt-oss-120b | **9.05 (5.12)** | 10.50 (6.88) | 0.00 (0.18) | 0.00 (0.47) | **0.20 (0.65)** | 0.05 (0.93) |
| gpt-oss-20b | **9.55 (3.10)** | 10.65 (5.88) | 0.00 (0.00) | 0.00 (0.18) | **0.25 (0.38)** | 0.05 (0.62) |
| Llama-70b | 8.55 (7.17) | **8.45 (10.00)** | 0.00 (0.30) | 0.00 (1.00) | 0.35 (1.00) | **0.40 (1.00)** |
| Qwen-14b | 11.00 (2.47) | 10.05 (6.67) | 0.00 (0.00) | 0.00 (0.33) | 0.00 (0.42) | 0.10 (0.78) |

## 4 Discussion

This study evaluates whether a epistemological model of medical reasoning can be used to shepherd LLM behavior during differential diagnosis. Overall, our epistemologically guided framework is competitive with a zero-shot baseline and shows model-dependent effects: it often matched or improved case-level median performance for larger gpt-oss models (gpt-oss-120B and gpt-oss-20B), particularly on rank-based prioritization and Top-10 accuracy, while performance was generally worse for Qwen3-14B. It is not surprising that zero-shot performs well, since we hypothesize that—because clinical notes are publicly available—models may have already encountered similar cases during pre-training. Moreover, the prompt used for the zero-shot baseline is more concise than our method, which relies on an incremental, node-by-node prompting strategy and per node LLM calling. This added "prompt load" may cause models, especially smaller ones, to become confused or to lose relevant information across steps and so propagating errors. Across settings, we also observed greater stability across cases (tighter IQRs), suggesting that structuring inference into explicit phases can reduce case-to-case variability in diagnostic prioritization. Crucially, interpretability and auditability are a key outcome: our approach provides intrinsic interpretability by producing an explicit, phase-structured reasoning trace—abstraction, abduction, ranking, deduction, and induction—persistently stored in per-run logs arising potential propagating error. This enables clinicians and auditors to reconstruct why a diagnosis was prioritized, which evidence supported competing hypotheses, and how hypotheses were corroborated, weakened, or rejected. In contrast, zero-shot prompting typically outputs only a final ranked list (and, at best, free-text justifications) without a standardized intermediate record, making auditing, validation, and post-hoc error analysis substantially harder. The fact that gains are apparently greater in larger LLMs is consistent with the idea that reasoning constraints do not add medical knowledge, but instead modulate how an LLM allocates capacity across generation, prioritization, and testing—an effect that can depend on task complexity and protocol "load" [16]. A key limitation is that the Differential Diagnosis task in CPC-Bench provides a fixed narrative, so the classic "request new information" step cannot be exercised interactively; our post-induction re-ranking only approximates the iterative refinement that conversational diagnostic systems emphasize [13]. Future work will therefore focus on implementing and evaluating the information-seeking loop in interactive settings, extending the evaluation to include error taxonomy analyses, and developing an interface that leverages the logged trace for clinician review and controlled refinement. In addition, we will conduct an ablation study to test different models (e.g. proprietary models) including future available clinical LLMs and prompt lengths, vary the inclusion of individual nodes, and evaluate multiple cycles of our framework.

## 5 Conclusion

We presented a novel way of guiding LLM clinical reasoning that operationalizes a epistemological model of medical reasoning, the ST-model, into explicit phases and produces a structured, auditable reasoning trace. On the Differential Diagnosis task of CPC-Bench, our framework was overall competitive with zero-shot baseline and, for larger gpt-oss models, often performed at parity or better on rank-based prioritization and Top-10 accuracy while showing greater stability across cases. Beyond performance, the framework's main added value is intrinsic interpretability: the explicit hypothesis-generation and testing steps are persistently logged, enabling clinicians and auditors to follow the model's reasoning in a way that is not available in standard zero-shot prompting. These results support the need for evaluation protocols that go beyond final-answer accuracy and motivate future work on interactive, reliability-aware, epistemically grounded clinical AI systems that can be safely reviewed and integrated into clinical decision support.

**Acknowledgments.** We would like to express our sincere gratitude to Professor Silvana Quaglini, for her valuable support and advice throughout this work.

## References

1. Chen, H., Fang, Z., Singla, Y., Dredze, M.: Benchmarking large language models on answering and explaining challenging medical questions. In: Chiruzzo, L., Ritter, A., Wang, L. (eds.) Proceedings of the 2025 Conference of the Nations of the Americas Chapter of the Association for Computational Linguistics: Human Language Technologies (Volume 1: Long Papers), pp. 3563–3599. Association for Computational Linguistics (2025). https://doi.org/10.18653/v1/2025.naacl-long.182

2. Hager, P., Jungmann, F., Holland, R., et al.: Evaluation and mitigation of the limitations of large language models in clinical decision-making. Nat. Med. **30**(9), 2613–2622 (2024). https://doi.org/10.1038/s41591-024-03097-1
3. Kanjee, Z., Crowe, B., Rodman, A.: Accuracy of a generative artificial intelligence model in a complex diagnostic challenge. JAMA. **330**(1), 78 (2023). https://doi.org/10.1001/jama.2023.8288
4. Johri, S., Jeong, J., Tran, B.A., et al.: An evaluation framework for clinical use of large language models in patient interaction tasks. Nat. Med. **31**(1), 77–86 (2025). https://doi.org/10.1038/s41591-024-03328-5
5. Shortliffe, E.H.: Mycin: a knowledge-based computer program applied to infectious diseases. In: Proceedings of the Annual Symposium on Computer Application in Medical Care, vol. 5, pp. 66–69 (1977)
6. Ramoni, M., Stefanelli, M., Magnani, L., Barosi, G.: An epistemological framework for medical knowledge-based systems. IEEE Trans. Syst. Man Cybern. **22**(6), 1361–1375 (1992). https://doi.org/10.1109/21.199462
7. Barosi, G., Magnani, L., Stefanelli, M.: Medical diagnostic reasoning: epistemological modeling as a strategy for design of computer-based consultation programs. Theor. Med. **14**(1), 43–55 (1993). https://doi.org/10.1007/BF00993987
8. Lanzola, G., Stefanelli, M., Barosi, G., Magnani, L.: A knowledge system architecture for diagnostic reasoning. In: Hunter, J., Cookson, J., Wyatt, J. (eds.) AIME 89 Lecture Notes in Medical Informatics, vol. 38, pp. 234–243. Springer, Berlin Heidelberg (1989). https://doi.org/10.1007/978-3-642-93437-7_27
9. Feldman, M.J., Hoffer, E.P., Conley, J.J., et al.: Dedicated AI expert system vs generative AI with large language model for clinical diagnoses. JAMA Netw. Open. **8**(5), e2512994 (2025). https://doi.org/10.1001/jamanetworkopen.2025.12994
10. McDuff, D., Schaekermann, M., Tu, T., et al.: Towards accurate differential diagnosis with large language models. Nature. **642** (2025). https://doi.org/10.1038/s41586-025-08869-4
11. Nori, H., Daswani, M., Kelly, C., et al.: Sequential diagnosis with language models. arXiv, arXiv: 2506.22405 (2025). https://doi.org/10.48550/arXiv.2506.22405
12. Liu, X., Liu, H., Yang, G., et al.: A generalist medical language model for disease diagnosis assistance. Nat Med. **31**, 1–11 (2025). https://doi.org/10.1038/s41591-024-03416-6
13. Tu, T., Schaekermann, M., Palepu, A., et al.: Towards conversational diagnostic artificial intelligence. Nature. **642**, 1–9 (2025). https://doi.org/10.1038/s41586-025-08866-7
14. Buckley, T.A., Conci, R., Brodeur, P.G., et al.: Advancing medical artificial intelligence using a century of cases. arXiv. (2025). https://doi.org/10.48550/ARXIV.2509.12194
15. Aronson, A.R., Lang, F.M.: An overview of MetaMap: historical perspective and recent advances. J. Am. Med. Inform. Assoc. **17**(3), 229–236 (2010). https://doi.org/10.1136/jamia.2009.002733
16. Shojaee, P., Mirzadeh, I., Alizadeh, K., Horton, M., Bengio, S., Farajtabar, M.: The illusion of thinking: understanding the strengths and limitations of reasoning models via the lens of problem complexity. arXiv, arXiv: 2506.06941 (2025). https://doi.org/10.48550/arXiv.2506.06941

# STRAGMED: Standardizing Retrieval-Augmented Generation Pipelines in Medical Domains

Leonardo Sanna(✉), Esin Ezgi Yildiz, and Mauro Dragoni

Center for Digital Health and Wellbeing, Fondazione Bruno Kessler, Trento, Italy
{lsanna,eyildiz,dragoni}@fbk.eu

**Abstract.** The design and evaluation of Retrieval-Augmented Generation (RAG) pipelines remain fragmented, with system components often tailored to specific datasets and tasks. In this paper, we propose STRAGMED, a simple yet effective RAG pipeline to provide a standardized baseline for system engineering and retrieval evaluation. Our experiments show that a hybrid pipeline combining a retriever, reranking at each step, and Reciprocal Rank Fusion (RRF), yields consistent improvements across medical datasets, outperforming retrieval-only and individually reranked outputs. These results highlight a robust and generalizable baseline configuration for medical RAG systems, enabling researchers to focus on task-specific optimizations such as query augmentation, model selection, and retrieval refinement.

**Keywords:** Retrieval-Augmented Generation · Information Retrieval · Reciprocal Rank Fusion

## 1 Introduction

Retrieval-Augmented Generation (RAG) systems have found prominent applications in healthcare by integrating Large Language Models (LLMs) with domain-specific knowledge bases such as PubMed, Electronic Health Records (EHRs), and clinical guidelines, thereby enhancing accuracy in high-stakes tasks. Key examples include Breast-CRAG [1], a specialized LLM for breast cancer diagnostics that retrieves multimodal data (e.g., mammograms and pathology reports) to generate precise risk assessments and treatment recommendations, and LAB-AI [17], a system designed for personalized lab test interpretation. More broadly, RAG systems are increasingly adopted to improve factual accuracy, transparency, and clinical trustworthiness.

The evaluation of medical RAG systems typically relies on a combination of quantitative metrics (e.g., accuracy, BLEU [13], ROUGE [12], and F1) and qualitative clinical assessments. Standard benchmarks such as PubMedQA [9] are widely used to evaluate medical reasoning and knowledge grounding. Despite extensive research on RAG evaluation, there is still no standardized practice for

© The Author(s), under exclusive license to Springer Nature Switzerland AG 2027
P. Andreev et al. (Eds.): AIME 2026, LNAI 16748, pp. 125–135, 2027.
https://doi.org/10.1007/978-3-032-30710-1_15

designing RAG pipeline components. However, the lack of a shared baseline pipeline negatively impacts on reproducibility and disperses research efforts. In particular, it remains unclear which components should be optimized for specific datasets and which should be considered fundamental elements of RAG architectures.

In this paper, we propose STRAGMED[1], a standard RAG pipeline composition for medical domains. For RAG pipeline we mean the composition that arises from the interaction of different retrieval modules. In particular, in this work we have: (i) a hybrid retriever integrating a vector-based component and a lexical retriever, (ii) a rereanker component and (iii) a fusion component to combine the output of different steps. The details on these components are explained in Sect. 3. The paper follows three research questions (RQ):

1. RQ1: What is the optimal number of reranking steps in a RAG pipeline?
2. RQ2: How should the fusion score be calculated in medical RAG systems?
3. RQ3: Can the same pipeline be applied with consistent performance across medical datasets of different complexity and language?

## 2 Related Work

RAG systems integrate external knowledge retrieval with LLMs to mitigate hallucinations and incorporate accurate and up-to-date information that extends beyond models' parametric knowledge.

RAG evolved significantly from 2023 onward, with a shift toward modular frameworks like RAGLAB [19], federated systems including knowledge graphs like FRAG [5], and iterative methods such as chain of verification [7] and chain of retrieval [16]

In the medical domain, RAG evaluation follows a modular sequence: retrieval metrics, generation metrics, and an end-to-end system assessment, ensuring clinical relevance. Retrieval evaluation precedes generation, using rank-based metrics such as Mean Reciprocal Rank (MRR), Mean Average Precision (MAP), and Hit Rate@K, and non-rank metrics such as Precision and Recall@K, often benchmarked against query-relevant documents or candidate sets to ensure context quality before feeding into the LLM. Retrieval quality is evaluated using LLM-as-judge or cosine similarity on retrieved chunks versus query [3].

In high-precision RAG systems, where it is crucial to retrieve the exact relevant document rather than a broad set of candidates to support the LLM reply, techniques range from fine-tuning to modular approaches, such as MGPRAG [15]. The latter explicitly aims to enhance the precision metric during retrieval by using fine-tuned embeddings and focuses on dense retrieval optimization and hybrid reranking, independent of generation evaluation. Similarly, ICA-RAG [8] employs fine-grained information-density guidance for adaptive retrieval in disease diagnosis, emphasizing Precision@5 via query reformulation and chunk filtering before any LLM involvement.

[1] https://github.com/IDA-FBK/STRAGMED--STandardizedRAGMEDical.

To the best of our knowledge, there is no consensus on a threshold value for determining the precision of an RAG system in medicine, as performance varies widely across datasets. One of the goals of this work is therefore to experiment whether it is possible to observe consistent performance across datasets, even without establishing reference values.

## 3 Methods

We use a RAG pipeline composed by different steps. The first one is a hybrid retriever. The step consists of a vector-based retriever that uses the embedding model *mxbai-embed-large-v1* [11] and a lexical retriever using BM25 [14]. This step takes as input two different queries: the original user query (henceforth Vector) and Hypothetical Document Embeddings (henceforth HyDE) [4], where a language model generates a synthetic answer that is used as an expanded retrieval query. The LLM used in the HyDE step is *mistral-small-24b-instruct-2501*, with a temperature of 0.6 and nucleus sampling set at 0.5. The LLM has been accessed via OpenRouter[2]. Document embeddings are stored and retrieved using the ChromaDB vector database.

The second step is a reranking step in which we use the cross-encoder model *bge-reranker-v2-m3*, which jointly encodes queries and candidate documents to produce final relevance scores.

Finally, we have a fusion step that combines multiple ranked lists. Here we adopt Reciprocal Rank Fusion (RRF) [2]. Given a document $d$ and a set of ranking systems $\mathcal{R}$, the RRF score is defined as:

$$\mathrm{RRF}(d) = \sum_{r \in \mathcal{R}} \frac{1}{k + \mathrm{rank}_r(d)} \tag{1}$$

where:

- $\mathrm{rank}_r(d)$ is the rank position of document $d$ in retrieval system $r$, and,
- $k$ is a smoothing constant controlling the contribution of lower-ranked documents.

In our experiments, we vary the constant $k$ to observe its effects on ranking stability and retrieval performance. The following ranking outputs are evaluated: raw retriever outputs, re-ranked retriever outputs, RRF-fused outputs, and final re-ranked fused outputs. We evaluate each ranking configuration on the top 50 retrieved documents using standard information retrieval metrics (see Sect. 3.1 that quantify both the presence and the quality of relevant results.

[2] https://openrouter.ai/.

### 3.1 Evaluation Metrics

We employ four common Information Retrieval (IR) metrics to test the soundness of the RAG pipeline: *Hit@3*, *Mean Reciprocal Rank*, *Mean Average Precision*, and *Normalized Discounted Cumulative Gain.*

Hit@3 measures the proportion of queries for which at least one relevant document is present within the top three results. For a single query $q$, the hit indicator is:

$$\text{Hit@3}(q) = \begin{cases} 1 & \text{if any relevant document appears in ranks 1..3} \\ 0 & \text{otherwise,} \end{cases} \tag{2}$$

and the overall Hit@3 score is:

$$\text{Hit@3} = \frac{1}{|Q|} \sum_{q \in Q} \text{Hit@3}(q), \tag{3}$$

where $Q$ is the set of all queries. A Hit@3 of 1 indicates that every query had at least one relevant document among the top three results.

Mean Reciprocal Rank (MRR) evaluates how early the first relevant document appears in the ranking. For each query $q$, let $\text{rank}_q$ denote the rank position of its first relevant document. MRR is then:

$$\text{MRR} = \frac{1}{|Q|} \sum_{q \in Q} \frac{1}{\text{rank}_q}. \tag{4}$$

Higher MRR values (closer to 1) indicate that relevant documents tend to appear higher in result lists.

Mean Average Precision at 50 (MAP@50) evaluates ranking quality by measuring how well relevant documents are retrieved and ordered within the top 50 results. The metric is especially useful when multiple documents may be relevant to the same query, as it rewards retrieving all relevant documents and ranking them highly:

$$\text{AP@50}(q) = \frac{1}{\min(R_q, 50)} \sum_{k=1}^{50} P@k(q) \cdot rel_k, \tag{5}$$

where $R_q$ is the total number of relevant documents for query $q$, $P@k(q)$ denotes the precision computed at rank $k$, and $rel_k$ is an indicator function equal to 1 if the document at rank $k$ is relevant and 0 otherwise. The normalization factor ensures that the score reflects how well relevant documents rank within the top 50 positions.

MAP@50 is then computed by averaging AP@50 across all queries:

$$\text{MAP@50} = \frac{1}{|Q|} \sum_{q \in Q} \text{AP@50}(q). \tag{6}$$

This metric rewards ranking systems that consistently retrieve relevant documents at higher positions in the result list.

Normalized Discounted Cumulative Gain at 50 (NDCG@50) measures ranking quality by comparing the predicted ranking with an ideal ordering of documents while accounting for the position of relevant results. The metric assigns greater weight to documents appearing earlier in the ranking via logarithmic discounting.

First, the Discounted Cumulative Gain at cutoff 50 is defined as:

$$\mathrm{DCG@50} = \sum_{i=1}^{50} \frac{2^{rel_i} - 1}{\log_2(i+1)}, \tag{7}$$

where $rel_i$ represents the relevance grade of the document at position $i$ (binary in our case). The exponential gain function increases the reward for retrieving relevant documents, while the logarithmic denominator reduces the contribution of documents appearing at lower ranks.

The Ideal Discounted Cumulative Gain (IDCG@50) is computed by ordering documents according to their true relevance and applying the same DCG formulation. The normalized score is then computed as:

$$\mathrm{NDCG@50} = \frac{\mathrm{DCG@50}}{\mathrm{IDCG@50}}, \tag{8}$$

resulting in a score between 0 and 1, where 1 indicates a perfectly ordered ranking.

### 3.2 Datasets

In this work, we evaluate the pipeline on three datasets. Two of them are biomedical research QA datasets from the MIRAGE benchmark [18], containing query-document pairs annotated for retrieval relevance across multiple domains. The third dataset is an internal proprietary set of domain-specific queries with manually annotated relevant documents, designed to assess system performance in a realistic production scenario.

The first set of questions is a subset of the biomedical question-answering (QA) benchmark, BioASQ Task B Y/N (2019–2023) [10], which is exactly the same dataset used in MIRAGE. It is designed to imitate actual questions created by the biomedical researchers; as a result, it is a realistic and challenging benchmark. The questions are paired with gold-standard relevant PubMed articles and snippets, and we use 618 Yes/No questions adopted in MIRAGE.

The second dataset is PubMedQA [9]. The questions are sourced from PubMed article titles. They are paired with article abstracts and answers, including the definitive answer Yes/No/Maybe. We use the full 1,000-question expert-annotated subset of PubMedQA (PQA-L), which extends beyond the 500 questions used in the MIRAGE benchmark for the test split. Since our pipeline does not require training, we used the largest dataset available to provide a more robust evaluation.

To evaluate the first two datasets, we created a corpus of 1 million PubMed abstracts from the MIRAGE dataset. The corpus includes 1,000 gold-standard reference documents for the PubMedQA questions and 3,554 for the BioASQ questions. The rest of the documents serve as negative documents, creating a 219:1 gold-to-negative ratio. To create a realistic retrieval task, we sampled half of the negative tasks from the MedRAG PubMed dataset on HuggingFace. The other half of the dataset was selected as hard negatives by querying PubMed using Medical Subject Headings (MeSH) terms that match the evaluation set's most common topics. The publication year distribution of the hard negatives was kept proportional to that of the gold-standard documents to ensure that the retrieval system could not rely on temporal cues to distinguish relevant from irrelevant abstracts. The bulk of the corpus (around 51.5% of documents) falls within the 2015–2021 range, with the gold docs following the same distribution.

The third dataset (henceforth ChatFAQ) consists of 1,000 Italian questions and their corresponding gold-standard documents. These documents are sourced from [6], totaling 1,512 verified documents focused on maternity and newborn care. This collection includes 953 documents from the UPPA website[3], 380 from the ISS-Salute website[4], and 179 informational materials provided by the Obstetrics Department of Trento Hospital.

## 4 Results

To answer **RQ1**, we examined the effect of reranking in the pipeline. While reranking clearly improves individual steps, it is unclear whether it is needed at each stage or if the pipeline can be simplified by reranking only after result fusion. We therefore compared final rankings under these two approaches. Table 1 shows that retrieving at each step provides a small but consistent advantage in all datasets, producing a better final ranked list.

**Table 1.** Final Hit@3 comparison between reranking only at the end (End RR) and reranking at each step of the pipeline (Multi RR). Delta indicates the improvement from per-retriever reranking.

| Dataset | End RR | Multi RR | Delta (%) |
|---|---|---|---|
| ChatFAQ | 0.670 | 0.770 | +10.0 |
| BioASQ | 0.910 | 0.915 | +0.49 |
| PubMedQA | 0.997 | 0.998 | +0.10 |

To answer **RQ2**, we experimented with the $k$ effect on the Hit@3 metric, shuffling from 0 to 200 across all datasets and fusing the reranked lists. As shown in Fig. 1, both ChatFAQ and BioASQ curves start to flatten around the

[3] https://www.uppa.it/.
[4] https://www.issalute.it/.

default value, while in PubMed, the plateau is reached around 150. However, we can observe that in all datasets the starting point (hence $k = 0$) reaches the best Hit@3. We therefore decided to keep the default value of 60 and experiment with $k = 0$ for comparison. It should be noted that in RRF formula (see Formula 1) $k = 0$ effectevely removes $k$ out of the calculation.

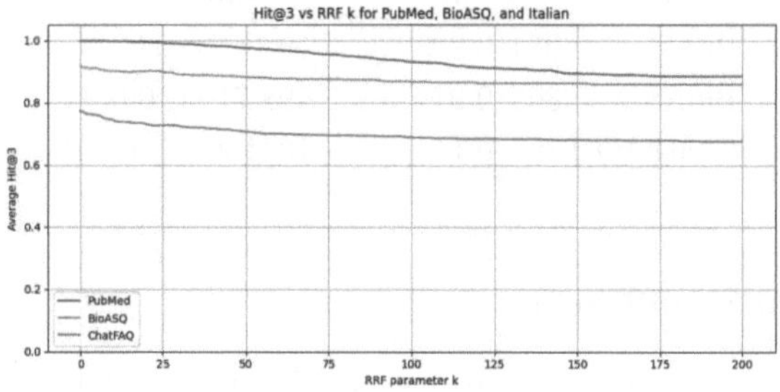


**Fig. 1.** Hit@3 vs different K values in calculating the RRF score

We then evaluated our pipeline on the selected datasets. The results are reported in Table 2. Regarding **RQ3**, we observe that RRF consistently improves RAG pipelines in all datasets. The most performing version of RRF seems to be RRF with $k = 0$, which is consistently the best fusing method. Final reranking steps seem necessary in for all datasets, although we see that they do not consistently modify RRF rankings, despite improving MRR, MAP@50, and NDCG@50, while having a negligible negative effect on HIT@3 (−0.001).

**Table 2.** Per-retriever evaluation metrics across datasets (PubMed, BioASQ, ChatFAQ). The best performance for each metric in each dataset is highlighted in **bold**.

| Retriever | PubMed | | | | BioASQ | | | | ChatFAQ | | | |
|---|---|---|---|---|---|---|---|---|---|---|---|---|
| | Hit@3 | MRR | MAP@50 | NDCG@50 | Hit@3 | MRR | MAP@50 | NDCG@50 | Hit@3 | MRR | MAP@50 | NDCG@50 |
| vector | 0.991 | 0.947 | 0.947 | 0.958 | 0.804 | 0.741 | 0.591 | 0.693 | 0.397 | 0.114 | 0.114 | 0.214 |
| vector reranked | 0.994 | 0.973 | 0.973 | 0.978 | 0.864 | 0.797 | 0.665 | 0.744 | 0.511 | 0.269 | 0.269 | 0.344 |
| BM25 | 0.984 | 0.940 | 0.940 | 0.953 | 0.839 | 0.785 | 0.660 | 0.761 | 0.647 | 0.207 | 0.207 | 0.343 |
| BM25 reranked | 0.996 | 0.984 | 0.984 | 0.987 | 0.899 | 0.842 | 0.737 | 0.814 | 0.725 | 0.335 | 0.335 | 0.455 |
| hyde | 0.989 | 0.949 | 0.949 | 0.960 | 0.865 | 0.798 | 0.646 | 0.745 | 0.548 | 0.169 | 0.169 | 0.296 |
| hyde reranked | 0.997 | 0.964 | 0.964 | 0.971 | 0.903 | 0.832 | 0.696 | 0.777 | 0.646 | 0.318 | 0.318 | 0.421 |
| RRF ($k = 60$) | 0.997 | 0.993 | 0.993 | 0.995 | 0.893 | 0.840 | 0.722 | 0.815 | 0.662 | 0.601 | 0.601 | 0.670 |
| RRF reranked ($k = 60$) | **0.998** | **0.996** | **0.996** | **0.997** | **0.916** | **0.861** | **0.765** | **0.844** | 0.750 | **0.690** | **0.690** | **0.741** |
| RRF ($k = 0$) | **0.998** | **0.996** | **0.996** | 0.996 | **0.917** | 0.860 | 0.751 | 0.835 | **0.751** | 0.670 | 0.670 | 0.727 |
| RRF reranked ($k = 0$) | **0.998** | **0.996** | **0.996** | **0.997** | **0.916** | **0.861** | **0.765** | **0.844** | 0.750 | **0.690** | **0.690** | **0.741** |

**Table 3.** Summary of retrieval performance and statistical significance per dataset. The Hit@3 (min–max) column reports the range of observed Hit@3 scores across pipeline steps, spanning from the initial vector retrieval stage to the final RRF + reranking. The Friedman ($p$) column reports the Friedman test statistic and corresponding $p$-value, assessing whether performance differences among pipeline's steps are statistically significant within each dataset.

| Dataset | Hit@3 (min–max) | Friedman ($p$) |
|---|---|---|
| PubMed | 0.984–0.998 | 59.11 ($< 0.001$) |
| BioASQ | 0.804–0.917 | 198.71 ($< 0.001$) |
| ChatFAQ | 0.397–0.751 | 1341.25 ($< 0.001$) |

### 4.1 Statistical Significance

We computed the Friedman test to assess whether overall performance differs across retrieval pipeline steps. The results indicate statistically significant differences among pipeline stages (see Table 3). For brevity, we report Hit@3; however, results are significant across all metrics, and stepwise comparisons show consistent performance improvements from simple vector retrieval up to the RRF-rerank stage across datasets.

To ensure that RRF-rerank is a necessary step, and superior to simple reranking, we also computed pairwise Wilcoxon signed-rank tests comparing the output of each reranker step (before RRF) with the output of RFF steps; the results are shown in Table 4. On the PubMed dataset, comparisons show small but consistent advantages for RRF variants over simple reranked outputs, although effect sizes are small due to near-ceiling performance (Hit@3 up to 0.998). On the BioASQ dataset, RRF outperforms individual rerankers, reflecting the benefit of aggregating the reranked outputs of our retrievers. Finally, the ChatFAQ dataset exhibits larger effect sizes overall, with further prove that RFF exceed the performance of single reranked lists.

Overall, these results indicate that while reranking is crucial for refining candidate rankings, RRF fusion provides an additional robust boost in retrieval

**Table 4.** Summary of Wilcoxon signed-rank tests comparing reranked outputs to RRF output. The $p$ column reports the range of observed $p$-values across pairwise comparisons, and the $|d|$ column instead shows the corresponding range of Cohen's $d$ effect size. Results indicate that while reranking improves retrieval, RRF variants often match or slightly exceed reranker performance, with effect sizes increasing on more challenging datasets.

| Dataset | $p$ | $\|d\|$ |
|---|---|---|
| PubMed | 0.041–0.083 | 0.055–0.071 |
| BioASQ | $<0.001$ | 0.185–0.255 |
| ChatFAQ | $<0.001$ | 0.615–0.735 |

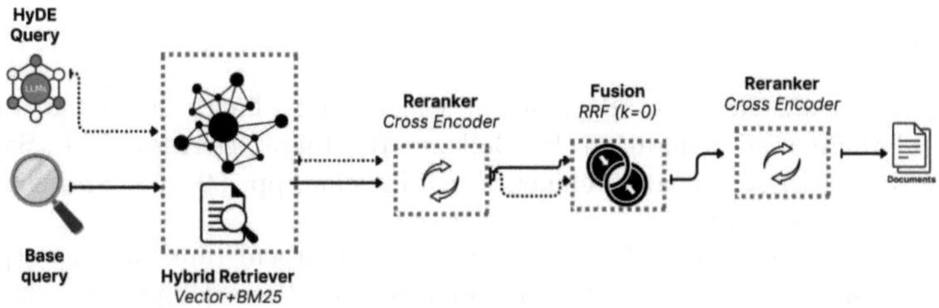


**Fig. 2.** The proposed STRAGMED pipeline. For each query, use a hybrid retriever and rerank the output. We also recommend using HyDE as base query augmentation. Finally, combine with RRF setting $K = 0$ and do a final re-ranking step.

precision, particularly on datasets where absolute performance is not saturated, underscoring the importance of combining multiple retrieval outputs rather than relying solely on reranking.

## 5 Conclusion

Our experiments confirm that the absolute performance of an RAG pipeline is dataset-dependent, consistent with previous studies. Nonetheless, we demonstrate that a pipeline structured as in our proposal (see Fig. 2) yields consistent results datasets, outperforming both retrieval-only and individually reranked outputs. Notably, augmenting queries with the HyDE methodology also proved consistently effective across datasets, and we recommend it as a baseline query augmentation strategy, although the optimal approach is likely dataset-dependent. We therefore propose this configuration (STRAGMED) as a standard RAG pipeline for medical systems, allowing researchers to focus on task-specific optimizations, such as query augmentation, selection of embedding and reranking models, and refinement of retrieval strategies. It should be noted that our pipeline achieved exceptionally high performance on the MIRAGE datasets, likely because these public data were included in the model's pretraining, which may limit their suitability as benchmarking datasets. Nevertheless, we also observed significant gains on the PubMed dataset, where, without reranking, we already obtained 0.98 for the Hit@3 metric. These results highlight the robustness of our pipeline while illustrating its sensitivity to dataset characteristics: gains are smaller on simpler datasets and more evident on complex ones.

Finally, our study was limited to a single configuration, i.e., one embedder, one reranker, and one LLM for HyDE. The components of the pipeline that are related to fusion and reranking are applicable to any other domain, however, elements such as HyDE prompt and model, and embedding model may introduce variability across domains and languages, and further experiments are necessary to validate the pipeline across different models and additional non-public datasets, such as ChatFAQ.

## References

1. Chen, Z., et al.: Breast-crag: a breast cancer large language model leveraging retrieval-augmented generation. In: Bellazzi, R., Juarez Herrero, J.M., Sacchi, L., Zupan, B. (eds.) Artificial Intelligence in Medicine, pp. 99–104. Springer Nature Switzerland, Cham (2025)
2. Cormack, G.V., Clarke, C.L., Buettcher, S.: Reciprocal rank fusion outperforms condorcet and individual rank learning methods. In: Proceedings of the 32nd International ACM SIGIR Conference on Research and Development in Information Retrieval, pp. 758–759 (2009)
3. Es, S., James, J., Espinosa Anke, L., Schockaert, S.: RAGAs: automated evaluation of retrieval augmented generation. In: Aletras, N., De Clercq, O. (eds.) Proceedings of the 18th Conference of the European Chapter of the Association for Computational Linguistics: System Demonstrations, pp. 150–158. Association for Computational Linguistics, St. Julians, Malta (2024). https://doi.org/10.18653/v1/2024.eacl-demo.16, https://aclanthology.org/2024.eacl-demo.16/
4. Gao, L., Ma, X., Lin, J., Callan, J.: Precise zero-shot dense retrieval without relevance labels. In: Rogers, A., Boyd-Graber, J.L., Okazaki, N. (eds.) Proceedings of the 61st Annual Meeting of the Association for Computational Linguistics (Volume 1: Long Papers), ACL 2023, Toronto, Canada, July 9-14, 2023, pp. 1762–1777. Association for Computational Linguistics (2023). https://doi.org/10.18653/V1/2023.ACL-LONG.99
5. Gao, Z., et al.: FRAG: a flexible modular framework for retrieval-augmented generation based on knowledge graphs. In: Che, W., Nabende, J., Shutova, E., Pilehvar, M.T. (eds.) Findings of the Association for Computational Linguistics: ACL 2025, pp. 6178–6192. Association for Computational Linguistics, Vienna, Austria (2025). https://doi.org/10.18653/v1/2025.findings-acl.321, https://aclanthology.org/2025.findings-acl.321/
6. Ghanbari Haez, S., et al.: A retrieval-augmented generation strategy to enhance medical chatbot reliability. In: Finkelstein, J., Moskovitch, R., Parimbelli, E. (eds.) Artificial Intelligence in Medicine, pp. 213–223. Springer Nature Switzerland, Cham (2024)
7. He, B., et al.: Retrieving, rethinking and revising: the chain-of-verification can improve retrieval augmented generation. In: Al-Onaizan, Y., Bansal, M., Chen, Y.N. (eds.) Findings of the Association for Computational Linguistics: EMNLP 2024, pp. 10371–10393. Association for Computational Linguistics, Miami, Florida, USA (2024). https://doi.org/10.18653/v1/2024.findings-emnlp.607, https://aclanthology.org/2024.findings-emnlp.607/
8. He, J., Jia, M., Jia, Z., Duan, J., Song, Y., Wang, J.: ICA-RAG: information completeness guided adaptive retrieval-augmented generation for disease diagnosis . In: 2025 IEEE International Conference on Bioinformatics and Biomedicine (BIBM). pp. 2219–2224. IEEE Computer Society, Los Alamitos, CA, USA (2025). https://doi.org/10.1109/BIBM66473.2025.11357045, https://doi.ieeecomputersociety.org/10.1109/BIBM66473.2025.11357045
9. Jin, Q., Dhingra, B., Liu, Z., Cohen, W., Lu, X.: PubMedQA: a dataset for biomedical research question answering. In: Inui, K., Jiang, J., Ng, V., Wan, X. (eds.) Proceedings of the 2019 Conference on Empirical Methods in Natural Language Processing and the 9th International Joint Conference on Natural Language Processing (EMNLP-IJCNLP), pp. 2567–2577. Association for Computational Linguistics, Hong Kong, China (2019). https://doi.org/10.18653/v1/D19-1259, https://aclanthology.org/D19-1259/

10. Krithara, A., Nentidis, A., Bougiatiotis, K., Paliouras, G.: BioASQ-QA: a manually curated corpus for biomedical question answering. Sci. Data **10**(1), 170 (2023). https://doi.org/10.1038/s41597-023-02068-4
11. Li, X., Li, J.: AoE: angle-optimized embeddings for semantic textual similarity. In: Ku, L.W., Martins, A., Srikumar, V. (eds.) Proceedings of the 62nd Annual Meeting of the Association for Computational Linguistics (Volume 1: Long Papers), pp. 1825–1839. Association for Computational Linguistics, Bangkok, Thailand (2024). https://doi.org/10.18653/v1/2024.acl-long.101, https://aclanthology.org/2024.acl-long.101/
12. Lin, C.Y.: ROUGE: a package for automatic evaluation of summaries. In: Text Summarization Branches Out, pp. 74–81. Association for Computational Linguistics, Barcelona, Spain (2004)
13. Papineni, K., Roukos, S., Ward, T., Zhu, W.J.: BLEU: a method for automatic evaluation of machine translation. In: Isabelle, P., Charniak, E., Lin, D. (eds.) Proceedings of the 40th Annual Meeting of the Association for Computational Linguistics, pp. 311–318. Association for Computational Linguistics, Philadelphia, Pennsylvania, USA (2002)
14. Robertson, S., Zaragoza, H., Taylor, M.: Simple BM25 extension to multiple weighted fields. In: Proceedings of the Thirteenth ACM International Conference on Information and Knowledge Management, pp. 42–49 (2004)
15. Shen, Y., Xu, D., Li, X., Fu, L., Liu, H.: MGPRAG: enhancing medical large language models via precision retrieval-augmented generation. IEEE Access **13**, 183225–183241 (2025). https://doi.org/10.1109/ACCESS.2025.3624887
16. Wang, L., Chen, H., Yang, N., Huang, X., Dou, Z., Wei, F.: Chain-of-retrieval augmented generation. In: NeurIPS 2025 (2025). https://www.microsoft.com/en-us/research/publication/chain-of-retrieval-augmented-generation/
17. Wang, X., et al.: Lab-AI: using retrieval augmentation to enhance language models for personalized lab test interpretation in clinical medicine. In: 2025 IEEE 13th International Conference on Healthcare Informatics (ICHI), pp. 359–368. IEEE (2025)
18. Xiong, G., Jin, Q., Lu, Z., Zhang, A.: Benchmarking retrieval-augmented generation for medicine. In: Ku, L.W., Martins, A., Srikumar, V. (eds.) Findings of the Association for Computational Linguistics: ACL 2024, pp. 6233–6251. Association for Computational Linguistics, Bangkok, Thailand (2024). https://doi.org/10.18653/v1/2024.findings-acl.372, https://aclanthology.org/2024.findings-acl.372/
19. Zhang, X., et al.: RAGLAB: a modular and research-oriented unified framework for retrieval-augmented generation. In: Hernandez Farias, D.I., Hope, T., Li, M. (eds.) Proceedings of the 2024 Conference on Empirical Methods in Natural Language Processing: System Demonstrations, pp. 408–418. Association for Computational Linguistics, Miami, Florida, USA (2024). https://doi.org/10.18653/v1/2024.emnlp-demo.43, https://aclanthology.org/2024.emnlp-demo.43/

# Detecting Silent Failures in Rare Tumor Segmentation: The Impact of Distributional Shift on Uncertainty-Aware Quality Assessment

Paula Alfken[1(✉)], Jacqueline Isabel Bereska[1,2], Robert Hemke[2], Henk Marquering[1,2], and Aneta Lisowska[3,4]

[1] Department of Biomedical Engineering and Physics, Amsterdam UMC, University of Amsterdam, Amsterdam, The Netherlands
p.l.alfken@amsterdamumc.nl
[2] Department of Radiology and Nuclear Medicine, Amsterdam UMC, University of Amsterdam, Amsterdam, The Netherlands
[3] Department of Computer Science, Vrije Universiteit Amsterdam and Amsterdam UMC, Amsterdam, The Netherlands
[4] Cancer Center Amsterdam, Amsterdam, The Netherlands

**Abstract.** Automated medical image segmentation often matches or exceeds segmentations by experts. However, clinical adoption remains limited due to the lack of reliable quality assessment methods that do not require ground-truth annotations. Quality assessment (QA) models estimate segmentation quality directly from imaging features, and recent approaches show improved performance by incorporating segmentation model uncertainty. Yet, these methods have primarily been evaluated on in-distribution data, leaving their reliability under distribution shift unclear. This limitation is particularly important for rare tumors, such as soft tissue tumors, which contain many subtypes often absent in training data. As a result, segmentation and QA models will encounter unseen tumor types at deployment, increasing the risk of silent failures—low-quality segmentations undetected by QA. We evaluate CNN-based uncertainty-aware QA models trained to predict Dice score categories using MRI, segmentation masks, and four uncertainty measures: Confidence, Entropy, Mutual Information (MI), and Expected Pairwise KL Divergence (EPKL). We assess QA performance on in-distribution and out-of- distribution (OOD) tumor subtypes using Cohen's kappa. The best QA configuration using MI achieved substantial in-distribution agreement ($\kappa_{quad} = 0.75$), which degraded on unseen tumor subtypes ($\kappa_{quad} = 0.24$). QA models trained with EPKL and MI showed overconfident behavior on OOD data, missing more than 40% of silent failures. In contrast, EPKL and MI achieved high AUROC when used to separate in- distribution from OOD tumors. These findings demonstrate that uncertainty-aware QA cannot be assumed safe under distributional shift. We propose OOD detection as a safety gate, flagging unreliable QA predictions and prompting manual review.

© The Author(s), under exclusive license to Springer Nature Switzerland AG 2027
P. Andreev et al. (Eds.): AIME 2026, LNAI 16748, pp. 136–146, 2027.
https://doi.org/10.1007/978-3-032-30710-1_16

**Keywords:** Segmentation Quality Assessment · Uncertainty Quantification · Out-of-Distribution Detection · Soft Tissue Tumors

# 1 Introduction

Quantitative analysis of magnetic resonance imaging (MRI) commonly relies on tumor segmentation to enable the assessment of volumetric and morphological features for downstream tasks such as subtype classification, treatment planning, and response monitoring [4]. Automated segmentation models often match or exceed segmentations by experts [7]. However, soft tissue tumors comprise 70 rare and heterogeneous histological subtypes [12], typically limiting training data to a subset and exposing models to unseen (out-of-distribution, OOD) subtypes at inference. Under such distributional shifts, models like nnU-Net [6] still generate segmentations despite increased epistemic uncertainty, risking silent failures - low-quality segmentations that are not accompanied by explicit failure signals (e.g. high uncertainty or low QA prediction) and may propagate unnoticed to downstream analysis and decision support systems [1].

Segmentation performance is typically evaluated using ground-truth metrics such as the Dice coefficient during development, but ground-truth annotations are rarely available in deployment, necessitating alternative quality assessment strategies to flag these silent failures. Learned quality assessment (QA) addresses this by predicting segmentation performance metrics (e.g., Dice score) from image and segmentation features [8]. In parallel, uncertainty estimation has been widely studied to quantify model reliability in medical image segmentation [5]. Common uncertainty quantification methods, such as Monte Carlo Dropout, generate multiple segmentations per image to capture predictive variability, which can be aggregated into voxel-wise uncertainty maps [5]. Incorporating these maps into QA models has been shown to improve performance compared to using image features alone [3]. More recently, Sikha et al. systematically compared several uncertainty estimation measures (confidence, entropy, mutual information (MI), and expected pairwise KL divergence (EPKL)) and uncertainty quantification strategies (Monte Carlo dropout, test-time augmentation, and ensembles) for uncertainty-aware QA, highlighting substantial variability in QA performance [10]. However, both studies evaluated uncertainty-aware QA performance exclusively on in-distribution data.

In this work, we evaluate the reliability of uncertainty-aware QA for soft tissue tumor segmentation when models are exposed to unseen tumor subtypes. Our main contributions are:

1. **Quantification of QA Degradation:** We demonstrate that uncertainty-aware QA agreement ($\kappa_{quad}$) degrades significantly from 0.75 in-distribution to 0.24 on unseen tumor subtypes.
2. **Silent Failure Risk Assessment:** We quantify the clinical risk of automated monitoring, showing that QA models fail to flag over 40% of poor-quality OOD segmentations.

3. **Identification of Task-Dependent Misalignment:** We identify a task-dependent misalignment in uncertainty estimates: while EPKL and MI are superior for OOD detection, their integration as features into learned QA models leads to the highest silent failure rates, suggesting the QA model fails to generalize the uncertainty-to-error mapping under distributional shift.
4. **Proposed Safety Framework:** We propose uncertainty-based OOD detection as safety gate flagging cases where QA model's quality estimates are no longer statistically reliable.

## 2 Methodology

### 2.1 Data and Distributional Shift

Two datasets were used. The publicly available Workflow for Optimal Radiomics Classification (WORC) dataset [11] from Erasmus MC (Rotterdam) contains 283 soft tissue tumor MRI scans with ground truth segmentations. The Amsterdam University Medical Center (AMC) dataset consists of 180 scans without segmentations. Ethical approval was obtained from the AMC Ethics Review Committee (METC number: 2025.0109). A distributional shift exists between the datasets, with only four shared tumor subtypes. UMC includes 15 additional subtypes absent from WORC. All lipoma cases (n=58) were withheld from WORC as a dedicated OOD validation set. The WORC dataset was split 40/60, with 40% used to train the segmentation models, and 60% reserved for training the QA models.

### 2.2 Experimental Design

Figure 1 separates the experimental design into three blocks: (I) segmentation and uncertainty quantification, (II) out-of-distribution detection, and (III) quality assessment.

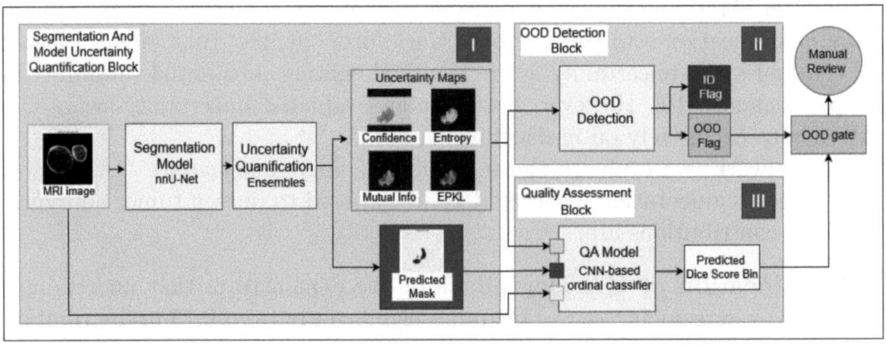


**Fig. 1.** Overview of the experimental design for segmentation, quality assessment and out-of-distribution detection.

*I. Segmentation and Uncertainty Quantification.* The 3D full-resolution nnU-Net v2 was used for all segmentation experiments [6]. One model was trained to convergence (85 epochs) for QA evaluation, while three additional models were trained for 5, 20, and 30 epochs to produce varying segmentation qualities for QA. Default nnU-Net v2 settings were used, except for five-fold cross-validation stratified by tumor subtype. Training employed stochastic gradient descent with polynomial learning rate decay, without architectural or hyperparameter changes.

As Sikha et al. [10] found ensembling to perform best on 3D data, the nnU-Net inference pipeline was modified to aggregate outputs from all five cross-validation models. Following [10], four uncertainty maps were computed. *Confidence* is defined as the maximum softmax probability averaged across ensemble members. *Entropy* is computed as the Shannon entropy of the ensemble mean. *Mutual information (MI)* captures epistemic uncertainty by quantifying disagreement among ensemble members. *Expected pairwise Kullback-Leibler divergence (EPKL)* represents the average divergence between individual predictions and the ensemble mean. Low confidence, high entropy, high MI, or high EPKL values indicate increased uncertainty in the segmentation predictions.

*II. Out-of-Distribution Detection.* For each uncertainty measure, a probability distribution was fitted to the per-sample mean uncertainties of the WORC dataset. At evaluation, sample log-likelihood were computed under the fitted distribution, and samples exceeding the 95th percentile threshold were identified as out-of-distribution.

*III. Quality Assessment.* A neural network was trained to predict Dice score bins, which divide segmentations into four quality categories based on Dice scores, using three input configurations: (1) MRI with uncertainty map, (2) predicted segmentation mask with uncertainty map, and (3) all three inputs. Following Sikha et al. [10], late fusion was implemented with separate 3D CNN branches encoding each input. Each branch consisted of three convolutional blocks with batch normalization, ReLU, and 3D max-pooling, followed by adaptive average pooling to generate a $[B, 64]$ feature vector. Features were concatenated and passed to a multilayer perceptron (MLP) classifier to predict the Dice bin.

To respect the natural ordering of Dice categories, we utilized the Conditional Ordinal Regression for Neural Networks (CORN) loss. Performance was evaluated with weighted Cohen's kappa ($\kappa_{quad}$), which penalizes predictions based on their distance from the true label. Kappa values of 0.60–0.80 are generally regarded as indicative of substantial agreement and strong performance [9]. We additionally monitored the *silent failure miss rate*, defined as the proportion of low-quality segmentations (Dice $< 0.70$) mislassified as "Good".

## 3 Results

*Segmentation and Uncertainty Validation.* The segmentation model achieved a mean Dice score of 0.52 across tumor subtypes, with comparable performance on OOD lipoma cases.

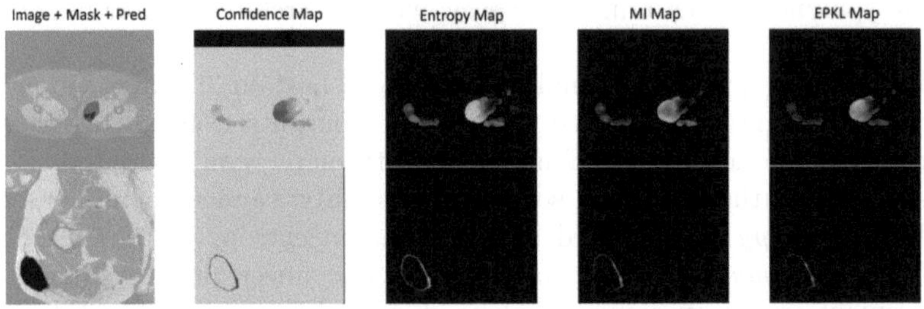


Dice: 0.047

Dice: 0.950

**Fig. 2.** Comparison of uncertainty maps for predicted segmentations with a very low and a very high dice score.

Confidence showed moderate positive correlations with Dice (Pearson 0.49, Spearman 0.58), while entropy exhibited moderate negative correlations (Pearson -0.54, Spearman -0.56). MI and EPKL showed no clear linear relationship. Visual validation of uncertainty maps confirmed their utility as quality indicators, with poor segmentations characterized by maps with multiple, irregularly shaped or patchy activated regions, and high-quality predictions reflected by maps focused on tumor boundaries (Fig. 2).

*Out-of-Distribution Detection.* As shown in Fig. 3, EPKL and MI show clear ID–OOD separation for low- and medium-quality segmentations (Dice bins 0–2), achieving AUROCs above 0.92 for bins 0 and 1. However, there is poor separation for high quality segmentations (bin 3), with AUROCs below 0.59. Confidence and entropy were ineffective for OOD flagging (AUROC $< 0.70$). On the UMC dataset, OOD detection remained moderate (EPKL up to 0.85). All unseen tumor subtypes were correctly flagged as OOD, though some samples from the seen tumor types Liposarcoma and Leiomyosarcoma were also flagged (Fig. 4).

To build a labeled QA dataset, each segmentation mask was paired with its uncertainty maps and the Dice score. Variation in segmentation quality was successfully generated by the three models (Fig. 5), but the Dice distribution remained bimodal, favoring very high or very low values. To capture this distributional structure, Dice scores were grouped into four bins (see Fig. 5b): *Complete Failure* (Dice $< 0.10$), *Poor* ($0.10 \leq$ Dice $< 0.50$), *Moderate* ($0.50 \leq$ Dice $< 0.70$), and *Good* (Dice $\geq 0.70$), with a wider poor bin to account for fewer mid-range scores. The 0.70 threshold is a common clinical cut-off for acceptable segmentations [2].

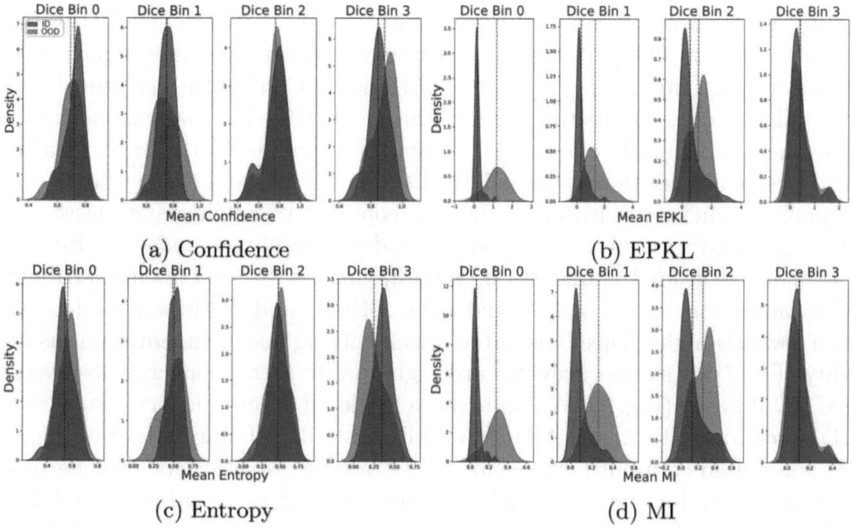


(a) Confidence (b) EPKL

(c) Entropy (d) MI

**Fig. 3.** ID vs OOD mean uncertainty distributions with the OOD lipoma set

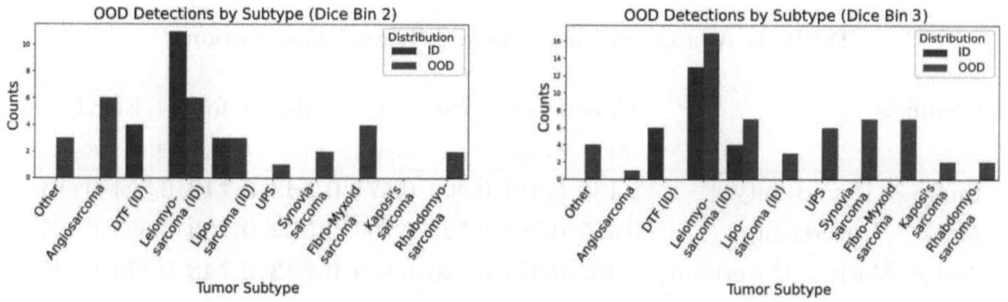


**Fig. 4.** Counts of flagged OOD samples per tumor subtype for Dice bins 2 (0.5–0.7) and 3 (>0.7) in the UMC dataset using EPKL mean uncertainty.

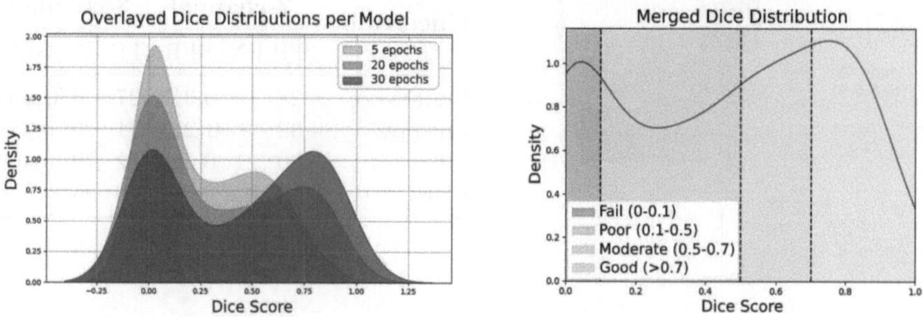


(a) Dice score distribution per model (after 5, 20, 30 epochs) (b) Merged Dice distribution from all models with bins

**Fig. 5.** Dice distribution per model for QA dataset construction, and the merged Dice distribution split into 4 dice bins or quality categories.

*Quality Assessment.* Across all uncertainty measures, MI achieved the highest in-distribution QA performance, particularly when combining image, mask, and uncertainty inputs ($\kappa_{\text{quad}} = 0.75$) (Table 1). Confidence performed worst across all settings, contrasting with Sikha et al. [10]. For two-channel inputs, the segmentation mask was more informative than the MRI image. Heatmap of the best configuration using MI (Fig. 6) show the model respects the ordinal quality structure, with errors largely confined to neighboring classes, and failed segmentations never predicted as good and rarely as moderate. However, performance degraded markedly on OOD lipomas, with the best in-distribution models achieving $\kappa_{\text{quad}} = 0.27$ and 0.24. EPKL- and MI-based models were biased towards higher Dice bins, often misclassifying poor segmentations as high quality (Fig. 7). A similar skew toward high-quality predictions was observed on the UMC dataset (Fig. 9). We observed a trade-off where metrics strongest for OOD detection (EPKL and MI) showed highest silent failure miss rates (up to 0.61) when used as input features for QA. Confidence-based models achieve the lowest miss rate for the 3 channel configuration and entropy-based models for the 2-channel configuration (Table 6), but these measures show to be ineffective for OOD detection. Figure 8 illustrates this divergence.

**Table 1.** Average $\kappa_{\text{lin}}/\kappa_{\text{quad}}$ across channel combinations

| Channels | Confidence | | Entropy | | Mut. Info | | EPKL | |
|---|---|---|---|---|---|---|---|---|
| | $\kappa_{\text{lin}}$ | $\kappa_{\text{quad}}$ | $\kappa_{\text{lin}}$ | $\kappa_{\text{quad}}$ | $\kappa_{\text{lin}}$ | $\kappa_{\text{quad}}$ | $\kappa_{\text{lin}}$ | $\kappa_{\text{quad}}$ |
| Image + Uncertainty | 0.156 | 0.219 | 0.402 | 0.574 | **0.543** | **0.713** | 0.524 | 0.691 |
| Mask + Uncertainty | 0.425 | 0.589 | 0.523 | 0.700 | **0.572** | **0.733** | 0.555 | 0.727 |
| Image, Mask + Uncertainty | 0.467 | 0.640 | 0.520 | 0.689 | **0.583** | **0.748** | 0.570 | 0.715 |

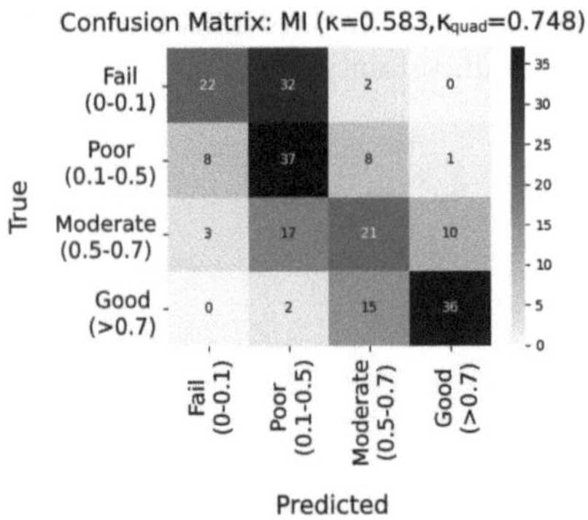


| Uncertainty | 2-channel | | | 3-channel | | |
|---|---|---|---|---|---|---|
| | TP | FN | SFR | TP | FN | SFR |
| Confidence | 28 | 13 | 0.317 | 27 | 14 | **0.341** |
| Entropy | 32 | 9 | **0.220** | 21 | 20 | 0.488 |
| MI | 20 | 21 | 0.512 | 22 | 19 | 0.463 |
| EPKL | 18 | 23 | 0.561 | 16 | 25 | 0.610 |

**Fig. 6.** Left: Heatmap of the best input configuration showing predicted vs. actual Dice scores. Right: Summary of QA failure detection on OOD lipoma cases. FN values capture missed silent failures. Silent Failure Miss Rate (SFR) is ratio of missed low quality flags.

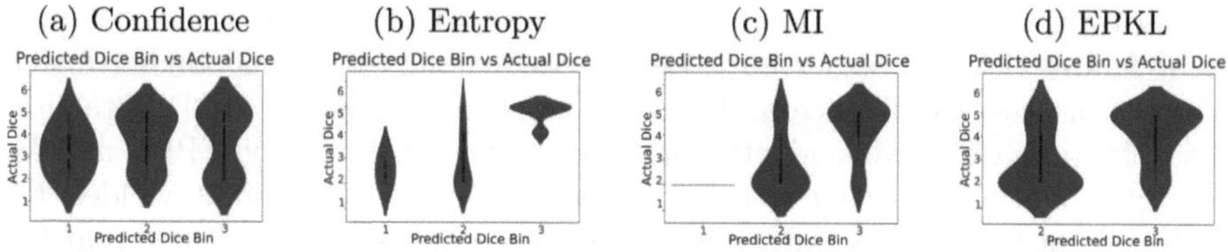


**Fig. 7.** Violin plots of predicted versus actual Dice scores for the OOD lipoma set (two-channel models with masks and uncertainty maps).

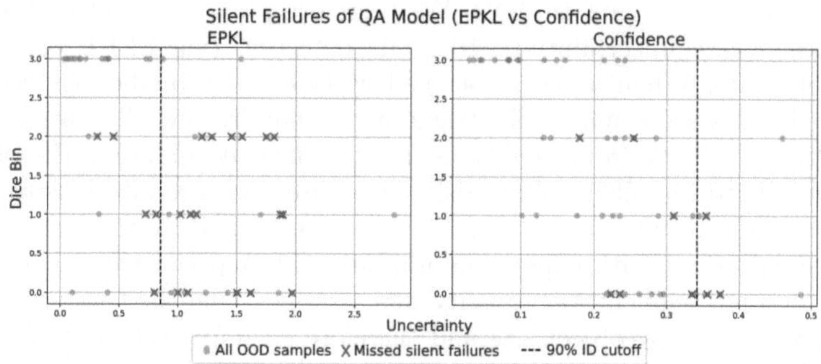


**Fig. 8.** Silent failures (true Dice bin < 3, predicted bin = 3; bins correspond to Dice score categories) in the OOD lipoma set (3-channel models), shown in uncertainty-Dice space. Confidence is inverted (higher values = more uncertainty). The 90th percentile ID threshold marks high-uncertainty cases.

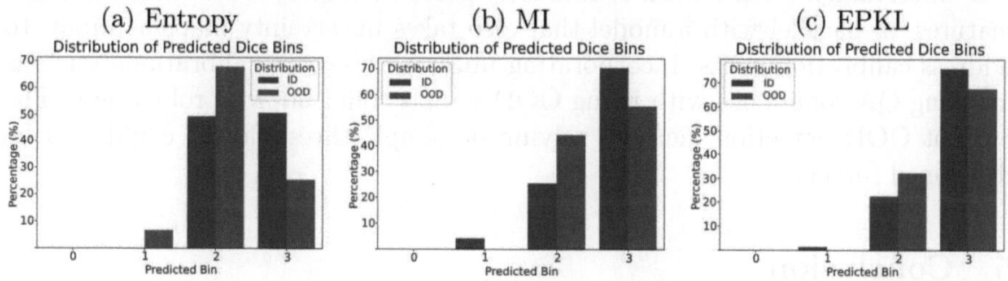


**Fig. 9.** Predicted Dice distributions for a subset of the UMC dataset, stratified by in-distribution (ID) and OOD tumors (two-channel mask + uncertainty models).

## 4 Discussion

The variability in segmentation quality was essential for evaluating the QA models, as focusing only on near-perfect predictions would provide limited insight. While prior work reported strong QA performance using uncertainty maps and imaging features [3,10], our findings reveal a critical AI safety vulnerability. QA achieved substantial in-distribution agreement ($\kappa_{quad} = 0.75$), but performance collapsed under distributional shift ($\kappa_{quad} = 0.24$), demonstrating severe QA degradation under OOD conditions. More concerning, QA models failed to flag over 40% of poor-quality OOD segmentations, revealing a substantial silent failure risk. We observed a task-dependent misalignment among uncertainty measures. Confidence and entropy were unsuitable for OOD detection, but were more effective at identifying silent failures. Conversely, EPKL and MI were effective measures for flagging unseen tumors as OOD, but yielded the highest silent failure miss rates when used as QA inputs. This indicates that QA models erroneously assume a stationary mapping between uncertainty patterns and segmentation quality, which does not hold for unseen tumor subtypes. From an AI safety perspective, a "Good" QA prediction is an insufficient safety signal if the underlying data is OOD. We therefore propose a multi-stage safety framework, where uncertainty-based OOD detection (via EPKL or MI) acts as a safety gate. When a case is flagged as OOD, QA predictions should be considered statistically unreliable, triggering manual review. This separation of distributional validity from quality estimation directly addresses the observed trade-off and reduces silent failure risk. There are several limitations to keep in mind. First, the results on the UMC dataset are limited by the lack of a dedicated validation set with expert annotations, so QA performance can only be inferred. Second, segmentation quality was assessed using the Dice score, which is strongly affected by object size and therefore an imperfect proxy for overall quality. Third, only tumor subtype shifts were evaluated; other clinical shifts, like scanner protocols or demographics, were not. Fourth, variations in segmentation quality were generated using early training epochs, which may not reflect real inference-time errors. Fifth, the segmentation model was trained on a small dataset, so uncertainty maps may partly reflect incomplete learning rather than true uncertainty. Future work could investigate training a model solely on image features, in parallel with a model that also takes uncertainty maps as input, to address calibration shifts. Incorporating uncertainty-aware calibration—such as lowering QA confidence with rising OOD signals could improve robustness. The current OOD detection method, relying on simple thresholding, could also be developed further.

## 5 Conclusion

Overall, our findings reveal a critical AI safety risk of QA under distributional shift, as models frequently overestimate segmentation quality, masking silent failures on unseen tumor types. We also identified a task-dependent misalignment in uncertainty measures. Although EPKL and MI reliably detect out-of-distribution (OOD) samples, their integration into learned QA models results in the highest silent failure miss rates. Future work should focus on distribution-aware recalibration strategies and safety-gating mechanisms to improve robustness and reliability under shift.

**Acknowledgements.** This work was supported by the EU Horizon Europe project COMBAT (grant agreement No. 101191315).

**Declaration of AI assistance.** The authors used ChatGPT for refinement, correction, editing or formatting of the manuscript to improve clarity. After using this technology, the authors reviewed the results and take full responsibility for the contents of the manuscript.

## References

1. Bungert, T., Kobelke, L., Jäger, P.: Understanding silent failures in medical image classification. In: Greenspan, H., et al. (eds.) Medical Image Computing and Computer-Assisted Intervention – MICCAI 2023. Lecture Notes in Computer Science, vol. 14222. Springer, Cham (2023). https://doi.org/10.1007/978-3-031-43898-1_39
2. DeSouza, N., Van der Lugt, A., Deroose, C., et al.: Standardised lesion segmentation for imaging biomarker quantitation: a consensus recommendation from ESR and EORTC. Insights Imaging **13**(1), 159 (2022). https://doi.org/10.1186/s13244-022-01287-4
3. DeVries, T., Taylor, G.: Leveraging uncertainty estimates for predicting segmentation quality. arXiv preprint arXiv:1807.00502 (2018)
4. Gao, Y., Jiang, Y., Peng, Y., Yuan, F., Zhang, X., Wang, J.: Medical image segmentation: a comprehensive review of deep learning-based methods. Tomography **11**(5), 52 (2025). https://doi.org/10.3390/tomography11050052
5. Gawlikowski, J., Basu, S., Rüger, S., Togelius, J., Tschannen, M.: A survey of uncertainty in deep neural networks. arXiv preprint arXiv:2107.03342 (2021). https://arxiv.org/abs/2107.03342
6. Isensee, F., Jaeger, P., Kohl, S., Petersen, J., Maier-Hein, K.: nnU-Net: a self-configuring method for deep learning-based biomedical image segmentation. Nat. Methods **18**(2), 203–211 (2021). https://doi.org/10.1038/s41592-020-01008-z
7. Kofler, F., Ezhov, I., Isensee, F.o.: Are we using appropriate segmentation metrics? identifying correlates of human expert perception for cnn training beyond rolling the dice coefficient. Mach. Learn. Biomed. Imag. **2**, 27–71 (2023). https://doi.org/10.59275/j.melba.2023-dg1f, https://melba-journal.org/2023:002
8. Kohlberger, T., Singh, V., Alvino, C., Bahlmann, C., Grady, L.: Evaluating segmentation error without ground truth. In: Ayache, N., Delingette, H., Golland, P., Mori, K. (eds.) Medical Image Computing and Computer-Assisted Intervention – MICCAI 2012. Lecture Notes in Computer Science, vol. 7510, pp. 528–536. Springer, Berlin, Heidelberg (2012). https://doi.org/10.1007/978-3-642-33415-3_65
9. Landis, J., Koch, G.: The measurement of observer agreement for categorical data. Biometrics **33**(1), 159–174 (1977)
10. Sikha, O., et al.: Uncertainty-aware segmentation quality prediction via deep learning bayesian modeling: Comprehensive evaluation and interpretation on skin cancer and liver segmentation. Computer. Med. Imaging Graph. **123**, 102547 (2025). https://doi.org/10.1016/j.compmedimag.2025.102547, https://www.sciencedirect.com/science/article/pii/S0895611125000564

11. Starmans, M., Timbergen, M., Vos, M., et al.: The worc database: Mri and ct scans, segmentations, and clinical labels for 930 patients from six radiomics studies. medRxiv (2021). https://doi.org/10.1101/2021.08.19.21262238, https://www.medrxiv.org/content/10.1101/2021.08.19.21262238v1.full, preprint, not peer-reviewed
12. Van Vliet, M., Kliffen, M., Krestin, G.P., Van Dijke, C.F.: Soft tissue sarcomas at a glance: clinical, histological, and MR imaging features of malignant extremity soft tissue tumors. Europ. Radiol. **19**(6), 1499–1511 (2009). https://doi.org/10.1007/s00330-008-1292-3, http://link.springer.com/10.1007/s00330-008-1292-3

# Unsupervised Anomaly Detection of Acute Health Events in Older Adults Using Longitudinal Wearable Sensor Data

Eldar Mukhtarov(✉) and Krzysztof Grudzień

Faculty of Electrical, Electronic, Computer and Control Engineering, Institute of Applied Computer Science, Lodz University of Technology, Lodz, Poland
eldar.mukhtarov.tech@gmail.com

**Abstract.** Monitoring the overall health status of independently living older adults is essential for ensuring their well-being and enabling the timely detection of acute incidents. A commonly used approach is remote health monitoring (telecare), which relies on wearable wristbands to continuously collect physiological and activity data. However, the frequent scarcity of event labels in such datasets significantly limits the effectiveness of supervised machine learning to predict health events. To address this challenge, we present an unsupervised Long Short-Term Memory Variational Autoencoder (LSTM-VAE), and we conduct a feasibility study applying it to real-world telecare data from 8,267 older adults monitored over 30 days. Training exclusively on 1.3 million windows of normal physiological patterns, the model achieved AUROC 0.68 (95% CI: 0.65–0.71) for detecting acute events on held-out test data. Comparison with a non-temporal Standard Autoencoder (AUROC 0.67, 95% CI: 0.64–0.71) revealed no statistically significant difference, indicating that the present model family provides a feasible baseline for unsupervised telecare monitoring rather than a production-ready detector. This work demonstrates the feasibility of unsupervised anomaly detection for telecare monitoring and provides a realistic performance baseline for future validation.

**Keywords:** Unsupervised anomaly detection · Wearable sensor data · Variational autoencoders · Acute event detection

## 1 Introduction

The global population aged 60 and older is expected to nearly double from 13.5% to 20% by 2050 [8], creating urgent demand for scalable solutions enabling older adults to age in place safely. While wearable sensors theoretically provide continuous monitoring for acute events like falls and cardiac incidents, real-world systems suffer from high false-positive rates and poor sensitivity, leading to alarm fatigue and device abandonment [4,9].

© The Author(s), under exclusive license to Springer Nature Switzerland AG 2027
P. Andreev et al. (Eds.): AIME 2026, LNAI 16748, pp. 147–152, 2027.
https://doi.org/10.1007/978-3-032-30710-1_17

The fundamental challenge is label scarcity: acute events constitute roughly 0.01% of monitoring data, preventing supervised classifiers from learning meaningful boundaries [3,11]. Labeling requires clinical expertise to distinguish genuine health crises from false alarms, making it expensive and time-consuming. Traditional threshold-based detectors show highly variable performance (sensitivity 19–100%, false-positives 30–40%) [4], while supervised deep learning [2] requires richly labeled datasets unavailable at such low event rates [1].

This gap motivates unsupervised anomaly detection. LSTM-based autoencoders [5] and VAE variants [6,10] have shown promise via reconstruction error, but healthcare presents unique challenges as physiological baselines vary between individuals and evolve with aging, medications, and comorbidities. We apply unsupervised LSTM-VAE to longitudinal data from 8,267 older adults, establishing a methodological baseline and identifying directions for improvement.

## 2 Methods

### 2.1 Dataset and Preprocessing

We obtained data from HRPCare Sp. z o. o., a telecare provider in Poland. The anonymized database includes 13,317 adults monitored continuously for 30 days in November 2025, yielding 72.6 million timestamped physiological measurements across five modalities: heart rate, systolic and diastolic blood pressure, body temperature, oxygen saturation, and step count. Ground truth labels came from 5,420 emergency alerts stratified by clinical staff into four severity levels, with Level 3 alerts corresponding to 73 confirmed acute crises requiring emergency services that serve as our positive class.

We retained 8,267 seniors with greater than 30% global data density. Raw streams were resampled into 15-minute intervals (mean aggregation for vitals, summation for steps) and imputed via forward-fill with a 1-hour tolerance. From these signals we engineered an 11-dimensional feature vector combining raw vitals with derived stability indicators: pulse pressure, shock index, heart rate volatility, blood pressure trend, step trend, and 6-hour rolling step sum. Static demographics (age, sex) were excluded after preliminary ablation showed negligible marginal predictive value. This may appear to differ from clinical risk frameworks such as SCORE2 [7], where age and sex are primary stratifiers, however, in a reconstruction-based setting these are time-invariant per-person constants rather than dynamic signals, with their effects partially absorbed into the learned latent space. Demographic conditioning remains a planned extension.

### 2.2 LSTM-VAE Architecture

The encoder LSTM processes 24-hour input sequences $X = \{x_1, \ldots, x_{96}\}$ at 15-minute resolution, producing latent parameters $\mu \in \mathbb{R}^{32}$ and $\log \sigma^2 \in \mathbb{R}^{32}$. The latent vector is sampled via $z = \mu + \sigma \odot \epsilon$, $\epsilon \sim \mathcal{N}(0, I)$, and a decoder LSTM reconstructs the sequence from $z$. The current architecture does not condition on time-varying covariates; extending the latent space to incorporate clinical context such as comorbidity burden is architecturally straightforward but beyond the scope of this feasibility study.

Training minimizes the Evidence Lower Bound (ELBO):

$$\mathcal{L} = \frac{1}{L \cdot D} \sum_{t=1}^{L} \sum_{d=1}^{D} (x_{t,d} - \hat{x}_{t,d})^2 + \beta D_{KL}(q(z|X) \| \mathcal{N}(0, I)) \tag{1}$$

where $L = 96$ is sequence length and $D = 11$ is feature dimensionality. The 24-hour window covers a full circadian cycle. Architecture hyperparameters were selected by grid search over $H \in \{64, 128\}$ and latent dimension $\in \{16, 32, 64\}$; $H = 64$, $D = 32$ yielded the best validation AUROC. $\beta = 0.001$ was chosen with linear KL annealing from 0 to $\beta$ over the first half of training to prevent posterior collapse while preserving reconstruction fidelity. Training used Adam at $10^{-3}$, batch size 512, 20 epochs, with gradient clipping.

### 2.3 Experimental Setup

Strict subject-level splits prevented data leakage: 70% training, 15% validation, 15% test. Training used only normal windows ($\approx$1.3 million sequences); validation and test sets were balanced at 50/50 normal/acute to assess discriminative capacity independent of prevalence. The detection threshold was optimized on validation data via G-Mean maximization and applied to the test set without modification. Performance was assessed by AUROC with 95% CIs from 1,000-iteration bootstrap resampling.

The primary comparison was a Standard Autoencoder with a symmetric five-layer dense encoder–decoder (dimensions 1056, 256, 64, 32 at the bottleneck, reversed for decoding) and ReLU activations, where input sequences are flattened to 1056-dimensional vectors, discarding temporal ordering. Standard AE has $\approx 10\times$ more parameters than LSTM-VAE ($\approx$580K vs. 60K) due to its fully-connected layers. Preliminary experiments with alternative approaches did not yield meaningful improvements over the reconstruction-based baseline, consistent with the extreme label scarcity that motivates the unsupervised setting. A comprehensive comparison with supervised deep-learning classifiers remains future work, as the available positive labels are too few to support such training.

## 3 Results and Discussion

Table 1 shows that LSTM-VAE (AUROC 0.68, 95% CI: 0.65–0.71) and Standard AE (AUROC 0.67, 95% CI: 0.64–0.71) achieved statistically equivalent discrimination. AUROC 0.68, while modest, represents a meaningful result for an entirely unsupervised model trained exclusively on normal data; the gap above chance (0.50) indicates the learned physiology embedding captures genuine signal. At true event prevalence of $\approx$0.01%, however, both models yield positive predictive values near 0.02%, clearly insufficient for clinical deployment.

**Table 1.** Performance on balanced test set ($N = 960$ windows).

| Model | AUROC (95% CI) | Sensitivity | Precision | PPV@0.01% |
|---|---|---|---|---|
| LSTM-VAE | 0.68 (0.65–0.71) | 0.58 | 0.64 | 0.0002 |
| Standard AE | 0.67 (0.64–0.71) | 0.71 | 0.56 | 0.0001 |

The most surprising result is that LSTM-VAE's recurrent architecture offered no advantage over Standard AE despite the latter having 10× more parameters. Figure 1 shows substantial reconstruction error overlap between classes. This suggests the engineered features may already encode relevant temporal structure, or that 24-hour windows are too coarse to capture acute deterioration onset. Standard AE's comparable performance offers additional practical advantages with 3–5× faster inference and simpler deployment on resource-constrained devices.

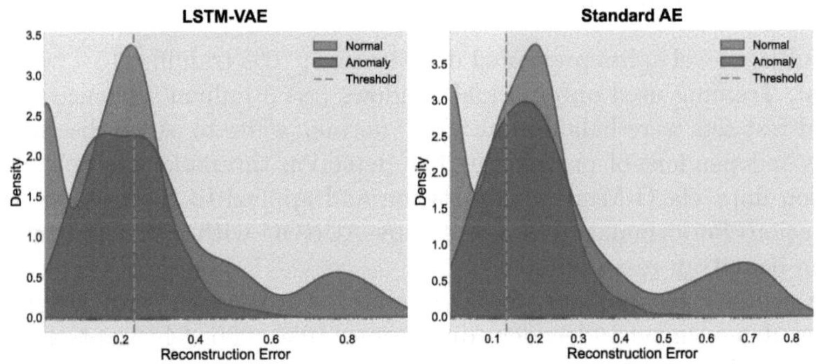


**Fig. 1.** Reconstruction error distributions for normal (blue, left-skewed) and acute (red/pink, right-spread) windows with detection thresholds (orange dashed lines). Substantial class overlap explains the modest AUROC values under the current feature set and windowing scheme. (Color figure online)

Several limitations warrant consideration. Ground truth derives from user-triggered alerts stratified by telecare staff rather than clinically confirmed diagnoses, introducing label noise that likely suppresses AUROC estimates. The model applies a universal detection threshold, which does not account for inter-individual physiological variation. Personalized thresholds calibrated to each subject's baseline physiology represent a more principled approach to reducing false alarms under realistic prevalence.

## 4 Conclusion and Future Work

We showed that unsupervised anomaly detection is feasible for acute health event monitoring, with LSTM-VAE (AUROC 0.68) statistically equivalent to

Standard AE (0.67). The equivalence suggests temporal recurrent processing offers no advantage under the current feature set and windowing scheme, though whether this reflects a genuine property of acute events or limitations of the 24-hour resolution remains open.

Performance remains well below clinical deployment thresholds. Future work will explore shorter temporal windows spanning 1–6 h to better capture acute deterioration patterns, implement attention mechanisms to identify which time segments are most critical for detection, and develop personalized detection thresholds calibrated to each individual's baseline. Most critically, prospective validation with clinically confirmed outcomes rather than user-triggered alerts is essential to establish real-world performance and guide the path toward reliable systems supporting aging-in-place.

**Acknowledgement.** This study was funded by the Polish Ministry of Science and Higher Education (grant FERS.01.05-IP.08-0217/23, offer N113). We thank HRPCare Sp. z o. o. for providing the anonymized dataset.

**Disclosure of Interests.** The authors have no competing interests to declare

**Declaration of AI Assistance Technologies During Manuscript Preparation.** The authors used Gemini 3.1 Pro for [A2] Drafting sections of text. After using this technology, the authors reviewed the results and take full responsibility for the contents of the manuscript.

## References

1. Chen, Z., Li, Q.: Anomaly detection of extremely rare events based on VAE-LSTM-SelfAttention. In: 2025 IEEE 7th International Conference on Communications, Information System and Computer Engineering (CISCE), pp. 477–482. IEEE (2025). https://doi.org/10.1109/CISCE65916.2025.11065862
2. García, E., Villar, M., Fáñez, M., et al.: Towards effective detection of elderly falls with CNN-LSTM neural networks. Neurocomputing **500**, 231–240 (2022). https://doi.org/10.1016/j.neucom.2021.06.102
3. Khan, S.S., Hoey, J.: Review of fall detection techniques: a data availability perspective. Med. Eng. Phys. **39**, 12–22 (2017). https://doi.org/10.1016/j.medengphy.2016.10.014
4. Lee, A., Lee, H., Lee, S.H.: Digital healthcare approaches for fall detection and prediction in older adults: A systematic review of evidence from hospital and long-term care settings. Medicina **61**(11), 1926 (2025). https://doi.org/10.3390/medicina61111926
5. Malhotra, P., Ramakrishnan, A., Anand, G., et al.: LSTM-based encoder-decoder for multi-sensor anomaly detection. arXiv:1607.00148 (2016). https://doi.org/10.48550/arXiv.1607.00148
6. Park, D., Hoshi, Y., Kemp, C.C.: A multimodal anomaly detector for robot-assisted feeding using an LSTM-based variational autoencoder. IEEE Robot. Autom. Lett. (2017). https://doi.org/10.1109/LRA.2018.2801475

7. SCORE2 working group and ESC Cardiovascular risk collaboration: Score2 risk prediction algorithms: new models to estimate 10-year risk of cardiovascular disease in Europe. Eur. Heart J. **42**(25), 2439–2454 (2021). https://doi.org/10.1093/eurheartj/ehab309
8. World Health Organization: Decade of Healthy Ageing: Baseline Report. Tech. rep, World Health Organization, Geneva (2021)
9. Wróbel-Lachowska, M., Dominiak, J., Wozniak, M.P., et al.: 'That's when I put it on': stakeholder perspectives in large-scale remote health monitoring for older adults. Pers. Ubiquit. Comput. **27**, 2193–2210 (2023). https://doi.org/10.1007/s00779-023-01753-w
10. Xu, H., Chen, W., Zhao, N., et al.: Unsupervised anomaly detection via variational auto-encoder for seasonal KPIs in web applications. In: Proceedings of the 2018 World Wide Web Conference, pp. 187–196 (2018). https://doi.org/10.1145/3178876.3185996
11. Zhao, Y., Wong, Z.S., Tsui, K.L.: A framework of rebalancing imbalanced healthcare data for rare events' classification: A case of look-alike sound-alike mix-up incident detection. J. Healthcare Eng. **2018**, 6275435 (2018). https://doi.org/10.1155/2018/6275435

# When to Adapt? Adapting the Model or Data in Federated Medical Imaging

Chamani Shiranthika(✉) and Parvaneh Saeedi

School of Engineering Science, Simon Fraser University, Burnaby, BC V5A 1S6, Canada
{csj5,psaeedi}@sfu.ca

**Abstract.** Federated learning enables collaborative model training across medical institutions without sharing raw data, but its performance is often limited by domain heterogeneity across clients. Existing approaches to address this challenge fall into two main paradigms: model-side personalization, which adapts model parameters to each client, and data-side harmonization, which reduces inter-client variation at the input level. Despite their widespread use, these strategies have not been systematically compared. In this work, we conduct a comprehensive study across six medical imaging settings—colon polyp, skin lesion, and breast tumor segmentation, and tuberculosis CXR, brain tumor, and breast tumor classification—covering diverse types of domain shift. We evaluate a broad set of state-of-the-art harmonization and personalization methods under a unified framework. Our results reveal a conditional trade-off driven by the nature of heterogeneity: harmonization is more effective when variation is primarily appearance-based (e.g., CXR classification), while personalization performs better when differences are structural (e.g., colon polyp segmentation). When inter-client variation is limited, both strategies perform similarly. These findings demonstrate that the effectiveness of adaptation in federated medical imaging depends on the type and magnitude of domain shift rather than the strategy alone. We provide practical guidelines for selecting between harmonization and personalization, and highlight directions for future hybrid approaches that combine both paradigms. Code is available at: https://github.com/ChamaniS/WhenToAdapt.

**Keywords:** data harmonization · model personalization · federated learning

## 1 Introduction

Federated learning (FL) [1] has emerged as a key paradigm for privacy-preserving medical imaging collaborations, enabling multiple institutions to jointly train models without sharing patients' data. However, its effectiveness is often limited by inter-client heterogeneity, differences in data acquisition protocols, patient demographics, and annotation practices. Such non-independent and identically

© The Author(s), under exclusive license to Springer Nature Switzerland AG 2027
P. Andreev et al. (Eds.): AIME 2026, LNAI 16748, pp. 153–163, 2027.
https://doi.org/10.1007/978-3-032-30710-1_18

distributed (IID) data distributions cause severe model bias and poor cross-site generalization. Therefore, managing data heterogeneity has become one of the most critical open challenges in federated medical learning [2,3].

Two broad research directions have evolved to address such heterogeneity challenge. *(1): Model-side personalization* focuses on adapting the model to each client through modularized layers, local fine-tuning, or adaptive optimization. Early personalized federated learning methods rely on local fine-tuning or partial model sharing (FedPer [4], FedRep [5], FedBN [6]), and on meta-learning or attention mechanisms (FedMeta [7], pFedMe [8], Per-FedAvg [9], FedAMP [10]). Some research treats clients as related tasks (MOCHA [11], VIRTUAL [12]), clusters of similar clients (IFCA [13], FedCluster [14], FedGroup [15]), or uses knowledge distillation (FedMD [16], FedDF [17]). Some other widely used methods include FedAdam [18], FedProx [19], SCAFFOLD [20], pFedMe [8], FedMeta [7], FedAMP [10], and Ditto [21]. *(2): Data-side harmonization* reduces appearance discrepancies caused by scanner hardware, acquisition protocols, or imaging settings while preserving clinically relevant anatomy and is commonly studied as protocol-level preprocessing (resampling, intensity/colour normalization) or image-level harmonization using learned cross-domain mappings [22]. State-of-the-art (SoTA) data-side harmonization methods include GANs and related generative models (CycleGAN [23], CUT [24], StarGAN, DeepHarmony [25], ImUnity [26], BlindHarmony [27]), attention/transformer-based approaches (AdaIN [28], CoMoGAN [29], QS-Attn [30], Harmonization Transformer [31]), and newer diffusion-based models, which align input distributions across sites while maintaining diagnostic content.

Despite substantial progress, prior work has largely studied personalization and harmonization in isolation, without analyzing when each is preferable under different domain shifts. We address this gap with a systematic comparison across six medical imaging tasks: colon polyp, skin lesion, and breast tumor segmentation, and tuberculosis CXR, brain tumor, and breast tumor classification. These tasks span diverse heterogeneity types, from strong structural variation (e.g., colon polyp segmentation) to predominantly appearance-driven shifts (e.g., tuberculosis CXR classification), as well as moderate or mixed variations (e.g., skin, brain, and breast tumor tasks).

Using a unified experimental protocol, we evaluate 18 SoTA harmonization and personalization methods under identical federated settings. Our results reveal a conditional trade-off: harmonization is more effective for appearance-driven variation, while personalization performs better under strong structural heterogeneity; when variation is limited or mixed, both approaches perform similarly. We contribute: (1) a comprehensive comparison of harmonization and personalization in federated medical imaging, (2) an empirical analysis of how the type and magnitude of domain shift affect their effectiveness, and (3) a modular codebase supporting both paradigms. Section 2 describes the methodology, Sect. 3 presents the results, and Sect. 4 concludes the paper.

# 2 Methodology

## 2.1 Problem Formulation

We consider a cross-silo FL setting with $k$ medical institutions (clients), each holding a local dataset: $D_k = \{(x_i^{(k)}, y_i^{(k)})\}_{i=1}^{n_k}$ drawn from an unknown distribution $\mathcal{P}_k$ over images $x$ and labels $y$. A standard FL objective learns a single global model $f_\theta$ by minimizing the weighted empirical risk:

$$\min_\theta \sum_{k=1}^{K} p_k \, \mathbb{E}_{(x,y)\sim\mathcal{P}_k} \big[\ell(f_\theta(x), y)\big], \tag{1}$$

where $p_k = n_k / \sum_j n_j$ and $\ell$ is a task-appropriate loss. In practice, the client distributions $\{\mathcal{P}_k\}$ are heterogeneous. In medical imaging collaborations, this heterogeneity arises from two distinct, qualitatively different sources:

1. **Input-level/style-level shift** $\Delta_{\text{style}}$: variations in scanner hardware, acquisition protocols, intensity scaling, contrast, noise level, padding, and background artifacts. These changes alter the global appearance statistics while largely preserving the anatomical layout and pathology of the data.

2. **Content-level/structural shift** $\Delta_{\text{content}}$: variations in anatomy, pathology morphology and prevalence, viewpoint, endoscope/camera pose, and scene context. These differences alter the spatial structure and semantic content that the model must segment or classify.

Let $\Delta_k = (\Delta_{\text{style},k}, \Delta_{\text{content},k})$ denote the domain shift of client $k$. A single global model $f_\theta$ may underperform when $\Delta_k$ is large and heterogeneous across clients. We empirically compare these two families of heterogeneity acting differently on:

- **Data harmonization**: learn or apply client-specific transformations $T_k$ in image or feature space such that the transformed data $T_k(x)$ are statistically aligned to a reference domain, and then train a *shared* model $f_\theta$ on harmonized data, and
- **Model personalization**: directly adapt the *shared* model $f_\theta$ per client, yielding client-specific parameters $\theta_k$, while leaving the raw images unchanged.

Formally, a harmonization-based system learns

$$\min_{\theta, \{T_k\}} \sum_{k=1}^{K} p_k \, \mathbb{E}_{(x,y)\sim\mathcal{P}_k} \big[\ell(f_\theta(T_k(x)) y)\big] \tag{2}$$

A personalization-based system instead learns client-specific models

$$\min_{\{\theta_k\}} \sum_{k=1}^{K} p_k \, \mathbb{E}_{(x,y)\sim\mathcal{P}_k} \big[\ell(f_{\theta_k}(x) y)\big] \tag{3}$$

Accordingly, our research question is:

*Under which types of domain shift does it pay to adapt the* ***data*** *(via harmonization), and under which types does it pay to adapt the* ***model*** *(via personalization)?*

To answer this, we design two federated medical imaging benchmarks that are deliberately dominated by different heterogeneity types: (i) colon polyp segmentation with large structural/contextual variation across four endoscopy datasets and (ii) Tuberculosis CXR classification with largely preserved anatomy but strong scanner/intensity variation across four CXR datasets.

## 2.2 Model Personalization and Data Harmonization Approaches Employed

We consider representative model personalization and data harmonization strategies commonly used in federated learning.

Model personalization methods adapt the global model to client-specific distributions. We group them into three categories: (1) layer-wise personalization, which shares a common backbone while keeping client-specific components local (e.g., FedPer [4], FedRep [5], FedBN [6]); (2) optimization-based approaches, which modify the training objective or update rules to handle heterogeneity (e.g., FedProx [19], SCAFFOLD [20], FedAdam [18]); and (3) bi-model and meta-learning approaches, which explicitly learn personalized client models alongside a global model (e.g., pFedMe [8], Ditto [21]).

Data harmonization methods aim to reduce inter-client appearance variation while preserving underlying structure. We consider: (1) basic preprocessing and augmentation to standardize resolution and intensity; (2) histogram-based methods that align intensity distributions across clients; (3) frequency-domain adaptation (FDA) to transfer low-frequency style information; (4) MixStyle-based approaches that interpolate feature or input statistics to simulate domain shifts; and (5) generative translation methods (e.g., CycleGAN [32], CUT [24], AdaIN [28], CoMoGAN [29]) that learn mappings between domains.

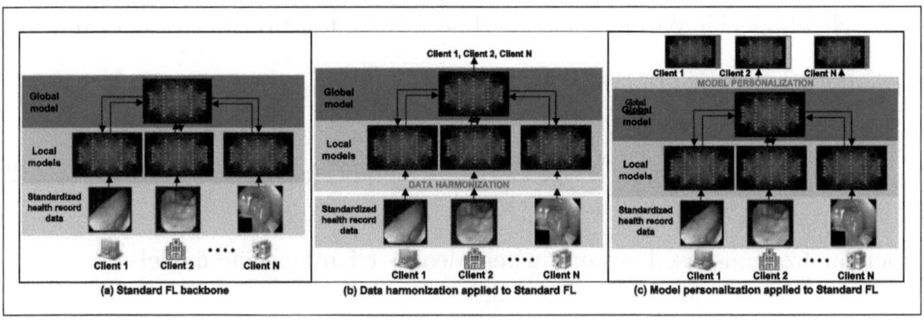


**Fig. 1.** Experimental methodology of the study.

### 2.3 Comparative Framework

As shown in Fig. 1, we instantiate model personalization and data harmonization strategies on top of a standard FL backbone (Flower [33]-based cross-silo FL with four clients per task). Each method uses the same base architecture for each task: a U-Net for colon polyp, skin lesion, and breast tumor segmentation; a DenseNet-based classifier for tuberculosis CXR; and an EfficientNet-based classifier for brain and breast tumor classification. All methods are trained with the same schedule and communication budget, ensuring that performance differences arise solely from the applied personalization or harmonization strategy.

*Tasks.* We design six FL settings using medical imaging tasks shown in Table 1:

*Baselines.* We include five non-personalized and non-harmonized baselines:

- **Locally-centralized**: each client trains its model solely on local data.
- **Centralized-globally tested**: a central model is trained on all clients' data and tested using all clients' pooled data.
- **Centralized-locally tested**: a central model is trained on all clients' data and tested using clients' local data separately in their local spaces.
- **Vanilla FedAvg-globally tested**: a single global model trained by standard FedAvg and tested using all clients' pooled data.
- **Vanilla FedAvg-locally tested**: a single global model trained by standard FedAvg and tested using clients' local data separately in their local spaces.

**Table 1.** Dataset composition across clients for the 6 tasks. Each client corresponds to a dataset with its sample size and fixed test split. Remaining data is split into 85% training and 15% validation.

(a) Segmentation tasks

| C# | Dataset | Modality | Total # | Test # |
|---|---|---|---|---|
| *Task 1: Colon polyp segmentation* | | | | |
| C1 | Kvasir-SEG [34] | Endoscopy | 1000 | 100 |
| C2 | ETIS-Larib [35] | Endoscopy | 196 | 19 |
| C3 | CVC-ColonDB [36] | Endoscopy | 380 | 38 |
| C4 | CVC-ClinicDB [37] | Endoscopy | 612 | 60 |
| *Task 2: Skin lesion segmentation* | | | | |
| C1 | HAM10K [38] | Dermoscopy | 10015 | 1001 |
| C2 | PH2 [39] | Dermoscopy | 200 | 20 |
| C3 | ISIC2017 [40] | Dermoscopy | 2000 | 200 |
| C4 | ISIC2018 [41] | Dermoscopy | 2594 | 259 |
| *Task 3: Breast tumor segmentation* | | | | |
| C1 | BUSBRA [42] | Ultrasound | 1875 | 81 |
| C2 | BUS_UC [43] | Ultrasound | 811 | 187 |
| C3 | BUSI [44] | Ultrasound | 437 | 43 |
| C4 | UDIAT [45] | Ultrasound | 163 | 16 |

(b) Classification tasks

| C# | Dataset | Modality | Total # | Test # |
|---|---|---|---|---|
| *Task 4: Tuberculosis CXR classification* | | | | |
| C1 | Shenzhen Hospital CXR [46] | X-ray | 662 | 65 |
| C2 | Montgomery County CXR [46] | X-ray | 138 | 13 |
| C3 | TBX11K [47] | X-ray | 1600 | 160 |
| C4 | Pakistan (local) | X-ray | 3008 | 300 |
| *Task 5: Brain tumor classification* | | | | |
| C1 | Sartajbhuvaji (Kaggle) [48] | MRI | 3160 | 314 |
| C2 | RM1000 (Kaggle) [49] | MRI | 7023 | 701 |
| C3 | thomasdubail (Kaggle) [50] | MRI | 3096 | 308 |
| C4 | Figshare [51] | MRI | 7200 | 720 |
| *Task 6: Breast tumor classification* | | | | |
| C1 | BUSBRA [42] | Ultrasound | 1875 | 186 |
| C2 | BUS_UC [43] | Ultrasound | 811 | 80 |
| C3 | BUSI [44] | Ultrasound | 647 | 64 |
| C4 | UDIAT [45] | Ultrasound | 163 | 15 |

## 3 Experimental Results

Table 2 shows one representative colon polyp sample per dataset after harmonization. Harmonized samples of other datasets are included in our code repository and are omitted here for space. We include the amplified difference, defined as the absolute per-pixel RGB difference between the original and harmonized images, scaled to highlight subtle color and contrast changes. Segmentation tasks use Dice as the primary metric (with IoU, pixel accuracy, precision, recall, and specificity), while classification tasks use Cohen's $\kappa$ (with accuracy, precision, recall, F1, and specificity). We compare harmonization and personalization methods and analyze trends by heterogeneity type (style vs. content). Results are reported in Tables 3 and 4.

**Table 2.** Examples of harmonized samples and amplified differences for Colon polyp (top), and skin lesion (bottom) datasets used for segmentation. H. = harmonized image; D. = amplified difference; Aug. = augmentation; Hist.mat. = histogram matching; ARI = average representative image; SRI = single representative image; FDA = Fourier domain adaptation.

| Image | | Aug. | Hist. mat. (SRI) | Hist. mat. (ARI) | FDA | Input level mixstyle | Feature level mixstyle | Cycle-GAN | CUT | AdaIN | CoMo-GAN |
|---|---|---|---|---|---|---|---|---|---|---|---|
| Colon polyp datasets | | | | | | | | | | | |

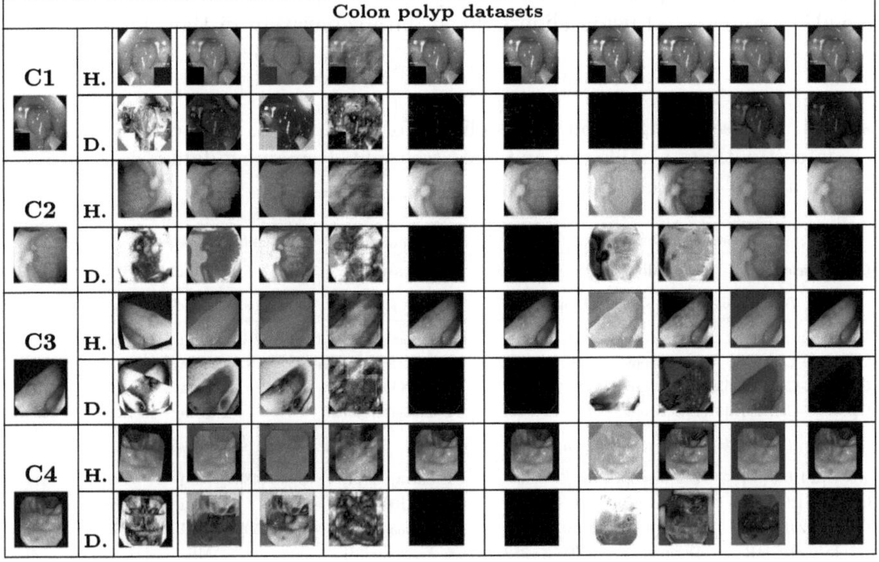


For colon polyp segmentation, where inter-client variation is large and primarily structural (e.g., shape and geometry), personalization methods consistently outperform harmonization, highlighting the need to adapt models to client-specific structures. In contrast, for skin lesion segmentation, where variation is more limited and largely appearance-driven, harmonization methods

**Table 3.** Data harmonization vs. model personalization across segmentation tasks. ARI = average representative image, SRI = single representative image. Best results are in **bold**.

| Method | Colon Polyp | | | | Skin Lesion | | | | Breast Tumor | | | |
|---|---|---|---|---|---|---|---|---|---|---|---|---|
| | C1 | C2 | C3 | C4 | C1 | C2 | C3 | C4 | C1 | C2 | C3 | C4 |
| *Baseline methods* | | | | | | | | | | | | |
| Locally centralized | 0.8297 | 0.7804 | 0.8857 | 0.8500 | 0.8920 | 0.8073 | 0.7692 | 0.8071 | 0.8367 | 0.9135 | 0.8049 | 0.7325 |
| Centralized – globally tested | 0.8499 | | | | 0.9250 | | | | 0.9008 | | | |
| Centralized – locally tested | 0.8024 | 0.7892 | 0.9121 | 0.8428 | 0.9178 | 0.8928 | 0.9374 | 0.9434 | 0.8998 | 0.9307 | 0.8419 | 0.9153 |
| Vanilla FedAvg – globally tested | 0.7286 | | | | 0.9355 | | | | 0.8933 | | | |
| Vanilla FedAvg – locally tested | 0.7559 | 0.4430 | 0.7508 | 0.8258 | 0.9283 | 0.9009 | 0.9448 | 0.9476 | 0.8964 | 0.9316 | 0.8027 | 0.9129 |
| *Harmonization methods* | | | | | | | | | | | | |
| Augmentations | 0.6698 | 0.3014 | 0.4714 | 0.6804 | 0.9217 | 0.8800 | 0.9322 | 0.9394 | 0.9351 | 0.9178 | 0.7424 | 0.9220 |
| Histogram matching (ARI) | 0.7149 | 0.3901 | 0.5892 | 0.7144 | 0.9153 | 0.8909 | 0.9322 | 0.9379 | 0.9145 | 0.8936 | 0.7997 | 0.8875 |
| Histogram matching (SRI) | 0.7749 | 0.6626 | 0.7336 | 0.7733 | 0.9141 | 0.9162 | 0.9307 | 0.9374 | 0.9193 | 0.8989 | 0.7747 | 0.8937 |
| FDA (SRI) | 0.7498 | 0.3888 | 0.6928 | 0.7233 | 0.8940 | 0.8465 | 0.9176 | 0.9216 | 0.8592 | 0.8807 | 0.7842 | 0.8477 |
| Input level MixStyle | 0.8296 | 0.6821 | 0.8270 | 0.8428 | 0.9114 | 0.8672 | 0.9324 | 0.9374 | 0.9173 | 0.8990 | 0.8073 | 0.9126 |
| Feature level MixStyle | 0.8336 | 0.6418 | 0.8273 | 0.8324 | 0.9237 | 0.8894 | 0.9375 | 0.9428 | 0.9237 | 0.8992 | 0.8022 | 0.9026 |
| Cycle-GAN | 0.8129 | 0.5506 | 0.6435 | 0.6685 | 0.9310 | 0.8926 | 0.9176 | 0.9355 | 0.8656 | 0.9174 | 0.7836 | 0.8390 |
| CUT | 0.6918 | 0.6069 | 0.8222 | 0.7056 | 0.9078 | 0.5536 | 0.4683 | 0.7853 | 0.5758 | 0.8600 | 0.3547 | 0.0421 |
| AdaIN | 0.7062 | 0.6282 | 0.8676 | 0.7679 | 0.7666 | 0.6694 | 0.7564 | 0.7484 | 0.9163 | 0.9025 | 0.8156 | 0.9062 |
| ComoGAN | 0.7774 | 0.5653 | 0.8498 | 0.8418 | 0.9204 | 0.9086 | 0.9362 | 0.9420 | 0.9185 | 0.9033 | 0.8014 | 0.9273 |
| *Personalization methods* | | | | | | | | | | | | |
| Local Finetuning | 0.8329 | 0.6914 | 0.8678 | 0.8311 | 0.9290 | 0.9100 | 0.9513 | 0.9501 | 0.9195 | 0.9087 | 0.8014 | 0.8875 |
| FedPer | 0.8085 | 0.4808 | 0.8212 | 0.8633 | 0.9206 | 0.9239 | 0.9427 | 0.9449 | 0.9233 | 0.9178 | 0.8270 | 0.8935 |
| FedRep | 0.8141 | 0.5503 | 0.8297 | 0.8775 | 0.9179 | 0.8984 | 0.9389 | 0.9423 | 0.9345 | 0.9073 | 0.8118 | 0.9093 |
| FedBN | 0.8200 | 0.6550 | 0.8287 | 0.8663 | 0.9229 | 0.8973 | 0.9366 | 0.9418 | 0.9341 | 0.9116 | 0.7887 | 0.9032 |
| FedProx | 0.8248 | 0.6829 | 0.7959 | 0.8173 | 0.8780 | 0.9307 | 0.9334 | 0.9156 | 0.9270 | 0.8955 | 0.8021 | 0.9138 |
| FedAdam | **0.8569** | **0.8332** | **0.9391** | **0.8906** | 0.9287 | 0.9124 | 0.9514 | 0.9511 | 0.9247 | 0.8975 | 0.8124 | 0.9043 |
| SCAFFOLD | 0.7368 | 0.3799 | 0.7083 | 0.7025 | 0.8715 | 0.8333 | 0.8940 | 0.9055 | 0.7006 | 0.7429 | 0.5701 | 0.5576 |
| pFedMe | 0.4564 | 0.1201 | 0.2354 | 0.4054 | 0.7233 | 0.8516 | 0.7843 | 0.7732 | 0.4158 | 0.1823 | 0.1654 | 0.1621 |
| Ditto | **0.8769** | **1.0000** | **1.0000** | **1.0000** | 0.9210 | 0.9232 | 0.9343 | 0.9416 | 0.9338 | 0.9026 | 0.8420 | 0.9089 |

(e.g., MixStyle, SRI, ComoGAN) perform comparably to personalization. Breast tumor segmentation follows a similar pattern, with both strategies achieving competitive performance, suggesting that when structural differences are moderate, neither approach has a clear advantage.

A similar trend is observed in classification tasks. For brain tumor classification, where inter-site variation is minimal, all methods reach near-ceiling performance, and neither harmonization nor personalization provides a clear benefit. Breast tumor classification shows comparable behavior, with both approaches yielding similar results across clients. In contrast, for tuberculosis CXR classification, where variation is dominated by appearance differences, harmonization consistently outperforms personalization by reducing input variability.

Overall, when inter-client differences are small or moderate, both strategies perform similarly regardless of task. When differences are large, the dominant type of variation determines the more effective approach: personalization is better suited for structurally heterogeneous segmentation tasks, whereas harmonization is more effective for appearance-driven classification tasks.

**Table 4.** Data harmonization vs. model personalization across classification tasks. ARI = average representative image, SRI = single representative image. Best results are in **bold**.

| Method | Tuberculosis CXR | | | | Brain Tumor | | | | Breast Tumor | | | |
|---|---|---|---|---|---|---|---|---|---|---|---|---|
| | C1 | C2 | C3 | C4 | C1 | C2 | C3 | C4 | C1 | C2 | C3 | C4 |
| *Baseline methods* | | | | | | | | | | | | |
| Locally centralized | 0.8462 | 0.6486 | 0.9750 | 0.9883 | 0.9563 | 0.9866 | 0.9690 | 0.9722 | 0.6353 | 0.6770 | 0.7764 | 0.7000 |
| Centralized – globally tested | 0.9656 | | | | 0.9941 | | | | 0.5872 | | | |
| Centralized – locally tested | 0.8768 | 0.6486 | 0.9875 | 0.9881 | 1.0000 | 0.9943 | 0.9911 | 0.9926 | 0.6398 | 0.4413 | 0.6513 | 0.5263 |
| Vanilla FedAvg – globally tested | 0.7763 | | | | 0.9974 | | | | 0.5466 | | | |
| Vanilla FedAvg – locally tested | 0.0000 | 0.0000 | 0.8500 | 0.9883 | 1.0000 | 0.9962 | 0.9956 | 0.9981 | 0.5645 | 0.3976 | 0.6074 | 0.6667 |
| *Harmonization methods* | | | | | | | | | | | | |
| Augmentations | 0.0901 | 0.0679 | 0.4631 | 0.6385 | 0.9956 | 0.9962 | 0.9956 | 0.9944 | 0.7251 | 0.4158 | 0.5320 | 0.6667 |
| Histogram matching (ARI) | 0.4937 | 0.4990 | 0.8625 | 1.0000 | 0.9956 | 0.9962 | 0.9823 | 0.9944 | 0.7451 | 0.4483 | 0.5412 | 0.6667 |
| Histogram matching (SRI) | 0.2536 | 0.3158 | 0.9000 | 1.0000 | 0.9956 | 0.9962 | 0.9603 | 0.9926 | 0.6385 | 0.3750 | 0.5412 | 0.6667 |
| FDA (SRI) | 0.1317 | 0.0000 | 0.8875 | 0.9542 | 0.9782 | 0.9790 | 0.9294 | 0.9778 | 0.3329 | 0.1832 | 0.3621 | 0.6667 |
| Input level MixStyle | 0.1898 | 0.0000 | 0.7750 | 1.0000 | 1.0000 | 1.0000 | 0.9734 | 0.9981 | 0.6596 | 0.3750 | 0.5218 | 0.6667 |
| Feature level MixStyle | 0.0634 | 0.0000 | 0.9250 | 1.0000 | 1.0000 | 1.0000 | 0.9823 | 0.9963 | 0.7359 | 0.3415 | 0.6177 | 0.6667 |
| Cycle-GAN | **0.5317** | **0.8158** | **0.7750** | **0.9883** | 0.9825 | 0.9867 | 0.9735 | 0.9648 | 0.6750 | 0.3077 | 0.5053 | 0.1429 |
| CUT | 0.0000 | 0.0000 | 0.7000 | 0.9883 | 1.0000 | 0.9962 | 0.9647 | 0.9926 | 0.6494 | 0.3333 | 0.2101 | 0.4706 |
| AdaIN | **0.5534** | **0.8434** | **0.8625** | **0.8606** | 0.9956 | 0.9962 | 0.9425 | 0.9889 | 0.4615 | 0.3671 | 0.3081 | 0.4706 |
| ComoGAN | 0.0000 | 0.0000 | 0.5250 | 1.0000 | 1.0000 | 0.9962 | 0.9734 | 0.9944 | 0.3654 | 0.2751 | 0.3932 | 0.7000 |
| *Personalization methods* | | | | | | | | | | | | |
| Local Finetuning | 0.0329 | 0.0914 | 0.8678 | 0.8217 | 0.9854 | 0.9760 | 0.9614 | 0.9340 | 0.5874 | 0.4476 | 0.5249 | 0.5682 |
| FedPer | 0.0634 | 0.0000 | 0.9125 | 0.9883 | 0.9956 | 0.9943 | 0.9911 | 0.9963 | 0.5994 | 0.4551 | 0.6074 | 0.6667 |
| FedRep | 0.0959 | 0.2041 | 0.9500 | 0.9883 | 0.9956 | 0.9943 | 0.9956 | 0.9926 | 0.6972 | 0.5280 | 0.6275 | 0.4000 |
| FedBN | 0.0000 | 0.0000 | 0.0000 | 0.0000 | 0.9826 | 0.9522 | 0.9297 | 0.8796 | 0.4639 | 0.5190 | 0.6456 | 0.4545 |
| FedProx | 0.3223 | 0.0990 | 0.9375 | 0.9883 | 0.9956 | 0.9981 | 0.9735 | 0.9963 | 0.3871 | 0.2298 | 0.4188 | 0.5263 |
| FedAdam | 0.0000 | 0.0000 | 0.0000 | 0.0000 | 0.0000 | 0.0000 | 0.0000 | 0.0000 | 0.0000 | 0.0000 | 0.0000 | 0.0000 |
| SCAFFOLD | 0.0000 | 0.0000 | 0.0000 | 0.0000 | 0.9869 | 0.9790 | 0.9691 | 0.9778 | 0.0000 | 0.0000 | 0.0000 | 0.0000 |
| pFedMe | 0.2547 | 0.1420 | 0.2847 | 0.4875 | 0.0890 | 0.0890 | 0.0305 | 0.1130 | 0.0000 | 0.0000 | 0.0000 | 0.0000 |
| Ditto | 0.7841 | 0.6486 | 1.0000 | 0.9268 | 0.9956 | 0.9943 | 0.9956 | 0.9926 | 0.6446 | 0.3191 | 0.5849 | 0.6667 |

## 4 Conclusions and Future Works

The results reveal a conditional trade-off rather than a strictly task-dependent pattern. When inter-client differences are large and primarily structural, as in colon polyp segmentation, personalization outperforms harmonization by adapting to client-specific geometry and context. In contrast, when variation is dominated by appearance and intensity differences, as in tuberculosis CXR classification, harmonization is more effective by reducing input variability and supporting a shared global model. However, this trend does not hold universally. When inter-client differences are small or moderate, both strategies perform similarly, as observed in skin lesion and breast tumor segmentation, as well as brain and breast tumor classification, where neither approach offers a clear advantage. Overall, the effectiveness of harmonization versus personalization is governed by the type and magnitude of dataset heterogeneity rather than the task alone. In practice, federated medical imaging systems should assess cross-site variation before selecting a strategy, rather than assuming a fixed preference. A key limitation is the assumption that inter-client heterogeneity is known a priori, whereas in practice it is unknown and dynamic. Future work should develop metrics to characterize heterogeneity directly from data and enable adaptive frameworks that combine harmonization and personalization at multiple levels. Extending this analysis to non-stationary settings and incorporating causal modeling are important directions. Standardized benchmarks and evaluation of performance–privacy–communication trade-offs are also needed.

**Disclosure of Interests.** The authors have no competing interests to declare that are relevant to the content of this article.

## References


1. McMahan, B., Moore, E., Ramage, D., Hampson, S., Aguera y Arcas, B.: Communication-efficient learning of deep networks from decentralized data. In: Proceedings of AISTATS, pp. 1273–1282. PMLR, Fort Lauderdale, FL, USA (2017)
2. Shiranthika, C., Saeedi, P., Bajić, I.V.: Decentralized learning in healthcare: a review of emerging techniques. IEEE Access **11**, 54188–54209 (2023). https://doi.org/10.1109/ACCESS.2023.3281832
3. Shiranthika, C., Hadizadeh, H., Saeedi, P., Bajić, I.V.: Adaptive asynchronous split federated learning for medical image segmentation. IEEE Access **12**, 182496–182515 (2024). https://doi.org/10.1109/ACCESS.2024.3511430
4. Arivazhagan, M.G., Aggarwal, V., Singh, A.K., Choudhary, S.: Federated Learning with Personalization Layers. arXiv preprint arXiv:1912.00818 (2019)
5. Collins, L., Hassani, H., Mokhtari, A., Shakkottai, S.: Exploiting shared representations for personalized federated learning. In: Proceedings of ICML, Proceedings of Machine Learning and Research, vol. 139, pp. 2089–2099. PMLR (2021)
6. Li, X., Jiang, M., Zhang, X., Kamp, M., Dou, Q.: FedBN: Federated Learning on Non-IID Features via Local Batch Normalization. arXiv preprint arXiv:2102.07623 (2021)
7. Chen, F., Luo, M., Dong, Z., Li, Z., He, X.: Federated Meta-Learning with Fast Convergence and Efficient Communication. arXiv preprint arXiv:1802.07876 (2018)
8. Dinh, C.T., Tran, N., Nguyen, J.: Personalized federated learning with Moreau envelopes. In: Proceedings of NeurIPS, vol. 33, pp. 21394–21405 (2020)
9. Fallah, A., Mokhtari, A., Ozdaglar, A.: Personalized federated learning with theoretical guarantees: a model-agnostic meta-learning approach. In: Proceedings of NeurIPS, vol. 33, pp. 3557–3568 (2020)
10. Huang, Y., et al.: Personalized cross-silo federated learning on non-IID data. In: Proceedings of AAAI, vol. 35, no. 9, pp. 7865–7873 (2021)
11. Smith, V., Chiang, C.-K., Sanjabi, M., Talwalkar, A.S.: Federated multi-task learning. In: Proceedings of NeurIPS, vol. 30 (2017)
12. Corinzia, L., Beuret, A., Buhmann, J.M.: Variational Federated Multi-Task Learning. arXiv preprint arXiv:1906.06268 (2019)
13. Ghosh, A., Chung, J., Yin, D., Ramchandran, K.: An efficient framework for clustered federated learning. In: Proceedings of NeurIPS, vol. 33, pp. 19586–19597 (2020)
14. Chen, C., Chen, Z., Zhou, Y., Kailkhura, B.: FedCluster: boosting the convergence of federated learning via cluster-cycling. In: IEEE BigData 2020, pp. 5017–5026. IEEE (2020)

15. Duan, M., et al.: FedGroup: efficient federated learning via decomposed similarity-based clustering. In: 2021 IEEE International Conference on Parallel and Distributed Processing with Applications, Big Data and Cloud Computing, Sustainable Computing and Communications, Social Computing and Networking (ISPA/BDCloud/SocialCom/SustainCom), pp. 228–237. IEEE (2021)
16. Li, D., Wang, J.: FedMD: Heterogenous Federated Learning via Model Distillation. arXiv preprint arXiv:1910.03581 (2019)
17. Zhang, H., Zhu, Y., Wu, T., Cheng, S., Liu, J.: Model-heterogeneous federated learning with bidirectional knowledge distillation. IEEE Trans. Mob. Comput. (2025). https://doi.org/10.1109/TMC.2025.3599315
18. Reddi, S., et al.: Adaptive federated optimization. In: Proceedings of ICLR (2021)
19. Li, T., Sahu, A.K., Zaheer, M., Sanjabi, M., Talwalkar, A., Smith, V.:Federated optimization in heterogeneous networks. In: Proceedings of MLSys, vol. 2, pp. 429–450 (2020)
20. Karimireddy, S.P., Kale, S., Mohri, M., Reddi, S., Stich, S., Suresh, A.T.: SCAFFOLD: stochastic controlled averaging for federated learning. In: Proceedings of the 37th International Conference on Machine Learning (ICML 2020), Proceedings of Machine Learning and Research, vol. 119, pp. 5132–5143. PMLR (2020)
21. Li, T., Hu, S., Beirami, A., Smith, V.: Ditto: fair and robust federated learning through personalization. In: Proceedings of ICML 2021, Proceedings Machine Learning and Research, vol. 139, pp. 6357–6368. PMLR (2021)
22. Mali, S.A., et al.: Making radiomics more reproducible across scanner and imaging protocol variations: a review of harmonization methods. J. Pers. Med. **11**(9), 842 (2021)
23. Liu, M., et al.: Alzheimer's Disease Neuroimaging Initiative: Style transfer generative adversarial networks to harmonize multisite MRI to a single reference image to avoid overcorrection. Hum. Brain Mapp. **44**(14), 4875–4892 (2023)
24. Park, T., Efros, A.A., Zhang, R., Zhu, J.-Y.: Contrastive learning for unpaired image-to-image translation. In: Vedaldi, A., Bischof, H., Brox, T., Frahm, J.-M. (eds.) ECCV 2020. LNCS, vol. 12354, pp. 319–345. Springer, Cham (2020). https://doi.org/10.1007/978-3-030-58545-7_19
25. Dewey, B.E., et al.: DeepHarmony: a deep learning approach to contrast harmonization across scanner changes. Magn. Reson. Imaging **64**, 160–170 (2019). https://doi.org/10.1016/j.mri.2019.05.041
26. Cackowski, S., Barbier, E.L., Dojat, M., Christen, T.: Imunity: a generalizable VAE-GAN solution for multicenter MR image harmonization. MIA **88**, 102799 (2023). https://doi.org/10.1016/j.media.2023.102799
27. Jeong, H., Byun, H., Kang, D.U., Lee, J.: BlindHarmony: "blind" harmonization for MR images via flow model. In: Proceedings of ICCV, pp. 21129–21139 (2023)
28. Huang, X., Belongie, S.: Arbitrary style transfer in real-time with adaptive instance normalization. In: Proceedings of ICCV, pp. 1501–1510. IEEE (2017)
29. Pizzati, F., Cerri, P., De Charette, F.: CoMoGAN: continuous model-guided image-to-image translation. In: Proceedings of CVPR, pp. 14288–14298. IEEE/CVF (2021)
30. Hu, X., Zhou, X., Huang, Q., Shi, Z., Sun, L., Li, Q.: QS-Attn: query-selected attention for contrastive learning in image-to-image translation. In: Proceedings of CVPR, pp. 18291–18300. IEEE/CVF (2022)
31. Guo, Z., Guo, D., Zheng, H., Gu, Z., Zheng, B., Dong, J.: Image harmonization with transformer. In: Proceedings of ICCV, pp. 14870–14879 (2021)

32. Zhu, J.-Y., Park, T., Isola, P., Efros, A.A.: Unpaired image-to-image translation using cycle-consistent adversarial networks. In: Proceedings of ICCV, pp. 2223–2232. IEEE (2017)
33. Beutel, D.J., et al.: Flower: a friendly federated learning research framework. arXiv preprint arXiv:2007.14390 (2020)
34. Jha, D., et al.: Kvasir-SEG: a segmented polyp dataset. In: Ro, Y.M., et al. (eds.) MMM 2020. LNCS, vol. 11962, pp. 451–462. Springer, Cham (2020). https://doi.org/10.1007/978-3-030-37734-2_37
35. Silva, J., Histace, A., Romain, O., Dray, X., Granado, B.: Toward embedded detection of polyps in WCE images for early diagnosis of colorectal cancer. IJCARS **9**(2), 283–293 (2014)
36. Bernal, J., Sánchez, J., Vilarino, F.: Towards automatic polyp detection with a polyp appearance model. Pattern Recogn. **45**(9), 3166–3182 (2012)
37. Bernal, J., Sánchez, F.J., Fernández-Esparrach, G., Gil, D., Rodriguez, C., Vilarino, F.: WMDOVA maps for accurate polyp highlighting in colonoscopy: validation vs. saliency maps from physicians. Comput. Med. Imaging Graph **43**, 99–111 (2015)
38. Tschandl, P., Rosendahl, C., Kittler, H.: The HAM10000 dataset, a large collection of multi-source dermatoscopic images of common pigmented skin lesions. Sci. Data **5**(1), 180161 (2018)
39. Mendonça, T., Ferreira, P.M., Marques, J., Marcal, A.R.S., Rozeira, J.: $PH^2$ - a dermoscopic image database for research and benchmarking. In: Proceedings of IEEE EMBC, Osaka, Japan (2013)
40. Codella, N.C.F., et al.: Skin lesion analysis toward melanoma detection: 2017 ISBI challenge. arXiv preprint arXiv:1703.00523 (2017)
41. Codella, N.C.F., et al.: Skin lesion analysis toward melanoma detection 2018: 2017 ISIC challenge. arXiv preprint arXiv:1807.07391 (2018)
42. Gómez-Flores, W., Gregorio-Calas, M.J., Coelho de Albuquerque Pereira, W.: BUS-BRA: a breast ultrasound dataset for assessing computer-aided diagnosis systems. Med. Phys. **51**(4), 3110–3123 (2024)
43. Rodrigues, P.S., et al.: BUS_UC: breast ultrasound dataset. Mendeley Data, V1 (2017). https://data.mendeley.com/datasets/3ksd7w7jkx/1
44. Al-Dhabyani, W., Gomaa, M., Khaled, H., Fahmy, A.: Dataset of breast ultrasound images. Data Brief **28**, 104863 (2020)
45. Yap, M.H., et al.: Automated breast ultrasound lesions detection using convolutional neural networks. IEEE JBHI **22**(4), 1218–1226 (2018)
46. Jaeger, S., Candemir, S., Antani, S., Wáng, Y.-X.J., Lu, P.-X., Thoma, G.: Two public chest X-ray datasets for computer-aided screening of pulmonary diseases. Quant. Imaging Med. Surg. **4**, 475–477 (2014)
47. Liu, Y., Wu, Y.-H., Ban, Y., Wang, H., Cheng, M.-M.: Rethinking computer-aided tuberculosis diagnosis. In: Proceedings of CVPR, pp. 2646–2655. IEEE/CVF (2020)
48. Bhuvaji, S.: Brain tumor classification (MRI). Kaggle dataset (2020). https://www.kaggle.com/datasets/sartajbhuvaji/brain-tumor-classification-mri
49. rm1000: Brain tumor MRI scans. Kaggle dataset. https://www.kaggle.com/datasets/rm1000/brain-tumor-mri-scans
50. Dubail, T.: Brain tumors (256x256). Kaggle dataset (2020). https://www.kaggle.com/datasets/thomasdubail/brain-tumors-256x256
51. Cheng, J., et al.: Enhanced performance of brain tumor classification via tumor region augmentation and partition. PLoS ONE **10**(10), e0140381 (2015)

# Action-Level Kinematic Analysis for Objective Performance Assessment in Microanastomosis

Yan Meng[1(✉)], Daniel A. Donoho[1], Robert D. M. Hutchinson[2], Marcelle Altshuler[3], and Omar Arnaout[3]

[1] Department of Neurosurgery, Children's National Hospital, Washington, DC 20010, USA
{mengy,ddonoho}@childrensnational.org

[2] School of Medicine and Health Sciences, George Washington University, Washington, DC 20052, USA
robert.hutchinson@gwu.edu

[3] Department of Neurosurgery, Brigham and Women's Hospital, Harvard Medical School, Boston, MA 02115, USA
{maltshuler,oarnaout}@bwh.harvard.edu

**Abstract.** Proficiency in microanastomosis is a critical surgical skill in neurosurgery to successful outcomes. There is a pressing need for automated and scalable assessment methods. To address this challenge, we introduce a novel AI-driven framework for automated action segmentation and performance assessment in microanastomosis procedures, designed to operate efficiently on edge computing platforms. The proposed system comprises three main components: (1) an object tracking and tip localization module; (2) an action segmentation module leveraging self-similarity matrix for action clustering; and (3) a supervised classification module to evaluate surgical gesture proficiency. Experimental validation on a dataset of 58 expert-rated microanastomosis videos demonstrates the effectiveness of our approach, achieving a frame-level action segmentation accuracy of 92.4% and an overall skill classification accuracy of 85.5% in replicating expert evaluations. These findings demonstrate the potential of the proposed method to provide objective, real-time feedback in microsurgical education, thereby enabling more standardized, data-driven training protocols and advancing competency assessment in surgical environments.

**Keywords:** Artificial intelligence · Computer vision · Action segmentation · Object detection and tracking · Surgical skill assessment

## 1 Introduction

In high-stakes environments, such as surgery, the ability to interpret fine-grained actions has direct implications for education, accreditation, and ultimately, patient safety. Among various surgical domains, microanastomosis procedures

© The Author(s), under exclusive license to Springer Nature Switzerland AG 2027
P. Andreev et al. (Eds.): AIME 2026, LNAI 16748, pp. 164–168, 2027.
https://doi.org/10.1007/978-3-032-30710-1_19

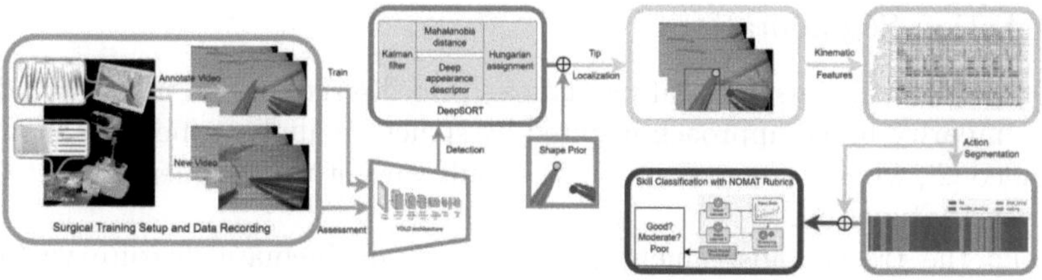


**Fig. 1.** Microanastomosis skill assessment framework overview.

exemplify the highest levels of technical difficulty. These tasks require precise manipulation, making them an ideal testbed for AI-driven video understanding.

Traditional methods for evaluating surgical performance rely heavily on expert raters using scoring rubrics such as Objective Structured Assessment of Technical Skill (OSATS) [4], and Northwestern Objective Microanastomosis Assessment Tool (NOMAT) [1]. While informative, such assessments are labor-intensive and subjective. There has been growing interest in using machine learning to automate surgical skill assessment [3,5], often by modeling instrument trajectories, motion dynamics, or gesture sequences. However, many existing approaches focus on coarse-grained scoring, lack interpretability, or fail to generalize across procedures.

In this paper, we focus on the problem of action segmentation and skill assessment in microanastomosis videos, where the goal is to segment surgical procedures into discrete action units and assess performance based on instrument handling behavior.

## 2 Method

We propose a framework for automated action segmentation and surgical skill assessment in microanastomosis videos as show in Fig. 1. The system consists of three primary components: (1) surgical instrument tip detection and tracking module adapted from YOLO and DeepSORT; (2) unsupervised action segmentation using a novelty function derived from a self-similarity matrix; and (3) supervised classification for action-level skill evaluation.

### 2.1 Instrument Tip Detection and Tracking

We adopt a hybrid detection-tracking strategy that integrates YOLO with an enhanced variant of DeepSORT, a multi-object tracker that associates detections using motion and appearance features [6]. The DeepSORT implementation is augmented with a ResNet-based appearance descriptor to enable robust identity preservation across frames.

We estimate the instrument tip position within each tracking bounding box by using a shape descriptor that captures local geometric features [6]. The position over time trajectories can be used for downstream tasks.

### 2.2 Action Segmentation

To segment continuous surgical procedures into discrete action units, we adopt a self-similarity based approach inspired by structure analysis methods in audio and video [2], where change points in the multivariant time sequence is detected with novelty function.

From the tracked instrument tip positions, a kinematic feature vector is extracted at each frame, comprising the velocity, acceleration, and jerk of each individual instrument, as well as inter-instrument distance, relative velocity, dot product, and angle. To partition the continuous video stream into discrete surgical actions, we construct a self-similarity matrix (SSM) $S$ by computing pairwise cosine similarity between the normalized kinematic feature vectors, then take $S^{'} = S^2$ to enhance the contrast of block-diagonal structures. We compute a novelty function over time with a Gaussian kernel in Eq. 1.

$$N(t) = \sum_{i=-h}^{h-1} \sum_{j=-h}^{h-1} G(i,j) \cdot C(i,j) \cdot S^{'}(t+i, t+j) \tag{1}$$

where $G(i,j)$ is a 2D Gaussian function, $C(i,j)$ is the checkerboard structure with alternating positive and negative quadrants, and $h$ is half of the kernel size.

Following the detection of temporal boundaries using the novelty function, descriptive features are then extracted from each segment to facilitate unsupervised clustering of meaning actions. For each segment $s_i$, we concatenate the mean and standard deviation of the segment with a indicator musk of instrument presence in the scene, which is semantically informative to the action classification. We apply K-means clustering to this feature summary matrix with an objective function that minimize within-cluster variance.

### 2.3 Microanastomosis Skill Classification

Each video captures a complete microanastomosis procedure, comprising three vessel cuts followed by eight suture placements. We adopt the NOMAT rubric as an evaluation standard and emulate expert grading using a supervised machine learning approach, where ground truth labels are provided by board-certified neurosurgeons. For skill classification, we employ a Gradient Boosting Classifier (GBC). It takes as input a feature vector constructed from each action, including the feature summary, action label, number of repetitions, and duration of each action. The output is a categorical skill label: Poor, Moderate, or Good, corresponding to the expert-rated performance levels.

## 3 Experiments

We conducted a comprehensive experimental study to evaluate the effectiveness of the proposed framework. All data collection procedures and study protocols were reviewed and approved by the Institutional Review Board of our collaborating institution.

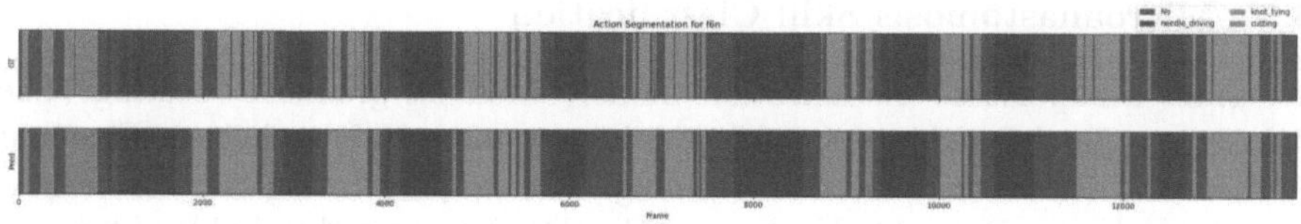


**Fig. 2.** An example of the action segmentation results compared with ground truth label.

### 3.1 Data Curation

Microanastomosis procedures were conducted within a controlled simulation environment using standardized microsurgical training kits. A total of nine medical practitioners (8 male, 1 female; average age of 30.5 years) participated in this study, representing a broad spectrum of microsurgical experience. Each participant performed between five to ten procedures, resulting in 58 recordings captured the entire procedure from start to finish, with an average duration of approximately 26 min.

Three board-certified neurosurgeons independently evaluated the videos using the NOMAT rubric and obtained average scores. Performance was rated on a five-point Likert scale, with higher scores reflecting better proficiency.

**Table 1.** Proposed action segmentation method performance.

| Test set | Acc | Prec | Rec | F1 | Jacc |
|---|---|---|---|---|---|
| 20 videos | 0.924 | 0.764 | 0.824 | 0.790 | 0.735 |

**Table 2.** Needle driving and knot tying action skill evaluation.

| Level | Needle Driving | | | Knot Tying | | |
|---|---|---|---|---|---|---|
| | Prec | Rec | F1 | Prec | Rec | F1 |
| Poor | 0.89 | 1.00 | 0.94 | 0.89 | 1.00 | 0.94 |
| Moderate | 0.80 | 0.97 | 0.88 | 0.80 | 0.97 | 0.88 |
| Good | 1.00 | 0.67 | 0.80 | 1.00 | 0.67 | 0.80 |

### 3.2 Kinematic-Based Action Segmentation

For the purpose of action segmentation and classification, we define three primary action classes corresponding to semantically meaningful microsurgical actions: **Cutting**, **Needle Driving**, and **Knot Tying**. In addition, we include a fourth class, labeled as **No Action** to group frames that have no instrument in the scene, or the instruments moving in the background with no clear actions.

To evaluate the performance of the unsupervised clustering algorithm, we manually annotated 20 videos with frame-level action labels. The quantitative results of the segmentation is reported in Table 1, where our method achieves an action segmentation accuracy of 92.41%. A qualitative comparison between the unsupervised action segmentation and ground truth annotations for an example video is illustrated in Fig. 2.

### 3.3 Microanastomosis Skill Classification

We train a supervised classification model based on gradient boosting. The dataset was partitioned into an 80% training set and a 20% testing set. Five-fold cross-validation was employed in training. The original rating was discretized into three classes: Poor, Moderate, and Good, using score thresholds of 2.5 and 3.5, resulted in class distributions of 32, 15, and 11 samples, respectively, for the needle driving action, and 37, 10, and 11 samples for the knot tying action. The classification results for each action type are summarized in Table 2. The gradient boosting classifier achieved an accuracy of 84% on needle driving actions and 88% on knot tying actions, resulting in an average classification accuracy of 85.5% across both action types. These findings demonstrate that the proposed system is capable of performing interpretable, action-level skill assessment.

## 4 Conclusion

In this paper, we present an AI-driven framework for automated action segmentation and skill assessment in microanastomosis procedures, addressing the need for objective, scalable, and fine-grained evaluation in surgical training. Experimental results demonstrate that our method offers grading outputs that align with established NOMAT rubrics, enabling interpretable feedback for trainees. The modularity of the framework allows for future extensions and generalization to other surgical tasks or procedural domains.

## References

1. Aoun, S.G., et al.: A pilot study to assess the construct and face validity of the northwestern objective microanastomosis assessment tool. J. Neurosurg. **123**(1), 103–109 (2015)
2. Funke, I., Mees, S.T., Weitz, J., Speidel, S.: Video-based surgical skill assessment using 3d convolutional neural networks. Int. J. Comput. Assist. Radiol. Surg. **14**, 1217–1225 (2019)
3. Lavanchy, J.L., et al.: Automation of surgical skill assessment using a three-stage machine learning algorithm. Sci. Rep. **11**(1), 5197 (2021)
4. Martin, J., et al.: Objective structured assessment of technical skill (OSATS) for surgical residents. Br. J. Surg. **84**(2), 273–278 (1997)
5. Meng, Y., Hahn, J.K.: An automatic grading system for neonatal endotracheal intubation with multi-task convolutional neural network. In: 2023 IEEE EMBS International Conference on Biomedical and Health Informatics (BHI), pp. 1–4. IEEE (2023)
6. Meng, Y., et al.: An AI framework for microanastomosis motion assessment (2025). Accepted to IEEE/EMBS 12th Annual International Conference on Neural Engineering, NER 2025 https://arxiv.org/abs/2601.21120

# Lesion-Preserving Multi-view Facial UV Texture Reconstruction

Sena Lee[1], Seungphil Hong[2], and Sejung Yang[1,3](✉)

[1] Department of Precision Medicine, Yonsei University Wonju College of Medicine, Wonju, Republic of Korea
syang@yonsei.ac.kr

[2] Department of Dermatology, Yonsei University Wonju College of Medicine, Wonju, Republic of Korea

[3] Department of Medical Informatics and Biostatistics, Yonsei University Wonju College of Medicine, Wonju, Republic of Korea

**Abstract.** Lesion-preserving facial UV textures are critical for quantitative 3D analysis of skin diseases such as vitiligo, yet conventional multi-view UV generation often blurs lesion boundaries. We propose PALM-UV, a pose-aware multi-view texture reconstruction framework that aligns inputs via landmark-based normalization and performs UV remapping using projection coordinates and visibility-guided soft blending to reduce lesion distortion. Evaluated on clinical images from 230 patients (690 images across three views), PALM-UV consistently improves perceptual and reconstruction quality, achieving lower LPIPS, higher PSNR, and reduced MAE. Improvements are particularly pronounced in lateral views, and all results are statistically significant ($p < 0.001$).

**Keywords:** 3D face reconstruction · Facial UV texture · Multi-view reconstruction · Lesion preservation · Reliability-aware blending · Vitiligo

## 1 Introduction

3D face reconstruction with UV texture mapping has been widely used in medical image analysis [1–4]. Recent multi-view methods (e.g., FFHQ-UV [6]) focus on visual realism using hard mask blending and template-based completion, which are not suitable for clinical analysis where preserving lesion boundaries is critical. To address this limitation, we propose PALM-UV, a lesion-preserving multi-view UV texture reconstruction framework that replaces hard mask fusion and template-based completion with visibility-guided soft blending, enabling reliability-aware integration of multi-view textures without distorting lesion structures. The method also incorporates pose-aware projection correction and Laplacian pyramid blending to improve geometric consistency while preserving fine lesion details.

© The Author(s), under exclusive license to Springer Nature Switzerland AG 2027
P. Andreev et al. (Eds.): AIME 2026, LNAI 16748, pp. 169–173, 2027.
https://doi.org/10.1007/978-3-032-30710-1_20

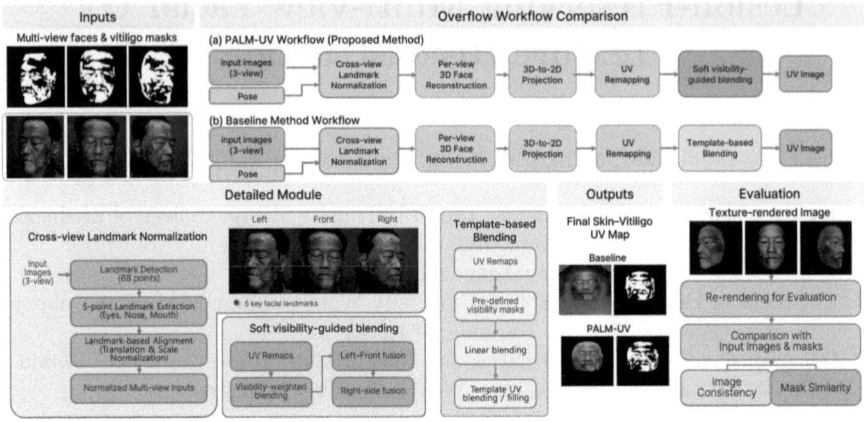


**Fig. 1.** Overview of the PALM-UV framework and baseline comparison.

## 2 Method

PALM-UV generates lesion-preserving UV textures from multi-view facial images. For pose-aware view assignment, yaw angles estimated from 3D face reconstruction coefficients are used to assign the inputs to left, front, and right views. For landmark-based normalization, 68 facial landmarks are detected, five key landmarks are extracted, and the inputs are aligned and cropped before UV remapping. The normalized inputs are then processed through mesh reconstruction, UV remapping, and reliability-aware soft blending, as shown in Fig. 1.

### 2.1 Mesh Generation and UV Remapping

Given the normalized three-view images, we reconstruct a 3D face mesh using ReconNet-based HIFI3D++ [7], which provides consistent topology and UV layout. Using the estimated camera parameters, projection coordinates (projXY) map UV pixels to image space, allowing each input image to be remapped onto the UV domain:

$$T^{(v)}(\mathbf{u}) = I^{(v)}\big(\mathbf{x}^{(v)}(\mathbf{u})\big), \tag{1}$$

where $v \in \{\text{left}, \text{front}, \text{right}\}$. This produces partial UV textures and corresponding visibility masks for each view.

### 2.2 Baseline Texture Generation

The baseline follows the FFHQ-UV pipeline [6]. Remapped textures are sequentially fused using predefined hard masks (left $\rightarrow$ right $\rightarrow$ front), and missing regions are completed using a template UV map. Unreliable areas such as eyes and mouth are further refined via Poisson blending. While this approach ensures

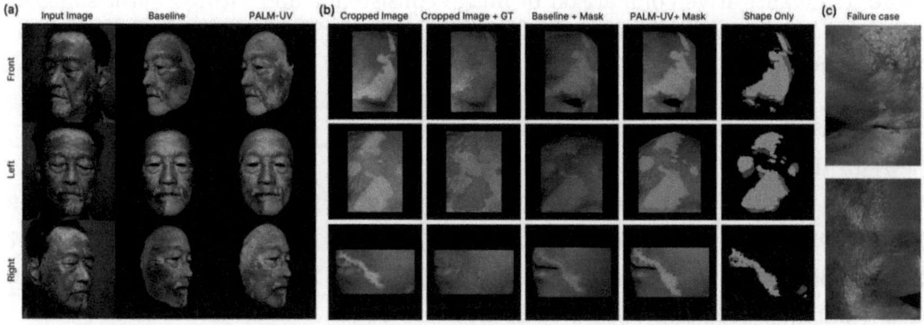


**Fig. 2.** Qualitative comparison between the baseline and PALM-UV for (a) image consistency, (b) vitiligo mask similarity, and (c) representative failure case caused by illumination inconsistency and glare across views.

full UV coverage, hard mask transitions and template-based completion often blur fine details and degrade lesion boundaries.

### 2.3 PALM-UV Texture Generation

PALM-UV replaces hard mask-based fusion with reliability-aware soft blending. For each view, the input image is remapped into the UV domain, producing a partial texture $T^{(v)}$ and a valid-region mask $M^{(v)}$. Reliability is defined as a soft visibility weight obtained by Gaussian smoothing of the valid-region mask:

$$W_{\text{front}}(\mathbf{u}) = \mathcal{G}_\sigma * M_{\text{front}}(\mathbf{u}), \tag{2}$$

where $\mathbf{u}$ denotes a UV pixel. In our implementation, an $11 \times 11$ Gaussian kernel with $\sigma = 7$ is used. The left and right textures are first combined within their valid regions, and the final UV texture is generated by six-level Laplacian pyramid blending between the front texture and the combined side texture using $W_{\text{front}}$ as the blending weight. The same reliability weight is applied to the remapped vitiligo masks, while side-view lesion regions are explicitly preserved outside the front-view valid region to prevent lesion loss.

### 2.4 Experimental Setup and Evaluation

We evaluate PALM-UV on a clinical vitiligo dataset (230 patients, 690 images across three views; IRB No. 2024-0193-001) from Yonsei University Wonju Severance Christian Hospital, with lesion masks annotated by board-certified dermatologists. The generated UV textures are rendered from a consistent viewpoint and compared with the input images. **Image consistency.** To assess image-level fidelity, we compare the rendered images with the input images using LPIPS (Learned Perceptual Image Patch Similarity), PSNR (Peak Signal-to-Noise Ratio), and MAE (Mean Absolute Error). LPIPS and MAE are lower-is-better metrics, whereas PSNR is a higher-is-better metric. **Vitiligo mask**

**Table 1.** Quantitative comparison of image consistency and vitiligo mask similarity. Values are presented as Baseline/PALM-UV (Mean ± SD for image metrics, Median for mask metrics).

| Image Consistency | | | |
|---|---|---|---|
| View | LPIPS ↓ | PSNR ↑ | MAE ↓ |
| Front | 0.211 ± 0.039/**0.205 ± 0.041** | 18.71 ± 1.77/**19.20 ± 1.78** | 23.21 ± 5.07/**21.10 ± 4.97** |
| Left | 0.291 ± 0.038/**0.247 ± 0.039** | 14.20 ± 1.39/**16.65 ± 1.55** | 42.47 ± 7.17/**29.79 ± 5.77** |
| Right | 0.266 ± 0.041/**0.223 ± 0.039** | 14.53 ± 1.51/**17.31 ± 1.68** | 41.06 ± 7.96/**27.36 ± 6.00** |
| Mask Similarity (Median) | | | |
| Metric | Compactness | LAR | Solidity |
| Mask | 0.267/**0.190** | 0.104/**0.070** | 0.080/**0.057** |

**similarity.** To quantitatively evaluate lesion preservation, we compute shape-based descriptors from the lesion mask in UV space. Let $\mathcal{M}$ denote the binary lesion mask, $A$ the total lesion area, and $A_{\text{largest}}$, $P_{\text{largest}}$, and $A_{\text{hull}}$ denote the area and perimeter of the largest connected component and its convex hull area, respectively. The metrics are defined as compactness ($4\pi A_{\text{largest}}/P^2_{\text{largest}}$), largest area ratio (LAR) ($A_{\text{largest}}/A$), and solidity ($A_{\text{largest}}/A_{\text{hull}}$). Compactness measures shape regularity, the largest area ratio reflects fragmentation, and solidity captures boundary smoothness. Statistical significance is evaluated using the Wilcoxon signed-rank test ($p < 0.001$).

# 3 Experimental Results and Analysis

## 3.1 Image Consistency Evaluation

Table 1 summarizes the image consistency results across three views. PALM-UV consistently outperforms the baseline, achieving lower LPIPS and MAE and higher PSNR. The improvements are more pronounced in side views, with notable gains in LPIPS, PSNR, and MAE, indicating more accurate reconstruction under challenging conditions. These results suggest that visibility-guided blending effectively reduces artifacts caused by hard mask transitions and template-based completion. As shown in Fig. 2(a), the baseline exhibits blurring and discontinuities near view boundaries, whereas PALM-UV produces smoother and more coherent textures. All improvements are statistically significant based on the Wilcoxon signed-rank test ($p < 0.001$).

## 3.2 Vitiligo Mask Similarity Evaluation

Table 1 compares shape-based lesion descriptors in UV space. PALM-UV yields lower compactness, largest area ratio, and solidity than the baseline. While higher values typically indicate more regular shapes, the baseline results are affected by template-based filling, which tends to oversmooth and expand lesion regions. In contrast, PALM-UV preserves lesion structures more faithfully, resulting in more consistent and less fragmented masks. This is also observed in Fig. 2(b), where PALM-UV better maintains lesion boundaries, especially in side-view regions.

## 4 Conclusion

We proposed PALM-UV, a visibility-guided UV texture generation framework for lesion-preserving facial reconstruction. By replacing hard mask fusion and template-based completion with soft visibility weighting and Laplacian pyramid blending, PALM-UV improves image consistency and lesion preservation, especially in side views. A representative failure case is shown in Fig. 2(c), where illumination differences and glare cause inconsistent reflections due to photometric mismatch or errors propagated from the FFHQ-UV reconstruction pipeline. Future work will focus on illumination normalization, glare-aware weighting, and more robust 3D reconstruction.

**Acknowledgments.** This research was supported in part by the National Research Foundation of Korea (NRF), funded by the Korean government (MSIT), under Grant Nos. 2022R1A2C2091160 and RS-2024-00440802, and in part by the Regional Innovation System & Education (RISE) Program through the Gangwon RISE Center, funded by the Ministry of Education (MOE) and Gangwon State (G.S.), Republic of Korea (2025-RISE-10-006).

## References

1. Blanz, V., Vetter, T.: A morphable model for the synthesis of 3D faces. In: Seminal Graphics Papers: Pushing the Boundaries, pp. 157–164 (1999)
2. Blanz, V., Vetter, T.: Face recognition based on fitting a 3D morphable model. IEEE Trans. Pattern Anal. Mach. Intell. **25**, 1063–1074 (2003)
3. Genova, K., Cole, F., Maschinot, A., Sarna, A., Vlasic, D., Freeman, W.T.: Unsupervised training for 3D morphable model regression. In: Proceedings of CVPR, pp. 8377–8386 (2018)
4. Sela, M., Richardson, E., Kimmel, R.: Unrestricted facial geometry reconstruction using image-to-image translation. In: Proceedings of ICCV, pp. 1576–1585 (2017)
5. Lei, B., Ren, J., Feng, M., Cui, M., Xie, X.: A hierarchical representation network for accurate and detailed face reconstruction from in-the-wild images. In: Proceedings of CVPR, pp. 394–403 (2023)
6. Bai, H., Kang, D., Zhang, H., Pan, J., Bao, L.: FFHQ-UV: normalized facial UV-texture dataset for 3D face reconstruction. In: Proceedings of CVPR, pp. 362–371 (2023)
7. Chai, Z., et al.: Realy: rethinking the evaluation of 3D face reconstruction. In: Avidan, S., Brostow, G., Cissé, M., Farinella, G.M., Hassner, T. (eds.) ECCV 2022. LNCS, vol. 13668, pp. 74–92. Springer, Cham (2022). https://doi.org/10.1007/978-3-031-20074-8_5
8. Zhang, R., Isola, P., Efros, A.A., Shechtman, E., Wang, O.: The unreasonable effectiveness of deep features as a perceptual metric. In: Proceedings of CVPR, pp. 586–595 (2018)

# The Critical Role of Model Selection in Causal Inference: A Comparative Analysis of Classification Models Within the InferBERT Framework for Pharmacovigilance

Csaba Kiss[1(✉)], Roland Molontay[1,2], and Gabriele Pergola[3]

[1] Department of Stochastics, Institute of Mathematics, Budapest University of Technology and Economics, Műegyetem rkp. 3., Budapest 1111, Hungary
kisscs@math.bme.hu

[2] Institute of Biostatistics and Network Science, Semmelweis University, Üllői út 26., Budapest 1085, Hungary

[3] Department of Computer Science, University of Warwick, Coventry CV4 7AL, UK

**Abstract.** Distinguishing true causal adverse drug events (ADEs) from spurious correlations is a core pharmacovigilance challenge. The InferBERT framework [12] combines a neural classifier with Judea Pearl's Do-calculus to address this, but the pipeline depends critically on the classification model's quality.

We compare four models: XGBoost (a strong tabular baseline), ALBERT (the original InferBERT implementation), BioBERT (a biomedical-domain transformer), and Med-LLaMA (an 8-billion-parameter medical LLM) on two FAERS benchmarks: Analgesics-induced Acute Liver Failure (AILF) and Tramadol-related Mortalities (TRAM). We evaluate accuracy, calibration (ECE before/after isotonic regression), and Jaccard concordance with PRR, ROR, and EBGM signals using 5-fold CV over 20 runs with paired t-tests.

BioBERT achieved significantly higher predictive accuracy than all other models on both datasets ($p < 0.0001$). Domain-specific pre-training proved essential, whereas the much larger Med-LLaMA performed worst. Post-hoc calibration reduced ECE but had inconsistent effects on accuracy and causal discovery. These results demonstrate that domain-specific pre-training offers a clear practical advantage over both simpler models and larger LLMs in computational pharmacovigilance.

**Keywords:** pharmacovigilance · causal inference · machine learning · transformer

## 1 Introduction

Pharmacovigilance forms the foundation of post-market drug safety. Regulatory agencies and pharmaceutical companies depend on large-scale spontaneous

© The Author(s), under exclusive license to Springer Nature Switzerland AG 2027
P. Andreev et al. (Eds.): AIME 2026, LNAI 16748, pp. 174–178, 2027.
https://doi.org/10.1007/978-3-032-30710-1_21

reporting systems such as the FDA Adverse Event Reporting System (FAERS) [1,11,14]. Although FAERS supplies an enormous volume of real-world evidence, separating genuine safety signals from observational noise continues to present a major computational difficulty [4,16].

The InferBERT framework [12] attempts to bridge this gap with a two-stage approach: a neural classifier first predicts the probability of a clinical endpoint from patient reports, after which Judea Pearl's Do-calculus [9] is applied to the model's probabilistic outputs to simulate interventions and uncover potential causal factors. This study systematically addresses whether: the choice of classifier materially influences causal conclusions; a tabular baseline (XGBoost) is sufficient; domain-specific pre-training (BioBERT) confers genuine benefit; model scale (Med-LLaMA) helps; and post-hoc calibration affects causal outputs.

# 2 Materials and Methods

## 2.1 Causal Inference Framework

Our methodology follows the two-stage InferBERT process illustrated in Fig. 1. In the first stage, a classification model is trained to predict the probability of a binary clinical endpoint. The three transformer models (ALBERT, BioBERT, Med-LLaMA) receive the structured FAERS features formatted as natural-language sentences using a fixed template, while XGBoost operates directly on multi-hot encoded tabular features. In the second stage, the predicted probabilities are used for Do-calculus interventions; statistically significant terms ($p < 0.05$) are identified via a one-tailed z-test [9].

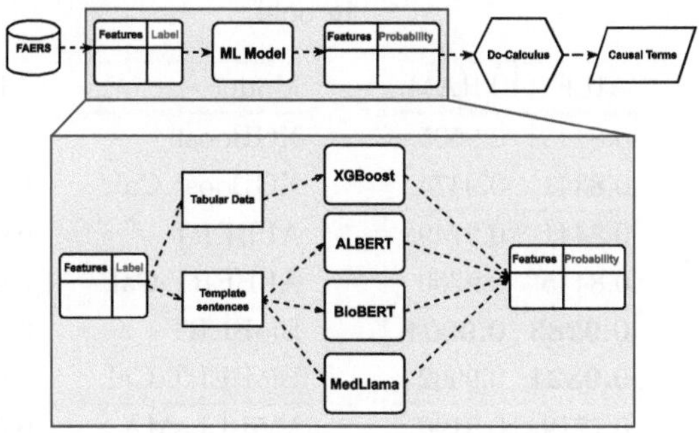


**Fig. 1.** InferBERT framework: full pipeline from FAERS data to causal term identification (upper), and model-specific input processing (lower).

## 2.2 Experimental Design, Metrics, and Implementation

Using 5-fold CV over 20 runs (3/5 train, 1/5 validation, 1/5 test), we compare XGBoost [2], ALBERT [6], BioBERT [8], and Med-LLaMA [15] on: (1) classification accuracy, (2) Expected Calibration Error (ECE) [10] before and after isotonic regression, and (3) Jaccard index measuring overlap between model-identified causal terms and Proportional Reporting Ratio (PRR), Reporting Odds Ratio (ROR), and Empirical Bayes Geometric Mean (EBGM) signals [12]. We report median values and assess significance with paired t-tests ($p < 0.05$).

All transformer models were fine-tuned for a maximum of three epochs with learning rate $\mu = 2 \times 10^{-5}$ and early stopping based on validation loss. ALBERT (~12M parameters) and BioBERT (~110M parameters) were fully fine-tuned. Med-LLaMA (~8B parameters) was adapted using PEFT with 4-bit quantization and LoRA [7].

Code and full experimental results (including AUC scores across all cross-validation splits and causal trees) are available at https://github.com/hsdslab/biomedical-causal-inference.git.

## 3 Results

### 3.1 Predictive Accuracy and Calibration

BioBERT attained the highest median accuracy on both datasets and significantly outperformed every other model ($p < 0.0001$), while Med-LLaMA performed worst overall (Table 1). Isotonic regression improved ECE for most models (Table 2), but had model-dependent and frequently negative effects on accuracy, and therefore cannot be regarded as a universally helpful post-processing step.

**Table 1.** Median accuracy (higher better). Best in bold.

| Model | AILF | TRAM |
|---|---|---|
| XGBoost | 0.8445 | 0.9535 |
| XGBoost Cal. | 0.8341 | 0.9474 |
| ALBERT | 0.8441 | 0.9749 |
| ALBERT Cal. | 0.8445 | 0.9760 |
| BioBERT | **0.9283** | **0.9904** |
| BioBERT Cal. | **0.9321** | 0.9902 |
| Med-LLaMA | 0.7719 | 0.9196 |
| Med-LLaMA Cal. | 0.7717 | 0.9196 |

**Table 2.** Median ECE (lower better). Best in bold.

| Model | AILF | TRAM |
|---|---|---|
| XGBoost | 0.0203 | 0.0125 |
| XGBoost Cal. | **0.0120** | 0.0095 |
| ALBERT | 0.0308 | 0.0137 |
| ALBERT Cal. | 0.0245 | 0.0071 |
| BioBERT | 0.0263 | 0.0068 |
| BioBERT Cal. | 0.0168 | **0.0040** |
| Med-LLaMA | 0.0178 | 0.0133 |
| Med-LLaMA Cal. | 0.0150 | 0.0115 |

### 3.2 Causal Discovery Performance

BioBERT also produced the highest Jaccard concordance with PRR and EBGM (Table 3), indicating that stronger predictions yield more reliable causal terms, though calibration's influence remained inconsistent.

**Table 3.** Median Jaccard index (higher better). Best in bold.

| Model | AILF | | | TRAM | | |
|---|---|---|---|---|---|---|
| | PRR | ROR | EBGM | PRR | ROR | EBGM |
| XGBoost | 0.0494 | 0.4665 | 0.0078 | 0.2977 | **0.7897** | 0.0749 |
| XGBoost Cal. | 0.0476 | 0.4616 | 0.0075 | 0.3069 | 0.7844 | 0.0753 |
| ALBERT | 0.0434 | 0.4722 | 0.0074 | 0.3044 | 0.7777 | 0.0757 |
| ALBERT Cal. | 0.0415 | 0.4800 | 0.0073 | 0.3046 | 0.7716 | 0.0753 |
| BioBERT | 0.0515 | 0.4296 | **0.0085** | **0.3166** | 0.7767 | **0.0761** |
| BioBERT Cal. | **0.0517** | 0.4338 | **0.0085** | 0.3132 | 0.7782 | 0.0757 |
| Med-LLaMA | 0.0418 | 0.4579 | 0.0072 | 0.2857 | 0.7447 | 0.0733 |
| Med-LLaMA Cal. | 0.0407 | **0.4686** | 0.0071 | 0.2842 | 0.7566 | 0.0729 |

## 4 Discussion and Conclusion

The experiments show that BioBERT, which incorporates domain-specific pre-training on biomedical literature (PubMed, PMC), substantially outperforms XGBoost, ALBERT, and Med-LLaMA in both predictive accuracy and the quality of causal discovery [3,5]. Med-LLaMA's underperformance is likely explained by the constraints of parameter-efficient fine-tuning. Better predictions lead directly to improved Do-calculus results and closer agreement with established pharmacovigilance signals (PRR, EBGM). Although isotonic regression reliably lowers ECE, its effects on accuracy and causal terms vary across models and should be evaluated case by case.

Limitations include reliance on traditional disproportionality metrics as a practical benchmark rather than definitive causal ground truth, and the templated conversion of structured data into natural language, which may limit relational pattern capture. Future work could explore multimodal architectures that process structured features and free-text narratives in parallel [13] and examine more effective ways to adapt large language models to tabular healthcare data.

**Acknowledgments.** R. Molontay was supported by the János Bolyai Research Scholarship of the Hungarian Academy of Sciences. C. Kiss was supported by the Cooperative Doctoral Programme of the National Research, Development, and Innovation Fund.

The authors used Gemini 3 Pro for language editing and take full responsibility for the manuscript.

**Disclosure of Interests.** The authors have no competing interests to declare that are relevant to the content of this article.

## References


1. Alomar, M., Tawfiq, A.M., Hassan, N., Palaian, S.: Post marketing surveillance of suspected adverse drug reactions through spontaneous reporting: current status, challenges and the future. Therapeut. Adv. Drug Saf. **11**, 2042098620938595 (2020)
2. Chen, T., Guestrin, C.: Xgboost: a scalable tree boosting system. In: Proceedings of the 22nd ACM SIGKDD International Conference on Knowledge Discovery and Data Mining (KDD '16), pp. 785–794. ACM (2016). https://doi.org/10.1145/2939672.2939785
3. Gu, Y., et al.: Domain-specific language model pretraining for biomedical natural language processing. ACM Trans. Comput. Healthc. (HEALTH) **3**(1), 1–23 (2021)
4. Hernán, M.A., Robins, J.M.: Causal inference (2010)
5. Huertas, C.: Gradient boosting trees and large language models for tabular data few-shot learning. arXiv preprint arXiv:2411.04324 (2024)
6. Lan, Z., Chen, M., Goodman, S., Gimpel, K., Sharma, P., Soricut, R.: Albert: a lite BERT for self-supervised learning of language representations. arXiv preprint arXiv:1909.11942 (2019)
7. Le, T.D., Ti Nguyen, T., Nguyen Ha, V.: The impact of LoRA adapters for LLMs on clinical NLP classification under data limitations. arXiv preprint arXiv:2407.19299 (2024)
8. Lee, J., et al.: BioBERT: a pre-trained biomedical language representation model for biomedical text mining. Bioinformatics **36**(4), 1234–1240 (2020). https://doi.org/10.1093/bioinformatics/btz682
9. Pearl, J.: Causal inference in statistics: an overview. Stat. Surv. **3**, 96–146 (2009). https://doi.org/10.1214/09-SS057
10. Posocco, N., Bonnefoy, A.: Estimating expected calibration errors (2021). https://arxiv.org/abs/2109.03480
11. Potter, E., Reyes, M., Naples, J., Dal Pan, G.: FDA adverse event reporting system (FAERS) essentials: a guide to understanding, applying, and interpreting adverse event data reported to FAERS. Clin. Pharmacol. Therapeut. (2025)
12. Wang, X., Xu, X., Tong, W., Roberts, R., Liu, Z.: InferBERT: a transformer-based causal inference framework for enhancing pharmacovigilance. Front. Artif. Intell. **4**, 659622 (2021)
13. Wang, Z., Sun, J.: Transtab: learning transferable tabular transformers across tables. In: Advances in Neural Information Processing Systems, vol. 35, pp. 2902–2915 (2022)
14. World Health Organization: Pharmacovigilance: ensuring the safe use of medicines. Technical report, World Health Organization (2004)
15. Xie, Q., et al.: Me-llama: foundation large language models for medical applications. arXiv preprint arXiv:2402.12749 (2024)
16. Zhao, Y., et al.: Machine learning in causal inference: application in pharmacovigilance. Drug Saf. **45**(5), 459–476 (2022)

# An Explainable Hybrid Framework for Automated Analysis of Bone Marrow Aspirates in Acute Myeloid Leukemia

Valentin Andral[1,4](✉), Jules Morata[2,4], Philippe Leleux[2], Pierre Brousset[3], Alban Canali[3], Jean-Baptiste Rieu[3], Sandrine Mouysset[1], and Sarah Bertoli[3,4]

[1] Institut de Recherche en Informatique de Toulouse, Toulouse, France
valentin.andral@irit.fr
[2] Laboratoire d'Analyse et d'Architecture des Systèmes, Toulouse, France
[3] Centre Hospitalier Universitaire de Toulouse, Toulouse, France
[4] Centre de Recherches en Cancérologie de Toulouse, Toulouse, France

**Abstract.** The diagnosis of Acute Myeloid Leukemia (AML) is based on the assessment of a Bone Marrow Aspirate Smear (BMAS) and the detection of an excess of immature malignant cells, called blasts by cytologists. In this paper, we exploit digitized BMAS stained from AML diagnosed at the Toulouse University Hospital. We have built an explainable hybrid pipeline to automatically segment and classify AML blasts that includes selection of regions of interest, cell segmentation, and cell classification without expert intervention by using deep learning and machine learning methods. Our pipeline allows the extraction of up to 5000 cells from a BMAS with a global accuracy of 92.4% for the correct prediction of AML. One of the main advantages of our approach is its interpretability with results competing with a foundation model, called DinoBloom, pretrained on hematological large dataset, which makes it an interactive tool to help cytologists in their diagnosis.

**Keywords:** Hematology · bone marrow aspirate smears · acute myeloid leukemia · diagnosis · explainability

## 1 Introduction

AML is a severe hematological disease resulting from the infiltration of the bone marrow and blood by immature malignant cells, called blasts. The diagnosis is delivered by cytologists, who perform microscopic examination of BMAS stained with May-Grünwald-Giemsa coloration through optical microscope. The assessment of bone marrow cells is central to this classification, relying on various morphological criteria such as the presence of Auer rods and the lineage differentiation of blast cells. Among these criteria, the blast count is the most crucial determinant for the diagnosis and the morphological classification of AML subtypes. The French-American-British system sets a threshold of at least 30% blast

© The Author(s), under exclusive license to Springer Nature Switzerland AG 2027
P. Andreev et al. (Eds.): AIME 2026, LNAI 16748, pp. 179–188, 2027.
https://doi.org/10.1007/978-3-032-30710-1_22

cells in the bone marrow to define AML, a criterion later refined by the WHO to 20% [1]. Given the fundamental role of blast enumeration in AML classification, our study focuses specifically on its automated assessment through the digital analysis of BMAS.

In clinical practice, the manual counting of differentiated cells in BMAS is performed under the microscope by a cytologist, who's analyzing a minimum of 500 cells. This process is time-consuming, heavily reliant on the expertise of the cytologists, and often lacks full reproducibility due to subjective interpretations. The advent of Machine Learning (ML) has opened new opportunities for automating this assessment, aiming to enhance efficiency and consistency. Developing explainable automatic tools for the segmentation and classification of cells in BMAS of patients with AML using ML and computer vision techniques is essential to reduce diagnostic variability and accelerate clinical workflows.

Despite the growing interest in Artificial Intelligence (AI) for BMAS analysis [2], only a limited number of studies address the fully automated processing of entire BMAS while explicitly prioritizing interpretability in the final decision-making stage. Most existing approaches focus either on isolated cell classification or rely on end-to-end Deep Learning (DL) pipelines that operate as black boxes, limiting their clinical transparency [3].

In this paper, we propose a hybrid framework designed to bridge this gap by leveraging the strengths of DL for tasks such as cell segmentation, while deliberately adopting feature-based ML methods for the classification and diagnostic decision stages. This design choice enables the exploitation of powerful deep representations where necessary, while maintaining an explainable and clinically meaningful classification process, better aligned with the morphological reasoning employed by cytologists when analyzing BMAS. While image feature extraction based on morphological, textural, and color descriptors is a well-established approach in cytological image analysis, the recent emergence of foundation models such as DinoBloom [4], pretrained on large-scale datasets of bone marrow and blood smear cells, introduces a new and compelling perspective. The feature representations learned by such models capture rich and discriminative cellular patterns. As a result, these deep features constitute an important point of comparison with traditional image-based features, enabling an evaluation of their respective ability to characterize cells in the context of BMAS analysis.

In the following of the paper, we first review related work in hematology addressing automated BMAS analysis. We then present our hybrid framework for the fully automatic processing of whole BMAS, before discussing the experimental results and a comparative evaluation with foundation models as based approaches.

## 2 Related Works

Several studies have explored different methodological approaches, leveraging DL models and digitized BMAS data. In [5], the authors developed a multi-stage DL framework for segmenting and classifying bone marrow cells, successfully distinguishing Acute Promyelocytic Leukemia (APL) from other AML subtypes.

Their model demonstrated high accuracy in a controlled dataset, highlighting the potential of AI in hematological diagnostics. Similarly, in [6], the authors employed Convolutional Neural Networks (CNNs) trained on a large dataset of digitized bone marrow images, achieving not only high AML classification accuracy but also the prediction of genetic mutations such as *NPM1*, emphasizing the potential of AI for genetic-informed diagnosis. Other studies, such as [7], have provided a broader perspective on AI applications in hematology, reviewing the state-of-the-art techniques for automated segmentation, classification, and diagnostic evaluation of bone marrow cells. Collectively, these studies highlight the effectiveness of DL for BMAS analysis. However, key challenges remain that we try to address in this paper: previous studies generally rely on manual manipulation of the digitized data before starting cell segmentation, and when the entire process is automatic, such as [8], the use of black box DL methods generally lacks explainability and/or interpretability in order to build a decision tool to help clinicians. Although several techniques, such as Grad-CAM [9] or saliency maps, have been proposed to provide visual explanations for DL models applied to cell images, they offer only limited interpretability [10]. These methods highlight image regions that contribute to a model's prediction, but they do not provide explicit, quantitative descriptors of the underlying morphological characteristics.

Previous works have demonstrated the use of shape, texture, and color descriptors extracted from segmented leukocytes combined with classical ML classifiers such as SVM to perform leukemia cell classification [11]. For example, classification methods based on manually extracted features achieved high performance when trained on shape and texture descriptors derived from segmented cells [12]. Hybrid pipelines that combine deep feature extraction using pretrained CNN backbones with classical classifiers (e.g., Random Forest, SVM, XGBoost) have also been proposed, showing robust performance for multiclass cell classification tasks [13]. These methods typically operate on pre-selected or manually cropped cells, without addressing the full slide context. As a result, they do not form complete, end-to-end pipelines capable of automatically selecting tiles of interest, segmenting cells across entire BMAS, and aggregating cell-level predictions into slide-level diagnoses. This limitation restricts their clinical applicability, particularly when handling whole-slide images where the distribution of cells and rare pathological events must be interpreted at a global scale, rather than in isolation.

## 3 Pipeline Description

To address the challenge of analyzing entire BMAS in a fully automated interpretable manner, our hybrid approach, illustrated in Fig. 1 (a), relies on a combination of both unsupervised and supervised learning strategies.

It starts by considering the BMAS as a whole slide image, digitized with a Panoramic 250 Flash II (3DHISTECH) scanner then stored in the *.mrxs* format, which supports multiple zoom levels - from level 0 (lowest magnification) to level

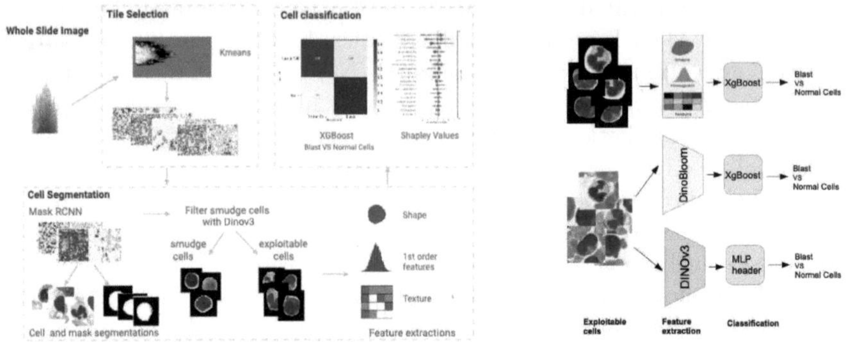


(a) Pipeline description (b) Feature-based cell classifications

**Fig. 1.** (a) Pipeline description of the hybrid automatic BMAS analysis; (b) Comparative study of feature-based cell classification.

19 (highest magnification), corresponding to a maximum zoom of ×823 (121 nm per pixel). At each level, the BMAS can be divided into a certain number of tiles, each being a section of the whole slide.

First, K-means clustering automatically selects relevant regions in whole-slide images, enabling scalable processing without manual input. Then, a deep learning instance-segmentation model (Mask R-CNN [15]) segments individual cells in those regions. After segmentation, the approach switches to interpretable, feature-based analysis: morphological, texture, and color features are extracted from each cell so classification aligns with cytologists' reasoning. This hybrid pipeline supports end-to-end whole-slide analysis while keeping final decisions transparent.

### 3.1 Tile Selection

The first step consists in selecting the Regions of Interest (RoI) in the BMAS. These RoI represent areas of the BMAS with the most information, i.e., the greatest number of exploitable cells. An exploitable cell is defined in this paper as a nucleated cell coming from the hematopoiesis, which lineage and maturation could be identified by a cytologist. Those tiles can be split into 3 distinct classes: sparse tiles found in the edges of the smear (few number of cells, low color saturation), dense tiles found near the starting point of the smear (high density of cells, high color saturation due to dye stains) and optimal tiles (good balance between number of red blood cells and exploitable cells).

So, from a cytological perspective, tile selection primarily relies on cell density, which is reflected by color variations in red blood cells and bone marrow cells. Therefore, an unsupervised clustering approach enables this filtering step to be performed efficiently and consistently. Clustering-based strategies have already been explored for tile selection in digital pathology [14], and the use of K-means is particularly relevant due to its numerical efficiency, robustness, and suitability for large-scale whole-slide analysis. Moreover, as mentioned earlier, the number of clusters used as a parameter is known: one for each tile class, for a total of three clusters.

From the clusters represented by its average RGB pixel value, the optimal tile exhibits a medium color level, revealing a balance between sparse and dense tiles. We use these optimal tiles as RoI in the remainder of the study.

### 3.2 Cell Segmentation

The selected RoI are input to a Mask R-CNN model, a DL architecture specifically designed for instance segmentation. This model simultaneously performs cell detection and segmentation, allowing each individual cell to be localized and segmented within the RoIs. For every detected cell, Mask R-CNN outputs a precise pixel-level segmentation mask, enabling the separation of overlapping or closely packed cells. This step is critical for downstream analysis, as it provides accurate cell boundaries required for reliable feature extraction and cell-level classification. DL is well suited for this step, as the automatic processing of numerous tiles and cells requires scalability and robustness, while explainability is not essential at this stage of the pipeline.

However, during testing, we noticed that, on average, 55% of the segmented cells are smudge cells, i.e. cells damaged during the smear preparation. These must be filtered out before the classification stage, as their distorted morphology does not provide meaningful features for cytologists. For this purpose, a DINOv3 model [16] was employed, leveraging its self-supervised feature representations to accurately distinguish and exclude these artifacts, while preserving both blasts and normal cells for the classification step. Its robust embeddings are particularly well-suited for our framework, as they enable automatic and generalizable artifact filtering. On the resulting set of exploitable cell images, we initiate the explainable analysis.

### 3.3 Explainable Cell Classification

To achieve explainability in the classification of bone marrow cells, we aim to identify which image features—such as average color, color variance, texture, and granularity—help to distinguish blasts from normal cells such as erythroblasts, lymphocytes, monocytes, and granulocytes. Using both the masks and images of cells, features are extracted with the feature extraction library pyradiomics [17]. Although the features are obtained with image processing techniques, they combine both texture descriptors (e.g., energy, entropy, GLCM features) and morphological descriptors (e.g., shape, area, sphericity), which are then used by an eXtreme Gradient Boosting (XGBoost) [18] classifier to classify the cells into blast or normal cell.

Finally, the SHAP-based method [19] is employed to extract the most discriminative features in cell classification, providing interpretability to the cytologists. This approach highlights which morphological characteristics drive the model's decisions, facilitating trust and clinical understanding through transparency.

# 4 Numerical Experiments

## 4.1 Datasets and Training Details

In this study, the Mask R-CNN model used in the cell segmentation part was trained on 5418 expert-annotate cells coming from 141 BMAS, all collected in Toulouse University Hospital.

The DINOv3 model, that filters the smudge cells, was trained on 7345 cells, 1282 of them being smudge cells, 4112 being normal cells and 1951 being blasts, extracted from 114 BMAS. Out of those 7345 cells, 820 cells were collected from microscope pictures and 117 cells from a public dataset [20].

The XGBoost model was trained on the same previous dataset, minus the 1282 smudge cells. To test both the DINOv3 model and the XGBoost model, 6 BMAS were removed from the dataset comprised of the 114 BMAS before training and used as a test dataset, for a total of 721 cells.

For the experimental evaluation and numerical experiments, our proposed pipeline is evaluated on a validation dataset comprised of 92 BMAS from the Toulouse University Hospital. Among those 92 BMAS, 23 were from non-AML patients and were used as control slides.

The XGBoost model hyperparameters have been tuned using a Tree-Structured Parzen Estimator [21] through the Optuna framework [22].

## 4.2 Results and Analysis

To evaluate the respective contributions of explainable and representation-based features, we compare three classification strategies trained on the same set of segmented bone marrow cells as illustrated in Fig. 1(b). First, we extract 271 handcrafted image features capturing explicit morphological and textural characteristics of the cells. After filtering out zero-variance and highly correlated features, we train an XGBoost classifier on 128 of those radiomics features. Second, we extract 781 latent embeddings from the DinoBloom foundation model and train a separate XGBoost classifier on these representations. Third, we use DINOv3 as a feature-based transfer learning approach as it requires relatively few labeled samples, enabling a fair comparison with other feature-based methods. We leverage features obtained from the DINOv3 architecture, using its MultiLayer Perceptron (MLP) classification head trained on the same cell-level dataset.

Furthermore, all cells segmented during the validation phase of our pipeline were saved and subsequently reused to evaluate both baselines approaches. This strategy ensures that identical cells are provided to each classification model, thereby eliminating potential biases introduced from differences in RoI selection.

After classifying cells as blasts or normal, the proportion of detected blasts is computed at the whole-slide level as described in Sect. 1: slides with a blast

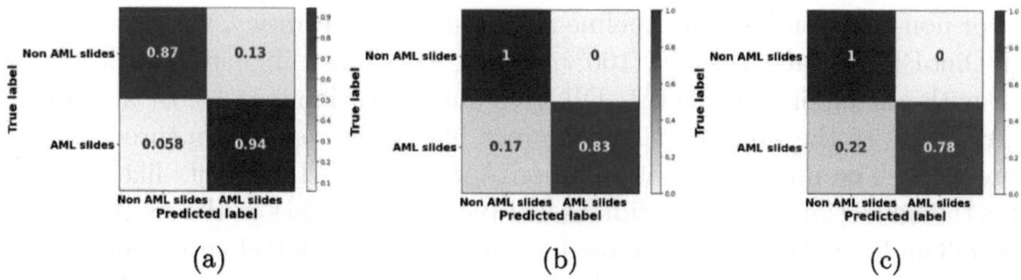


**Fig. 2.** Confusion matrices from (a) our pipeline, (b) DINOv3 and (c) DinoBloom to diagnose AML on the validation dataset consisting of 92 BMAS.

**Table 1.** Mean difference between ground-truth blast percentage and predicted blast percentage with associated standard deviation for each approach.

| Model | Mean difference | Standard deviation |
|---|---|---|
| **Pipeline** | **16.52** | 18.90 |
| DINOv3 | 30.50 | 21.45 |
| DinoBloom | 27.88 | **17.28** |

percentage above 20% are labeled AML, whereas those below this threshold are labeled non-AML. Results on validation dataset are respectively given by Fig. 2(a) for our pipeline, Fig. 2(b) for DINOv3 and Fig. 2(c) for DinoBloom. The mean difference between the ground-truth blast percentage and the predicted blast percentage was computed for each slide and averaged across all slides. In addition, the standard deviation of these differences was calculated to evaluate the variability of the prediction. All computed means and standard deviations are shown in Table 1.

**Table 2.** Score metrics for each model used in our study.

| Model | Accuracy (weighted) | F1-macro | Recall macro |
|---|---|---|---|
| **Pipeline** | **0.924** | **0.900** | 0.906 |
| DINOv3 | 0.869 | 0.848 | **0.913** |
| DinoBloom | 0.837 | 0.816 | 0.891 |

As can be seen in Tables 1 and 2 and Fig. 2, our evaluation demonstrates comparable performance between feature-based radiomics and foundation-model approaches for BMAS classification. Our pipeline achieved 92.4% accuracy, 90.0% macro-F1, and 90.6% macro-recall, compared with accuracies of 86.9% and 83.7%, macro-F1 scores of 84.8% and 81.6%, and macro-recalls of 91.3% and 89.1% for DINOv3 and DinoBloom, respectively.

For non-AML slides, our pipeline achieved 87.0% accuracy, whereas DINOv3 and DinoBloom each reached 100%. For AML slides, all methods performed well, with our pipeline at 94.0%, DINOv3 and DinoBloom at 83.0% and 78.0%, respectively, as the abundant and distinct blasts are readily captured by both approaches. The imbalance between non-AML and AML patients likely exacerbates the limitations of foundation model-based approaches in the results such as DINOv3 and DinoBloom. These models, pre-trained to detect subtle morphological patterns in large and diverse haematological datasets, appear to be slightly less effective at detecting blast cells. Indeed, our pipeline misclassified 4 AML patients as healthy, whereas the foundation models DinoBloom and DINOv3 misclassified 12 and 15 patients, respectively.

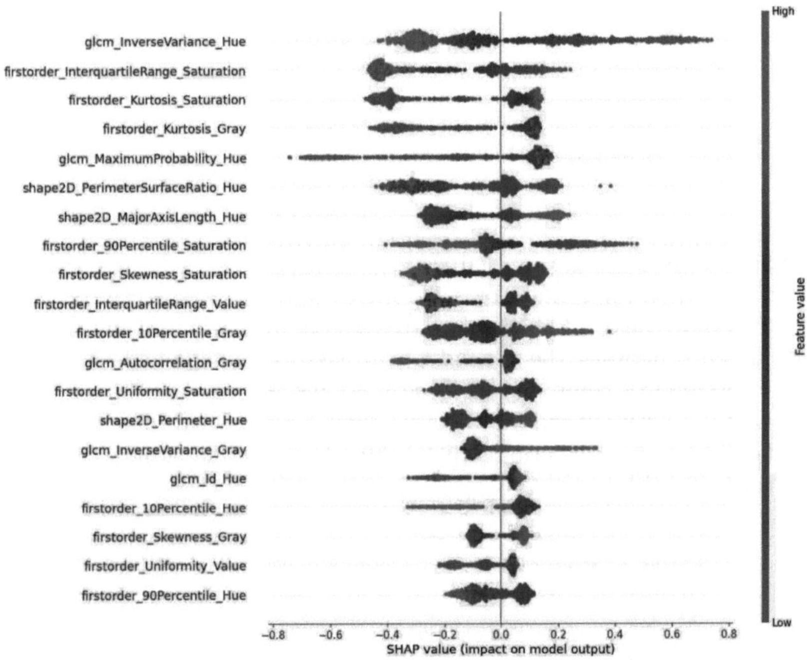


**Fig. 3.** Top 20 most impactful features for blast diagnosis using SHAP values. Each dot represents a value. The further right the dot is from the center, the more this value helped to predict a blast. A blue dot means a lower numerical value and a red dot means a higher numerical value. (Color figure online)

## 4.3 Explainability

Using Shapley values, features that were important for the identification of blasts were compared with the elements used by cytologists during their diagnosis.

First-order descriptors (kurtosis, skewness, interquartile range, saturation) capture differences in nuclear size, chromatin density, and cytoplasm clarity between blasts and normal cells. GLCM features, such as maximum probability, reflect nuclear texture patterns, while Shape2D features, including the perimeter-to-surface ratio, describe geometric differences. Together, these interpretable features enable discrimination of blasts from normal cells while maintaining a direct link to cytologists' morphological reasoning. Those features, presented in Fig. 3, correlate with morphological characteristics of a blast: a high nucleus-to-cytoplasm ratio with a stippled nucleus [23]. This observation is then confirmed by the first three features: a low inverse variance indicates that most pixels have the same value, indicating a high nucleus-to-cytoplasm ratio, while a low interquartile range with high kurtosis indicates that few pixels differ greatly from others (the stippled aspect).

## 5 Conclusion and Future Work

We introduce a hybrid approach in which DL is leveraged for highly controlled tasks such as cell segmentation and smudge cell filtering, while the final decision-making relies on well-established, robust, and explainable feature-based methods. This fully automatic processing of BMAS achieves performance comparable to foundation model-based approaches (DinoBloom, DINOv3).

The proposed pipeline demonstrates promising capabilities in distinguishing blast cells, uncovering discriminative features that reflect the analytical approach used by expert cytologists. Future research will focus on developing further cell lineages predictions while emphasizing the adaptation of the pipeline to work primarily on BMAS from other national centers. Moreover, incorporating more slides from multiple centers and different scanners would improve generalizability.

## References


1. Vardiman, James W., et al.: The 2008 revision of the World Health Organization (WHO) classification of myeloid neoplasms and acute leukemia: rationale and important changes. Blood **114**(5), 937–951 (2009)
2. Ghete, T., Kock, et al.: Models for the marrow: A comprehensive review of AI-based cell classification methods and malignancy detection in bone marrow aspirate smears. HemaSphere **8**(12), e70048 (2024)
3. Lewis, J.E., Pozdnyakova, O.: Advances in bone marrow evaluation. Clin. Lab. Med. **44**(3), 431–440 (2024)
4. Koch, V., Wagner, et al.: DinoBloom: a foundation model for generalizable cell embeddings in hematology. In: International Conference on Medical Image Computing and Computer-Assisted Intervention, pp. 520–530 (2024)
5. Eckardt, J.-N., et al.: Deep learning identifies acute promyelocytic leukemia in bone marrow smears. BMC Cancer **22**(1), 201 (2022)
6. Eckardt, J.-N., et al.: Deep learning detects acute myeloid leukemia and predicts NPM1 mutation status from bone marrow smears. Leukemia **36**(1), 111–118 (2022)

7. Ghete, T., et al.: Models for the marrow: a comprehensive review of AI-based cell classification methods and malignancy detection in bone marrow aspirate smears. HemaSphere **8**(12), e70048 (2024)
8. Wei, B.-H., et al.: Annotation-free deep learning for predicting gene mutations from whole slide images of acute myeloid leukemia. NPJ Precis. Oncol. **9**(1), 35 (2025)
9. Selvaraju, R.R., et al.: Grad-cam: visual explanations from deep networks via gradient-based localization. In: Proceedings of the IEEE International Conference on Computer Vision, pp. 618–626 (2017)
10. Zhang, H., et al.: Saliency maps give a false sense of explanability to image classifiers: an empirical evaluation across methods and metrics. In: The 16th Asian Conference on Machine Learning (Conference Track) (2024)
11. El Houby, E.M.: Acute lymphoblastic leukemia diagnosis using machine learning techniques based on selected features. Sci. Rep. **15**(1), 28056 (2025)
12. Putzu, L., et al.: Leucocyte classification for Leukaemia detection using image processing techniques. Artif. Intell. Med. **62**(3), 179–191 (2014)
13. Kasim, S., et al.: Multiclass leukemia cell classification using hybrid deep learning and machine learning with CNN-based feature extraction. Sci. Rep. **15**(1), 23782 (2025)
14. Li, J., et al.: A multi-resolution model for histopathology image classification and localization with multiple instance learning. Comput. Biol. Med. **131**, 104253 (2021)
15. He, K., et al.: Mask R-CNN. In: Proceedings of the IEEE International Conference on Computer Vision, pp. 2961–2969 (2017)
16. Siméoni, O., et al.: DINOv3. arXiv preprint arXiv:2508.10104 (2025)
17. Van Griethuysen, J.J.M., et al.: Computational radiomics system to decode the radiographic phenotype. Can. Res. **77**(21), e104–e107 (2017)
18. Chen, T.: XGBoost: A Scalable Tree Boosting System. Cornell University (2016)
19. Sundararajan, M., Najmi, A.: The many Shapley values for model explanation. In: International Conference on Machine Learning, pp. 9269–9278. PMLR (2020)
20. Matek, C., et al.: A single-cell morphological dataset of leukocytes from AML patients and non-malignant controls (AML-Cytomorphology-LMU). The Cancer Imaging Archive (TCIA) [Internet] (2019)
21. Watanabe, S.: Tree-structured Parzen estimator: understanding its algorithm components and their roles for better empirical performance. arXiv preprint arXiv:2304.11127 (2023)
22. Akiba, T., et al.: Optuna: a next-generation hyperparameter optimization framework. In: Proceedings of the 25th ACM SIGKDD International Conference on Knowledge Discovery and Data Mining, pp. 2623–2631 (2019)
23. Arber, D.A., et al.: The 2016 revision to the World Health Organization classification of myeloid neoplasms and acute leukemia. Blood, J. Am. Soc. Hematol. **127**(20), 2391–2405 (2016)

# Is Heavier Better? Benchmarking Optical Flow Time-Series vs. Video Transformers for In Vitro Fertilization Counseling

Lorenzo Corso[1(✉)], Andrea Fantinato[2], Emirhan Kayar[1], Margherita Isernia[2], Giulia Fiorentino[2], Marilena Taggi[3], Federica Innocenti[3], Marcos Meseguer[4], Alberto Vaiarelli[5], Laura Rienzi[3,6], Maurizio Zuccotti[2], Giovanni Coticchio[3], Riccardo Bellazzi[1], Danilo Cimadomo[2,3], and Giovanna Nicora[1]

[1] Department of Computer, Electrical and Biomedical Engineering, University of Pavia, Pavia, Italy
lorenzo.corso01@universitadipavia.it
[2] Department of Biology and Biotechnology 'Lazzaro Spallanzani', Pavia, Italy
[3] IVIRMA Global Research Alliance, IVIRMA Italia, Rome, Italy
[4] IVIRMA Global Research Alliance, IVI Valencia, Valencia, Spain
[5] IVIRMA Global Research Alliance, Genera, Clinica Valle Giulia, Rome, Italy
[6] Department of Biomolecular Sciences, University of Urbino, Urbino, Italy

**Abstract.** Early prediction of embryo developmental competence is crucial for In Vitro Fertilization counseling. Time-lapse microscopy technologies allow for continuous monitoring of embryo development, enabling AI systems to support clinical decision-making. However, state-of-the-art systems for image and video analysis, such as Video Transformers (ViViT), suffer from high computational costs and opacity, thus hampering their deployment in clinical routine. We investigate if lightweight optical-flow classifiers can match heavy vision models in predictive accuracy while adhering to "Green AI" principles. We analyzed 5,011 human embryo videos (3.1 M frames), benchmarking (1) a resource-intensive ViViT on raw video against (2) a lightweight time-series model (ConvTran) on extracted optical-flow signals. Performance was evaluated at 24, 72 and 120 h post-insemination (hpi), alongside computational footprint (latency, FLOPs, $CO_2$). ConvTran significantly outperforms ViViT at 24 hpi (AUC 0.62 [0.58–0.66] vs 0.57 [0.53–0.62]) and 72 hpi (0.70 [0.66–0.74] vs 0.66 [0.61–0.70]); at 120 hpi ViViT modestly leads (0.91 [0.88–0.93] vs 0.88 [0.85–0.90]) but at ~2,500× the inference cost, a trade-off we argue against for clinical deployment. ConvTran reduces model-only inference latency from 13.6 s to 5.5 ms per embryo and estimated $CO_2$ emissions by >99%. Interpretability analysis uncovers a novel prognostic window in the first 5 hpi of development. Domain-specific feature engineering coupled with efficient time-series transformers provides a sustainable alternative to large foundation models for low-latency clinical deployment.

**Keywords:** Clinical Decision Support Systems (CDSS) · Medical Imaging · Explainable AI (XAI) · Ethics · Embryoscope

© The Author(s), under exclusive license to Springer Nature Switzerland AG 2027
P. Andreev et al. (Eds.): AIME 2026, LNAI 16748, pp. 189–193, 2027.
https://doi.org/10.1007/978-3-032-30710-1_23

# 1 Introduction

Time-Lapse Monitoring (TLM) has transformed In Vitro Fertilization (IVF) embryology into a data-intensive video discipline, driving the adoption of resource-intensive Deep Learning architectures (3D-CNNs, Video Vision Transformers, and Foundation Models trained on millions of frames [1, 2]) that exemplify "Red AI" [3]: most fertility clinics lack the high-performance GPU infrastructure required for real-time inference, and these models' opacity obscures the biological events driving predictions. We challenge the assumption that "heavier is automatically better" and propose a "Green AI" alternative that decouples diagnostic accuracy from computational cost. Instead of processing raw video tensors, we extract domain-specific motion signals via dense optical flow [4], compressing the data dimensionality by orders of magnitude. We benchmark this lightweight approach against a ViViT baseline. Our contributions are: (1) *Sustainability*: lightweight time-series transformers (ConvTran [5]) match or exceed ViViT accuracy at clinically decisive early timepoints with ~2,500× lower latency and > 99% lower $CO_2$; (2) *Early Prediction*: motion-based signals significantly outperform raw-pixel video models in the earliest developmental window [Day 1, 24 h post-insemination (hpi)]; (3) *Discovery*: interpretability uncovers a novel prognostic window in the first 5 hpi of development.

# 2 Methods

## 2.1 Dataset and Automated Preprocessing

We used a dataset of 5,011 embryo videos (3.1 M frames) collected between 2013 and 2020 at an Italian fertility center. The cohort was approximately balanced (2,537 blastocysts, 2,474 arrested embryos; ratio ≈1.03:1) and stratified by patient and outcome into training (n = 3,506), validation (n = 743), and test (n = 762) sets, with class proportions preserved across splits. We adopted a held-out patient-stratified test split rather than k-fold cross-validation to guarantee strict patient-level separation between training and evaluation. To standardize inputs for the ViViT model, we developed an automated Region of Interest (RoI) pipeline (see Fig. 1).

## 2.2 The Green Stream and Architectures

To decouple diagnostic accuracy from computational cost, we implemented a dimensionality reduction pipeline using Farneback's dense optical flow [4]. Between consecutive frames we computed dense motion fields and aggregated the pixel-wise magnitudes of horizontal and vertical velocity components into a univariate Sum of Mean Magnitude (SMM) signal over a sliding window of size n, reducing input dimensionality by a factor of $\sim 2.5 \times 10^5$ while preserving global morphokinetic energy. On the SMM signal we employed ConvTran [5], a lightweight time-series transformer with convolutional embeddings. As a baseline we used ViViT with factorized self-attention [1], which processes video as a sequence of spatio-temporal tokens at substantial compute and memory cost.

### 2.3 Sustainability Metrics and Interpretability

We measured: (1) theoretical complexity in Floating Point Operations (FLOPs); (2) model-only inference latency per embryo on CPU, since fertility clinics typically lack GPU infrastructure; (3) Carbon Footprint, estimated using the CodeCarbon methodology [6] as $E \times C_{intensity}$ ($C_{intensity}$ is the carbon intensity of the local grid, $\approx 250 gCO2/kWh$). Upstream preprocessing is excluded symmetrically from both pipelines (Farneback flow extraction: 5.4 s/video for ConvTran; RoI cropping and resizing: 9.9 s/video for ViViT), since in time-lapse deployment it is streamed frame-by-frame during image acquisition and is therefore off the critical path of inference at the clinical decision timepoint. We note that this symmetric exclusion, if anything, favors ViViT, whose preprocessing is nominally heavier. Uncertainty was quantified via non-parametric bootstrap (B = 2000) on the test set; between-model differences were assessed via Welch's t-test on the bootstrap distributions. Interpretability was assessed using Signal-GradCAM [7] to map attention weights to developmental hours.

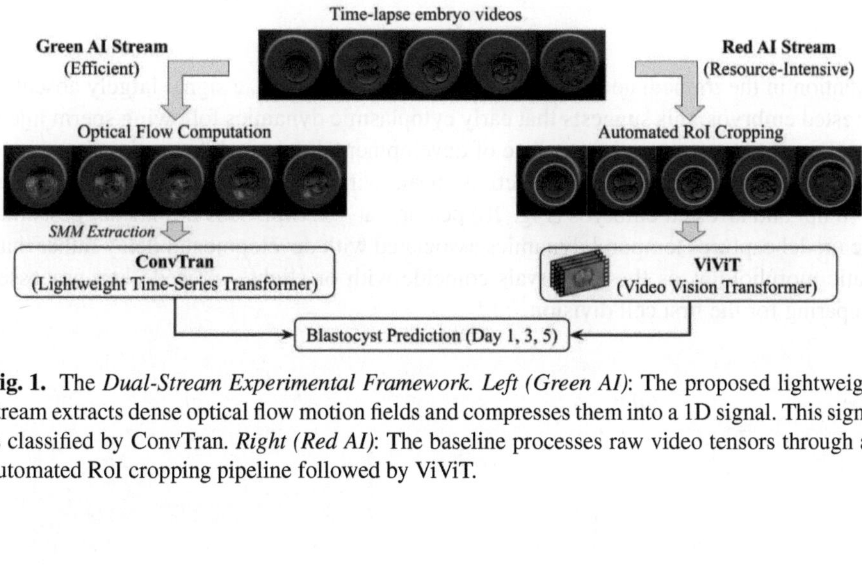


**Fig. 1.** The *Dual-Stream Experimental Framework. Left (Green AI)*: The proposed lightweight stream extracts dense optical flow motion fields and compresses them into a 1D signal. This signal is classified by ConvTran. *Right (Red AI)*: The baseline processes raw video tensors through an automated RoI cropping pipeline followed by ViViT.

## 3 Results

**Performance.** Table 1 details the accuracy–efficiency trade-off. ConvTran significantly outperformed ViViT at Day 1 (24 hpi; $p < 0.001$) and Day 3 (72 hpi; $p < 0.001$), suggesting that explicit motion signals are more robust than raw pixels against early background noise. At Day 5 (120 hpi), ViViT modestly surpassed ConvTran by 0.03 AUC at ~2,500× the inference cost—a trade-off we argue does not justify heavy-model deployment in clinical routine.

**Biological Discovery.** Signal-GradCAM analysis (Fig. 2) revealed two morphokinetic signatures. First, embryos reaching the blastocyst stage (Fig. 2a) triggered consistent

**Table 1.** The Green AI Trade-off. AUC and F1 with bootstrap 95% CIs (B = 2000); all between-model differences are significant (Welch's t-test, $p < 0.001$). [a]Train/Inference at Day 5.

| Model | Params (M) | FLOPs | Latency (ms) | AUC [95% CI] | F1 [95% CI] | kgCO2 Train/Inf[a] |
|---|---|---|---|---|---|---|
| *ViViT* | 42.40 | 2,477 G | 13,638 | **D1:** 0.57 [0.53–0.62] **D3:** 0.66 [0.61–0.70] **D5:** 0.91 [0.88–0.93] | **D1:** 0.59 [0.54–0.63] **D3:** 0.65 [0.61–0.70] **D5:** 0.84 [0.81–0.88] | 1.09 / 0.008 |
| *ConvTran* | 0.20 | 0.12 M | 5.5 | **D1:** 0.62 [0.58–0.66] **D3:** 0.70 [0.66–0.74] **D5:** 0.88 [0.85–0.90] | **D1:** 0.63 [0.59–0.67] **D3:** 0.69 [0.66–0.72] **D5:** 0.79 [0.76–0.82] | 0.005 / ~0 |

attention in the immediate post-fertilization period (0–5 hpi), a signal largely absent in arrested embryos; this suggests that early cytoplasmic dynamics following sperm injection may represent an early correlate of developmental potential. Second, we observed a temporal shift in the subsequent activity peak, with blastocysts triggering attention at ~18 hpi and arrested embryos (Fig. 2b) peaking at ~20 hpi. This 2-h lag suggests that the model captures temporal dynamics associated with developmental delay rather than static morphology, as these intervals coincide with or slightly precede key processes preparing for the first cell division.

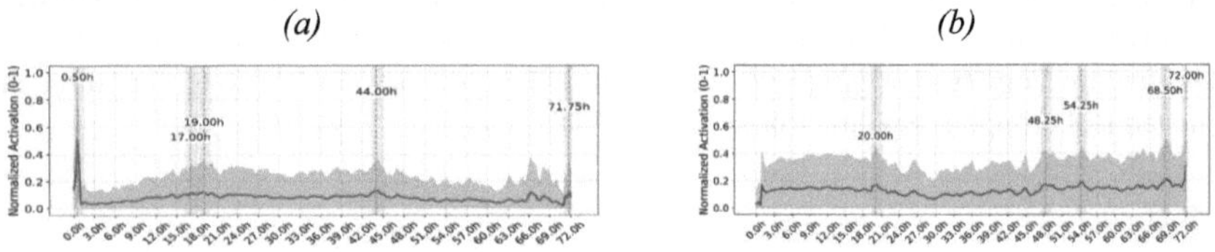


**Fig. 2.** *Temporal Attention Maps (Signal-GradCAM).* Mean normalized attention weights ± standard deviation over the first 72 h. (a) True Positives (embryos correctly predicted as blastocysts). (b) True Negatives (correctly predicted arrested embryos).

## 4 Discussion and Conclusion

Our findings challenge the assumption that "heavier is automatically better" in medical AI. A lightweight optical-flow classifier significantly outperformed a Video Vision Transformer at the earliest and clinically most valuable decision timepoints (Day 1 and Day 3), while using <0.001% of the compute, and closed to within 0.03 AUC of ViViT at Day 5—a gap that the ~2,500-fold efficiency advantage and > 99% lower $CO_2$ footprint render uncompelling for clinical deployment. Our pipeline enables privacy-preserving, local inference on standard workstations, aligned with the call to address the sustainability crisis in deep learning [3]. Interpretability analysis (Fig. 2) further surfaced a prognostic window in the first 5 hpi and a 2-h peak shift between blastocysts and arrested embryos, indicating that the model captures temporal dynamics rather than static morphology.

*Limitations and Future Work.* This study is limited by a single-center retrospective design; a multi-center external validation is already underway. Our benchmark includes a single SOTA video transformer baseline, and an extended comparison against 3D-CNNs, CNN-LSTMs, and compressed (quantized or distilled) video transformers is planned—heavy architectures may be made more cost-effective, but our results suggest that motion-based feature engineering is a simpler and more directly interpretable route. Optical-flow summarization necessarily discards fine-grained spatial appearance information; we are developing a hybrid segmentation-plus-flow model to recover morphological cues. Demographic fairness analysis is constrained by available metadata; an age-stratified analysis (point-biserial $r = -0.110$, $p < 0.01$ with outcome) is in preparation.

*Code Availability:* upon request at https://github.com/prontoSoCorso/blastoGreenAI.

**Acknowledgments.** Work supported by ESHRE Grant 2024 for research in reproductive medicine. Lorenzo Corso is enrolled in the National PhD Program in Artificial Intelligence (XL cycle) – Health and Life Sciences, organized by Università Campus Bio-Medico di Roma.

**Disclosure of Interests** The authors have no competing interests to declare.

## References

1. Arnab, A., et al.: ViViT: a video vision transformer. In: Presented at the 2021 IEEE/CVF International Conference on Computer Vision (ICCV), pp. 6816–6826. IEEE Computer Society (2021). https://doi.org/10.1109/ICCV48922.2021.00676
2. Rajendran, S., et al.: A foundational model for in vitro fertilization trained on 18 million time-lapse images. Nat. Commun. **16**(1), 6235 (2025). https://doi.org/10.1038/s41467-025-61116-2
3. Schwartz, R., et al.: Green AI. Commun. ACM. **63**(12), 54–63 (2020). https://doi.org/10.1145/3381831
4. Farneback, G.: Fast and accurate motion estimation using orientation tensors and parametric motion models. In: Proceedings 15th International Conference on Pattern Recognition. ICPR-2000, vol. 1, pp. 135–139 (2000). https://doi.org/10.1109/ICPR.2000.905291
5. Foumani, N.M., et al.: Improving position encoding of transformers for multivariate time series classification. Data Min. Knowl. Discov. **38**(1), 22–48 (2024). https://doi.org/10.1007/s10618-023-00948-2
6. Lacoste, A., et al.: Quantifying the Carbon Emissions of Machine Learning. arXiv, 1910.09700 (2019). https://doi.org/10.48550/arXiv.1910.09700
7. Pe, S., et al.: SignalGrad-CAM: beyond image explanation. In: Joint Proceedings with the 3rd World Conference on eXplainable Artificial Intelligence, Istanbul, Turkey (2025) [Online]. Available: https://ceur-ws.org/Vol-4017/paper_27.pdf

# Image-Based EEG Representations for Convolutional Neural Networks: A Task-Dependent Analysis

Izabela Rejer[1](✉) and Aleksandra Kawala-Sterniuk[2]

[1] West Pomeranian University of Technology in Szczecin, Żołnierska 49, 71-210 Szczecin, Poland
izabela.rejer@zut.edu.pl
[2] Wroclaw University of Science and Technology, Wyb. Wyspianskiego 27, 50-380 Wroclaw, Poland
aleksandra.kawala-sterniuk@pwr.edu.pl

**Abstract.** The increasing adoption of Convolutional Neural Networks (CNNs) for EEG signal classification has emphasized the need for effective image-based representations of those inherently one-dimensional signals. This study investigates how different transformation strategies for converting a matrix of EEG signals into two-dimensional images influence classification performance. In particular, we examine time–space, frequency–space, and time–frequency representations, evaluating their ability to preserve discriminative signal characteristics. To improve the generalizability of our findings, experiments are conducted on four datasets representing distinct neurophysiological paradigms, including blink-related transients, steady-state visual evoked potentials, motor imagery, and activity associated with Alzheimer's disease. The results demonstrate that, contrary to the widespread assumption that CNNs can autonomously extract all relevant information from minimally processed inputs, providing task-adapted representations substantially improves the network performance. Hence, these findings highlight the critical role of using representation methods aligned with the characteristics of the signal and the target task in EEG-based classification.

**Keywords:** CNN · EEG · Signal-to-image representation

## 1 Introduction

Deep learning methods, and convolutional neural networks (CNNs) in particular, have become a dominant approach in EEG-based classification across a wide range of applications. In many recent studies, CNNs are applied either directly to raw EEG signals or to their transformed representations, often under the implicit assumption that sufficiently deep and highly parameterized models will automatically learn task-relevant features regardless of the chosen input encoding. As noted in the systematic review by Roy et al. [7], one of the frequently

© The Author(s), under exclusive license to Springer Nature Switzerland AG 2027
P. Andreev et al. (Eds.): AIME 2026, LNAI 16748, pp. 194–204, 2027.
https://doi.org/10.1007/978-3-032-30710-1_24

cited motivations for applying deep learning to EEG analysis is precisely its ability to perform automatic feature learning. While more recent architectures, including transformer-based and hybrid models, have been increasingly explored, convolutional neural networks remain a strong and widely used baseline due to their efficiency and suitability for structured signal representations [2,7].

However, EEG recordings exhibit fundamentally different properties depending on the underlying physiological context. For instance, in steady-state visual evoked potential (SSVEP) paradigm, the signal is dominated by stable, narrowband oscillatory components synchronized with the stimulation frequency [4]. In contrast, motor imagery (MI) is characterized by event-related desynchronization/synchronization (ERD/ERS) in sensorimotor rhythms, manifested as task-dependent modulations of band power rather than persistent frequency-specific oscillations [5]. Eye blink activity appears in EEG as high-amplitude, low-frequency transients that introduce strong spectral components predominantly in the delta and theta bands [6], while neurodegenerative conditions such as Alzheimer's disease are associated with long-term alterations in the distribution of spectral power across frequency bands [1]. These differences raise a fundamental question: does a universal EEG representation exist for CNN-based classification, or is the optimal representation inherently task-dependent?

To address this question, we investigate the influence of input representation on CNN-based EEG classification across four conceptually different problems: (i) SSVEP-based frequency discrimination, (ii) motor imagery classification, (iii) blink detection, and (iv) Alzheimer's disease detection. For each task, we evaluate several input representations, including time-domain, frequency-domain, and time–frequency representations. In the SSVEP setting, we further analyze the impact of spectral density and explicitly test whether incorporating phase information improves classification performance.

Our central hypothesis is that the optimal EEG representation depends on the dominant properties of the signal, and that CNN performance cannot be assumed invariant to representation choice. The results provide strong evidence supporting this hypothesis, indicating that (1) no single image-based EEG representation is universally optimal for CNNs, (2) sufficient spectral density is required when narrowband responses are encoded as frequency-domain images, and (3) explicit phase encoding can enhance CNN performance. These findings emphasize that, when EEG signals are transformed into image-like representations for CNN-based classification, aligning the representation with the underlying neurophysiological characteristics of the task is crucial for achieving reliable performance. Thus, we challenge the notion that deep architectures alone can compensate for suboptimal signal encoding.

## 2 Methods

### 2.1 Datasets

Four EEG datasets were analyzed to cover distinct signal structures and neurophysiological contexts: *An Open Dataset for Wearable SSVEP-Based Brain-Computer Interfaces* (SSVEP) [9], *EEG Motor Movement/Imagery Dataset*

(MI) [8], *A dataset of EEG recordings from: Alzheimer's disease, Frontotemporal dementia and Healthy subjects* (AD) [3], and *Blink detection dataset* (BLINK) [6]. The selected datasets, whose key characteristics are summarized in Table 1, differ substantially in temporal dynamics and spectral structure.

**The SSVEP dataset** comprises EEG recordings from 8 occipital and parieto-occipital channels acquired during a steady-state visual evoked potential experiment involving twelve stimulation frequencies at sub-Hz intervals (9.25–14.75 Hz). The original dataset includes recordings from 102 subjects under wet and dry electrode conditions. In this study, only wet-electrode recordings were considered. To ensure reliable stimulus synchronization, subjects with weak frequency locking were excluded using canonical correlation analysis (CCA). Specifically, only subjects achieving a mean CCA accuracy of at least 50% were retained, resulting in a subset of 61 subjects. For reference, the average CCA accuracy within the selected group was 74.81%. Each of the 61 selected subjects completed 10 trials per stimulation frequency (120 trials per subject), resulting in a total of 7,320 trials used in this study. From the original 2.84-second recordings, the 2-second stimulation interval was extracted for analysis.

**Table 1.** Summary of analyzed EEG datasets.

| Dataset | Task type | Subjects | Channels | Fs | Trial length | Classes |
|---|---|---|---|---|---|---|
| SSVEP | Frequency discrimination | 61 | 8 | 250 Hz | 2 s | 12 |
| MI | Motor imagery classification | 107 | 64 | 160 Hz | 4 s | 2 |
| BLINK | Blink detection | 1 | 19 | 500 Hz | 1 s | 2 |
| AD | Alzheimer detection | 63 | 19 | 500 Hz | 10 s | 2 |

**The MI dataset** comprises EEG recordings from 109 subjects performing motor execution and motor imagery tasks involving upper and lower limbs. Each subject participated in 14 sessions: two baseline sessions and twelve main-task sessions. The main-task sessions included four different two-class cue-based paradigms alternated with rest periods and repeated three times. Each non-baseline session consisted of 30 trials, each lasting 4 seconds. In this study, a reduced two-class subset was constructed using only one of the four main paradigms, namely actual left- and right-fist movements. Each subject completed three sessions of this task, yielding 90 trials per subject (45 rest trials and 45 movement trials, unevenly distributed between left and right conditions). Two subjects (S088 and S092) were excluded due to irregular trial durations. After removing rest trials, the final dataset consisted of 4,815 trials from 107 subjects.

**The BLINK dataset** comprises EEG recordings from 10 subjects participating in a cognitive experiment designed to collect blink episodes of varying characteristics. The experiment lasted approximately 45 min and included five tasks with different levels of cognitive load. For the purpose of this study, the continuous recordings acquired during the experiment were segmented into 1-second trials. Each trial was assigned to one of two classes: blink (single or multiple blink episode) or non-blink, based on the event marker channel indicating blink occurrence at the sample level. Due to the highly imbalanced distribution of trials, with substantially more non-blink than blink segments, i) data augmentation (noise addition and temporal shifting) was applied to the blink class, ii) 90% of non-blink trials were randomly removed. This strategy, however; was applied only for the training data, the test data retained the natural distribution of blink events. For the study presented in this paper, one representative subject (S6) was randomly selected, resulting in 17,055 trials used for analysis.

Finally, **the AD dataset** comprises resting-state, eyes-closed EEG recordings from participants diagnosed with Alzheimer's disease (AD; n = 36), frontotemporal dementia (FTD; n = 23), and cognitively normal controls (CN; n = 29). In this study, only the AD and CN cohorts were considered. Two participants (one AD and one CN) were excluded due to substantially shorter recordings. The final dataset therefore included 35 AD and 28 CN participants. To ensure consistent data contribution across subjects, recordings were truncated to a common duration (554 seconds per participant). These segments were further divided into 10-second trials with no overlap. This segmentation resulted in 55 trials per participant (3,465 trials in total).

## 2.2 Representations

**Time-Domain Representation (Channel × Time).** Let $X \in \mathbb{R}^{C \times T}$ denote a single EEG trial, where $C$ is the number of channels and $T$ the number of temporal samples. The time-domain representation is defined directly as

$$I_{\text{time}} = X. \tag{1}$$

When required, temporal resampling is applied:

$$\tilde{X} = \mathcal{R}_t(X), \qquad \tilde{X} \in \mathbb{R}^{C \times T'}, \tag{2}$$

where $\mathcal{R}_t(\cdot)$ denotes a temporal resampling operator and $T'$ is the target number of temporal samples.

**Frequency-Domain Representation (channel × frequency).** For each channel $c$, the complex spectral coefficient at frequency $f_k$ is defined as

$$S_c(f_k) = \sum_{t=0}^{T-1} x_c(t)\, e^{-j2\pi f_k t}, \tag{3}$$

where $x_c(t)$ denotes the temporal signal and $f_k$ the $k$-th frequency. In the FFT setting, $f_k$ corresponds to the discrete Fourier grid. In the Goertzel-based projection, $S_c(f_k)$ is evaluated directly for arbitrarily selected frequencies. When Welch's method is used, $S_c(f_k)$ denotes the averaged spectral estimate obtained from windowed segments. The frequency-domain image is constructed from logarithmic magnitude:

$$I_{\text{freq}}(c,k) = \log(|S_c(f_k)| + \epsilon)\,, \tag{4}$$

yielding an image of size $C \times K$, where $K$ is the number of frequency bins. For phase-aware encoding, magnitude and phase are retained as separate channels:

$$I_{\text{freq}}(c,k) = \Big[\ \log(|S_c(f_k)| + \epsilon),\ \arg(S_c(f_k))\Big]. \tag{5}$$

**Time-Frequency Representation (Frequency × Time).** For each channel $c$, the continuous wavelet transform (CWT) is defined as

$$W_c(f,\tau) = \int_{-\infty}^{\infty} x_c(t)\,\psi^*_{f,\tau}(t)\,dt, \tag{6}$$

where $\psi_{f,\tau}(t)$ denotes the scaled and shifted mother wavelet, $f$ represents frequency and $\tau$ time localization. The time–frequency image is constructed directly from logarithmic power:

$$I_{\text{tf}}(f,\tau) = \log\big(|W_c(f,\tau)|^2 + \epsilon\big)\,, \tag{7}$$

yielding an image of size $K \times T$. If a dimension decrease is required, temporal resampling is applied according to Eq. (2).

### 2.3 CNN Architectures and Experimental Protocol

All models follow a relatively lightweight and standardized CNN architecture designed to ensure fair comparison across representations and to isolate the effect of input encoding from architectural complexity. Accordingly, the focus of this study is on representation design rather than architectural optimization. The network consists of convolutional blocks (convolution, batch normalization, LeakyReLU, average pooling, dropout with rate 0.3) followed by one or more fully connected layers and a final softmax classification layer trained with cross-entropy loss. Convolutional layers use stride = 1 and zero-padding. Dataset-specific architectural details are summarized in Table 2.

**Training and Validation Strategy.** For each dataset, an independent test set was defined prior to training. In SSVEP, MI, and AD, subject-wise splits were applied, with seven, five, and nine randomly selected subjects reserved for independent testing, respectively. In BLINK, data from one of the five experimental tasks were used exclusively for testing. The remaining data were further divided into training/validation subsets. Models were trained using the Adam optimizer with a learning rate of 0.001 for up to 100 epochs, with early stopping (patience = 20) based on validation loss. Elastic net regularization (L1 and L2) was applied with regularization coefficients set to 0.1. Batch size was set to 128.

**Table 2.** Dataset-specific CNN architectures; "Filters" denotes the number of kernels per layer, "Kernel" - the kernel sizes, "Pool" - the pooling sizes; "FC" column lists the number of neurons in successive fully connected layers; "Arch" stands for Architecture.

| Dataset | Arch | Convolution blocks | | | FC |
|---|---|---|---|---|---|
| | | Filters | Kernel | Pool | |
| SSVEP | S1 | 16,32,64 | 1x7,1x5,1x3 | 1x2,1x2,1x2 | 128 |
| | S2 | 16,32,64 | 3x1,3x1,3x1 | 2x1,2x1,2x1 | 64 |
| | S3 | 16,32,64,128 | 3x3,3x3,3x3,3x3 | 1x2,1x2,1x2,1x2 | 128 |
| MI | M1 | 16,32,64 | 3x7,3x5,3x3 | 1x2,1x2,2x2 | 128 |
| | M2 | 16,32,32 | 5x3,3x3,3x3 | 2x2,2x2,1x2 | 128 |
| | M3 | 16,32,64 | 8x15,1x9,1x5 | 2x2,1x2,1x2 | 128 |
| BLINK | B1 | 16,32 | 3x5,3x3 | 1x2,1x2 | 64 |
| | B2 | 16,32,64 | 3x3,3x3,3x3 | 2x2,2x2,2x2 | 64 |
| | B3 | 3,3,3,3 | 3x3,3x3,3x3,3x3 | 2x2,2x2,1x2,1x2 | 5,5,5 |
| AD | A1 | 32,64,128 | 3x3,3x3,3x3 | 2x2,1x2,1x2 | 40,30 |
| | A2 | 16,32,64 | 3x3,3x3,3x3 | 2x2,2x2,2x2 | 128 |
| | A3 | 16,32 | 3x5,3x3 | 1x2,2x2 | 64 |

**Experimental Procedure.** For each dataset, all defined architectures were trained for each representation. Each configuration was trained 10 times with different random initializations. Classification performance was evaluated using class-wise (balanced) accuracy, computed as the mean accuracy across classes to ensure equal contribution of each class regardless of class distribution. This metric was adopted due to the severe class imbalance present in the BLINK test set: 9689 non-blink vs. 2042 blink trials (all remaining datasets were class-balanced). Statistical significance of pairwise differences between representations was assessed using the Wilcoxon signed-rank test ($p < 0.05$).

## 3 Results and Discussion

The objective of this study was to determine whether a single EEG image representation can generalize across tasks, or whether representation choice must be aligned with task-specific signal characteristics. To this end, each dataset was evaluated using time-domain, frequency-domain, and time–frequency representations under multiple CNN architectures and repeated training runs. Table 3 summarizes the best-performing architecture within each representation type for every dataset. For all datasets, the difference between the best- and worst-performing representations was found to be statistically significant; additionally, significant differences between the best and second-best representations were observed for SSVEP, MI, and AD, but not for BLINK.

The results reveal two complementary observations. First, each representation type achieves top performance for at least one dataset. Second, none of the

**Table 3.** Best-performing architectures within each representation type for all datasets. Reported values correspond to mean class-wise accuracy (± standard deviation) over 10 independent runs. Bold values indicate the top accuracy for each dataset.

| | Time-domain | Frequency-domain | Time–frequency |
|---|---|---|---|
| SSVEP | 81.35±0.35 (S2) | **83.34**±0.54 (S2) | 63.89±0.72 (S3) |
| MI | **80.62**±2.06 (M3) | 68.27±2.85 (M1) | 75.13±3.36 (M2) |
| BLINK | 91.13±2.65 (B3) | **99.31**±0.11 (B1) | 98.37±1.25 (B3) |
| AD | 75.52±1.64 (A1) | 91.85±0.64 (A1) | **94.15**±2.76 (A1) |

representations performs consistently well across all tasks. Time-domain encoding dominates in motor imagery, frequency-based representations lead in SSVEP and blink detection, and time–frequency encoding achieves the best performance in Alzheimer detection. However, each representation also exhibits at least one clear performance drop, highlighting the absence of a universally optimal encoding strategy. These findings reinforce the central premise of this study: representation effectiveness is inherently task-dependent and must be aligned with the properties of the EEG signal under analysis. In the following, we examine the results for each of the four analyzed datasets in greater detail.

**SSVEP**. For the SSVEP dataset, multiple image representations were constructed within the 8–16 Hz band containing the stimulation frequencies. These included: time-domain encoding, FFT-based spectral representation, CWT-based time–frequency representation, and three variants of Goertzel projection (with amplitude, amplitude+phase, and real+imaginary components). Figure 1 presents image representations obtained from a single trial using 0.1 Hz resolution.

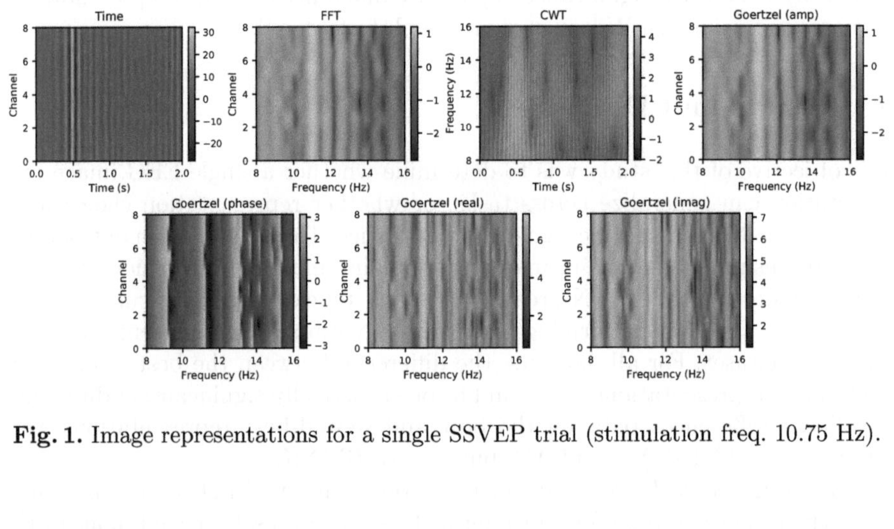


**Fig. 1.** Image representations for a single SSVEP trial (stimulation freq. 10.75 Hz).

Since discriminative information in the SSVEP paradigm is concentrated within a narrow frequency range, this dataset provides a controlled scenario for analyzing the influence of representation design, particularly in frequency- and time–frequency-based encodings. In this setting, spectral resolution emerges as a critical factor, as shown in Table 4, which summarizes the classification accuracy obtained for different spectral resolutions and representation variants.

Table 4 shows that for amplitude-only frequency representations (FFT and Goertzel), performance improved substantially when moving from the native 0.5 Hz resolution (FFT: 63.89%, Goertzel: 63.53%) to sub-Hz sampling (77-78%). However, since increasing spectral density beyond 0.25 Hz did not produce further gains, this suggests that resolving closely spaced stimulation frequencies is sufficient, while excessively dense sampling provides limited additional benefit. Notably, FFT with zero-padding achieved results comparable to Goertzel-based projection at 0.1 Hz, suggesting that dense spectral interpolation is sufficient for CNN-based discrimination, even without explicit targeting exact frequencies. The most pronounced improvement was observed when phase information was included into representation. Goertzel with amplitude and phase encoding reached around 83% accuracy at both 0.25 and 0.1 Hz resolutions, outperforming amplitude-only representations by approximately 5 percentage points. In contrast, representing the complex coefficient directly (real and imaginary parts) did not yield comparable gains (79.09% at 0.1 Hz).

**Table 4.** SSVEP accuracy (%) for different spectral resolutions and representations. Values denote mean class-wise accuracy (v standard deviation) over 10 runs. The highest accuracy is highlighted in bold.

| Method | 0.5 Hz | 0.25 Hz | 0.1 Hz |
|---|---|---|---|
| FFT (S2) | 63.89±0.42 | 77.94±0.99 | 77.02±1.04 |
| Goertzel (amp) (S2) | 63.53±1.01 | 77.06±1.08 | 77.82±0.59 |
| Goertzel (amp+phase) (S2) | 77.03±0.83 | 82.52±0.84 | **83.34**±0.54 |
| Goertzel (complex) (S2) | 64.76±1.15 | 77.27±0.73 | 79.09±1.01 |
| CWT (S3) | 63.89±0.72 | 57.98±0.84 | 53.30±0.91 |

For the time-domain and CWT representations, the temporal dimension was downsampled from 500 to 100 samples prior to constructing the final representations. The time-domain representation achieved 81.35% accuracy, making it the second-best performing approach and outperforming all amplitude-only frequency representations. This result suggests that, in the case of narrowband oscillatory signals such as SSVEP, CNNs are capable of implicitly extracting both frequency-specific and phase-related structure directly from spatio-temporal inputs, even without explicit spectral decomposition. Despite preserving joint temporal and spectral information, the CWT-based representation performed markedly worse (53–64%), likely because the limited frequency resolution of wavelet scales in the low-frequency range prevents reliable separation of closely spaced stimulation frequencies.

**MI.** For the MI dataset, representations were constructed within the 0.5–40 Hz range. In contrast to the SSVEP experiments, spectral resolution was not artificially increased: both FFT and CWT were computed using their native frequency resolution. Moreover, for time-domain and CWT encodings, the temporal dimension was resampled from 640 to 160 samples to obtain compact image representations. For this dataset, the time-domain representation achieved the highest performance (80.62%), outperforming both CWT (75.13%) and FFT-based encodings (68.27%). This outcome is consistent with the neurophysiological nature of motor imagery. ERD/ERS patterns are not stationary oscillations but time-limited modulations of band power that emerge after cue onset and evolve throughout the trial. When FFT is computed over the entire 4-second segment, these temporal dynamics are averaged into a single spectral estimate per frequency bin. As a result, transient desynchronization and resynchronization effects become attenuated, reducing class separability. The CWT-based representation partially preserves temporal evolution and therefore performs significantly better than FFT. In contrast, the direct channel × time encoding retains the full spatio-temporal evolution of ERD/ERS dynamics, allowing the CNN to learn both when and where discriminative changes occur.

**BLINK.** For the blink detection dataset, representations were constructed within the 1–30 Hz range using native spectral resolution (1 Hz). For time-domain and CWT encodings, the temporal dimension was resampled from 500 to 100 samples. In contrast to the previous datasets, the CNNs trained on all representation types built from blink data, achieved very high performance, with FFT reaching 99.31%, CWT 98.37%, and the time-domain representation 91.13%. This consistently strong performance reflects the inherent simplicity of blink-related activity: eye blinks manifest as high-amplitude, low-frequency transients that produce pronounced and easily separable patterns across both temporal and spectral domains. Frequency-based encodings achieve slightly higher accuracy likely because blink events generate strong low-frequency spectral peaks that remain invariant with respect to their temporal position within the trial. In contrast, in the time-domain representation the peak may occur at different temporal locations across trials. Although CNNs are translation-tolerant, variability in the temporal position of a single high-amplitude event may introduce additional learning complexity.

**AD.** Representations were constructed within the 0.5–40 Hz range. Spectral features were obtained using Welch's method (2-second segments, 75% overlap). Prior to constructing time-domain and CWT representations, the temporal dimension was downsampled to 100 samples. The time–frequency representation achieved the highest performance (94.15%), followed by the frequency-domain encoding (91.85%), whereas the time-domain representation performed substantially worse (75.52%). These results reflect a fundamental difference between the AD dataset and the three remaining paradigms. In SSVEP, MI, and BLINK, the analyzed signals correspond to activity that is temporally aligned with stimulus onset or behavioral events. In contrast, the AD dataset consists of spontaneous resting-state activity, where no external event defines a temporal reference point. Consequently, discriminative information is not tied to specific temporal segments but is instead reflected in global alterations of spectral power distribution. In this setting, the raw time-domain signal lacks consistent temporal structure across trials, which likely explains its markedly inferior performance. On the other hand, representations that explicitly encode spectral characteristics are better suited to capture these, long-term spectral alterations.

## 4 Conclusion

The study reported in this paper tested the hypothesis that the optimal EEG representation depends on the dominant properties of the signal and that CNN performance is not invariant to representation choice. The results across four fundamentally different datasets provide clear support for this claim. Each representation type achieved top performance in at least one task, yet each also failed in another. No universal encoding emerged. Instead, narrowband oscillations (SSVEP), spatially localized short-term alterations (MI), transient artifacts (BLINK), and long-term spectral modulations (AD) each required a representation aligned with their intrinsic signal properties. These findings demonstrate that representation design is not a neutral preprocessing step but a primary determinant of CNN effectiveness in EEG-based classification. Architectural variation alone cannot compensate for a misaligned signal encoding. Consequently, representation selection should be treated as a task-specific modeling decision rather than a fixed pipeline component.

*Declaration of AI Assistance Technologies During Manuscript Preparation.* The authors used ChatGPT 5.2 for refinement, correction, editing or formatting the manuscript to improve clarity of language (AI activity class no. 1). After using this technology, the authors reviewed the results and take full responsibility for the contents of the manuscript.

**Acknowledgments.** This study was financially supported by Minister of Science under the 'Regional Initiative of Excellence' (RID) programme.

## References

1. Babiloni, C., et al.: Resting state EEG rhythms in Alzheimer's disease: toward EEG biomarkers for clinical applications. Clin. Neurophysiol. **131**(2), 427–443 (2020)
2. Hallal, L., et al.: Efficient feature extraction for EEG-based classification: a review of deep learning approaches. Signals **7**(2), 50 (2026)
3. Miltiadous, A., et al.: A dataset of scalp EEG recordings of Alzheimer's disease, frontotemporal dementia and healthy subjects from routine EEG. Data **8**(6), 95 (2023)

4. Norcia, A.M., Appelbaum, L.G., Ales, J.M., Cottereau, B.R., Rossion, B.: The steady-state visual evoked potential in vision research: a review. J. Vis. **15**(6), 4 (2015)
5. Pfurtscheller, G., Neuper, C.: Motor imagery and direct brain-computer communication. Proc. IEEE **89**(7), 1123–1134 (2001)
6. Rejer, I., Gago, I.: A CNN-based approach for detecting eye blink episodes in EEG signals. J. Neural Eng. **22**(3), 036017 (2025)
7. Roy, Y., Banville, H., Albuquerque, I., Gramfort, A., Falk, T.H., Faubert, J.: Deep learning-based electroencephalography analysis: a systematic review. J. Neural Eng. **16**(5), 051001 (2019)
8. Schalk, G., McFarland, D.J., Hinterberger, T., Birbaumer, N., Wolpaw, J.R.: BCI 2000: a general-purpose brain-computer interface (BCI) system. IEEE Trans. Biomed. Eng. **51**(6), 1034–1043 (2004)
9. Zhu, F., Jiang, L., Dong, G., Gao, X., Wang, Y.: An open dataset for wearable SSVEP-based brain-computer interfaces. Sensors **21**(4), 1256 (2021)

# C2W-Tune: Cavity-to-Wall Transfer Learning for Thin Atrial Wall Segmentation in 3D LGE-MRI

Yusri Al-Sanaani[1(✉)], Rebecca Thornhill[1,2], and Sreeraman Rajan[1]

[1] Systems and Computer Engineering, Carleton University, Ottawa, ON, Canada
YusriAlSanaani@cmail.carleton.ca

[2] Department of Radiology, University of Ottawa, Ottawa, ON, Canada

**Abstract.** Accurate segmentation of the left atrial (LA) wall in 3D late gadolinium-enhanced MRI (LGE-MRI) is essential for wall thickness mapping and fibrosis quantification, yet it remains challenging due to the wall's thin geometry, complex anatomy, and low contrast. We propose C2W-Tune, a two-stage cavity-to-wall transfer framework that leverages a high-accuracy LA cavity model as an anatomical prior to improving thin-wall delineation. Using a 3D U-Net with a ResNeXt encoder and instance normalization, Stage 1 pre-trains the network to segment the LA cavity, learning robust atrial representations. Stage 2 transfers these weights and adapts the network to LA wall segmentation using a progressive layer-unfreezing schedule to preserve cavity features while enabling wall-specific refinement. On the 2018 LA Segmentation Challenge dataset, C2W-Tune outperformed an architecture-matched baseline trained from scratch. The wall Dice score increased from 0.623 to 0.814, surface Dice at 1 mm increased from 0.553 to 0.731, 95th-percentile Hausdorff distance (HD95) decreased from 2.95 mm to 2.55 mm, and average symmetric surface distance (ASSD) decreased from 0.71 mm to 0.63 mm. Under reduced supervision using 70 training volumes sampled from the same training set, C2W-Tune achieved a Dice of 0.78, remaining competitive with recent multi-class bi-atrial benchmarks (typically 0.6–0.7). These results show that anatomically grounded task transfer with controlled fine-tuning improves accuracy for thin LA wall segmentation in 3D LGE-MRI.

**Keywords:** Left atrial wall segmentation · LGE-MRI · Transfer learning · Atrial fibrillation

## 1 Introduction

Late gadolinium-enhanced MRI (LGE-MRI) is widely used to assess and quantify scarring within the left atrium (LA). The spatial distribution and severity of these fibrotic regions may offer key insights into the underlying mechanisms and clinical progression of atrial fibrillation (AF). Consequently, robust computational methods for processing and analyzing LA LGE-MRI data are important for supporting image-guided diagnosis and guiding personalized treatment strategies for patients with AF [1]. For example,

© The Author(s), under exclusive license to Springer Nature Switzerland AG 2027
P. Andreev et al. (Eds.): AIME 2026, LNAI 16748, pp. 205–214, 2027.
https://doi.org/10.1007/978-3-032-30710-1_25

LGE-MRI can enable measurement of LA wall thickness, which is a predictor of ablation outcome and safety, while delineation of the endocardial (inner) and epicardial (outer) surfaces enables quantification of scar transmurality (full-thickness injury), which correlates with AF recurrence [1]. However, automatically segmenting the LA wall from 3D LGE-MRI is extremely challenging. The LA wall is very thin and has a complex geometry with multiple discontinuities (e.g., pulmonary veins (PV) and the mitral valve (MV)), making it difficult to distinguish it from surrounding structures. LGE-MRI images often suffer from low contrast and heterogeneous enhancement; the atrial wall and nearby tissues can exhibit similar intensity, complicating boundary identification [1–4]. These factors lead to severe class imbalance and segmentation ambiguity because the LA wall is very thin, and even expert, fellowship-trained cardiothoracic radiologists struggle to provide reproducible manual delineations [5].

As a result, most prior work has focused on the more tractable task of segmenting the LA cavity. For instance, the 2018 LA Segmentation Challenge benchmark demonstrated that a two-step pipeline (localization followed by refinement) achieved a Dice score of 93.2% and a mean surface distance of approximately 0.7 mm on the test set [2]. Rapid left atrial cavity segmentation in 3D LGE-MRI was achieved by fine-tuning an ImageNet-pretrained VGG-16 fully convolutional network on the 2018 LA Segmentation Challenge dataset using a pseudo-3D slice-stacking input in [6]. These works indicate that with sufficient training data and appropriate architecture, the LA cavity (blood pool) can be segmented with high accuracy from LGE-MRI.

While deep learning has advanced cavity segmentation [2] and joint cavity-scar frameworks [7], automating thin atrial wall segmentation remains a major bottleneck. The recent multi-class bi-atrial segmentation challenge (MBAS) further highlights this performance gap. It evaluated a wide spectrum of architectures, including 3D nnU-Nets with residual encoders such as [8, 9], Mamba-style state-space models such as [9, 10], transformer-augmented networks such as [9, 11], and various multi-stage pipelines such as [12, 13]. Across these methods, the left and right cavities consistently achieve Dice scores above 0.90, whereas the bi-atrial (left and right) wall typically remains in the ~0.6–0.7 Dice range. Although most MBAS approaches formulate the problem as the joint prediction of the LA cavity, right atrium (RA) cavity, and bi-atrial wall within a single model, this shared-parameter training induces multi-task-like interactions among outputs. In practice, atrial wall delineation remains the most challenging target, with consistently lower Dice than the cavity classes across challenge reports, suggesting that simultaneous optimization may be biased toward the easier cavity classes.

Several methods implicitly address this imbalance through coarse-to-fine pipelines that refine wall predictions after an initial joint segmentation, such as [12, 13]. Recent work, such as [14], similarly adopts a two-stage ResNeXt-based architecture using a coarse-to-fine spatial cropping strategy for bi-atrial segmentation, but the left and right walls are segmented separately. Conventional deep learning workflows in medical imaging, such as [6], often rely on transfer learning, in which a model is pre-trained on a large, unrelated natural-image dataset (e.g., ImageNet) and then fine-tuned on the target medical task [15]. While this strategy can effectively initialize low-level feature detectors (e.g., edges and blobs), it does not necessarily encode the domain-specific anatomical priors needed for robust medical image analysis.

In this work, we propose C2W-Tune (Cavity-to-Wall Tune), a two-stage 3D segmentation approach that leverages the strong performance of cavity segmentation by initializing wall segmentation from a high-quality cavity model via task-specific anatomical transfer learning. Instead of learning wall segmentation from scratch, C2W-Tune uses the pre-trained LA cavity segmentation model as an anatomical prior, which is subsequently fine-tuned for the thin-wall segmentation task by replacing the final segmentation head and progressively adapting the transferred network for wall segmentation. By transferring the learned encoder features from the cavity task, we prime the network to recognize the LA region, while the progressive fine-tuning avoids catastrophic forgetting of these features.

## 2 Methodology

Our C2W-Tune approach consists of two stages. First, we use a 3D U-Net to produce a coarse segmentation that localizes the atrial region. We then compute the center of mass of the coarse atrial mask and extract a fixed patch around it to define the region of interest (ROI). Stage 1 trains a second 3D U-Net to segment the LA cavity from these ROIs. This model provides a robust encoder pre-trained on the anatomical region of interest. Stage 2 fine-tunes this model to segment the LA wall by introducing a new segmentation head and employing a progressive layer-unfreezing schedule. Figure 1 illustrates the pipeline.

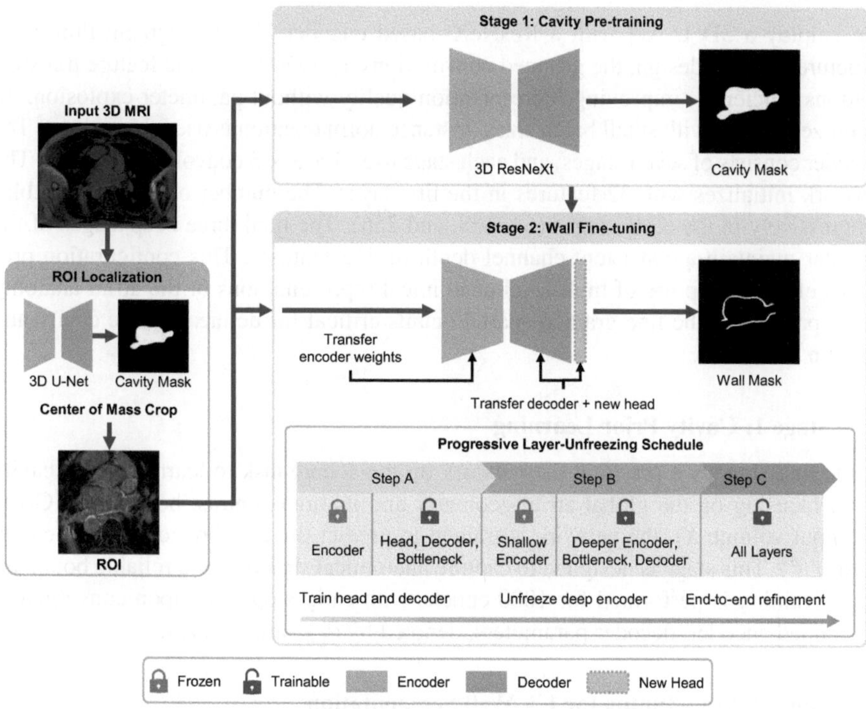


**Fig. 1.** C2W-Tune pipeline: atrial ROI localization, cavity pre-training, and wall fine-tuning.

### 2.1 Dataset

Let $\mathcal{D} = \{(X_i, Y_i^{cav}, Y_i^{wall})\}_{i=1}^{N}$ be the dataset of N 3D LGE-MRI volumes. $X_i \in R^{D \times H \times W}$ is the input LGE-MRI volume. $Y_i^{cav} \in \{0, 1\}^{D \times H \times W}$ is the binary ground truth for the LA cavity. $Y_i^{wall} \in \{0, 1\}^{D \times H \times W}$ is the binary ground truth for the LA wall. We utilize the 2018 LA Segmentation Challenge dataset [2]. The dataset consists of 154 LGE-MRI 3D volumes of patients with AF, acquired at an isotropic voxel spacing of approximately 0.625 mm. Each volume has an expert manual segmentation of the LA cavity and LA wall as ground truth masks.

To reduce background interference and mitigate class imbalance, we first apply a coarse 3D U-Net to each input volume $X_i$ to obtain a preliminary cavity prediction $\hat{Y}_i^{cav}$. We then compute the center of mass of $\hat{Y}_i^{cav}$ and crop $X_i$ to a fixed ROI patch of size $256 \times 256 \times 44$ voxels (and cropping $Y_i^{cav}$ and $Y_i^{wall}$ identically during training). The ROI size is chosen to preserve sufficient spatial context around the atrial wall, consistent with findings of the 2018 LA Segmentation Challenge benchmark [2], which reported performance degradation for ROIs smaller than $240 \times 160$. Therefore, this ROI restricts subsequent cavity/wall prediction to an anatomically relevant subvolume, reducing the effective search space and encouraging the model to focus on left atrial structures rather than surrounding tissue.

### 2.2 Network Architecture

We employ a 3D U-Net with a ResNeXt-based encoder [16] to segment thin atrial structures. In this design, the grouped convolutions aggregate multiple feature transformations efficiently, improving representation quality without parameter explosion. To stabilize training with small batch sizes, instance normalization is used throughout. The encoder consists of seven stages, and each stage uses $3 \times 3 \times 3$ convolution kernels. The network initializes with 32 features in the first layer. The number of features doubles progressively in the early stages (64, 128, and 256). The final three deep stages of the encoder maintain a consistent channel depth of 512 features. This configuration promotes effective capture of high-level anatomical representations of the atrial anatomy while preserving the fine-grained spatial details critical for delineating the cavity and the thin atrial wall.

### 2.3 Stage 1: Cavity Prior Learning

In the first stage, we pre-train the network on the source task to learn a robust cavity prior, focusing on the global atrial geometry and its high-contrast boundaries. Given the input volume $X_i$, the network is trained to predict the corresponding atrial cavity mask $\hat{Y}_i^{cav}$. This stage is designed to capture anatomical structure and reliable boundary cues. Training is performed for 1000 epochs with early stopping. Upon convergence, the trained encoder–decoder parameters, denoted by $\theta_{\text{cav}}$, are retained.

### 2.4 Stage 2: Fine-Tuning for LA Wall Segmentation

In the second stage, we initialize the wall-segmentation network ($\theta_{wall}$) by transferring anatomical representations learned during cavity pre-training ($\theta_{cav}$). This transfer provides a strong starting point for wall prediction by preserving the learned global atrial geometry and contextual features. We then fine-tune the model for atrial wall segmentation using the progressive layer-unfreezing schedule described below.

### 2.5 Progressive Unfreezing Schedule

To mitigate catastrophic forgetting during the transfer from cavity to wall segmentation, we adopt a three-step progressive layer-unfreezing schedule strategy. This strategy leverages layer-wise fine-tuning [17] to incrementally adapt the network, thereby preserving learned feature representations and reducing the risk of losing global atrial geometry during optimization.

**Step A (Head/Decoder Remapping; Epochs 0–60).** We freeze the entire encoder and train the wall segmentation head, decoder, and bottleneck, allowing the decoder to remap transferred atrial features from cavity to wall prediction. In this stage, the encoder serves as a fixed feature extractor, while the decoder is adapted to reinterpret the transferred atrial features for wall prediction rather than cavity prediction.

**Step B (Deep Fine-Tuning; Epochs 61–180).** We keep the shallow encoder layers frozen and unfreeze the deeper encoder stages, together with the bottleneck and decoder. This allows higher-level semantic representations to adapt to wall-specific appearance and geometry, while maintaining stable low-level edge and intensity features learned during pre-training.

**Step C (Full Optimization; Epochs 181–Max 1000).** Finally, all layers are unfrozen for end-to-end refinement. Early stopping is applied during Step C based on validation performance, and the best-performing checkpoint is retained.

The epoch boundaries (e.g., 60 and 180) are validation-selected hyperparameters rather than fixed constants.

### 2.6 Training Setup

The LGE-MRI images were normalized using z-score normalization. The dataset was split into 30 independent test cases (held-out for final evaluation) and 124 development cases. To optimize hyperparameters and assess model stability without data leakage, we performed five-fold cross-validation on the 124 development cases. All splits were performed at the patient level. Following hyperparameter optimization via cross-validation, the final model was retrained once using a fixed 100/24 train/validation split from the 124 development cases and evaluated on the held-out test set. Data augmentation was applied on-the-fly to improve generalization. We used geometric augmentations (random elastic deformations to simulate anatomical variability, and random rotations and axis-constrained flips to reflect plausible pose and orientation differences) and intensity augmentations (intensity scaling and histogram matching to mitigate scanner- and protocol-dependent intensity variability in LGE-MRI [18]). These augmentations help reduce overfitting given the dataset size and address potential domain shifts. Training used the AdamW optimizer with $\beta_1 = 0.9, \beta_2 = 0.999$, and a weight decay of $1 \times 10^{-4}$. We used DiceFocal loss [19] to mitigate class imbalance for both stages, and a batch size of 4. For Stage 1, we utilized a cosine annealing schedule with a 50-epoch linear warmup to stabilize the grouped convolutions, decaying the learning rate from $1 \times 10^{-3}$ to $1 \times 10^{-6}$. For Stage 2, given the constraint of small batch sizes, we employed a stage-wise cosine annealing scheduler with linear warmup. Consistent with our progressive unfreezing strategy, the maximum learning rate was decayed by a factor of 10 at each restart ($1 \times 10^{-3} \rightarrow 1 \times 10^{-4} \rightarrow 1 \times 10^{-5}$) to avoid disrupting the transferred spatial representations during the transition from cavity to wall segmentation. Hyperparameters were selected empirically based on validation Dice score (five-fold cross-validation).

### 2.7 Evaluation Metrics

We report the Dice Similarity Coefficient to measure global volumetric overlap between the predicted and reference masks. To emphasize boundary accuracy, we additionally compute surface Dice at 1 mm, defined as the fraction of surface points on the predicted and ground-truth masks that lie within 1 mm of each other; this is particularly informative for thin-wall segmentation [20]. Finally, we report HD95 (95th-percentile Hausdorff distance) to capture near-worst-case boundary deviations while reducing sensitivity to extreme outliers, together with average symmetric surface distance (ASSD) to summarize the average symmetric surface error.

## 3 Results and Discussion

To quantify the difficulty of LA wall segmentation, we trained an architecture-matched 3D U-Net baseline from scratch using the same loss, data split, and training protocol, but without cavity pre-training. Stage 1 produced a strong cavity model, achieving a Dice score of 0.921 on the cavity test set, comparable to published results [2, 14]. These weights were then transferred for wall segmentation in Stage 2. As shown in Table 1, the baseline had difficulty delineating the thin atrial wall, yielding a Dice score of 0.623, often producing fragmented boundaries. In contrast, C2W-Tune effectively leveraged the anatomical features learned during Stage 1 to guide the wall segmentation. This resulted in a substantial performance gain: wall Dice increased to 0.814 (paired two-sided Wilcoxon signed-rank, $p = 0.001$ vs. baseline model), surface Dice increased from 0.55 to 0.73, HD95 decreased from 2.95 mm to 2.55 mm, and ASSD decreased from 0.71 mm to 0.63 mm. Together, the improved means and lower standard deviations indicate better, more consistent overlap and boundary agreement than the baseline. These gains produced more continuous, anatomically realistic surfaces than the fragmented baseline predictions. Figure 2 shows representative axial slices from challenging cases, including thin low-contrast walls and complex geometry near the pulmonary vein ostia and appendage. In these examples, the baseline often exhibits fragmentation or missing segments, whereas C2W-Tune better preserves boundary continuity.

These results indicate that using a well-resolved anatomical target (the LA cavity) to guide the more difficult wall segmentation helps address the challenges of thin LA wall delineation. Stage 1 provides a strong anatomical prior by identifying the atrial region and approximating the endocardial boundary. The progressive layer-unfreezing

**Table 1.** LA wall segmentation performance on the held-out test set (mean ± standard deviation across test cases).

| Method | Wall Dice ↑ | Surface Dice ↑ | HD95 (mm) ↓ | ASSD (mm) ↓ |
|---|---|---|---|---|
| 3D U-Net (baseline) | 0.623 ± 0.042 | 0.553 ± 0.061 | 2.95 ± 0.88 | 0.71 ± 0.24 |
| C2W-Tune | **0.814 ± 0.028** | **0.731 ± 0.045** | **2.55 ± 0.55** | **0.63 ± 0.17** |

fine-tuning strategy then preserves this anatomical context while enabling adaptation to better capture the epicardial boundary (outer wall border).

A direct numerical comparison with prior studies is contextual due to differences in task definitions and data partitions. As detailed in Table 2, the majority of recent benchmarks [8, 9, 11–13] target a combined bi-atrial wall class (LA + RA) within a multi-class framework, whereas our method focuses specifically on the clinically relevant LA wall. Furthermore, many of these approaches were evaluated using restricted training sets (typically $N \approx 70$). To ensure a fair comparison regarding supervision size, we performed a controlled ablation by retraining C2W-Tune using 70 randomly selected volumes from the 100-volume training pool, while keeping the validation and test sets fixed. Results are reported as mean ± standard deviation across multiple 70-volume subsets; prior methods are reported as published because variance was unavailable (Table 2). Under matched supervision, C2W-Tune (N = 70) achieved 0.78 Dice and 3.15 mm HD95, compared with published Dice values of 0.62–0.71 for recent multi-class bi-atrial methods and 0.617 for LA wall in [14].

These results suggest that C2W-Tune benefits from leveraging the cavity prior through progressive fine-tuning, rather than from training-set size alone. Consequently, our LA wall performance remains competitive in reduced supervision settings and compares favorably to reported ranges, while our primary comparison against the scratch baseline remains a fully controlled evaluation (Table 1).

**Table 2.** Contextual comparison with state-of-the-art bi-atrial segmentation methods.

| Method | Target Label | Train N | Wall Dice ↑ | HD95 (mm) ↓ |
|---|---|---|---|---|
| 3D nnU-Net Ensemble [8] | bi-atrial | 70 | 0.672 | 4.24 |
| 3D MambaBot [9] | bi-atrial | 70 | 0.712 | 3.21 |
| 3D nnU-Net [11] | bi-atrial | 70 | 0.670 | 4.53 |
| 3D nnU-Net [12] | bi-atrial | 70 | 0.626 | 5.21 |
| SegBAW-Net [13] | bi-atrial | 70 | 0.620 | 6.32 |
| 3D U-Net [14] | LA wall | 80 | 0.617 | 3.42 |
| C2W-Tune (ours) | LA wall | **70** | **0.78 ± 0.02** | **3.15 ± 0.21** |

**Limitations and Future Work.** Evaluation used a single public dataset with a fixed split, so generalization to external cohorts, scanners, and protocols remains to be

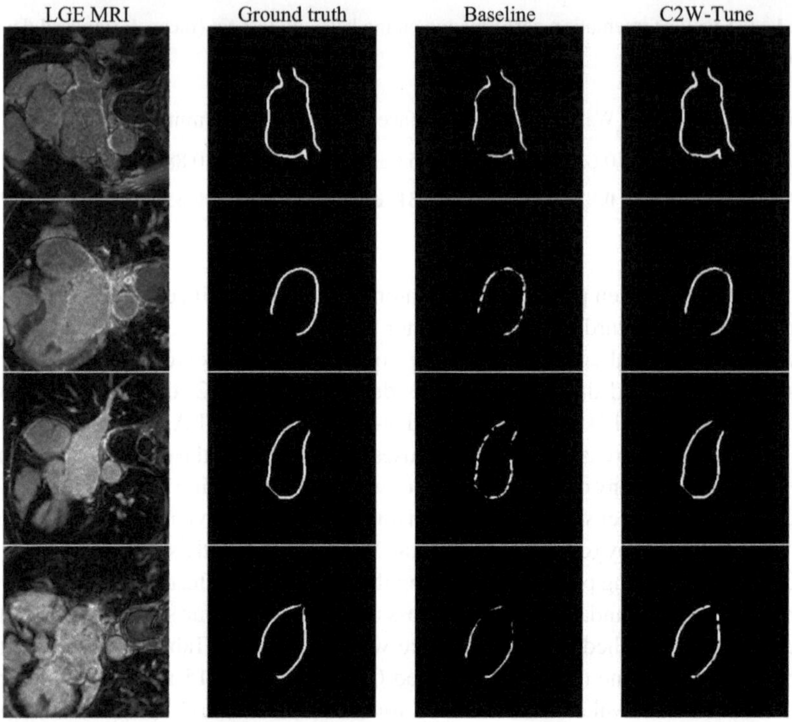


**Fig. 2.** Representative axial slices comparing ground truth, baseline, and C2W-Tune.

assessed. In addition, C2W-Tune was evaluated only for LA wall segmentation, and its extension to the RA wall or to combined bi-atrial wall targets requires further validation because of anatomical and appearance differences. Although the progressive layer-unfreezing strategy improved boundary quality, residual errors may still occur in challenging regions such as the pulmonary vein ostia and LA appendage, where boundaries are ambiguous and inter-observer variability is high. Future work will focus on external multi-center validation, domain-shift analysis, extension to bi-atrial and multi-class settings, and explicit boundary-aware refinements, including inner/outer wall-surface supervision and boundary-sensitive objectives.

## 4 Conclusion

We presented C2W-Tune, a two-stage cavity-to-wall transfer framework for thin LA wall segmentation in 3D LGE-MRI. The method first learns robust atrial representations via LA cavity pre-training and then adapts the same architecture to wall segmentation using a progressive layer-unfreezing curriculum, which preserves informative endocardial features while enabling wall-specific refinement. On the held-out test set, C2W-Tune achieved higher overlap and improved boundary accuracy than an architecture-matched baseline trained from scratch and remained competitive under reduced supervision settings. Furthermore, this work suggests that hierarchical task transfer, in which an easier anatomical target guides a more difficult one, is a promising strategy for addressing extremely thin anatomical structures. These improvements in surface fidelity and topological continuity may enhance patient-specific wall analysis and atrial remodeling assessment, supporting more precise image-guided ablation planning, and AF recurrence risk stratification.

**Acknowledgments.** This research was enabled in part by the Natural Sciences and Engineering Research Council of Canada (NSERC) Discovery Grant, and by computational resources provided by the Digital Research Alliance of Canada (https://alliancecan.ca).

## References

1. Li, L., Zimmer, V.A., Schnabel, J.A., Zhuang, X.: Medical image analysis on left atrial LGE MRI for atrial fibrillation studies: a review. Med. Image Anal. **77**, 102360 (2022). https://doi.org/10.1016/j.media.2022.102360
2. Xiong, Z., et al.: A global benchmark of algorithms for segmenting the left atrium from late gadolinium-enhanced cardiac magnetic resonance imaging. Med. Image Anal. **67**, 101832 (2021). https://doi.org/10.1016/j.media.2020.101832
3. Maceira, A.M., Cosín-Sales, J., Roughton, M., Prasad, S.K., Pennell, D.J.: Reference left atrial dimensions and volumes by steady state free precession cardiovascular magnetic resonance. J. Cardiovasc. Magn. Reson. **12**, 65 (2010). https://doi.org/10.1186/1532-429X-12-65
4. Wang, Y., et al.: A robust computational framework for estimating 3D bi-atrial chamber wall thickness. Comput. Biol. Med. **114**, 103444 (2019). https://doi.org/10.1016/j.compbiomed.2019.103444
5. Petitjean, C., Dacher, J.-N.: A review of segmentation methods in short axis cardiac MR images. Med. Image Anal. **15**(2), 169–184 (2011). https://doi.org/10.1016/j.media.2010.12.004
6. Puybareau, É., et al.: Left atrial segmentation in a few seconds using fully convolutional network and transfer learning. In: Pop, M., et al. (eds.) Statistical Atlases and Computational Models of the Heart. Atrial Segmentation and LV Quantification Challenges. LNCS, vol. 11395, pp. 339–347. Springer, Cham (2019). https://doi.org/10.1007/978-3-030-12029-0_37
7. Li, L., Zimmer, V.A., Schnabel, J.A., Zhuang, X.: AtrialJSQnet: a new framework for joint segmentation and quantification of left atrium and scars incorporating spatial and shape information. Med. Image Anal. **76**, 102303 (2022). https://doi.org/10.1016/j.media.2021.102303
8. Zolotarev, A., Johnson, K., Khan, A., Slabaugh, G., Roney, C.: An ensemble of 3D residual encoder UNet models for solving multi-class bi-atrial segmentation challenge. In: Camara, O., et al. (eds.) Statistical Atlases and Computational Models of the Heart. Workshop, CMRxRecon and MBAS Challenge Papers. LNCS, vol. 15448, pp. 209–213. Springer, Cham (2025). https://doi.org/10.1007/978-3-031-87756-8_21
9. Thesing, C., Bueno-Orovio, A., Banerjee, A.: Evaluating convolution, attention, and Mamba based U-Net models for multi-class bi-atrial segmentation from LGE-MRI. In: Camara, O., et al. (eds.) Statistical Atlases and Computational Models of the Heart. Workshop, CMRxRecon and MBAS Challenge Papers. LNCS, vol. 15448, pp. 214–225. Springer, Cham (2025). https://doi.org/10.1007/978-3-031-87756-8_22

10. Almar-Munoz, E., et al.: Multi-loss 3D segmentation for enhanced bi-atrial segmentation. In: Camara, O., et al. (eds.) Statistical Atlases and Computational Models of the Heart. Workshop, CMRxRecon and MBAS Challenge Papers. LNCS, vol. 15448, pp. 236–244. Springer, Cham (2025). https://doi.org/10.1007/978-3-031-87756-8_24
11. Zhang, Y., Cheng, Y., Qi, Y.: Exploring CNN and transformer architectures for multi-class bi-atrial segmentation from late gadolinium-enhanced MRI. In: Camara, O., et al. (eds.) Statistical Atlases and Computational Models of the Heart. Workshop, CMRxRecon and MBAS Challenge Papers. LNCS, vol. 15448, pp. 390–397. Springer, Cham (2025). https://doi.org/10.1007/978-3-031-87756-8_38
12. Merino-Caviedes, S., Nnadozie, E.C., Moya-Sáez, E., Martín-Fernández, M., Alberola-López, C.: CavityBASNet: cavity-focused biatrial automatic segmentation on LGE-MRI with augmented input channel and left-right myocardium splitting. In: Camara, O., et al. (eds.) Statistical Atlases and Computational Models of the Heart. Workshop, CMRxRecon and MBAS Challenge Papers. LNCS, vol. 15448, pp. 53–63. Springer, Cham (2025). https://doi.org/10.1007/978-3-031-87756-8_6
13. Lefebvre, A.L., et al.: SegBAW-Net: segmentation of bi-atria and wall network offering valuable insights into challenge data. In: Camara, O., et al. (eds.) Statistical Atlases and Computational Models of the Heart. Workshop, CMRxRecon and MBAS Challenge Papers. LNCS, vol. 15448, pp. 345–356. Springer, Cham (2025). https://doi.org/10.1007/978-3-031-87756-8_34
14. Gunawardhana, M., Trew, M.L., Sands, G.B., Zhao, J.: Segmenting bi-atrial structures using ResNext based framework. arXiv preprint arXiv:2503.02892 (2025). https://doi.org/10.48550/arXiv.2503.02892
15. Raghu, M., Zhang, C., Kleinberg, J., Bengio, S.: Transfusion: understanding transfer learning for medical imaging. In: Wallach, H.M., Larochelle, H., Beygelzimer, A., d'Alché-Buc, F., Fox, E.A., Garnett, R. (eds.) Advances in Neural Information Processing Systems, vol. 32, pp. 3342–3352. Curran Associates, Inc. (2019)
16. Xie, S., Girshick, R., Dollar, P., Tu, Z., He, K.: Aggregated residual transformations for deep neural networks. In: 2017 IEEE Conference on Computer Vision and Pattern Recognition (CVPR), pp. 5987–5995. IEEE, Honolulu, HI (2017). https://doi.org/10.1109/CVPR.2017.634
17. Tajbakhsh, N., et al.: Convolutional neural networks for medical image analysis: full training or fine tuning? IEEE Trans. Med. Imaging. **35**(5), 1299–1312 (2016). https://doi.org/10.1109/TMI.2016.2535302
18. Sendra-Balcells, C., et al.: Domain generalization in deep learning for contrast-enhanced imaging. Comput. Biol. Med. **149**, 106052 (2022). https://doi.org/10.1016/j.compbiomed.2022.106052
19. Ma, J., et al.: Loss odyssey in medical image segmentation. Med. Image Anal. **71**, 102035 (2021). https://doi.org/10.1016/j.media.2021.102035
20. Zhang, Z., Wang, Z., Wang, X., Wang, K., Yuan, Y., Li, Q.: A novel network with enhanced edge information for left atrium segmentation from LGE-MRI. Front. Physiol. **15**, 1478347 (2024). https://doi.org/10.3389/fphys.2024.1478347

# Automated Pulmonary Hypertension Subtype Discrimination from CTPA Scans

Matteo Dallera[1(✉)], Carlotta Pairazzi[2], Riccardo Bellazzi[1], Stefano Ghio[3], Adele Valentini[2], and Lucia Sacchi[1]

[1] Department of Electrical, Computer and Biomedical Engineering, University of Pavia, Pavia, Italy
matteo.dallera01@universitadipavia.it
[2] Radiology Unit-Diagnostic Imaging I, Department of Diagnostic Medicine, IRCCS Fondazione Policlinico San Matteo, Pavia, Italy
[3] Division of Cardiology, IRCCS Fondazione Policlinico San Matteo, Pavia, Italy

**Abstract.** Accurate differentiation between Arterial Pulmonary Hypertension (PAH) and Chronic Thromboembolic Pulmonary Hypertension (CTEPH), two subtypes of Pulmonary Hypertension (PH), from CT Pulmonary Angiography (CTPA) scans may facilitate earlier diagnosis and improve patient prognosis. In this work, we reimplemented an existing framework originally developed for the identification of chronic thrombi in CTPA scans and adapted it to the differentiation between PAH and CTEPH. The original framework was based on generating Maximum Intensity Projections (MIP) of the CTPA scans from different spatial positions, which were then embedded and classified using a neural network architecture. Furthermore, we introduce a variant of the approach that allows ranking MIP projections and generating relevance maps in the original CT image space, thereby improving explainability. The two methods exhibited comparable classification performance. However, a preliminary radiologist assessment of the relevance maps generated by the proposed variant suggests an ability to focus on regions of abnormal pulmonary perfusion that are characteristic of thromboembolic disease.

**Keywords:** Artificial Intelligence Explainability · Deep Learning · CTPA Scans Classification

## 1 Introduction

The correct differentiation between Pulmonary Arterial Hypertension (PAH) and Chronic Thromboembolic Pulmonary Hypertension (CTEPH) by evaluating CTPA scan is an important clinical task. It may reduce the delay which often characterizes the diagnosis of PAH and CTEPH [2,3], leading to an improvement of patient prognosis by ensuring subtype-specific treatment. The identification of the radiological signs of CTEPH still represents a challenging task, highly dependent on the radiologist's expertise [4]. The feasibility of identifying chronic

© The Author(s), under exclusive license to Springer Nature Switzerland AG 2027
P. Andreev et al. (Eds.): AIME 2026, LNAI 16748, pp. 215–219, 2027.
https://doi.org/10.1007/978-3-032-30710-1_26

pulmonary embolism using deep learning has already been investigated in the literature. The work by Tuomas Vainio et al. [5] proposes a classification framework that uses Maximum Intensity Projections (MIP) of CTPA scans. These projections are acquired by rotating around the patient's volume, and then embedded using a 121-layer DenseNet trained on ImageNet [1]. The embeddings are subsequently aggregated via element-wise mean pooling and classified using an MLP-based architecture. Using average pooling, however, has two main drawbacks: (i) the contribution of each MIP projection to the model's final decision is lost, and (ii) the projections are assumed to have equal weight in the generation of the final feature vector. Since radiological signs of CTEPH may not be visible in every MIP projection, it may be useful to understand which projections drive the model towards its prediction, with the aim of gaining a deeper insight into the model's decision-making process. In this work, we reimplemented the approach proposed by [5], and we adapted it to the task of discriminating between PAH and CTEPH. In addition, we propose a variation of the algorithm that classifies each CTPA scan by taking into account the weight of each projection and its individual prediction. Finally, we introduce an explainability module that, based on the extracted projections, highlights the regions in the original CTPA image space that exhibit radiological signs of the disease.

## 2 Material and Methods

The dataset used in this work was collected at the Department of Radiology, IRCCS Policlinico San Matteo (Pavia, Italy) and consists of 168 CTPA scans, including 130 scans from patients diagnosed with CTEPH and 38 from patients with PAH. The study obtained the approval of the Ethics Committee (CET Lombardia 6). The volumes were acquired using different CT scanners and exhibit variability in the number of voxels and in their physical spacing. CTPA scans underwent a set of preprocessing operations prior to MIP extraction. First, lungs segmentation was performed on each volume using the *TotalSegmentator* Python library [6]. Then, both volumes and segmentation masks underwent interpolation to achieve consistent voxel spacing across subjects. Finally, regions outside lungs were removed. Since separate labels for each lung were not available, we decided to analyze the lungs jointly rather than considering them separately. For each volume, 11 2-D MIP projections were generated by rotating around the volume along the longitudinal and transverse axes. In the framework by Vainio et al. [5], each MIP projection was embedded into a 1024-feature vector using a 121-layer DenseNet pretrained on ImageNet. To create the final embedding of the CT scan for classification, element-wise mean pooling was performed on the 11 feature vectors coming from the projections. In this work we propose a modification of the original pipeline aimed at taking into account the separate contribution of each projection. In details, each MIP projection is embedded using the same approach as [5] and then, exploiting a low-depth neural network, mapped into a bidimensional unit vector into what we refer to as *Decision Space* (Fig. 1).

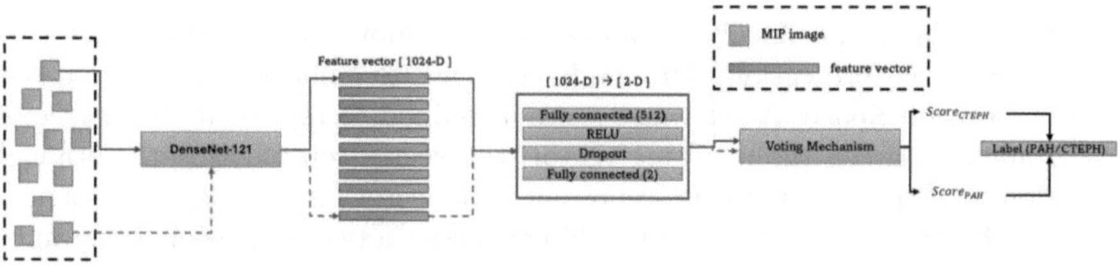


**Fig. 1.** Schematic representation of the proposed classification system architecture

As shown in Fig. 2, the Decision Space is a two-dimensional plane, where two unit vectors (CTEPH vector and PAH vector) encode the semantic representation of the two classes. The direction orthogonal to the one identified by these vectors divides the Decision Space into two half-planes, corresponding to CTEPH and PAH, respectively. When a projection is mapped into the decision space, the half-plane where it lies determines the vote associated with the projection (CTEPH or PAH). Each vote is also associated to a weight, computed as the cosine similarity between the projection vector and the unit vector representing the selected class.

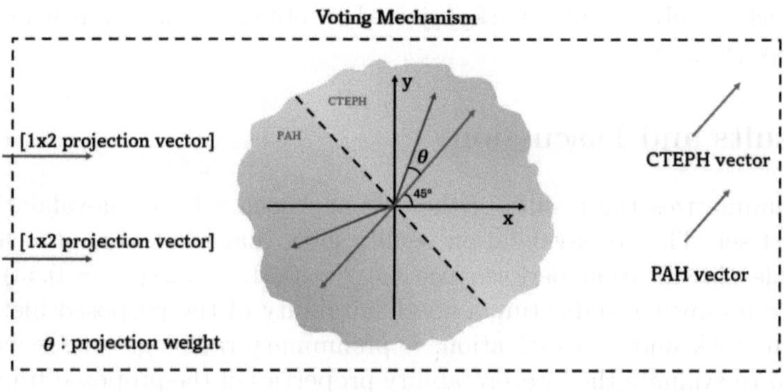


**Fig. 2.** Visualization of the voting mechanism: $\theta$ represents the angle between the MIP projection in the Decision Space and the vector associated to the class it votes for.

The model's final prediction is given by the class that results in the highest weighted sum of votes across the 11 projections. With this strategy the algorithm takes into account the contribution of the individual projections. The validation of the frameworks was performed by splitting the dataset at the patient-level into training and test sets, with an 80/20 ratio. Parameter optimization and comparison between the two approaches were carried out using a 6-fold cross-validation procedure applied to the training data. Both training and test set maintained the original proportion of classes. To assess whether the model focuses on radiological signs of CTEPH when this class is predicted and to support radiologists in their assessment, we propose the construction of relevance maps. To generate such maps, an occlusion analysis is performed for each projection voting for the CTEPH class. Specifically, a sliding patch is moved across the image corresponding to the projection. The modified image is embedded and remapped into the Decision Space. A relevance score is defined to represent the degree of misalignment between the resulting vector, the vector representing the original projection, and the CTEPH class-representative vector (see Fig. 3) and assigned to the patch. After completing the patching process, a two-dimensional relevance map including the relevance scores for each patch region is obtained.

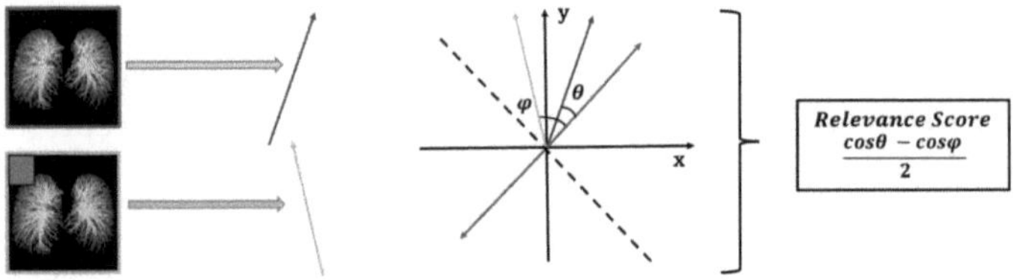


**Fig. 3.** Definition of the relevance score to be assigned to each patch

The resulting bidimensional relevance maps are then used to compute a sinogram, which is subsequently backprojected to obtain a three-dimensional relevance map. (Fig. 4).

## 3 Results and Discussion

Table 1 summarizes the results of the two approaches for cross-validation and on the test set. The cross-validation results show that the two approaches have comparable classification performance ($p_{F_1} = 0.31$, $p_{\text{PR-AUC}} = 0.43$). These results are promising, indicating a good suitability of the proposed methodologies for the task under investigation. A preliminary radiologist assessment was conducted to evaluate the interpretability properties of the proposed framework. One relevance map was evaluated by an expert radiologist, who observed that the classification system appears to focus on regions characterized by abnormal pulmonary perfusion (Fig. 4). However, a more in-depth analysis is required to understand why the model prioritizes certain regions of the CTPA scan over others that appear similar from a radiological perspective.

**Table 1.** Classification performance of the proposed frameworks

| | Cross-validation | | Test set | |
|---|---|---|---|---|
| Model | F1-macro | PR-AUC | F1-macro | PR-AUC |
| Mean Pooling | $0.86 \pm 0.05$ | $0.87 \pm 0.12$ | 0.91 | 0.93 |
| Weighted Voting | $0.88 \pm 0.06$ | $0.82 \pm 0.18$ | 0.95 | 0.98 |

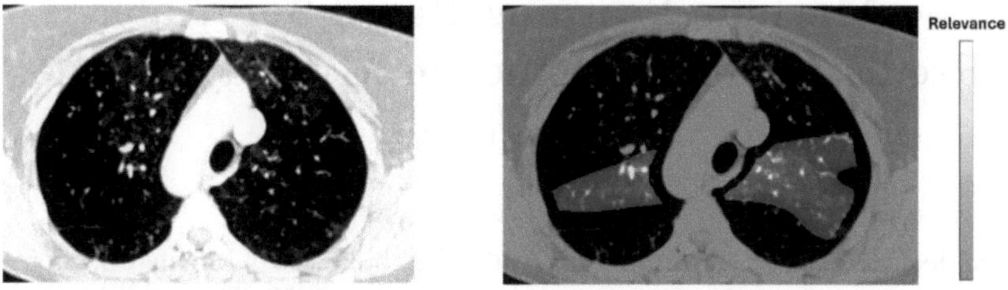


**Fig. 4.** Axial CTPA slice of a CTEPH patient (left) and corresponding slice with superimposed relevance map (right), highlighting abnormal pulmonary perfusion regions.

## 4 Conclusion

In this paper we compared two frameworks based on MIP projections to differentiate CTPA scans of CTEPH and PAH patients. The first framework is adapted from an approach existing in the literature that uses MIP projections embedding and mean-pooling, whereas the second proposes a solution that allows taking into account the contribution of single projections through weighted voting. Furthermore, it integrates a method to reconstruct relevance maps in the original CTPA space. The results show comparable performance between the two frameworks, and the preliminary explainability analysis motivates further investigation of relevance maps. Nevertheless, the small, imbalanced dataset limits generalizability and requires validation on larger datasets.

**Disclosure of Interests.** The authors have no competing interests to declare.

## References


1. Deng, J., Dong, W., Socher, R., et al.: ImageNet: a large-scale hierarchical image database. In: 2009 IEEE Conference on Computer Vision and Pattern Recognition, pp. 248–255 (2009). https://doi.org/10.1109/CVPR.2009.5206848
2. Didden, E.M., Lee, E., Wyckmans, J., et al.: Time to diagnosis of pulmonary hypertension and diagnostic burden: a retrospective analysis of nationwide US healthcare data. Pulm. Circ. **13**(1), e12188 (2023)
3. Pepke-Zaba, J., Delcroix, M., Lang, I., et al.: Chronic thromboembolic pulmonary hypertension (CTEPH): results from an international prospective registry. Circulation **124**(18), 1973–1981 (2011)
4. Rogberg, A.N., Gopalan, D., Westerlund, E., et al.: Do radiologists detect chronic thromboembolic disease on computed tomography? Acta Radiol. **60**(11), 1576–1583 (2019)
5. Vainio, T., Mäkelä, T., Arkko, A., et al.: Leveraging open dataset and transfer learning for accurate recognition of chronic pulmonary embolism from CT angiogram maximum intensity projection images. Eur. Radiol. Exp. **7**(1), 33 (2023)
6. Wasserthal, J., Breit, H.C., Meyer, M.T., et al.: TotalSegmentator: robust segmentation of 104 anatomic structures in CT images. Radiol. Artif. Intell. **5**(5), e230024 (2023)

# Machine Learning-Based Survival Prediction of Outcomes in Myelodysplastic Syndromes

Fayeq Jeelani Syed[1,2], Ziming Cui[3], Dulat Bekbolsynov[1], Michael S. Sloma[1], Stanislaw Stepkowski[1], and Kevin S. Xu[3(✉)]

[1] University of Toledo, Toledo, OH 43606, USA
[2] Indiana University, Indianapolis, IN 46202, USA
[3] Case Western Reserve University, Cleveland, OH 44106, USA
ksx2@case.edu

**Abstract.** Myelodysplastic syndromes (MDS) are a rare group of bone marrow disorders. Survival analysis techniques have been used to develop prognostic scoring systems to assist clinicians in making personalized treatment choices. In this paper, we explore the potential of machine learning-based survival prediction models to predict MDS outcomes. We find that two deep learning-based models trained on molecular genetic features yield the highest prediction accuracy, achieving gains of 4–6% in concordance index (C-index) compared to the latest Molecular International Prognostic Scoring System (IPSS-M).

**Keywords:** MDS · International Prognostic Scoring System · IPSS

## 1 Introduction

Myelodysplastic syndromes (MDS) are a rare group of bone marrow disorders where the body does not produce enough healthy blood cells. Patients diagnosed with MDS may progress into acute myeloid leukemia (AML). Estimates suggest that 10,000 to 15,000 new cases of MDS are diagnosed in the U.S. every year, with about 1/3 eventually progressing into AML [15].

Survival analysis techniques have been used to develop prognostic scoring systems to help clinicians make informed and personalized decisions regarding the patients with MDS. The International Prognostic Scoring System (IPSS) and its revised version, IPSS-R [6] have been popular for decades as a global standard for stratification of MDS. More recently, Bernard et al. [2] proposed to incorporate patient molecular features, resulting in the development of IPSS-M.

Machine learning (ML)-based approaches for modeling MDS remain relatively limited. A previous study [11] using a random survival forest model trained on over 7,000 patients achieved accuracy comparable to IPSS-M while using only routine clinical variables. In this paper, we develop predictive models for MDS

F. J. Syed and Z. Cui—Equal contribution.

© The Author(s), under exclusive license to Springer Nature Switzerland AG 2027
P. Andreev et al. (Eds.): AIME 2026, LNAI 16748, pp. 220–225, 2027.
https://doi.org/10.1007/978-3-032-30710-1_27

endpoints using five machine learning-based survival prediction algorithms. We create four different feature sets from MDS data to predict three different clinical endpoints and investigate the following key *research questions (RQs)*:

**RQ1.** What is the impact of different feature sets and outcomes on prediction accuracy of the models for different clinical endpoints?
**RQ2.** How do the different models compare in terms of prediction accuracy?
**RQ3.** Can we achieve better prediction accuracy than the IPSS-M system?

## 2 Materials and Methods

### 2.1 Data Description and Pre-processing

The dataset we use in this study was provided by Bernard et al. [2]. It has 3,323 patients. We use the same inclusion criteria as Awada et al. [1], namely patients with blasts at least 20% and white blood cell count less than $13 \times 10^9/l$.

We aim to predict three clinical endpoints in our analysis: *leukemia-free survival (LFS)*, the time till a patient with MDS remains free of leukemia after receiving treatment for MDS; *overall survival (OS)*, the time a person survives after being diagnosed with MDS, regardless of whether they develop leukemia; and *acute myeloid leukemic transformation (AMLt)*, the time from the diagnosis of MDS to transformation into AML. The time to event was measured in months from the time of sample collection to the time of the clinical endpoint.

We use one-hot encoding for clinical categorical variables. Patients with missing targets (clinical endpoints) or cytogenetic values are dropped, which reduces the dataset to 2,496 patients. Missing values are imputed using the mean value for that feature over all other patients. Non-binary features are standardized, while binary features are not scaled.

### 2.2 Feature Sets

We categorized the features into four sets:

**Clin.** This feature set contains only the clinical features of the patient, including age, sex, and MDS type. A subset of these features contains information about the treatment and are thus used to predict overall survival (OS) only.
**Clin+Cyt.** This feature set combines clinical and cytogenetic features. Greenberg et al. [6] divided these features into 5 categories as part of the IPSS-R score calculation. We use these categories rather than the raw cytogenetic events, the same as Bernard et al. [2], and one-hot encode the 5 categories.
**Clin+MG.** This feature set combines clinical and molecular genetic features. Bernard et al. [2] appropriately coded these features and tested each genetic mutation for contribution to predictions.
**All** This feature set combines all of the above features.

**Table 1.** Survival prediction accuracy for different models and feature sets using C-index. Higher values denote greater accuracy, with most the accurate model in bold.

| Outcome | Features | Coxnet | DeepSurv | L-MTLR | N-MTLR | PC Hazard |
|---|---|---|---|---|---|---|
| OS | Clin | 0.702 | 0.698 | 0.695 | 0.708 | 0.715 |
| | Clin+Cyt | 0.720 | 0.759 | 0.717 | 0.717 | 0.729 |
| | Clin+MG | 0.718 | 0.727 | 0.691 | 0.737 | 0.732 |
| | All | 0.723 | 0.738 | 0.687 | **0.777** | 0.749 |
| LFS | Clin | 0.706 | 0.703 | 0.697 | 0.694 | 0.703 |
| | Clin+Cyt | 0.727 | 0.733 | 0.725 | 0.734 | 0.728 |
| | Clin+MG | 0.720 | **0.793** | 0.699 | 0.745 | 0.750 |
| | All | 0.725 | 0.729 | 0.702 | 0.732 | 0.758 |
| AMLt | Clin | 0.781 | 0.738 | 0.725 | 0.763 | 0.792 |
| | Clin+Cyt | 0.802 | 0.824 | 0.787 | 0.862 | 0.852 |
| | Clin+MG | 0.817 | 0.874 | 0.788 | 0.874 | 0.851 |
| | All | 0.824 | 0.866 | 0.778 | **0.875** | 0.823 |

### 2.3 Survival Prediction Model Training

We consider two linear models and three non-linear models for survival prediction in this paper. The linear models are CoxPH with elastic net (Coxnet) [14] and linear multi-task logistic regression (L-MTLR) [16]. The non-linear models are a neural network (NN)-based extension of CoxPH (DeepSurv) [8], an NN-based extension of multi-task logistic regression (N-MTLR) [3], and an NN-based model with piecewise constant hazard function (PC Hazard) [10].

The data was split into proportions of 0.6/0.2/0.2 for train/validation/test, respectively. We use the Coxnet implementation from the `scikit-survival` package [12]. We use the implementations of DeepSurv, N-MTLR and PC Hazard from `pycox` [9]. We use the L-MTLR implementation from `pysurvival` [4]. Finally, we use the `SurvivalEVAL` package [13] that gives flexibility to evaluate the survival prediction models from all available packages.

We tune hyperparameters (HPs) using a random search over 1,000 configurations, except for the value of $\alpha$ for Coxnet, where we use 11 evenly-spaced values on a log grid as its regularization path and then use a random search for the $l_1$-ratio $r$. For all NN-based methods, we vary the number of hidden layers from 1 to 10 with 1 to 256 nodes in each layer. For all discrete-time methods, we vary the number of time bins from 5 to 100. For L-MTLR, we vary the two $l_2$ regularization parameters $C_1, C_2$ on a log uniform scale between $10^{-6}$ and 1. Each model with the most accurate HP configuration evaluated on the validation set is then trained on the combined train and validation sets.

We use the concordance index (C-index) [7] as the evaluation metric for prediction accuracy. We note that it measures only discrimination ability (how well its predictions order patients by their actual survival times), so a model with high C-index may still be poorly calibrated.

## 3 Results and Discussion

The prediction accuracy values for the different models are shown in Table 1. While the prediction accuracy varies across models, outcomes, feature sets, and evaluation metrics, we do observe some trends, which we investigate through the three research questions posed in the introduction.

*RQ1: What is the impact of different feature sets and outcomes on prediction accuracy of the models?* For most models, we find that including cytogenetic features generally improves prediction accuracy, but not as much as including molecular genetic features. The highest C-indices are all achieved using molecular genetic features, both without cytogenetic features (for LFS) and with (for OS and AMLt). Overall, we find that the use of molecular genetic features is important for maximizing prediction accuracy, regardless of the MDS outcome.

*RQ2: How do the constructed models compare in terms of prediction accuracy?* We find that the deep learning-based models (DeepSurv, N-MTLR, and PC Hazard) generally achieve much higher C-indices compared to the linear models (Coxnet and L-MTLR). Among the deep learning-based models, accuracy varies depending on the outcome and feature sets. The highest C-indices are achieved by DeepSurv for LFS and N-MTLR for OS, while they are very similar for AMLt.

*RQ3: Can we achieve better prediction accuracy than the IPSS-M scoring system?* Previous research on prognostic scoring systems was based on quantifying the relative risk of adverse outcomes for each patient variable [2,6]. In Table 2, we compare the predictive ability of our models against IPSS-R and IPSS-M. When using only cytogenetic features, we find that Coxnet, DeepSurv, and N-MTLR models all achieve superior discrimination compared to IPSS-R. When using molecular genetic features, the DeepSurv and N-MTLR are both more accurate than IPSS-M on all three outcomes, while Coxnet performs slightly worse than IPSS-M.

**Table 2.** Comparison of C-index of our models with IPSS-R and IPSS-M. Models in the top half of the table do not use molecular features. Bold quantity denotes most accurate predictor in each half.

| Model | Features | OS | LFS | AMLt |
|---|---|---|---|---|
| Coxnet | Clin+Cyt | 0.720 | 0.727 | 0.802 |
| DeepSurv | Clin+Cyt | **0.759** | 0.733 | 0.824 |
| N-MTLR | Clin+Cyt | 0.717 | **0.734** | **0.862** |
| IPSS-R | Clin+Cyt | 0.686 | 0.697 | 0.774 |
| Coxnet | All | 0.723 | 0.725 | 0.824 |
| DeepSurv | Clin+MG | 0.727 | **0.793** | 0.874 |
| N-MTLR | All | **0.777** | 0.732 | **0.875** |
| IPSS-M | All | 0.732 | 0.746 | 0.837 |

## 4 Conclusion

Machine learning-based survival prediction models have the potential to enhance outcome prediction in MDS patients, facilitating patient-specific decision-making. We found that deep learning-based survival prediction models, particularly DeepSurv and N-MTLR, generally achieved the highest prediction accuracy, resulting in improvements of 4–6% in C-index compared to IPSS-M.

A limitation of our study is that C-index measures only discrimination ability, not calibration. Our preliminary results using the integrated Brier score [5], which measures both discrimination and calibration, show the same patterns as we found with C-index, albeit with a smaller gap between deep learning and linear models. Nonetheless, we see potential for deep learning-based prognostic models such as the ones we investigate in this paper, to be used clinically. For example, improved risk prediction could enable better selection of candidates for allogeneic hematopoietic stem cell transplantation (allo-HCT) [11].

**Declaration of AI assistance technologies during manuscript preparation** The authors used ChatGPT for AI activity class 2 (writing or drafting manuscript content) to rewrite some sections more concisely. After using this technology, the authors reviewed the results and take full responsibility for the contents of the manuscript.

**Disclosure of Interests** The authors have no competing interests to declare that are relevant to the content of this article.

## References

1. Awada, H., et al.: Personalized risk schemes and machine learning to empower genomic prognostication models in myelodysplastic syndromes. Int. J. Mol. Sci. **23**(5), 2802 (2022)
2. Bernard, E., et al.: Molecular international prognostic scoring system for myelodysplastic syndromes. NEJM Evid. **1**(7), EVIDoa2200008 (2022)
3. Fotso, S.: Deep neural networks for survival analysis based on a multi-task framework. arXiv preprint arXiv:1801.05512 (2018)
4. Fotso, S., et al.: PySurvival: Open source package for survival analysis modeling (2019). https://www.pysurvival.io/
5. Graf, E., et al.: Assessment and comparison of prognostic classification schemes for survival data. Stat. Med. **18**(17–18), 2529–2545 (1999)
6. Greenberg, P.L., et al.: Revised international prognostic scoring system for myelodysplastic syndromes. Blood **120**(12), 2454–2465 (2012)
7. Harrell, F.E., et al.: Evaluating the yield of medical tests. JAMA **247**(18), 2543–2546 (1982)
8. Katzman, J.L., et al.: DeepSurv: personalized treatment recommender system using a Cox proportional hazards deep neural network. BMC Med. Res. Methodol. **18**, 24 (2018)
9. Kvamme, H., et al.: HAVAKV/PYCOX: Survival analysis with PyTorch (2024). https://github.com/havakv/pycox
10. Kvamme, H., Borgan, Ø.: Continuous and discrete-time survival prediction with neural networks. Lifetime Data Anal. **27**(4), 710–736 (2021)
11. Mosquera Orgueira, A., et al.: Machine learning improves risk stratification in myelodysplastic neoplasms: an analysis of the Spanish group of myelodysplastic syndromes. Hemasphere **7**(10), e961 (2023)
12. Pölsterl, S.: scikit-survival: a library for time-to-event analysis built on top of scikit-learn. J. Mach. Learn. Res. **21**(212), 1–6 (2020)
13. Qi, S., et al.: SurvivalEVAL: a comprehensive open-source Python package for evaluating individual survival distributions. In: Proceedings AAAI Symposium Series , vol. 2, pp. 453–457 (2024)

14. Simon, N., et al.: Regularization paths for Cox's proportional hazards model via coordinate descent. J. Stat. Softw. **39**(5), 1–13 (2011)
15. The MDS Foundation: What is MDS? (2026). https://www.mds-foundation.org/mds-and-treatments/what-is-mds/
16. Yu, C.N., et al.: Learning patient-specific cancer survival distributions as a sequence of dependent regressors. In: Advances in Neural Information Processing Systems (NeurIPS), vol. 24 (2011)

# Nutrilyzer: Vision-Based Nutritional Estimation for Postprandial Glucose Response Prediction

El Arbi Belfarsi(✉), Ahmed Amarak, Maria Valero, Valentina Nino, and Katherine Ingram

Kennesaw State University, Kennesaw, GA, USA
{ebelfars,aamarak}@students.kennesaw.edu,
{mvalero2,lvallad1,kingra14}@kennesaw.edu

**Abstract.** Nutrilyzer is a vision-based pipeline replacing manual food diaries with AI-derived nutritional estimates for postprandial glucose prediction. Validated on Menu-Match, the vision component achieves macronutrient MAPEs of 17.6%, 13.4%, 24.7%, and 19.4% for calories, protein, carbs, and fats respectively, using Claude—the best of three evaluated VLMs. On CGMacros (45 participants, dual Abbott Libre Pro / Dexcom G6 Pro CGMs), a 13-model comparison reaches $R^2 = 0.831$ (Voting Ensemble) with MyFitnessPal (MFP) labels plus biometrics; replacing MFP with AI estimates and confidence filtering raises $R^2$ from 0.70 to 0.783 (Random Forest), recovering 94.2% of manual-label performance. Glucose targets in both tracks are sensor-measured—AI labels feed only inputs. Clarke Error Grid shows 96.0% A+B and 0% Zone E.

**Keywords:** Continuous Glucose Monitoring · Postprandial Glucose Prediction · Food Image Recognition · Vision-Language Models

## 1 Introduction

Continuous glucose monitors (CGMs) enable real-time glycemic tracking [1], and predicting postprandial response has clear clinical value [2], but nutritional data acquisition is a bottleneck: manual MyFitnessPal (MFP) logging is time-consuming and error-prone [3]. Vision-language models (VLMs) offer an alternative by estimating nutrients from meal photographs [4].

Using CGMacros [5]—45 participants, dual CGMs, meal images—we ask: (i) *How does substituting AI-derived for manually logged data influence postprandial glucose prediction?* (ii) *How does CGM sensor choice shift downstream performance?* (iii) *How does confidence-based filtering trade dataset size against label noise?*

**Contributions.** (i) Strong baselines: $R^2 = 0.831$ (Voting Ensemble, 13 architectures). (ii) Sensor comparison ($R^2$ 0.767 vs. 0.718, Libre vs. Dexcom). (iii) AI labels with confidence filtering ($\tau$=0.8) reach $R^2 = 0.783$, recovering 94.2% of

© The Author(s), under exclusive license to Springer Nature Switzerland AG 2027
P. Andreev et al. (Eds.): AIME 2026, LNAI 16748, pp. 226–230, 2027.
https://doi.org/10.1007/978-3-032-30710-1_28

manual-label performance. (iv) Clarke Error Grid: 96.0% clinical acceptability. Code released on publication. Prior CGMacros work [5] and personalized glucose prediction [6] has not systematically compared AI-derived against manual labels. Tree ensembles dominate tabular health data [7,8,10]; VLMs achieve competitive zero-shot nutritional estimation on Menu-Match [4,9].

## 2 Dataset and Method

*CGMacros.* 45 free-living participants wore both CGMs concurrently, photographed meals, and logged macros via MFP [5]. Within a 120-min post-meal window we extract **max glucose** (target), time-to-peak, slope, and pre-meal baseline. Age 18–69, BMI 20.7–49.1, HbA1c 4.6–8.5%; 1,644 meals have valid Libre responses for Track 1.

*Track Sizes.* Track 2 ($n$=1,156) is smaller because the VLM must *see* food: 488 images are blurred, beverage-only, packaging, or partially-eaten and cannot yield meaningful estimates. MFP-logged meals are usable regardless of image quality.

*Sensor Selection.* Table 1 shows Libre's $R^2$ advantage is consistent across Linear, RF, and GB regressors, suggesting tighter coupling between arm-placed interstitial readings and macronutrient excursions rather than model misfit. We adopt **max postprandial Libre glucose** as the target.

*Test Labels are CGM-Measured.* In both tracks the target $y$ is the sensor-measured peak from the Libre CGM. AI estimates appear *only* as input features replacing MFP macros; ground truth is physiological—Track 2 thus measures real-world utility, not agreement with Claude.

**Table 1.** Sensor comparison: Test $R^2$ for predicting max postprandial glucose. Libre's advantage is consistent across model families.

| Model | Libre | Dexcom |
|---|---|---|
| Linear Regression | 0.578 | 0.503 |
| Random Forest | 0.608 | 0.583 |
| Gradient Boosting | **0.767** | 0.718 |

*AI Labeling.* Claude (selected via Menu-Match validation against Gemini and GPT-4V; MAPEs 17.6/13.4/24.7/19.4% for calories/protein/carbs/fats) labels each identifiable image with five macros and a confidence score, yielding 1,156 labels with confidence 0.60–1.00 (mean 0.795).

*Tracks and Models. Track 1:* MFP + biometrics, $n$=1,644, 21 features (5 macros + 2 pre-meal glucose + 14 biometrics). *Track 2:* MFP macros replaced by AI estimates plus confidence, $n$=1,156, 22 features, threshold $\tau \in \{0.0, \ldots, 0.9\}$. 13 regressors: trees (GB, RF, XGBoost [7], LightGBM [8]); linear (Ridge, Lasso, Elastic Net); non-linear (SVR, KNN, MLP); meta-ensembles (Voting GB+RF+LGB; Stacking GB+RF+XGB with Ridge); and a PyTorch TabularNet with Huber loss [10]. 80/20 splits, seed 42. Metrics: $R^2$, RMSE, MAE (mg/dL), Clarke Error Grid [11].

## 3 Results

### 3.1 Track 1: MFP Labels

Table 2 shows three tiers: trees ($R^2$ = 0.818–0.831), non-linear (0.732–0.752), and linear/KNN (0.661–0.693). The Voting Ensemble leads ($R^2$ = 0.831, MAE = 16.88 mg/dL); deep learning ($R^2$ = 0.738) does not surpass tree ensembles, consistent with [10]. The GB feature ranking (Fig. 1) shows HbA1c (32.9%) and pre-meal glucose (31.4%) jointly account for 64.3% of importance, outweighing any meal feature by an order of magnitude—GB models baseline shifts and uses macros (carbs largest at 6.5%) to refine the excursion. A reduced 9-feature Stacking model retains $R^2$ = 0.821. Clarke Error Grid on GB: 76.9% Zone A, 19.1% B (96.0% A+B), 0% E (Fig. 2).

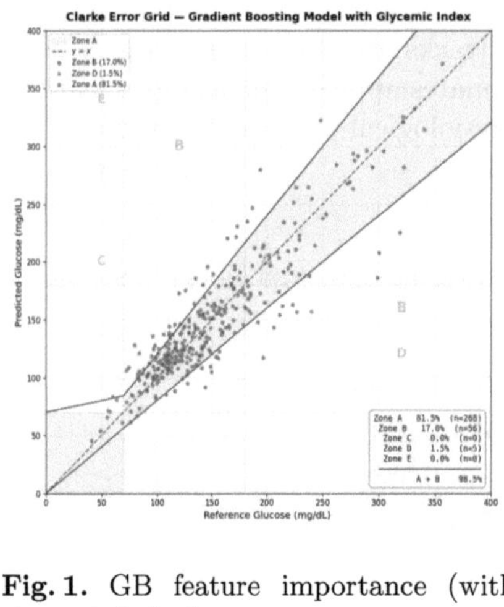


**Fig. 1.** GB feature importance (with glycemic index).

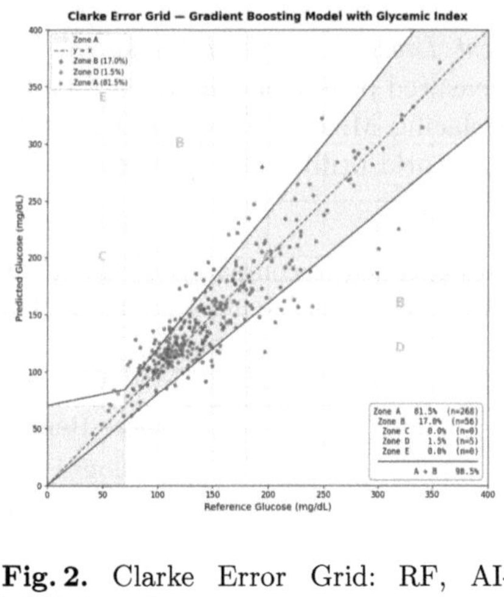


**Fig. 2.** Clarke Error Grid: RF, AI-labeled track.

### 3.2 Track 2: AI Labels with Confidence Filtering

At $\tau = 0.8$ ($n$ = 866), RF achieves $R^2$ = 0.783 (MAE = 18.39 mg/dL), reversing Track 1's GB lead—we attribute this to bagging's variance reduction being more

**Table 2.** Model comparison using MFP labels with biometric enrichment ($n$=1,644, 21 features). Sorted by test $R^2$.

| Model | $R^2$ | RMSE | MAE | Model | $R^2$ | RMSE | MAE |
|---|---|---|---|---|---|---|---|
| Voting Ens. | **0.831** | **23.08** | **16.88** | Deep Learning | 0.738 | — | — |
| Stacking Ens. | 0.830 | 23.18 | 16.98 | MLP | 0.732 | 29.10 | 23.17 |
| Gradient Boost. | 0.826 | 23.45 | 17.01 | Ridge | 0.693 | 31.13 | 23.18 |
| Random Forest | 0.825 | 23.51 | 17.36 | Lasso | 0.693 | 31.14 | 23.15 |
| XGBoost | 0.821 | 23.81 | 17.26 | Elastic Net | 0.692 | 31.18 | 23.18 |
| LightGBM | 0.818 | 24.01 | 17.21 | KNN | 0.661 | 32.75 | 24.30 |
| SVR | 0.752 | 27.98 | 19.38 | | | | |

robust to noisier AI labels. XGBoost (0.777), LightGBM (0.759), GB (0.754) follow. The confidence score itself enters RF's top-10 features (1.2%), indicating the model exploits label quality. Figure 3 shows the sweep: $\tau \leq 0.6$ retains all 1,156 samples ($R^2 \approx 0.68$–$0.70$); $\tau = 0.8$ jumps sharply to $R^2 = 0.75$–$0.78$ on 75% of samples (the lowest-confidence quartile is noisy); $\tau = 0.9$ collapses to 148 samples and models degrade (LGB $R^2 = -0.02$).

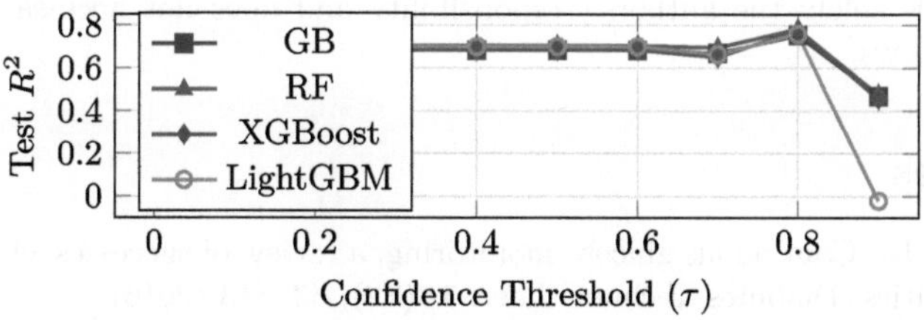


**Fig. 3.** Test $R^2$ vs. confidence threshold. All models peak at $\tau = 0.8$ ($n = 866$) before collapsing at $\tau = 0.9$ ($n = 148$).

## 4 Discussion

**Vision-Based Labeling is Viable.** The best AI model ($R^2 = 0.783$) approaches the best MFP model ($R^2 = 0.831$) and exceeds the basic-feature baseline ($R^2 = 0.767$). Deployment still requires human-in-the-loop safeguards—96% A+B is not a substitute for clinical oversight, especially for insulin users. Nutrilyzer is a logging-burden reducer, not an autonomous decision-maker.

**Confidence Filtering Works.** The sharp jump at $\tau = 0.8$ and collapse at $\tau = 0.9$ indicate VLM confidence scores flag a noisier quartile whose removal improves training, until data scarcity dominates.

**Metabolic State Dominates Meal Composition.** The dominance of HbA1c and pre-meal glucose, consistent with [6], shows postprandial peaks are governed by chronic control and the immediate baseline, with meals modulating—not driving—the response. This explains the AI track's tolerance for noisier inputs: the dominant signal is biometric.

**Limitations.** The 45-participant cohort limits generalizability; random splits (vs. patient-level CV) may inflate $R^2$ via leakage. Other determinants (exercise, sleep, stress, meal interval) are unmodeled, and we treat meals independently rather than modeling CGM dynamics temporally. Neither MFP nor AI labels are weighed-food ground truth, and we used a single VLM.

## 5 Conclusion

Nutrilyzer's AI labels with confidence filtering achieve $R^2 = 0.783$ on CGMacros, recovering 94.2% of MFP-label performance ($R^2 = 0.831$) while eliminating manual logging. Clarke Error Grid confirms 96.0% clinical acceptability, suggesting automated meal photography can approach food-diary accuracy in postprandial glucose prediction.

**Acknowledgments.** This work was supported in part by the NIH/NIA (Award P30AG073105) and by the Georgia Research Alliance (Award GRA.25.016.KSU.01.a). The content is solely the authors' responsibility and does not necessarily represent official NIH views.

## References

1. Rodbard, D.: Continuous glucose monitoring: a review of successes, challenges, and opportunities. Diabetes Technol. Ther. **18**(S2), S3–S13 (2016)
2. Ceriello, A.: Postprandial hyperglycemia and diabetes complications. Diabetes **54**(1), 1–7 (2005)
3. Evenepoel, C., et al.: Accuracy of nutrient calculations using MyFitnessPal. J. Acad. Nutr. Diet. **120**(3), 452–461 (2020)
4. Beijbom, O., et al.: Menu-Match: restaurant-specific food logging from images. In: IEEE WACV, pp. 844–851 (2015)
5. Chaspari, T., et al.: CGMacros: a multimodal dataset for CGM with dietary and activity data. Sci. Data **10**, 567 (2023)
6. Zeevi, D., et al.: Personalized nutrition by prediction of glycemic responses. Cell **163**(5), 1079–1094 (2015)
7. Chen, T., Guestrin, C.: XGBoost: a scalable tree boosting system. In: ACM SIGKDD, pp. 785–794 (2016)
8. Ke, G., et al.: LightGBM: a highly efficient gradient boosting decision tree. In: NeurIPS **30**, 3146–3154 (2017)
9. Official Nutrilyzer Paper: Validation of vision models for nutritional estimation using the Menu-Match dataset (2024)
10. Grinsztajn, L., et al.: Why do tree-based models still outperform deep learning on typical tabular data? In: NeurIPS, vol. 35, pp. 507–520 (2022)
11. Clarke, W.L., et al.: Evaluating clinical accuracy of systems for self-monitoring of blood glucose. Diabetes Care **10**(5), 622–628 (1987)

# Missing-Aware Evolving Fuzzy Learning for MASLD Risk Prediction from Irregular Time Series

Zhuoxuan Zhan[1], Hong Sheng Cheng[2], Ian Yang Liew[2], Hwee Pin Phua[3], Angela Li Ping Chow[4], Eng Sing Lee[2], Kuo Chao Yew[5(✉)], and Xiuyi Fan[1,2,6(✉)]

[1] College of Computing and Data Science, Nanyang Technological University, Singapore, Singapore
xyfan@ntu.edu.sg

[2] Lee Kong Chian School of Medicine, Nanyang Technological University, Singapore, Singapore

[3] Ministry of Health (MOH) Holdings Pte Ltd, Singapore, Singapore

[4] Department of Preventive and Population Health, Tan Tock Seng Hospital, Singapore, Singapore

[5] Tan Tock Seng Hospital, National University Health System, Singapore, Singapore
kuo.chao.yew@nhghealth.com.sg

[6] Centre of AI in Medicine, Nanyang Technological University, Singapore, Singapore

**Abstract.** Metabolic dysfunction-associated steatotic liver disease (MASLD) affects a large and growing population worldwide, and a subset of patients progress to clinically significant liver outcomes, creating a need for longitudinal risk monitoring from routinely collected follow-up data. In this work, we study a monitoring-style prediction problem: given an irregular history of follow-up laboratory measurements for a MASLD patient, predict whether the patient will develop severe liver outcomes in the near future. We study a previously underexplored monitoring-style risk prediction formulation for MASLD progression risk prediction using irregular follow-up laboratory records, and show that a missing-aware evolving neuro-fuzzy classifier (MEF-Classifier) is well suited to this setting. MEF-Classifier explicitly encodes both observed and missing states without ad hoc imputation, activates interpretable fuzzy rules that accumulate positive and negative evidence, and aggregates evidence into probabilistic risk estimates using imbalance-aware class weighting to stabilize learning under rare outcomes. Evaluated on a large public cohort and a local Singapore cohort, MEF-Classifier demonstrates improved performance over diverse baseline models while providing transparent explanations in the form of if–then rules that support clinical inspection and hypothesis generation.

Code is available at https://github.com/zzx0001/MEF-Classifier.

**Keywords:** Metabolic dysfunction-associated steatotic liver disease · Irregular time series · Fuzzy logic

© The Author(s), under exclusive license to Springer Nature Switzerland AG 2027
P. Andreev et al. (Eds.): AIME 2026, LNAI 16748, pp. 231–241, 2027.
https://doi.org/10.1007/978-3-032-30710-1_29

# 1 Introduction

Metabolic dysfunction-associated steatotic liver disease (MASLD), the recently adopted umbrella term replacing non-alcoholic fatty liver disease nomenclature in the context of cardiometabolic dysfunction, is now a major driver of chronic liver disease worldwide [19]. With an estimated global prevalence around 38% and substantial burden in Asia (28–32%), MASLD presents an escalating public-health challenge and a large population requiring longitudinal follow-up [8,23]. Clinically, the central need is early identification of the minority of patients who will progress to severe liver outcomes (advanced fibrosis/cirrhosis, hepatocellular carcinoma, or liver failure) to enable intensified surveillance and timely intervention [28]. In routine practice, MASLD risk assessment relies heavily on cross-sectional "snapshot" tools such as serum-based noninvasive tests (e.g., FIB-4) and vibration-controlled transient elastography. While useful for staging, these tools are less suited for continuous monitoring of evolving risk [29].

In this work, we study severe liver outcome risk assessment for MASLD patients from irregular time series. Using irregularly spaced laboratory records collected during patient follow-ups, we predict whether an MASLD patient is likely to progress to severe liver outcomes. Although artificial intelligence (AI) has demonstrated strong performance in general time-series prediction tasks [17], real-world follow-up data are often irregularly sampled and incomplete [26]. Clinically significant liver outcomes are also relatively rare, meaning that class imbalance can substantially distort both model training and evaluation [20]. In addition, models trained in one health system may experience substantial distribution shift when deployed elsewhere, and robustness under external validation is increasingly recognized as a core requirement for clinically credible AI [14].

We study a previously underexplored monitoring-style risk prediction formulation for MASLD progression risk prediction from irregular follow-up laboratories, and show that a missing-aware evolving neuro-fuzzy classifier (MEF-Classifier) is well suited to this setting. MEF-Classifier encodes irregular laboratory records and their associated liver outcomes into fuzzy rules, performs inference by matching queries to the most applicable rules and aggregating their consequents, and continuously updates its rule set as new observations become available. We evaluated MEF-Classifier on two large datasets, MIMIC-IV [13] (n = 2,358) and a proprietary MASLD cohort (n = 3,025), achieving AUROC values of 0.817 and 0.831 and AUPRC values of 0.419 and 0.452, respectively. These results represent a 5%–20% improvement in AUROC and a 54%–82% improvement in AUPRC over the second-best model.

# 2 Related Work

**MASLD.** Recent work has applied machine learning to predict MASLD progression to severe outcomes. Most approaches employ tree-based ensembles (e.g., Random Forest) or neural networks trained on routine electronic health records, reporting superior discrimination compared to traditional non-invasive tests like FIB-4 [9]. However, a major limitation is that these models predominantly rely on cross-sectional representations (single-visit labs, snapshot scores, or coarse summary statistics), leaving the use of serial follow-up laboratories as trajectory-level evidence less systematically explored in monitoring-style prediction [6,21].

**Irregular-Time Models.** In machine learning literature, to address the irregularity of time series without obscuring missingness patterns, specialized model architectures have been developed. Recurrent models such as GRU-D [2] and BRITS [1] introduce time-decay mechanisms to handle non-uniform intervals and missing values directly. Continuous-time approaches, including Neural ODEs [3], model latent dynamics using differential equations. Attention-based, graph-guided, and set-function methods, including mTAN [22], Raindrop [30], and SeFT [10], have demonstrated strong performance on sparse, asynchronous medical data. However, these models function as opaque black boxes, lacking the interpretability required for medicine, motivating our proposed approach.

## 3 Methodology

The prediction problem is defined as follows:

> *Given irregularly spaced laboratory records spanning $T$ months, whether a severe liver outcome (advanced fibrosis, cirrhosis, hepatocellular carcinoma, or liver failure) will occur within the subsequent $K$ months.*

Practically, each patient is represented as a set of instances, where each instance consists of a $T$-month observation window and its corresponding outcome label (positive or negative). Given $F$ laboratory variables, each instance is represented as a $F \times T$ matrix. The prediction is to learn a mapping $\mathbb{R}^{F \times T} \mapsto \{0, 1\}$.

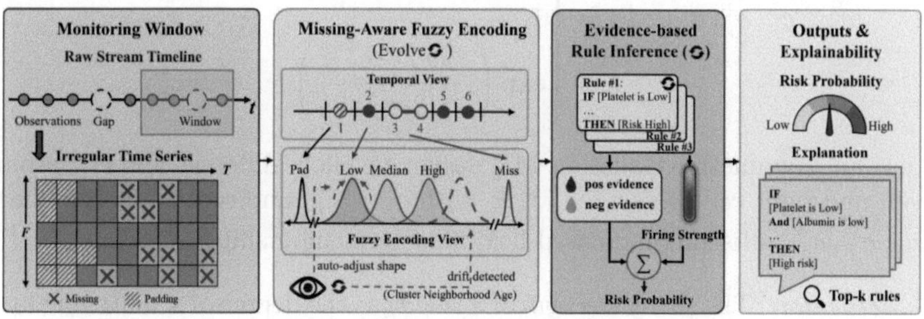


**Fig. 1.** The Conceptual Map of MEF-Classifier. Model converts irregular windows with explicit states into a probabilistic risk via missing-aware fuzzy encoding and evidence-based rule inference. Activated rules provide interpretable IF–THEN explanations.

As illustrated in Fig. 1, MEF-Classifier makes predictions through: (1) observation encoding, (2) clustering and rule-based inference, and (3) online adaptation. During encoding, each instance is represented by a matrix $\mathbf{X} \in \mathbb{R}^{F \times T}$, where $\mathbf{X}[i,j]$ is either the observed value of feature $i$ at time $j$, $-\infty$ if there is no observation for feature $i$ at or before time $j$, or $\infty$ if there is no observation for feature $i$ at time $j$, but at least one earlier observation exists for this feature. For efficient processing, $\mathbf{X}$ is flattened into a vector $\mathbf{x} \in \mathbb{R}^D$, where $D = F \cdot T$.

Once encoded, the model derives a set of interpretable prediction rules through a clustering-based procedure. Intuitively, clustering groups similar observations together, and each group forms a rule that links a characteristic observation pattern (the antecedent) to an associated outcome tendency (the consequent), estimated from the data. Given $\mathbf{x} = [x_1, \ldots, x_D]$, a fuzzy rule has the form:

*IF* $x_1$ is $A_1$, $x_2$ is $A_2$, ..., $x_D$ is $A_D$ *THEN* $y$ is positive/negative.

At query time, a new instance is matched against these rules, and the prediction is obtained by combining the outcomes derived from relevant rules. The rules are updated as new observations become available, enabling online adaptation and improved robustness when the data distribution evolves over time.

**Neuro-Fuzzy Inference.** [11,12] Prediction proceeds in three steps: (1) fuzzification, (2) rule activation, and (3) aggregation. An instance $\mathbf{x}$ is first fuzzified into a set of membership values, which are used to activate rules. The consequents of rules are subsequently aggregated to produce the final prediction.

*Fuzzification.* For an instance $\mathbf{x} = [x_1, \ldots, x_D]$, given a rule with antecedent $(A_1, \ldots, A_D)$, for each dimension $j = 1 \ldots D$, we compute a match value $v_j = \mu_{A_j}(x_j)$ with $\mu_{A_j}(\cdot)$ a *membership function (MF)* of $A_j$ that maps $x_j$ to $[0,1]$:

$$\mu(x_j; c_j^-, c_j^+, \sigma_j^-, \sigma_j^+) = \begin{cases} \exp\left(-\dfrac{(x_j - c_j^-)^2}{2(\sigma_j^-)^2}\right), & x_j < c_j^-, \\ 1, & c_j^- \le x_j \le c_j^+ \\ \exp\left(-\dfrac{(x_j - c_j^+)^2}{2(\sigma_j^+)^2}\right), & x_j > c_j^+. \end{cases} \tag{1}$$

We use an asymmetric Gaussian MF design to allow different spreads around the left and right *centroids* $c_j^-, c_j^+ \in \mathbb{R}$, with $c_j^- \le c_j^+$, and corresponding *cluster widths* $\sigma_j^-, \sigma_j^+$, affording increased flexibility in membership.

*Rule Activation.* The *firing strength* of a rule $r_k$ is the degree of $\mathbf{x}$ matching $r_k$. It is defined as an aggregation of memberships: $f_k(\mathbf{x}) = \min_{j=1..D} v_{k,j}$. Intuitively, $r_k$ is strongly activated only when all members in the antecedent of $r_k$ are "well matched". For each inference using a rule $r_k$,

$$p_k(\mathbf{x}) = \frac{e_k^+ + 1}{e_k^+ + e_k^- + 2} \tag{2}$$

is the *consequent probability* of applying $\mathbf{x}$ to $r_k$, where $e_k^+, e_k^- \in \mathbb{R}$ are *positive* and *negative evidences*, respectively, learned with online adaptation (see blow).

*Aggregation.* With $p_k$ the consequent probability obtained by applying $\mathbf{x}$ to rule $r_k$, and $g_k = f_k \cdot w_k \cdot e^{-\zeta}$, with $f_k$ denoting the firing strength of $r_k$, $w_k$ the *rule weight*, and $\zeta$ the number of missing observations in $\mathbf{x}$, i.e., $\zeta = |\{j : x_j \in \{\infty\}\}|$, the final prediction is

$$\hat{p} = \frac{\sum_k p_k \cdot g_k}{\sum_k g_k}. \tag{3}$$

We present rule creation and estimation of evidences and rule weight next.

**Rule Creation and Evolution.** Rule creation incrementally constructs and updates the rule base from incoming instances. Given an instance $\mathbf{x} = [x_1, \ldots, x_D]$, rule creation and update are performed as follows.

*Rule Creation.* We first construct a *candidate antecedent* by selecting, for each dimension $j$, the MF that best matches $x_j$ from the $l$ MFs for dimension $j$. This yields a candidate antecedent $A^*$:

$$A^* = (A_1, \ldots, A_D), \text{ where } A_j = \arg\max_l \mu_j^l(x_j).$$

We then compare $A^*$ against all existing rules using a *matching score* $\rho_k$ computed from the memberships of the rule-selected MFs under $\mathbf{x}$, and identify the best-matching rule $r_k^*$:

$$\rho_k = \min_j \mu_{A_{k,j}(x_j)} \text{ and } k^* = \arg\max_k \rho_k.$$

If $\rho_k^*$, the matching score of $r_k^*$, is greater than threshold $\tau$, then $\mathbf{x}$ is considered covered by existing rules. Otherwise, a new rule is created with antecedent $A^*$.

*Parameter Update.* To compute the consequent probability for $\mathbf{x}$, we update the positive and negative evidences $(e^+, e^-)$ using a firing-weighted increment, and the rule weight $w$ is recomputed as a function of total evidence:

$$e^+ \leftarrow e^+ + \alpha f(\mathbf{x}) \cdot y, \quad e^- \leftarrow e^- + f(\mathbf{x}) \cdot (1 - y), \quad w \leftarrow \frac{e^+ + e^-}{e^+ + e^- + 2}, \tag{4}$$

where $y$ is the true prediction label of $\mathbf{x}$, and $\alpha$ is an *evidence factor* designed to counter data imbalance. Finally, rules with persistently low rule weights $w$ are pruned to keep the active rule base compact.

In addition to updating rule parameters, MF parameters, especially the centroids $(c^+, c^-)$ and widths $(\sigma^+, \sigma^-)$, are also updated online. Specifically, for each MF, we apply an exponential-forgetting update that gives higher weight to recent observations while retaining long-term stability: centroids are adjusted via a weighted moving average toward newly observed inputs, and widths are updated in the same spirit. This allows the fuzzy partition to adapt smoothly over time, supporting robust tracking under gradual distribution shifts. Algorithm 1 details the evolution process.

**Algorithm 1:** Rule Base Evolution

**Input:** $\mathbf{x}$, $y$; MF set $\{\mu_{j,\ell}\}$ with stability $s_{j,\ell}$ for all $\ell$ MFs on dim $j$; Rule base $\mathcal{R}$
**Input:** Hyperparams: $\tau_{\text{mf}}$, $\tau_{\text{match}}(=\tau_{\text{mf}})$, $\tau_{\text{prune}}$, $h$, $K$, $\epsilon$, $\gamma = 0.5^{1/h}$, $\gamma_q = 0.5^{1/(10h)}$
**1. Membership Evolution (per dim $j$)**
$\text{max\_mf}_j \leftarrow \max_\ell \mu_{j,\ell}(x_j)$
$a_j \leftarrow a_j + (1 - \text{max\_mf}_j)$ // Update cluster age, inspired by rule-age[16]
$\text{is\_drift} \leftarrow (\Delta^2 a_j(t-1) > \Delta^2 a_j(t-2)) \wedge (\text{max\_mf}_j < \tau_{\text{mf}})$
**if** is_drift **then**
  Create a new MF on dim $j$ centered at $x_j$
**end**
$s_{j,\ell} \leftarrow \gamma s_{j,\ell} + \mu_{j,\ell}(x_j)$ // Update stability
$c^-_{j,\ell} \leftarrow \frac{\gamma s_{j,\ell} c^-_{j,\ell} + \mu_{j,\ell}(x_j)\, x_j}{\gamma s_{j,\ell} + \mu_{j,\ell}(x_j)}$, $\sigma^-_{j,\ell} \leftarrow \frac{s_{j,\ell-1}}{s_{j,\ell} + s_{j,\ell-1}} |c^-_{j,\ell} - c^+_{j,\ell-1}|$ // $(c^+_{j,\ell}, \sigma^+_{j,\ell})$ similarly
**2. MF Merging (per dim $j$)**
Compute adaptive $d^{st}_j$ as in [24], set $\theta_j = d^{st}_j / K$
**for** neighbor MFs pair $(\ell, \ell+1)$ **do**
  $\Delta_{j,\ell} = |c_{j,\ell+1} - c_{j,\ell}|$
  **if** $\Delta_{j,\ell} < \theta_j$ **then** // Merge redundant MFs
    $c_{j,\text{merge}} \leftarrow \frac{s_{j,\ell} c_{j,\ell} + s_{j,\ell+1} c_{j,\ell+1}}{s_{j,\ell} + s_{j,\ell+1}}$, $\sigma_{j,\text{merge}} \leftarrow \frac{\sigma_{j,\ell} + \sigma_{j,\ell+1}}{2}$
  **end**
**end**
**3. Rule Evolution**
Instantiate candidate antecedent $A^*_j \leftarrow \arg\max_\ell \mu_{j,\ell}(x_j)$
$\rho_k \leftarrow \min_j \mu_{j,A_{k,j}}(x_j)$, $k^* = \arg\max_k \rho_k$
**if** $\rho_{k^*} < \tau_{match}$ **then** // Soft matching
  Create new rule with antecedent $A^*$
**end**
// Evidence/Weight Update & Pruning
$q_{pos} \leftarrow \gamma_q q_{pos} + y$, $q_{total} \leftarrow \gamma_q q_{total} + 1$ // Global stats
$\omega^+ \leftarrow (q_{total} - q_{pos} + \epsilon)/(q_{pos} + \epsilon)$ // Imbalance weight
$e^+ \leftarrow e^+ + \omega^+ f y$, $e^- \leftarrow e^- + f(1-y)$ // Evidence update
$w \leftarrow (e^+ + e^-)/(e^+ + e^- + 2)$ // Rule weight update
Normalize $\{w\}_\mathcal{R}$; Pseudo-prune if $w_k < \tau_{\text{prune}}$

# 4 Experiments

The MIMIC-IV dataset [13] and an MASLD dataset from Tan Tock Seng Hospital (TTSH) in Singapore are used in our experiments. The MIMIC-IV dataset contains 5,976 instances collected from 2,358 patients with a 9% positive rate, while the TTSH dataset contains 6,398 instances from 3,025 patients with a 11% positive rate. Specifically, the MIMIC-IV cohort has a mean age of $57.4 \pm 14.3$ years, with a near-equal gender distribution (48.8% male). The selected patients in MIMIC-IV are followed for $2.92 \pm 3.02$ years on average. In TTSH, the mean age is $54.7 \pm 15.1$ years; the gender distribution is also near equal (50.3% male); and the follow-up duration is $3.23 \pm 3.06$ years on average.

Both cohorts adopt a patient-level train-test split (80% for train, 20% for test) and a sliding-window monitoring setup with a 12-month window ($T = 12$), and we predict whether a composite liver outcome will occur within the next 12 months ($K = 12$). We only consider the first onset of a severe liver outcome and each patient is associated with at most one positive event.

The laboratory feature set includes eight variables: Albumin ($g/L$), Basophils ($K/\mu L$), Eosinophils (%), Lymphocytes ($K/\mu L$), Neutrophils ($K/\mu L$), Platelets

($K/\mu L$), Total protein ($g/L$), and White blood cell count (WBC) ($K/\mu L$). We also include two static features, age and gender in our modeling.

We report AUROC and AUPRC (mean ± std over 5 random seeds) on three cohort settings: (1) MIMIC-IV, (2) TTSH, and (3) MIMIC-IV + TTSH. We additionally performed a pre-specified formal comparison of AUROC between MEF-Classifier and the strongest baseline in Table 1 (SeFT) on a fixed held-out test split for each cohort, using DeLong's test for paired ROC curves.

All methods use z-score normalization based on training data. Static features are handled in a baseline-specific manner: models with dedicated static inputs use them directly; otherwise, we concatenate them to each time step. For MEF-Classifier, we append static features to the flattened representation. The hyperparameters of MEF-Classifier are: $\tau_{mf} = 0.7$, $\tau_{prune} = 0.6$, and $h = 100$.

**Table 1.** Per-instance performance on MIMIC-IV and TTSH cohorts. Results are mean ± std over 5 seeds. Best results are in **bold** and second-best are underlined. Baselines include irregular-time models (†), regular-time models (‡), and classic RNN/ML models (⋆), where models required fix-grid is treated with MICE imputation [25].

| Model | MIMIC-IV | | TTSH | | MIMIC-IV + TTSH | |
|---|---|---|---|---|---|---|
| | AUROC | AUPRC | AUROC | AUPRC | AUROC | AUPRC |
| MEF-Classifier | **0.817 ± 0.040** | **0.419 ± 0.064** | **0.831 ± 0.040** | **0.452 ± 0.061** | **0.813 ± 0.023** | **0.426 ± 0.039** |
| mTAN [22] † | 0.685 ± 0.061 | 0.124 ± 0.039 | 0.637 ± 0.034 | 0.178 ± 0.030 | 0.615 ± 0.032 | 0.136 ± 0.030 |
| SeFT [10] † | 0.779 ± 0.027 | 0.272 ± 0.087 | 0.694 ± 0.044 | 0.248 ± 0.086 | 0.728 ± 0.027 | 0.257 ± 0.067 |
| Neural ODE [3] † | 0.504 ± 0.030 | 0.066 ± 0.013 | 0.497 ± 0.005 | 0.109 ± 0.009 | 0.491 ± 0.007 | 0.088 ± 0.005 |
| GRU-D [2] † | 0.703 ± 0.015 | 0.159 ± 0.033 | 0.640 ± 0.029 | 0.172 ± 0.023 | 0.656 ± 0.032 | 0.152 ± 0.022 |
| Raindrop [30] † | 0.683 ± 0.043 | 0.161 ± 0.050 | 0.606 ± 0.048 | 0.158 ± 0.031 | 0.639 ± 0.039 | 0.145 ± 0.027 |
| BRITS [1] † | 0.658 ± 0.047 | 0.121 ± 0.025 | 0.588 ± 0.038 | 0.140 ± 0.019 | 0.632 ± 0.036 | 0.137 ± 0.025 |
| iTransformer [15] ‡ | 0.696 ± 0.022 | 0.145 ± 0.018 | 0.607 ± 0.034 | 0.161 ± 0.027 | 0.642 ± 0.027 | 0.147 ± 0.020 |
| PatchTST [18] ‡ | 0.695 ± 0.023 | 0.131 ± 0.012 | 0.600 ± 0.040 | 0.153 ± 0.030 | 0.632 ± 0.025 | 0.144 ± 0.022 |
| TimesNet [27] ‡ | 0.692 ± 0.060 | 0.143 ± 0.036 | 0.578 ± 0.049 | 0.140 ± 0.032 | 0.629 ± 0.025 | 0.133 ± 0.019 |
| GRU [5,7] ⋆ | 0.762 ± 0.042 | 0.239 ± 0.069 | 0.652 ± 0.053 | 0.224 ± 0.079 | 0.694 ± 0.027 | 0.215 ± 0.049 |
| LSTM [5,7] ⋆ | 0.757 ± 0.041 | 0.242 ± 0.084 | 0.657 ± 0.044 | 0.215 ± 0.065 | 0.698 ± 0.024 | 0.213 ± 0.049 |
| XGBoost [4] ⋆ | 0.773 ± 0.012 | 0.270 ± 0.026 | 0.664 ± 0.033 | 0.208 ± 0.052 | 0.703 ± 0.016 | 0.231 ± 0.060 |

Table 1 reports per-instance performance on MIMIC-IV and TTSH. Across both individual datasets and the combined cohort, MEF-Classifier shows consistently strong discrimination, with a notable relative improvement in AUPRC, suggesting improved identification of high-risk patients under severe class imbalance. These findings support the potential suitability of neuro-fuzzy approaches for processing irregular clinical data in the presence of pronounced class imbalance. As shown in Table 2, MEF-Classifier achieved significantly higher AUROC than SeFT on all three cohorts.

Figure 2 shows that the rule base size remains bounded over time (left), and a few rules can cover most positive scenarios (right). We also conducted an ablation study and external validation, as shown in Table 4, which demonstrates that each component in MEF-Classifier contributes to the desirable performance.

**Table 2.** DeLong's test on per-instance prediction. Results are computed on fixed held-out test splits using MEF-Classifier and the best baseline (SeFT).

| Cohort | AUROC (MEF-Classifier) | AUROC (SeFT) | $\Delta$AUROC | p-value |
|---|---|---|---|---|
| MIMIC-IV | 0.872 | 0.715 | 0.157 | 0.0025 |
| TTSH | 0.866 | 0.793 | 0.073 | 0.0051 |
| MIMIC-IV + TTSH | 0.870 | 0.794 | 0.076 | <0.001 |

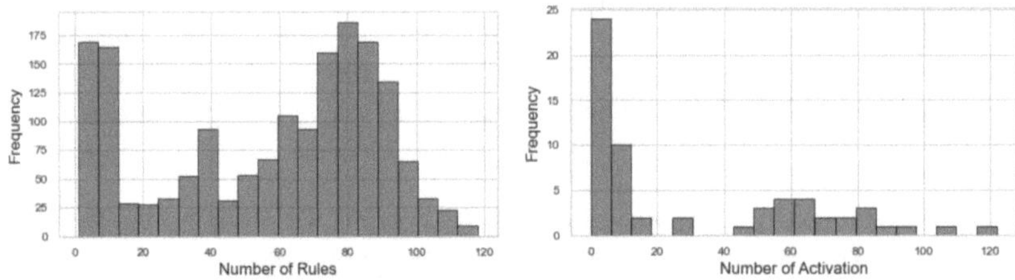


**Fig. 2.** Rule-base size throughout online learning and activations of rules with $e^+ > 0$. The left plot shows that the number of rules remains bounded throughout online learning; the right plot shows that a few rules can cover most positive scenarios.

Table 3 reports the per-patient performance of MEF-Classifier alongside strong baselines, where instance-level predictions are aggregated for each patient using max pooling (i.e., the patient-level score is defined as the maximum predicted risk across all instances) to reflect a conservative clinical monitoring scenario where any high-risk window warrants attention.

**Interpretability Analysis.** MEF-Classifier affords a transparent rule-based representation because each prediction is a weighted aggregation of fuzzy rules, each encoding an explicit antecedent pattern that can be translated into natural language (Fig. 3). The top rules highlight two complementary high-risk trajectories: an acute inflammatory/stress "hit" on a vulnerable baseline marked by low Platelets and low/unstable Albumin, and a progressive deterioration pattern marked by declining Platelets and persistently low/worsening Albumin. While

**Table 3.** Per-patient performance on MIMIC-IV and TTSH cohorts. Results are mean ± std over 5 seeds. Best results are in **bold** and second-best are underlined.

| Model | MIMIC-IV | | TTSH | | MIMIC-IV + TTSH | |
|---|---|---|---|---|---|---|
| | AUROC | AUPRC | AUROC | AUPRC | AUROC | AUPRC |
| MEF-Classifier | **0.821 ± 0.064** | **0.507 ± 0.099** | **0.791 ± 0.053** | **0.534 ± 0.077** | **0.759 ± 0.009** | **0.453 ± 0.010** |
| SeFT | 0.791 ± 0.042 | 0.355 ± 0.072 | 0.682 ± 0.028 | 0.296 ± 0.048 | 0.719 ± 0.035 | 0.289 ± 0.054 |
| GRU-D | 0.720 ± 0.060 | 0.199 ± 0.041 | 0.618 ± 0.019 | 0.195 ± 0.004 | 0.672 ± 0.019 | 0.191 ± 0.005 |
| GRU | 0.751 ± 0.040 | 0.282 ± 0.048 | 0.648 ± 0.047 | 0.285 ± 0.052 | 0.693 ± 0.038 | 0.267 ± 0.042 |
| XGBoost | 0.777 ± 0.061 | 0.333 ± 0.061 | 0.657 ± 0.049 | 0.299 ± 0.084 | 0.706 ± 0.050 | 0.304 ± 0.071 |

**Table 4.** Ablation Study. For w/o missing-aware, MICE imputation is used to fill the gaps; for w/o imbalance weight, we set $\omega^+ = 1$; for w/o evolving, we force the model to stop updating its rule base with TTSH, using only the rules generated from MIMIC-IV.

| Model | AUROC | AUPRC |
|---|---|---|
| MEF-Classifier (on MIMIC) | 0.872 | 0.568 |
| w/o missing-aware (on MIMIC) | 0.833 | 0.479 |
| w/o imbalance weight (on MIMIC) | 0.643 | 0.289 |
| *External Validation* | | |
| with evolving (MIMIC → TTSH) | 0.817 | 0.434 |
| w/o evolving (MIMIC → TTSH) | 0.599 | 0.136 |

MASLD monitoring often focuses on Albumin and inflammatory markers (e.g., WBC/Neutrophils), these rules repeatedly identify Platelets as a key longitudinal signal that may warrant explicit attention. Clinicians can inspect the top-contributing rules to see which patterns drive an elevated risk estimate, though formal user studies are left to future work. Beyond explanation, the evolving rule base can surface recurring, previously unrecognized risk phenotypes from longitudinal follow-ups, offering hypotheses for further clinical investigation.

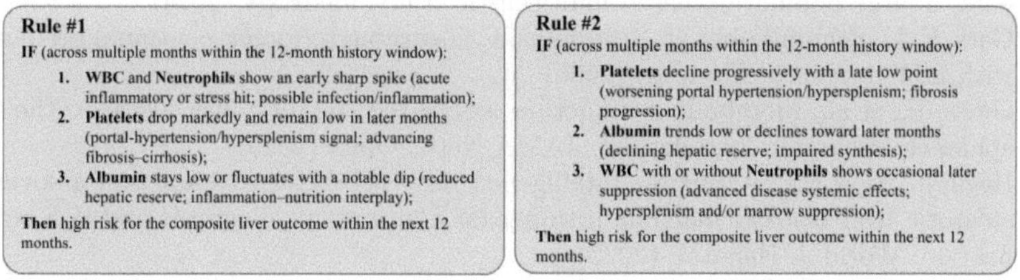


**Fig. 3.** Explainable Rules. Rules are extracted from MEF-Classifier after evaluation on the MIMIC-IV. The two presented rules are the top-2 with the highest rule weights, with $e_k^+ > 0$. For simplicity, we report only the dominant clauses.

## 5 Conclusion

We studied longitudinal risk prediction for MASLD progression using irregular follow-up records. We investigate MASLD progression risk prediction through a monitoring-style lens and find that MEF-Classifier, a missing-aware evolving neuro-fuzzy approach with evidence-based rule inference and imbalance-aware weighting, delivers strong discrimination while retaining transparent rule-based explanations. We evaluated the approach on MIMIC-IV and a local Singapore cohort, as well as a pooled setting, and conducted ablation studies, observing consistently strong discrimination performance. Future work will conduct a formal user study and evaluate clinical utility prospectively.

**Acknowledgements.** This project is supported by the Ministry of Education, Singapore (Grant RS15/23).

**Declaration of AI Assistance Technologies During Manuscript Preparation.** The author(s) used GPT 5.2 for Refinement, correction, editing or formatting the manuscript to improve clarity of language. After using this technology, the author(s) reviewed the results and take(s) full responsibility for the contents of the manuscript.

## References

1. Cao, W., et al.: BRITS: bidirectional recurrent imputation for time series. Adv. Neural Inf. Process. Syst. (2018)
2. Che, Z., et al.: Recurrent neural networks for multivariate time series with missing values. Sci. Rep. (2018)
3. Chen, R.T., et al.: Neural ordinary differential equations. Adv. Neural Inf. Process. Syst. (2018)
4. Chen, T., Guestrin, C.: XGBoost: a scalable tree boosting system. In: KDD (2016)
5. Cho, K., et al.: Learning phrase representations using RNN encoder-decoder for statistical machine translation. In: EMNLP (2014)
6. Clusmann, J., et al.: Machine learning predicts liver cancer risk from routine clinical data: a large population-based multicentric study. medRxiv (2024)
7. Gers, F.A., Schmidhuber, J., Cummins, F.: Learning to forget: continual prediction with LSTM. Neural Comput. (2000)
8. Ginès, P., et al.: Metabolic dysfunction–associated steatotic liver disease—the new epidemic of chronic liver disease. JAMA Netw. Open (2025)
9. Hegazy, M.A.E.: Artificial intelligence in metabolic dysfunction-associated steatotic liver disease: machine learning for non-invasive diagnosis and risk stratification. World J. Hepatol. (2025)
10. Horn, M., et al.: Set functions for time series. In: International Conference on Machine Learning. PMLR (2020)
11. Ishibuchi, H., Yamamoto, T.: Rule weight specification in fuzzy rule-based classification systems. IEEE Trans. Fuzzy Syst. (2005)
12. Jang, J.S.: ANFIS: adaptive-network-based fuzzy inference system. IEEE Trans. Syst. Man Cybernet. (1993)
13. Johnson, A., et al.: MIMIC-IV. PhysioNet (2024)
14. Koch, L.M., Baumgartner, C.F., Berens, P.: Distribution shift detection for the postmarket surveillance of medical AI algorithms: a retrospective simulation study. NPJ Digit. Med. (2024)
15. Liu, Y., et al.: itransformer: inverted transformers are effective for time series forecasting. In: ICLR (2024)
16. Lughofer, E., Angelov, P.: Handling drifts and shifts in on-line data streams with evolving fuzzy systems. Appl. Soft Comput. (2011)
17. Morid, M.A., Sheng, O.R.L., Dunbar, J.: Time series prediction using deep learning methods in healthcare. ACM Trans. Manage. Inf. Syst. (2023)
18. Nie, Y., et al.: A time series is worth 64 words: long-term forecasting with transformers. In: ICLR (2023)

19. Rinella, M.E., et al.: A multisociety Delphi consensus statement on new fatty liver disease nomenclature. Hepatology (2023)
20. Salmi, M., et al.: Handling imbalanced medical datasets: review of a decade of research. Artif. Intell. Rev. (2024)
21. Sarkar, S., et al.: A machine learning model to predict risk for hepatocellular carcinoma in patients with metabolic dysfunction-associated steatotic liver disease. Gastro Hep Adv. (2024)
22. Shukla, S.N., Marlin, B.M.: Multi-time attention networks for irregularly sampled time series. arXiv preprint arXiv:2101.10318 (2021)
23. Stefan, N., Yki-Järvinen, H., Neuschwander-Tetri, B.A.: Metabolic dysfunction-associated steatotic liver disease: heterogeneous pathomechanisms and effectiveness of metabolism-based treatment. Lancet Diabetes Endocrinol. (2025)
24. Tan, J., Quek, C.: A BCM theory of meta-plasticity for online self-reorganizing fuzzy-associative learning. IEEE Trans. Neural Netw. (2010)
25. Van Buuren, S., Groothuis-Oudshoorn, K.: mice: multivariate imputation by chained equations in R. J. Stat. Softw. (2011)
26. Weerakody, P.B., et al.: A review of irregular time series data handling with gated recurrent neural networks. Neurocomputing (2021)
27. Wu, H., et al.: TimesNet: temporal 2D-variation modeling for general time series analysis. In: ICLR (2023)
28. Younossi, Z.M., Kalligeros, M., Henry, L.: Epidemiology of metabolic dysfunction-associated steatotic liver disease. Clin. Mol. Hepatol. (2024)
29. Younossi, Z.M., et al.: Global consensus recommendations for metabolic dysfunction-associated steatotic liver disease and steatohepatitis. Gastroenterology (2025)
30. Zhang, X., et al.: Graph-guided network for irregularly sampled multivariate time series. In: ICLR (2022)

# Validation of an Interpretable AI System for Localizing the SubThalamic Nucleus During DBS Neurosurgery

Fabrizio Sciscenti[1,2](✉), Valentina Agostini[1,2], Laura Rizzi[3,4], Michele Lanotte[3,4], and Marco Ghislieri[1,2]

[1] PolitoBIOMed Lab, Politecnico di Torino, Turin 10129, Italy
fabrizio.sciscenti@polito.it
[2] Department of Electronics and Telecommunications, Politecnico di Torino, Turin 10129, Italy
[3] Department of Neuroscience "Rita Levi Montalcini", University of Turin, Turin 10126, Italy
[4] AOU Città della Salute e della Scienza di Torino, Turin 10126, Italy

**Abstract.** Accurate localization of the SubThalamic Nucleus (STN) during Deep Brain Stimulation (DBS) surgery is critical for therapeutic efficacy and is commonly supported by intraoperative MicroElectrode Recordings (MERs). While deep learning approaches have shown promising performance in automatic STN identification, their limited transparency hinders their clinical adoption. In this work, we present an interpretable deep learning pipeline for MERs classification coupled with a structured validation framework aimed at assessing the clinical relevance of the model reasoning. To this aim, the classification output from a patch-based convolutional neural network with self-attention is combined with Grad-CAM relevance maps. Alignment between relevance maps and manual annotations from 3 expert neurologists with 27, 20, and 11 years of experience was quantified using overlap-based metrics, while perceived transparency, usefulness, and trustworthiness were assessed through Likert-scale questionnaires. Results show competitive classification performance (0.92 ± 0.07 AUC) and consistent agreement between automatic explanations and expert reasoning, with a maximum Dice Score of 0.77 ± 0.11, alongside high clinician acceptance and perceived interpretability. These findings suggest that structured, expert-centred validation of XAI can provide a meaningful contribution toward trustworthy AI-assisted decision support systems in intraoperative neurosurgery.

**Keywords:** explainable artificial intelligence · expert-centred validation · pilot study · deep brain stimulation · microelectrode recordings · Parkinson's disease

## 1 Introduction

Deep Brain Stimulation (DBS) of the SubThalamic Nucleus (STN) is an established electroceutical therapy for treating motor symptoms in patients with advanced Parkinson's Disease (PD) [1]. The therapeutic efficacy of DBS strongly depends on the accurate

© The Author(s), under exclusive license to Springer Nature Switzerland AG 2027
P. Andreev et al. (Eds.): AIME 2026, LNAI 16748, pp. 242–247, 2027.
https://doi.org/10.1007/978-3-032-30710-1_30

placement of the stimulating electrode. For this reason, neurosurgeons rely on intra-operative MicroElectrode Recordings (MERs), acquired along a pre-planned trajectory, to refine anatomical localization and identify the stimulation target, the STN. In recent years, Machine Learning (ML) [2] and Deep Learning (DL) [3] approaches have shown promising performance in the automatic identification of the STN. However, their adoption into clinical practice remains limited due to the insufficient transparency of data-driven models. In this context, eXplainable Artificial Intelligence (XAI) has been proposed as a potential solution. Nevertheless, in clinical contexts, explanations are frequently evaluated only qualitatively [4].

In this work, we present an interpretable DL-based pipeline for the automatic identification of the STN from MERs, coupled with a structured validation framework for its generated explanations.

## 2 Materials and Methods

### 2.1 Datasets and Data Harmonization

We retrospectively analysed MERs from 168 bilateral DBS surgeries collected from two publicly available datasets (Dataset A: 46 patients [3]; Dataset B: 36 patients [2]), and one proprietary dataset (Dataset C: 86 patients, age of $59.1 \pm 7.2$, disease duration of $13.5 \pm 5.1$, 45 males and 41 females), collected at the Stereotactic and Functional Neurosurgery Unit of the University of Turin, Italy [5]. Each surgery included recordings from approximately $-10$ mm to $+5$ mm with respect to the estimated STN position. Each recording was labelled as in-STN (class 1) or out-STN (class 0). Dataset A provided three simultaneously recording electrodes (Central, Anterior, and Medial), while Datasets B and C included a single electrode. Sampling frequencies were 24 kHz, 20 kHz, and 12 kHz for Datasets A, B, and C, respectively, with hardware high-pass filtering at 200 Hz (Dataset B) and 100 Hz (Dataset C). To harmonize the data, only the Central electrode from Dataset A was considered; all signals were down-sampled to 10 kHz, and a 250 Hz high-pass filter was applied. Recordings were divided into 1-s overlapping segments, with a patient- and class-dependent overlap (0%–75%) to balance intra-patient and inter-dataset class distributions. The final dataset comprised 48114 in-STN and 44437 out-STN segments. For evaluation, a patient-wise split was adopted. The test set included 30 randomly selected patients (10 per dataset; 10280 in-STN and 10224 out-STN segments). The remaining patients were randomly divided into training (125 patients; 33948 in-STN, 31046 out-STN) and validation sets (13 patients; 3886 in-STN, 3167 out-STN). Finally, each segment was z-score normalized.

### 2.2 MERs Classification

We adopted a hybrid patch-based Convolutional Neural Network (CNN), integrated with Multi-Head self-Attention (MHA). Each input signal is divided into 50 non-overlapping patches (200 samples). Each patch is encoded by three CNN blocks, each with a convolutional layer (kernel size 5, stride 1, 32 output channels), ReLU activation, and pooling (two max-pooling layers, and one adaptive average pooling layer). Patch embeddings are processed by a two-head MHA (embedding dimension 32), then concatenated and classified by a multi-layer perceptron with two hidden layers (32 and 16 neurons) and a two-neuron output layer. The network was implemented in Python 3.10, with PyTorch 2.9, and trained on a workstation with Intel Core i7 and RTX 3060 GPU, using AdamW optimizer (learning rate $10^{-4}$, batch size 32) and cross-entropy loss.

Classification performance on the test set was evaluated using Area Under the ROC Curve (AUC), Precision, and Recall, computed at the patient level by aggregating the binary predictions of all signal segments belonging to the same patient.

**Explainability Method.** Gradient-weighted Class Activation Mapping (Grad-CAM) [6], adapted to one-dimensional signals, was used to generate patch-level relevance scores that were min–max normalized at the segment level. For visualization, relevance maps were superimposed onto the raw MERs as heatmaps, concatenated across 1-s segments, smoothed with a Gaussian kernel ($\sigma = 250$ samples), and scaled by the classifier's output probability. A representative example of superimposed Grad-CAM relevance heatmaps is shown in Fig. 1, where warmer colours highlight the regions that most strongly influenced the AI's decision.

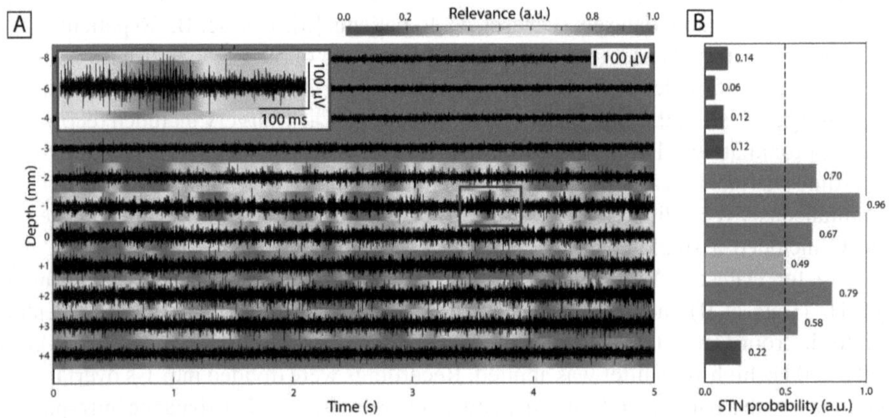


**Fig. 1. XAI validation interface.** (A) Example microelectrode recordings trajectory, with superimposed Grad-CAM relevance heatmaps. The inset shows a zoomed-in segment of the recording at −1 mm, highlighted by a magenta box. (B) Average probability of belonging to the SubThalamic Nucleus (STN). The dashed vertical line mark probability threshold.

### 2.3 XAI Validation Protocol

Three neurologists from the "Rita Levi Montalcini" Department of Neuroscience of the University of Turin (Turin, Italy), with 27 (Expert 1), 20 (Expert 2), and 11 years (Expert 3) of experience participated in the study. Each clinician was presented with 10 trajectories, each with 9 to 15 MERs (5-s segments) arranged by depth. For each depth, the average in-STN probability was provided, alongside Grad-CAM-generated heatmaps. Figure 1 shows the interface developed for the validation phase.

The validation protocol consisted of four sequential phases, each performed independently by each neurologist:

1. *Blind Annotation.* Neurologists were shown the trajectories without any annotation and were asked to manually highlight the signal portions they considered representative of STN activity;
2. *Explanation-Informed Evaluation.* Neurologists were presented with the model's classification output and relevance heatmaps, enabling them to revise their initial annotations based on the model's automatic classification and explanation;
3. *Ongoing Questionnaire.* After completing the annotation phases, neurologists completed a short Likert-scale questionnaire to assess the perceived quality and plausibility of the provided explanations. The specific questionnaire items are reported in Fig. 2C;
4. *Final Questionnaire.* At the end of the session, neurologists completed a final Likert-scale questionnaire summarizing their overall assessment of the system. The specific questionnaire items are reported in Fig. 2D.

Phases 1, 2, and 3 were repeated for each trajectory [7].

**Explanation Validation.** Explanations were evaluated qualitatively using 6-point Likert questionnaires and quantitatively by measuring the agreement between relevance maps and clinician annotation masks. The overlap was quantified using the Dice Similarity Coefficient (DSC), by binarizing relevance maps using 15% of the maximum as a threshold [6], and the Area Under the masked relevance Curve (AUmC), computed as the ratio between the sum of relevance values falling within the expert-annotated mask, and the total sum of relevance values.

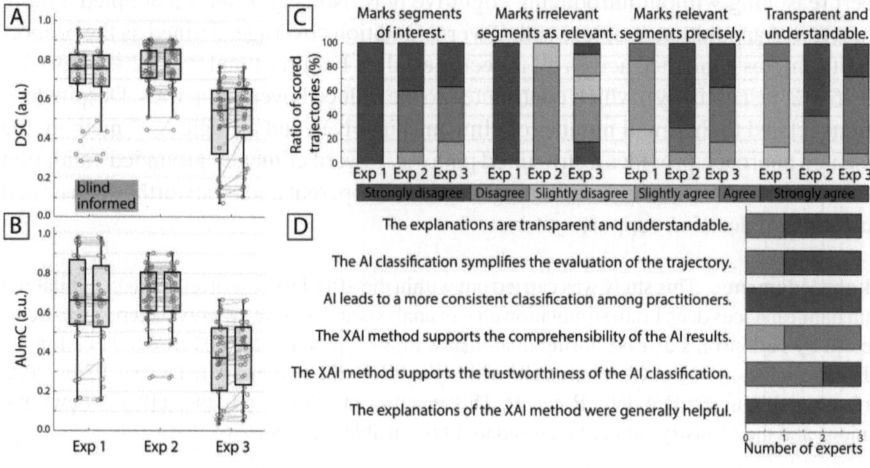


**Fig. 2. XAI validation results.** (A-B) Distribution of overlap metrics (DSC: Dice Similarity Coefficient; AUmC: Area Under the masked relevance Curve). Boxplots represent the central tendency and dispersion, while scatter points represent individual recordings; corresponding recordings across annotation phases (blind vs. informed) are connected by grey lines. (C) Results of the ongoing questionnaires. (D) Results of the final questionnaire.

## 3 Results

The proposed hybrid CNN-MHA model achieved competitive performance in the automatic identification of STN activity at the patient level with an AUC of 0.92 ± 0.07 (mean ± standard deviation), Precision of 0.86 ± 0.09, and Recall of 0.81 ± 0.15 [2, 3]. The per-dataset AUC values, each computed on the 10 test patients in each dataset, were 0.88 ± 0.04, 0.94 ± 0.07, and 0.92 ± 0.07 for datasets A, B, and C, respectively.

Figure 2 summarizes the results of the XAI-validation phase. Across neurologists, the explanations showed moderate to high alignment with annotated regions (Fig. 2A, B). Expert 1 achieved a DSC of 0.71 ± 0.18 during the blind annotation phase, and 0.70 ± 0.18 after annotation refinement (AUmC of 0.65 ± 0.24 and 0.64 ± 0.24, respectively). Expert 2 reported the highest agreement, with DSC of 0.77 ± 0.11 in both conditions (AUmC of 0.69 ± 0.15). Expert 3 showed lower scores (DSC of 0.48 ± 0.21 and 0.50 ± 0.19; AUmC of 0.36 ± 0.19 and 0.38 ± 0.18). The ongoing questionnaires revealed a positive perception of the explanations (Fig. 2C). All experts reported that the XAI effectively highlighted segments of interest. The relevance of highlighted portions was high for Experts 1 and 2, while Expert 3 exhibited occasional disagreement. Perceived transparency and understandability increased with decreasing years of experience (Fig. 2D).

## 4 Discussion and Conclusion

This pilot study validated an interpretable AI system for intraoperative MER-based STN localization. Grad-CAM relevance maps achieved moderate to high agreement with expert annotations, while the minimal changes after review suggest alignment with expert reasoning without introducing cognitive bias. Notably, Expert 3 adopted a more conservative annotation strategy, with lower annotation coverage, defined as the proportion of samples annotated across all trajectories, than Experts 1 and 2 (13.2% vs. 30.3% and 26.3%, respectively), which contributed to the reduced overlap metrics. Despite limitations related to the small number of clinicians involved and a single XAI method, the presented approach provides a structured pathway toward clinically grounded validation of interpretable AI, thereby contributing to more transparent and trustworthy AI-assisted neurosurgical decision support systems.

**Acknowledgments.** This study was carried out within the «PD-DBS» project ("Effect of bilateral subthalamic nucleus deep brain stimulation on gait analysis and muscle synergy patterns of patients affected by Parkinson's disease during dual-task walking", protocol No 2022KWSJJT) – funded by European Union – Next Generation EU within the PRIN 2022 program (D.D. 104 - 02/02/2022 Ministero dell'Università e della Ricerca). This manuscript reflects only the authors' views and opinions and the Ministry cannot be considered responsible for them.

**Disclosure of Interests** The authors have no competing interests to declare that are relevant to the content of this article.

## References


1. Ghislieri, M., et al.: Improved dual-task interference in Parkinson's disease following deep brain stimulation. IEEE Trans. Neural Syst. Rehabil. Eng. **33**, 4624–4635 (2025)
2. Sciscenti, F., Agostini, V., Rizzi, L., Lanotte, M., Ghislieri, M.: ML-STIM: machine learning for SubThalamic nucleus intraoperative mapping. J. Neural Eng. **22**(4), 046041 (2025)
3. Ciecierski, K., Mandat, T.: Classification of DBS microelectrode recordings using a residual neural network with attention in the temporal domain. Neural Netw. **170**, 18–31 (2024)
4. Longo, L., et al.: Explainable artificial intelligence (XAI) 2.0: a manifesto of open challenges and interdisciplinary research directions. Inf. Fusion. **106**, 102301 (2024)
5. Lanotte, M., Rizzone, M., Bergamasco, B., Faccani, G., Melcarne, A., Lopiano, L.: Deep brain stimulation of the subthalamic nucleus: anatomical, neurophysiological, and outcome correlations with the effects of stimulation. J. Neurol. Neurosurg. Psychiatry. **72**(1), 53–58 (2002)
6. Selvaraju, R., Cogswell, M., Das, A., Vedantam, R., Parikh, D., Batra, D.: Grad-CAM: visual explanations from deep networks via gradient-based localization. Int. J. Comput. Vis. **128**(2), 336–359 (2020)
7. Manz, R., et al.: Do explainable AI (XAI) methods improve the acceptance of AI in clinical practice? An evaluation of XAI methods on Gleason grading. J Pathol Clin Res. **11**(2), e70023 (2025)

# Predicting Fibromyalgia Pain From Self-reported Health Data Using Time-Series and Deep Learning Models

Delnia Alipour[1(✉)], Olga Perepelkina[2], Alessandro Vinciarelli[1], Tahir Janmohamed[3], Binh Nguyen[3], and Simone Stumpf[1]

[1] School of Computing Science, University of Glasgow, Glasgow, UK
2937762a@student.gla.ac.uk,
{alessandro.vinciarelli,simone.stumpf}@glasgow.ac.uk
[2] Intel, Munich, Germany
olga.perepelkina@intel.com
[3] ManagingLife, Inc., Toronto, Canada
{tahir.janmohamed,binh.nguyen}@managinglife.com

**Abstract.** People with Fibromyalgia (FM) suffer from variable, day-to-day pain that complicates self-management and timely clinical support. This study investigates whether pain severity can be predicted from self-reported health data using statistical and time-series foundation models (TSFMs) compared to standard deep learning models. We used a dataset obtained through the Manage My Pain (MMP) app of users who self-report FM, splitting them into *Dense* (N = 681) and *Sparse* (N = 333) cohorts based on their frequency of pain logging. We conducted an analysis of temporality and seasonality, which showed consistent short-term temporal dependence and some seasonality. We then evaluated the error of predicting pain scores for next-day and next-week horizons using statistical and foundation time-series models alongside their covariate variants, compared with a CNN baseline. Overall, TSFMs achieved the lowest errors. Statistical time-series models offered only limited gains and, in some cases, were worse than CNN. These findings suggest that TSFMs are a feasible choice for personalised pain prediction from FM self-reported health data.

**Keywords:** Fibromyalgia · Pain Prediction · Time-series prediction · self-reported health data · Digital health · mHealth · Foundation models

## 1 Introduction

Fibromyalgia (FM) is a chronic, heterogeneous pain condition characterised by widespread musculoskeletal pain, fatigue, sleep disturbance, and cognitive difficulties [12]. A challenge in FM is substantial day-to-day fluctuation in pain severity, which complicates clinical management and everyday planning. Anticipating these changes could support self-management, personalised feedback, and

© The Author(s), under exclusive license to Springer Nature Switzerland AG 2027
P. Andreev et al. (Eds.): AIME 2026, LNAI 16748, pp. 248–257, 2027.
https://doi.org/10.1007/978-3-032-30710-1_31

earlier clinical review. Conventional assessments based on periodic appointments or retrospective questionnaires are poorly suited to capturing rapid symptom dynamics. In contrast, self-reported health data from mobile health (mHealth) tools can provide frequent, ecologically valid measurements in everyday life [6]. In this work, we study self-reports from the Manage My Pain (MMP)[1] app, where users log pain symptoms and its impact over time. The MMP dataset provides a setting that is both clinically relevant and methodologically challenging, including large amounts of varied data coupled with irregular self-reporting.

Time-series prediction, using historical data to predict future values, is widely used in healthcare for tasks such as predicting expenditure or estimating disease cases [5]. In pain prediction, however, most existing studies focus on oncology settings and rely primarily on task-trained deep learning models, such as CNN [3]. Prior work using MMP data has focused on longer-term outcome prediction in chronic pain using fixed observation windows, rather than time-series prediction [10]. This is the first study to perform time-series pain prediction for FM using self-reported data for two horizons, compared to a CNN baseline. We address the following research questions: **RQ1:** *How well can we predict a user's pain severity for the next day* ($H{=}1$)*from their previous pain records?* and **RQ2:** *How well can we predict a user's pain severity trajectory over the next week* ($H{=}7$) *from their previous pain records?*

## 2 Related Work

Prior work on pain prediction can be grouped into three broad families: task-trained deep learning, classical statistical time-series models, and time-series foundation models (TSFMs). Deep learning models can capture non-linear patterns and temporal dependencies but are sensitive to long horizons and irregular sampling [8]. Nonetheless, deep models have been used for short-horizon prediction of cancer pain exacerbation, with performance varying by the amount of recent history and the temporal binning/aggregation used [2]. More broadly, cancer symptom prediction performs best at short windows, with accuracy degrading as aggregation windows lengthen and effective sample size decreases [3].

Statistical time-series approaches such as Autoregressive Integrated Moving Average (ARIMA) have been applied to healthcare domains where trends and seasonality are prominent [5]; however, there is comparatively limited work on pain prediction using self-reported data. Previous work employing ARIMAX, a covariate approach extending ARIMA, to predict weekly pain and treatment response achieved good accuracy [4]. A study investigating daily pain prediction in the workplace compared Gaussian process and ARIMA models, with the Gaussian process achieving lower error, especially with limited data [9]. Overall, this shows that statistical time-series methods can be effective for short-term pain prediction but struggle when data are irregular and sparse.

A relatively new approach are TSFMs, which are pretrained models that learn reusable temporal representations from corpora drawn from many domains and

[1] https://managemypainapp.com.

sampling frequencies and can be applied to new datasets via zero-shot inference or lightweight adaptation [7]. In this family, Chronos and its covariate extension, Chronos-2, enable prediction using group attention for in-context learning across related series [1]. While foundation-model approaches have shown strong potential in healthcare across language, vision, and multimodal integration of clinical data [11], evidence for TSFMs on self-reported health data remains limited, particularly under substantial missingness and variable logging density.

## 3 Methods

**Dataset.** Manage My Pain (MMP) is a digital health app that enables users to log pain episodes throughout the day, track symptoms over time, and generate reports for clinical communication. The core functionality of MMP centres around two types of user entries: Pain Records (PRs) and Daily Reflections (DRs). Pain Records capture momentary pain experiences and can be completed multiple times per day. Users are prompted with "How is your pain right now?" and rate their severity on a visual analogue scale from 0 (no pain) to 10 (worst ever). Following this rating, users can complete seven optional fields to describe the pain episode: Location, Symptoms, Characteristics, Aggravating Factors, Medications, Interventions, and Environmental Context. Daily Reflections are daily self-reports of the user's functional and psychological state on a 0–10 scale, with optional entries on meaningful activities. For this research, we focus on Pain Records. The study received ethical approval from the College of Science and Engineering Ethics Committee, University of Glasgow.

Data were obtained from the MMP platform[2]. We identified 26,564 users who self-reported FM in their profiles between August 2012 and June 2025. For each user, we identified their starting point of logging and used this to extract user data that met three criteria: (i) an observation span of at least 60 d, (ii) at least 60% day-level coverage (approximately 3–4 d per week), and (iii) a maximum inter-report gap of 15 d. These criteria resulted in 282,995 Pain Records from 1,014 users. On average, daily pain scores were 5.64, with 279.1 PRs per user. Observations spanned on average 279.6 d, with an average maximum gap of 5.62 d. We then split this dataset into two cohorts, based on their logging behaviour. Users with a maximum log gap of $\leq 5$ d were defined as the *Dense* cohort (N = 681). Users with $5 <$ gaps $\leq 15$ days were defined as the *Sparse* cohort (N = 333).

The availability of demographic information was limited. Missingness exceeded 50% for age, height, and weight; gender was available for only 513 out of 1,014 users. Therefore, demographics were not included in the models.

**Models.** Preprocessing was intentionally kept conservative to preserve the real-world characteristics of self-reported data. Days without pain reports were retained as unobserved rather than globally imputed. Continuous features were

[2] The dataset is not publicly available and is accessible only under a data licensing agreement with ManagingLife.

standardised using training-split statistics only, while binary indicators and missingness flags were left unscaled. Where necessary, we applied minimal short-gap interpolation.

We designed two feature representations: the first used only lagged pain severity scores, while the second augmented it with contextual covariates derived from pain descriptors, engagement, and calendar variables. PRs were aligned to a daily calendar and aggregated using median pain severity. Additional daily summaries included number of PRs, within-day pain range and standard deviation, and a missingness indicator. For each pain descriptor (Locations, Symptoms, Character, Aggravating Factors, Effective Factors, Ineffective Factors, and Environment), we derived a binary indicator of presence, along with richness measures counting distinct items reported. Descriptors with <5% prevalence were removed to reduce sparsity. For engagement, we derived two indicators: days since the most recent PR and proportion of days in the previous week with at least one PR. Finally, we included day-of-week as a calendar feature to capture weekly rhythms.

We used the following models over two horizons (H = 1 and H = 7), selected as representative examples of convolutional, statistical and TSFM families rather than an exhaustive benchmark of all prediction architectures. We trained a global CNN on pooled user-anchor samples. Each instance is a multivariate tensor $X \in \mathbb{R}^{C \times 180}$ (180 prior days; $C$ channels = pain plus covariates). The model comprised two 1D convolution layers with 64 filters and kernel size 3, followed by batch normalisation, global average pooling, and a two-layer fully connected head to predict the target horizon. Training used Adam optimiser (learning rate $10^{-3}$, batch size 64) for 15 epochs at $H = 1$ and 20 epochs at $H = 7$, with the same settings across Dense and Sparse cohorts. We used two versions of statistical time-series models, one which investigated predicting pain from pain severity alone (ARIMA), and one which included contextual covariates in addition to lagged pain (ARIMAX). For ARIMA, we fitted an autoregressive integrated moving average model separately per user using only the daily pain series, where $p$ is the autoregressive order, $d$ the differencing order, and $q$ the moving-average order. Orders were selected by grid search over $p, q \in \{0, 1, 2, 3\}$ and $d \in \{0, 1\}$, with $d$ determined using the KPSS stationarity test. The final $(p^*, d^*, q^*)$ was chosen by minimising AICc subject to stationarity and invertibility constraints. For ARIMAX, we extended ARIMA by adding exogenous regressors (PR summaries, descriptor indicators, compliance features, and calendar effects). Model orders were selected using the same procedure as ARIMA. For TSFMs, we used two configurations, Chronos, evaluated on pain severity only, and Chronos-2, evaluated on pain severity with additional covariates, both applied in a zero-shot setting with their respective pipelines. For Chronos-2, we used a 180-day context window containing pain and covariates. Only calendar variables were provided as known-future covariates; diary-derived covariates were restricted to the historical window. Predictions used the median (0.5-quantile) and were evaluated per anchor, then aggregated to per-user metrics.

**Analysis.** Before fitting predictive models, we assessed short-term temporal dependence in daily pain scores using pairwise-complete autocorrelation functions at lags 1–7 and user-level autoregressive models of order three. Distributions of autocorrelations, regression coefficients, and adjusted $R^2$ were summarised across users. Longer-range cyclic structure was assessed at weekly (lag 7) and approximately monthly (lag 30) intervals. A user was classified as exhibiting seasonality at a given lag if at least 15 observation pairs were available and the correlation was significant ($p < 0.05$).

Models were evaluated at predefined anchor days within each user's time-series, using only observations available up to each forecast origin to prevent information leakage. For $H{=}1$, anchors with a missing next-day target were excluded; for $H{=}7$, anchors were retained if at least one target in the $[t+1, t+7]$ window was observed, and errors were computed on observed days only. Statistical and foundation models used a rolling-origin protocol, while the CNN used a temporal holdout with sliding-window inputs. Preliminary experiments with a within-user rolling-origin CNN showed weaker results, so we retained the pooled configuration as the primary baseline. Performance is summarised per user using Mean Absolute Error (MAE) and Mean Absolute Scaled Error (MASE), which normalises MAE by a naïve persistence baseline. User-level metrics are aggregated using the median and interquartile range (IQR).

We tested performance differences using a mixed ANOVA with Model as a within-subject factor and Cohort (Dense vs Sparse) as a between-subject factor, run separately for each horizon, to estimate main effects and their interaction while accounting for repeated measures. As sphericity was violated in all analyses (Mauchly's test), within-subject effects used Greenhouse–Geisser-corrected degrees of freedom and p-values. Raw MASE values were right-skewed; inferential analyses involving MASE were therefore performed on a log1p-transformed scale, with descriptive summaries reported on the original scale. Follow-up pairwise comparisons for significant effects used Holm correction to control the family-wise error rate. Effect sizes are reported as partial ($\eta_p^2$) for omnibus effects and Hedges' g for pairwise comparisons.

## 4 Results

**Investigating Temporal Aspects of Fibromyalgia Pain.** We investigated both temporal dependence and seasonality of pain scores across *Dense* and *Sparse* cohorts. In the *Dense* cohort, lag-1 autocorrelation was predominantly positive (mean $r$ = 0.30; 94.5% positive, 67% significant) and decayed with lag. AR(3) models were driven mainly by the first-order term, with $\beta_1$ positive in 91.3% and significant in 52% of users, and weaker higher-order effects; the model was significant in 56% of users (median adjusted $R^2 = 0.095$). The *Sparse* cohort showed a similar pattern, with lag-1 autocorrelation typically positive (mean $r = 0.30$; 89.9% positive, 68% significant) and gradual decay across lags. AR(3) models again showed a dominant first-order term ($\beta_1$ positive in 86.5%, significant in 47%), were significant in 52% of users, and achieved a median $R^2$ of

0.085. While short-term autoregressive dynamics (Lag-1) were pervasive across the population, fixed seasonal periodicities were observed in a smaller subset of the cohort. A significant weekly cycle (Lag-7) was detected in approximately 23% of users in both cohorts, likely reflecting weekend or work-week effects, and a monthly cycle (Lag-30) in 10%, possibly linked to hormonal or environmental rhythms. Our findings support modelling pain as an individualised time series with short-term memory and weak seasonal components.

**Predicting Fibromyalgia Pain.** We first investigated predicting the next pain severity from self-reported data ($H$=1). Table 1 summarises user-level prediction accuracy for next-day pain across models and cohorts. In the *Dense* cohort, Chronos-based models achieved the lowest prediction errors, with the covariate variant providing the strongest overall performance and clear improvements over the CNN baseline. In the *Dense* cohort, the covariate Chronos achieved the lowest median MAE (0.86), followed by univariate Chronos (0.88), CNN (0.90), ARIMAX (0.97), and ARIMA (0.99). The covariate Chronos significantly outperformed all other models, with small-to-moderate effects ($g$ = 0.07–0.34). Univariate Chronos also significantly outperformed the three remaining models ($g$ = 0.14–0.26). CNN and ARIMAX did not differ from each other but both outperformed ARIMA, albeit with small effects ($g$ = 0.06–0.11). A similar ordering was observed in the *Sparse* cohort, although absolute performance was generally weaker, reflecting the greater challenge posed by irregular reporting. ARIMAX performed comparably to ARIMA, indicating limited incremental benefit from contextual covariates in this setting. In contrast, the CNN showed competitive performance in the *Dense* cohort but underperformed in the *Sparse* cohort, suggesting reduced robustness to data sparsity. In the *Sparse* cohort, both Chronos models achieved similarly low MAE (0.91 for both), substantially outperforming CNN (1.08), ARIMAX (1.00), and ARIMA (1.01). Covariate Chronos again significantly outperformed all models ($g$ = 0.09–0.41), with the largest effect observed against CNN. Notably, CNN performed worse than all other models in this cohort, a reversal from the Dense cohort pattern that likely drove the significant interaction. ARIMA and ARIMAX did not differ significantly from each other. For MAE, there was a significant main effect of Model ($F(2.02, 2048.66) = 92.06$, $p < .001$, $\eta_p^2 = .083$; GG-corrected, $\varepsilon = 0.506$) and a small main effect of Cohort ($F(1, 1012) = 4.15$, $p = .042$, $\eta_p^2 = .004$). The significant Model × Cohort interaction ($F(2.02, 2048.66) = 15.70$, $p < .001$, $\eta_p^2 = .015$) warranted separate Holm-corrected post-hoc comparisons within each cohort. Due to right-skew, MASE analyses were conducted on log(1 + MASE). There was a significant main effect of Model ($F(1.21, 1226) = 28.19$, $p < .001$, $\eta_p^2 = .027$; GG-corrected, $\varepsilon = 0.303$), while neither Cohort ($p = .560$) nor the interaction ($p = .686$) reached significance. The absence of an interaction indicates that relative model performance on this scale-independent metric was consistent across reporting-density groups. Pooled post-hoc comparisons showed all pairwise differences were significant ($g$ = 0.06–0.26). Notably, ARIMA was the only model with a median MASE above 1.0, whereas covariate Chronos reduced error by approximately 16%.

**Table 1.** Next-day prediction performance ($H$=1). Values are median across users.

| Model | Features | Dense ($N$=681) | | Sparse ($N$=333) | |
|---|---|---|---|---|---|
| | | MAE | MASE | MAE | MASE |
| ARIMA | pain-only | 0.99 [0.74–1.32] | 1.00 [0.90–1.23] | 1.01 [0.77–1.31] | 1.01 [0.90–1.17] |
| Chronos | pain-only | 0.88 [0.65–1.20] | 0.91 [0.84–0.97] | 0.91 [0.71–1.26] | 0.91 [0.84–0.96] |
| ARIMAX | pain-only + contextual | 0.97 [0.71–1.28] | 0.96 [0.89–1.06] | 1.00 [0.77–1.37] | 0.94 [0.87–1.03] |
| Chronos-2 | pain-only + contextual | **0.86** [0.65–1.12] | **0.84** [0.78–0.93] | **0.91** [0.70–1.20] | **0.84** [0.77–0.91] |
| CNN | pain-only + contextual | 0.90 [0.67–1.25] | 0.96 [0.81–1.24] | 1.08 [0.76–1.40] | 0.98 [0.78–1.34] |

**Table 2.** Next-week prediction performance ($H$=7). Values are median across users.

| Model | Features | Dense ($N$=681) | | Sparse ($N$=333) | |
|---|---|---|---|---|---|
| | | MAE | MASE | MAE | MASE |
| ARIMA | pain-only | 1.00 [0.75–1.34] | 0.87 [0.80–1.02] | 1.03 [0.78–1.38] | 0.85 [0.79–0.97] |
| Chronos | pain-only | 0.95 [0.71–1.29] | 0.84 [0.78–0.90] | 0.98 [0.75–1.34] | 0.84 [0.80–0.90] |
| ARIMAX | pain-only + contextual | 1.05 [0.75–1.39] | 0.93 [0.84–1.01] | 1.05 [0.80–1.45] | 0.90 [0.83–0.97] |
| Chronos-2 | pain-only + contextual | **0.90** [0.68–1.21] | **0.79** [0.74–0.86] | **0.94** [0.72–1.30] | **0.79** [0.75–0.85] |
| CNN | pain-only + contextual | 0.93 [0.68–1.12] | 0.87 [0.75–1.10] | 1.01 [0.71–1.40] | 0.88 [0.76–1.33] |

We then investigated whether it is possible to predict pain scores for the following week ($H$=7). Table 2 reports performance for predicting the 7-day horizon. Across both cohorts, Chronos-based approaches again achieved the strongest accuracy, with covariate Chronos attaining the lowest errors. In the *Dense* cohort, covariate Chronos achieved the lowest median MAE (0.90), followed by CNN (0.93), Chronos (0.95), ARIMA (1.00), and ARIMAX (1.05). Most pairwise comparisons were significant; only CNN vs Chronos did not differ. In the *Sparse* cohort, covariate Chronos again achieved the lowest MAE (0.94), followed by univariate Chronos (0.98), CNN (1.01), ARIMA (1.03), and ARIMAX (1.05). However, the differences between ARIMA, ARIMAX and CNN were non-significant, reflecting CNN's diminished advantage in this cohort, consistent with the interaction pattern observed at $H$=1. For MAE, there was a significant main effect of Model ($F(1.98, 1991.08) = 64.26$, $p < .001$; GG-corrected, $\varepsilon$=0.49, $\eta_p^2$=0.06), while the Cohort main effect was not significant ($F(1, 1008) = 1.96$, $p = .161$). A small but significant interaction was observed ($F(1.98, 1991.08) = 6.29$, $p = .002$; GG-corrected, $\eta_p^2$=0.006), therefore Holm-corrected paired post-hoc tests were conducted within each cohort. Relative-to-baseline performance (MASE) indicated modest but consistent gains over ARIMA at $H$=7, whereas ARIMAX did not improve upon pain-only models, and CNN showed weaker robustness in the Sparse cohort. For MASE, the main effect of Model was significant ($F(1.23, 1237.99) = 22.55$, $p < .001$; GG-corrected, $\varepsilon$=0.307, $\eta_p^2$=0.022), while Cohort ($F(1, 1008) = 0.88$, $p = .349$) and Model×Cohort ($F(1.23, 1237.99) = 1.61$, $p = .206$; GG-corrected) were not significant. Chronos-2 achieved the lowest median MASE of 0.79, representing a 21% improvement over the naïve persistence baseline. Accordingly, pooled Holm-corrected post-hoc tests across all users showed that CNN exhibited significantly higher MASE than each of the other models, with small effect sizes (Hedges' $|g| \approx 0.13$–$0.15$). No other pairwise model differences remained significant after Holm correction.

## 5 Discussion and Conclusion

Using real-world, self-reported health data in FM, we found clear temporal and some seasonal patterns. We also showed that TSFMs in general outperformed statistical time-series models and CNN; their simplicity using zero-shot approaches makes them a suitable alternative for pain prediction. However, caution is advised with employing statistical time-series models; in most cases, ARIMA performed worse than even the baseline CNN, consistent with prior evidence that statistical models struggle under irregular and limited data [9]. A related finding concerns the ability of model families to exploit contextual information to minimise error. ARIMAX offered negligible improvement over pain-only ARIMA, suggesting that covariates added little information. In contrast, covariate Chronos achieved gains from the same feature set. This indicates that contextual signals in patient-generated data might carry predictive value, but are possibly too noisy and sparse for statistical models to exploit reliably. Foundation models, with temporal priors learned from large-scale pretraining, are possibly better positioned to extract these weak signals. Our findings revealed that irregular self-reporting leads to some degradation of model performance but is not a fundamental barrier to prediction. This shows that pain prediction could be applied to larger segments of users than perhaps previously anticipated.

These results suggest that mHealth applications could serve not only as digital diaries but as platforms supporting near real-time predictive analytics. The zero-shot capability of foundation models and their robustness to irregular reporting lower the barrier to deployment, as they require no per-user training and tolerate the variable logging adherence typical of real-world use. From a clinical standpoint, integrating pain prediction into digital therapeutics or clinical decision support systems could enable more proactive and personalised pain management. For example, predictions could trigger automated recommendations for self-management strategies tailored to anticipated symptom trajectories, or flag high-risk periods for clinician review. Such systems could complement traditional clinical encounters with continuous monitoring and early intervention, potentially reducing patients visiting their healthcare provider and improving patient outcomes. However, realising these benefits will require careful attention to clinical workflow integration, user interface design, and the ethical implications of algorithmic prediction in healthcare. These include risks of over-reliance on AI, patient anxiety induced by predicted symptom worsening, and the need for transparency around model uncertainty. Additionally, while model differences were statistically significant, the practical magnitude of these gains remains to be established.

**Limitations and Future Work.** This work has four main limitations. First, FM status, symptoms and pain scores were self-reported within the app, without clinical verification, which may introduce some inconsistencies in the data. Second, the cohorts were defined using minimum span, coverage, and maximum-gap criteria to enable reliable time-series evaluation. However, this meant that many users of the app with very short or highly intermittent logging were not included in our modelling. Third, while foundation models such as Chronos showed strong zero-shot performance, we did not explore fine-tuning or few-shot adaptation strategies that might further improve accuracy for specific user subgroups or clinical contexts. Last, the comparison set could also be broadened to include XGBoost, ROCKET, and LSTM-based models.

Three avenues for future research emerge from this work. First, investigating strategies beyond zero-shot foundation models represents a promising direction. Few-shot adaptation, where models are lightly fine-tuned on the first weeks of an individual's data before prediction, could improve accuracy. Meta-learning approaches that optimise for rapid adaptation to new users may be suitable for personalised prediction with minimal per-user data requirements. At the same time, it could be investigated how to extend our approaches to users with sparser data, possibly employing better data imputation methods. An initial next-day sensitivity analysis we conducted suggests that shorter-window variants improve CNN performance, whereas Chronos-2 generally benefits from the longer 180-day window. Second, it could be explored whether the foundation model–based prediction generalises across other conditions with differing temporal dynamics. Third, evaluations in clinical settings are needed to investigate how delivering pain predictions to patients or clinicians affects user acceptance, behavioural responses to predictions, and downstream effects on interactions with healthcare professionals and quality of life. Understanding how individuals interpret and act upon algorithmic predictions will be critical for ethical and responsible implementation. This also goes hand in hand with making these models and predictions more interpretable and therefore more trustworthy, employing approaches from Explainable AI (XAI) and ablation studies to determine how important features are to predictions beyond the dense–sparse cohort comparison already examined here.

This study showed that TSFMs consistently achieved the lowest errors across both next-day and next-week horizons and across both Dense and Sparse reporting cohorts, largely unencumbered by noisy, sparse inputs. These findings position pretrained TSFMs as practical solutions for real-world chronic pain data, offering personalised prediction without requiring idealised data collection behaviour.

**Acknowledgement.** This work was supported by the UKRI Centre for Doctoral Training in Socially Intelligent Artificial Agents, Grant Number EP/S02266X/1.

**Disclosure of Interests.** The authors have no competing interests to declare that are relevant to the content of this article.

## References

1. Ansari, A.F., et al.: Chronos-2: from univariate to universal forecasting (2025). https://doi.org/10.48550/arXiv.2510.15821
2. Chae, S., Street, W.N., Ramaraju, N., Gilbertson-White, S.: Prediction of cancer symptom trajectory using longitudinal electronic health record data and long short-term memory neural network. JCO Clin. Cancer Inf. **8**, e2300039 (2024). https://doi.org/10.1200/CCI.23.00039
3. Finkelstein, J., Smiley, A., Echeverria, C., Mooney, K.: AI-driven prediction of symptom trajectories in cancer care: a deep learning approach for chemotherapy management. Bioengineering **11**(11), 1172 (2024)
4. Alexander Jr., J., et al.: Using time series analysis approaches for improved prediction of pain outcomes in subgroups of patients with painful diabetic peripheral neuropathy. PLoS ONE **13**(12), e0207120 (2018). https://doi.org/10.1371/journal.pone.0207120
5. Kaushik, S., et al.: AI in healthcare: time-series forecasting using statistical, neural, and ensemble architectures. Front. Big Data **3**, 4 (2020). https://doi.org/10.3389/fdata.2020.00004
6. Khatiwada, P., Yang, B., Lin, J.C., Blobel, B.: Patient-generated health data (PGHD): understanding, requirements, challenges, and existing techniques for data security and privacy. J. Personal. Med. **14**(3), 282 (2024). https://doi.org/10.3390/jpm14030282
7. Liang, Y., et al.: Foundation models for time series analysis: a tutorial and survey. In: Proceedings of the 30th ACM SIGKDD Conference on Knowledge Discovery and Data Mining, pp. 6555–6565 (2024). https://doi.org/10.1145/3637528.3671451
8. Morid, M.A., Sheng, O.R.L., Dunbar, J.: Time series prediction using deep learning methods in healthcare. ACM Trans. Manage. Inf. Syst. **14**(1), 2:1–2:29 (2023). https://doi.org/10.1145/3531326
9. Puri, C., et al.: Daily pain prediction in workplace using Gaussian processes. In: 16th International Conference on Health Informatics, pp. 239–247 (Sep 2025)
10. Skoric, J., et al.: Predicting clinical outcomes at the toronto general hospital transitional pain service via the manage my pain app: machine learning approach. JMIR Med. Inform. **13**(1), e67178 (2025). https://doi.org/10.2196/67178
11. Timilsina, M., Buosi, S., Razzaq, M.A., Haque, R., Judge, C., Curry, E.: Harmonizing foundation models in healthcare: a comprehensive survey of their roles, relationships, and impact in artificial intelligence's advancing terrain. Comput. Biol. Med. **189**, 109925 (2025). https://doi.org/10.1016/j.compbiomed.2025.109925
12. Walitt, B., Fitzcharles, M.A., Hassett, A.L., Katz, R.S., Häuser, W., Wolfe, F.: The longitudinal outcome of fibromyalgia: a study of 1555 patients. J. Rheumatol. **38**(10), 2238–2246 (2011). https://doi.org/10.3899/jrheum.110026

# Agentic AI for Automated Value-Set Construction in a Guideline Driven Clinical Knowledge Graph

Elizabeth Nicholson(✉), Orlando Buendia, Matthew Rallison, Catriona Baker, Jeff Lai, Ravi Bajracharya, and Chris Wroe

BMJ Digital Health, BMJ Group, 5th floor, 90 Whitfield Street, London W1T 4EZ, UK
{enicholson,obuendia,mrallison,cbaker,jlai,rbajracharya,cwroe}@bmj.com

**Abstract.** Clinical decision-support systems increasingly rely on structured knowledge representations such as knowledge graphs, yet a major bottleneck persists upstream: constructing consistent, standards-linked clinical value sets. These value sets define the semantic boundaries of clinical concepts by mapping them to standardised terminology codes, but manual construction is labour-intensive, error-prone, and difficult to scale. We present an automated pipeline that combines dense semantic retrieval over embedded terminologies, adaptive statistical thresholding, structural expansion through SNOMED CT hierarchies, and LLM-based semantic review to construct clinical value sets from a knowledge graph derived from BMJ Best Practice. We evaluate this pipeline across 22 conditions spanning five clinical specialties (cardiology, dermatology, endocrinology, gastroenterology, and neurology), comprising 6,603 tagged terms requiring SNOMED CT value sets. Cross-specialty analysis demonstrated that the adaptive thresholding stage generalised without domain-specific tuning, while variation in final value set size was driven by entity type composition rather than clinical domain. Clinical validation using 66 scenario-based patient vignettes (1,122 expected concepts) confirmed within-specialty recall of 72.4–89.3%, with cross-specialty matching patterns that were clinically coherent. External validation against published reference standards from the US Value Set Authority Center confirmed a median precision of 91.7%. These results suggest that agentic AI can substantially reduce the manual burden of value set construction while maintaining clinical validity across diverse clinical domains.

**Keywords:** Clinical value sets · Agentic AI · Knowledge graphs · SNOMED CT · Clinical decision support

## 1 Introduction

Knowledge graphs provide a structured representation of relationships between entities in a domain, encoding semantic connections that can support reasoning,

© The Author(s), under exclusive license to Springer Nature Switzerland AG 2027
P. Andreev et al. (Eds.): AIME 2026, LNAI 16748, pp. 258–267, 2027.
https://doi.org/10.1007/978-3-032-30710-1_32

retrieval, and inference [1,2]. In healthcare, knowledge graphs populated with standardised clinical terminology codes can represent the relationships between disorders, diagnostic findings, procedures, and interventions in a computationally tractable form. A critical prerequisite for deploying such graphs is the construction of clinical value sets: curated collections of coded terms from standard terminologies such as SNOMED CT, LOINC, RxNorm, and ICD-10 that define the semantic boundaries of each clinical concept referenced by the graph and support integration with electronic healthcare record systems [3,4].

In current practice, value set construction remains predominantly manual, requiring authors to translate clinical concepts into precise lists of terminology codes where each individual code is explicitly included or excluded [5]. This process is difficult to scale, error-prone, and characterised by substantial inter-author variability. Analysis of user-reported errors in the US Value Set Authority Center (VSAC) found that 42% involved missing codes, 14% involved extraneous codes, and 72% were present at initial creation [5]. Independent studies have reached comparable conclusions: a median of 45% of codes appeared in only some but not all theoretically equivalent value sets for the same conditions [6], and manually curated extensional SNOMED CT value sets included a median of only 35% of concepts captured by intensional hierarchy-based definitions [7]. These limitations directly affect downstream clinical decision support, quality measurement, and research.

In this paper, we present an automated pipeline for clinical value set construction that combines dense semantic retrieval over embedded terminologies, adaptive statistical thresholding, structural expansion through SNOMED CT hierarchies, and LLM-based semantic review with explainable inclusion decisions. We evaluate this pipeline across 22 conditions spanning five clinical specialties (cardiology, dermatology, endocrinology, gastroenterology, and neurology), comprising 6,603 knowledge graph nodes requiring SNOMED CT value sets. We demonstrate that the pipeline generalises across clinical domains without specialty-specific tuning, and validate the generated value sets against independently constructed clinical scenarios.

## 2 Methods

### 2.1 Data Structure

Our pipeline operates over a clinical knowledge graph derived from BMJ decision support dataset (BMJ Dataset) that also underpins BMJ Best Practice, a point-of-care clinical decision support resource covering over 1000 medical conditions. Domain experts have annotated six clinical sections: treatment options, investigations, differentials, risk factors, diagnostic factors, and complications, tagging individual instances with structured roles (e.g., risk-factor, complication, treatment) and encoding their relationships using RDF ontologies. Each condition yields references to hundreds of granular concepts, each requiring mapping to standardised terminology codes to deploy the knowledge graph. It is this mapping task, constructing a value set for each concept, that our pipeline automates.

## 2.2 Pipeline Structure

Prior to value set construction, an LLM-based classification step filters out non-clinical terms (e.g., pure numeric values, administrative labels, treatment intensity modifiers), retaining only terms that represent standalone clinical concepts suitable for SNOMED CT value sets. The pipeline then proceeds in four stages:

**Dense Semantic Retrieval Over Embedded Terminologies.** We embed the complete active content of SNOMED CT into a dense vector space using OpenAI's "text-embedding-3-large" and encode each source term in the knowledge graph. We retrieve the $k = 40$ nearest neighbours using cosine similarity, deduplicating by concept identifier to handle SNOMED CT's multiple descriptions per concept. Post-hoc analysis confirmed that $k = 40$ functions as a generous ceiling: a median of 30 out of 40 candidates were excluded by the adaptive thresholding stage, and 95.3% of terms had 20 or more candidates excluded.

**Adaptive Statistical Thresholding.** Rather than applying a fixed similarity cutoff, we compute multiple threshold candidates using complementary statistical methods: gap-based detection, elbow-point detection, absolute domain thresholds (0.85 and 0.70), and score compression detection. These candidates and the full ranked list are passed to an LLM (GPT-5.2, temperature 0, seed 42) via a single-turn prompt. The LLM selects a final threshold by analysing distributional patterns to identify the natural boundary between relevant and tangential candidates.

**Structural Expansion Through Terminology Hierarchies.** Candidates passing the threshold are expanded through SNOMED CT's "is-a" hierarchy to include relevant child concepts that may not be close in embedding space but are clinically relevant through formal ontological relationships.

**LLM-based Semantic Review.** All candidates are passed through an LLM-based reasoning agent that receives: the full set of 40 nearest neighbours with similarity scores, the thresholded subset, the hierarchy-expanded candidates, and the source concept with its clinical context. The core decision criterion is whether each candidate can be semantically interchanged with the source concept in its clinical context. The review is performed via a single-turn LLM call with structured inclusion and exclusion criteria; the agent returns a JSON response containing a binary inclusion/exclusion decision, a confidence score (high, medium, or low), and a natural-language reasoning trace for each candidate. High-confidence decisions can be accepted automatically, while medium and low-confidence decisions are flagged for clinical editor review.

We characterise this pipeline as agentic in that the LLM components exercise autonomous, context-dependent reasoning, selecting thresholds based on distributional properties and making inclusion decisions with calibrated confidence, rather than applying fixed classification rules. The pipeline does not incorporate iterative feedback loops; this is a deliberate design choice discussed in Sect. 4

### 2.3 Evaluation

We evaluated the pipeline in five ways: (1) cross-specialty comparison of pipeline behaviour using Kruskal–Wallis tests across five specialties, (2) analysis of pipeline stage contributions by entity type, (3) ablation analysis comparing six pipeline configurations from fixed-threshold baselines to the full pipeline, and (4) clinical validation using 66 scenario-based patient vignettes whose expected SNOMED CT concepts were mapped to SNOMED CT using the same embedding model and FAISS index used in the pipeline itself, then matched against generated value sets. A cosine similarity of 0.70 was selected via sensitivity analysis across thresholds 0.50–0.90. Recall was assessed using two denominators: all vignette concepts (reflecting full coverage including terminology gaps) and SNOMED-resolvable concepts only (evaluating pipeline performance within its intended scope). The vignettes were generated independently using an LLM prompted with condition names only, without access to the pipeline output. (5) External precision validation comparing pipeline outputs against independently constructed SNOMED CT value sets from VSAC, retrieved programmatically via the FHIR API. Nine clinical concepts were selected for external precision evaluation by a clinical informaticist, chosen to represent a range of clinical domains (cardiovascular, respiratory, metabolic, renal, hepatic), value set size (34 to 1,396), and concept specificity (from focused clinical findings to broad disease categories).

## 3 Results

### 3.1 Description of Knowledge Graph Data to Be Mapped

We evaluated the pipeline across five clinical specialties, each comprising four to five conditions drawn from BMJ Best Practice (Table 1). For each condition, five guideline sections (excluding treatment algorithms) were included, yielding a total of 6,603 tagged terms requiring value sets across 22 conditions. Entity type composition varied across specialties, explaining differences in pipeline behaviour across domains.

### 3.2 Pipeline Behaviour Across Different Concepts Mapped to SNOMED CT

The relative contribution of each pipeline stage varies with concept specificity. Broad procedural concepts (e.g. "surgery") are dominated by hierarchy expansion. Mid-specificity concepts (e.g. "atrial fibrillation") rely on dual evidence from both semantic and hierarchical sources. Highly specific concepts (e.g. "advanced age") are resolved by thresholding alone, with LLM review serving as a filter. No single stage is sufficient across all concept types.

**Table 1.** Overview of the evaluation dataset.

| Specialty | Conditions | Topics | Nodes |
|---|---|---|---|
| Cardiology | Established AF, New-onset AF, Essential | 5 | 1,584 |
| | hypertension, Pericarditis, STEMI | | |
| Dermatology | Acne vulgaris, Atopic dermatitis, Contact | 4 | 1,125 |
| | dermatitis, Cutaneous larva migrans | | |
| Endocrinology | DKA, Diabetic kidney disease, Diabetic | 4 | 1,473 |
| | retinopathy, Type 1 diabetes | | |
| Gastroenterology | Gastroparesis, GERD, Hiatal hernia, | 5 | 1,070 |
| | Intra-abdominal abscess, Small bowel obstruction | | |
| Neurology | Alzheimer's disease, Cerebral aneurysm, | 5 | 1,351 |
| | Parkinson's disease, Restless leg syndrome | | |

### 3.3 Pipeline Behaviour Across Specialties and Entity Types

The number of candidates passing the adaptive similarity threshold was remarkably consistent, with a median of 1 (IQR 1–2) across all specialties and no significant difference between them (Kruskal–Wallis $H = 3.51$, $p = 0.48$). Although the LLM-set similarity thresholds themselves showed a statistically significant difference across specialties ($H = 17.48$, $p = 0.002$), the practical difference was minimal (median range 0.668–0.679). All subsequent pipeline stages differed significantly across specialties: hierarchy expansion ($H = 29.38$, $p < 0.001$), final value set size ($H = 21.27$, $p < 0.001$), and exclusion rates ($H = 46.66$, $p < 0.001$), though exclusion rate medians remained narrow (33–35).

Table 2 reveals that this downstream variation is driven by entity type rather than specialty. Within every specialty, entity types differed significantly in final value set size (Kruskal–Wallis $p < 0.001$ in all five cases, $H$ ranging from 45.9 to 190.0). Broad clinical concepts such as complication conditions (median final value set: 28, IQR 6–121) and risk factors (median 44, IQR 9–128) expanded substantially through hierarchy traversal, while constrained types such as characteristics (median 2, IQR 1–21) and investigation results (median 5, IQR 1–24) showed minimal expansion and high LLM exclusion rates. This entity-type effect was replicated independently within each specialty, confirming it is a property of the concepts themselves rather than an artefact of any single clinical domain.

### 3.4 Ablation Analysis

To quantify the marginal contribution of each pipeline stage, we evaluated six configurations against the same 66 scenario-based vignettes using embedding-based concept matching (cosine similarity $\geq 0.70$). Table 3 reports recall over SNOMED-resolvable concepts for each configuration.

Pure embedding retrieval with the strictest fixed threshold ($\geq 0.85$) achieved mean recall of 45.8%, rising to 52.4% at $\geq 0.80$ and 67.7% at $\geq 0.70$, demon-

**Table 2.** Pipeline stage behaviour across the seven most frequent entity types ($n \geq 250$). Values are median (IQR).

| Entity type ($n$) | Above threshold | Hierarchy & Top40 | Hierarchy expansion | Final value set | Excluded |
|---|---|---|---|---|---|
| Patient factor (2,153) | 1 (1–2) | 5 (0–12) | 4 (0–46) | 14 (2–64) | 32 (26–38) |
| Investigation result (821) | 1 (1–2) | 2 (0–7) | 0 (0–12) | 5 (1–24) | 36 (30–39) |
| Diagnostic action (518) | 1 (1–2) | 4 (1–10) | 1 (0–42) | 7 (3–51) | 34 (28–38) |
| Complication (413) | 1 (1–1) | 9 (3–14) | 17 (0–105) | 28 (6–121) | 29 (24–36) |
| Diagnostic factor (309) | 1 (1–1) | 9 (1–14) | 9 (0–46) | 22 (3–68) | 30 (22–37) |
| Characteristic (288) | 1 (1–2) | 0 (0–9) | 0 (0–9) | 2 (1–21) | 38 (29–39) |
| Risk factor (255) | 1 (1–2) | 9 (2–14) | 0 (1–116) | 44 (9–128) | 29 (25–35) |

strating that retrieval alone is insufficient regardless of threshold. Replacing the fixed threshold with the LLM-selected adaptive threshold improved recall by 3.3% points (67.7% to 71.0%), reflecting recovery of dual-evidence concepts that fall below fixed cutoffs but are confirmed by hierarchy membership. Hierarchy expansion provided the largest single contribution, adding 9.4% points (71.0% to 80.4%) while increasing the mean value set from 4,670 to 115,460 codes. The LLM semantic review stage reduced recall by 3.9% points (84.3% to 80.4%) while removing approximately 4,246 codes per specialty, a deliberate precision trade-off that excludes contradictory or off-target concepts. Overall, the full pipeline achieved 1.8 times the recall of the strictest fixed-threshold baseline.

**Table 3.** Ablation study: mean within-specialty recall (%) across five specialties. Recall is measured over SNOMED-resolvable vignette concepts.

| | Cardio | Derma | Endo | Gastro | Neuro | Mean | VS codes |
|---|---|---|---|---|---|---|---|
| Fixed threshold $\geq 0.85$ | 53.8 | 31.6 | 58.0 | 49.3 | 36.2 | 45.8 | 415 |
| Fixed threshold $\geq 0.80$ | 60.0 | 41.2 | 61.6 | 56.5 | 42.6 | 52.4 | 724 |
| Fixed threshold $\geq 0.70$ | 73.1 | 60.5 | 71.4 | 69.6 | 63.8 | 67.7 | 2,987 |
| No hierarchy | 73.1 | 66.7 | 76.8 | 73.2 | 65.2 | 71.0 | 4,670 |
| No LLM review | 81.2 | 80.7 | 84.8 | 87.7 | 87.2 | 84.3 | 119,706 |
| Full pipeline | 80.0 | 75.4 | 80.4 | 85.5 | 80.9 | 80.4 | 115,460 |

### 3.5 Clinical Validation Using Scenario-Based Vignettes

Each specialty's complete set of generated value sets was matched against expected concepts from all five specialties' scenarios (Table 4). Among

SNOMED-resolvable concepts, within-specialty recall ranged from 72.4% (dermatology) to 89.3% (gastroenterology). When including all vignette concepts regardless of SNOMED resolvability, recall ranged from 59.8% to 78.6%; the 90 unresolvable concepts (8.0% of total) were predominantly treatments, investigations and management goals outside the current pipeline scope. The cross-specialty matching pattern was clinically coherent: matching was highest between gastroenterology and cardiology (67.5%) and lowest between cardiology and dermatology (28.4%), confirming that the value sets are both sensitive to their target domain and appropriately specific.

**Table 4.** Cross-specialty validation: percentage of SNOMED-resolvable vignette concepts matched. Rows = scenario specialty; columns = value set specialty.

| Scenario ↓ / Value set → | Cardio | Derma | Endo | Gastro | Neuro |
|---|---|---|---|---|---|
| Cardio | **82.0** | 28.4 | 65.2 | 64.0 | 48.8 |
| Derma | 46.2 | **72.4** | 57.7 | 51.9 | 58.3 |
| Endo | 60.1 | 36.6 | **83.1** | 64.5 | 42.6 |
| Gastro | 67.5 | 32.5 | 63.6 | **89.3** | 66.0 |
| Neuro | 50.3 | 29.5 | 61.7 | 51.4 | **79.8** |

**Table 5.** Precision/Recall evaluation against VSAC reference standards.

| Concept | Pipeline | VSAC | Union | Precision | Recall |
|---|---|---|---|---|---|
| CKD | 1,396 | 22 | 1,070 | 72.1 | 94.0 |
| Dyspnea | 44 | 6 | 61 | 100.0 | 72.1 |
| Heart failure | 127 | 21 | 170 | 95.3 | 71.2 |
| Hypertension | 218 | 38 | 925 | 91.7 | 21.6 |
| Obesity | 64 | 13 | 119 | 100.0 | 53.8 |
| Sleep apnea | 34 | 8 | 47 | 61.8 | 44.7 |
| Thyroid dysfunction | 264 | 19 | 376 | 84.5 | 59.3 |
| Median | | | | **91.7** | **59.3** |

### 3.6 External Precision Validation

To assess precision, pipeline outputs were compared against independently constructed SNOMED CT value sets from VSAC. For each concept, all active VSAC value sets were retrieved via the FHIR API using the concept name and clinical synonyms, and the union of SNOMED CT codes across matching sets was used as the reference standard. Seven of nine concepts had matching VSAC sets; complete blood count (primarily LOINC-encoded) and hepatic toxicity (no matching sets) were excluded.

Median precision against the VSAC union was 91.7% (range 61.8–100.0%). Recall against the union was lower (median 59.3%), but this reflects the aggregation of VSAC sets built for heterogeneous purposes; per-individual-set analysis showed substantially higher recall against focused reference sets (e.g., 96.4% against "Diagnosis of Hypertension" vs. 12.3% against the broad "relatedconditions_hypertension" set containing 742 codes). For heart failure, the pipeline converged with five independently constructed VSAC sets from four stewards at 91–93% precision and recall, suggesting the automated pipeline reaches a similar clinical consensus to expert curation (Table 5).

# 4 Discussion

This study demonstrates that a multi-stage pipeline combining dense semantic retrieval, adaptive thresholding, SNOMED CT hierarchy expansion, and LLM-based semantic review can automate clinical value set construction across diverse clinical domains. Three principal findings emerged.

First, the pipeline generalises across clinical specialties without domain-specific tuning. The adaptive thresholding stage produced consistent outcomes across all five specialties, with no significant difference in the number of candidates passing the threshold. Although the LLM-selected similarity thresholds themselves differed statistically across specialties, the effect size was minimal (median range 0.668–0.679). Downstream variation in value set size is driven by entity type rather than specialty: broad clinical concepts such as risk factors and complication conditions produce large value sets through hierarchy expansion, while specific concepts such as characteristics and investigation results produce small, tightly filtered sets. This suggests that pipeline performance should be evaluated and optimised at the entity type level rather than the specialty level.

Second, each pipeline stage makes a distinct and necessary contribution. The ablation analysis confirms that embedding retrieval with a strict fixed threshold captures fewer than half of expected concepts, while hierarchy expansion accounts for the largest recall gain (+9.4% points). The LLM semantic review stage reduces recall by 3.9% points, but serves a deliberate precision role, filtering off-target inclusions. External validation against VSAC reference standards confirmed that this trade-off is well calibrated: the pipeline achieved median precision of 91.7% across 7 clinical concepts evaluated against independently curated value sets. For heart failure, the pipeline converged with 5 value sets from 4 independent stewards at 91–93% precision and recall, suggesting the automated approach reaches a similar clinical consensus to expert curation.

Third, clinical validation confirmed that the generated value sets capture the expected clinical content. Within-specialty recall ranged from 72.4–89.3% among SNOMED-resolvable concepts, with cross-specialty matching patterns that were clinically coherent. The unmatched concepts among SNOMED-resolvable vignettes were predominantly broad or ambiguous terms where the embedding-based matching could not identify a sufficiently close SNOMED equivalent, while the 90 concepts (8.0%) that could not be resolved to SNOMED

CT at all were predominantly treatments, investigations and management goals outside the current pipeline scope.

Our findings complement existing work on value set quality. Zahn et al. [5] identified missing codes (42%) and extraneous codes (14%) as the dominant error types in manually authored value sets. The within-specialty recall of 72.4–89.3% observed in our scenario validation suggests the pipeline addresses the missing code problem, while median precision of 91.7% against VSAC reference standards indicates that extraneous inclusion is also well controlled. Lukyanchikov and Kawamoto [6] reported that a median of 45% of codes appeared in only some but not all theoretically equivalent value sets for the same conditions. An automated pipeline eliminates this inter-author variability by producing deterministic output for any given input concept.

Several limitations should be acknowledged. Although the clinical scenarios were generated independently of the pipeline, both the vignette generation and the concept-to-SNOMED mapping rely on LLM and embedding-based methods, introducing a risk of circular validation. The external precision evaluation against VSAC reference standards partially mitigates this concern by providing a fully independent validation source; however, the 9 concepts evaluated were chosen purposefully to ensure meaningful comparison with VSAC, which has variable coverage across clinical domains, and future work should extend this analysis to a broader sample of pipeline outputs. The VSAC-based precision evaluation also provides a conservative estimate, as the reference sets were constructed for clinical quality measurement rather than knowledge graph retrieval; pipeline codes absent from VSAC may therefore represent appropriate expansions for the retrieval task rather than erroneous inclusions.

The reproducibility of the agentic decisions was not assessed in this study; although temperature 0 and a fixed seed were used throughout to maximise determinism, formal inter-run agreement was not measured. During development, reflection-based architectures were found to degrade performance, introducing inconsistency without correcting first-pass errors while increasing latency and cost. The single-pass design reflects this empirical finding.

Although the pipeline is designed to reduce manual effort, quantitative comparison of time and cost between automated and manual value set construction was not performed in this study and remains future work.

The current evaluation focuses on SNOMED CT; extending the analysis to LOINC and RxNorm is ongoing work. The pipeline is currently in an experimental phase within BMJ Digital Health.

## 5 Conclusion

We have presented an automated pipeline for clinical value set construction that combines semantic retrieval, adaptive thresholding, terminology hierarchy expansion, and LLM-based review. Evaluation across 22 conditions spanning five clinical specialties and 6,603 knowledge graph nodes demonstrates that the pipeline generalises across domains without specialty-specific tuning, with adaptive thresholding behaving consistently (Kruskal–Wallis $p = 0.48$) while producing appropriately varied value sets driven by the semantic properties of each concept. Scenario-based clinical validation confirmed within-specialty recall of 72.4–89.3%. External validation against published VSAC reference standards confirmed a median precision of 91.7%. These results suggest that agentic AI can substantially reduce the manual burden of value set construction while maintaining clinical validity, supporting scalable, standards-linked knowledge graph development.

**Acknowledgements.** The authors would like to thank the BMJ Digital Health team and the BMJ Best Practice clinical editors for their work in tagging and quality-assuring the clinical content that underpins this study. We also thank the BMJ data engineering team for integrating and debugging the tagged content within the knowledge-graph infrastructure.

**Disclosure of Interests.** All the authors on this paper are employees of BMJ Group, which is developing and intends to commercialise the Clinical Intelligence Knowledge Graph described in this work.

**Declaration of AI Assistance Technologies During Manuscript Preparation.** The authors used Claude Opus 4.6 for writing or drafting manuscript content and assisting with gathering references. After using this technology, the authors reviewed the results and take full responsibility for the contents of the manuscript.

## References

1. Wang, Z., Shi, D., Zhao, J., Diao, X., Tang, X., Qin, Y.: Automated construction of medical indicator knowledge graphs using retrieval augmented large language models. arXiv:2511.13526 (2025). https://doi.org/10.48550/arXiv.2511.13526
2. Cui, H., et al.: A review on knowledge graphs for healthcare: resources, applications, and promises. J. Biomed. Inform. **169**, 104861 (2025). https://doi.org/10.1016/j.jbi.2025.104861
3. Gold, S., et al.: Clinical concept value sets and interoperability in health data analytics. AMIA Annu. Symp. Proc. **2018**, 480–489 (2018)
4. Rossander, A., Karlsson, D.: Structure of health information with different information models: evaluation study with competency questions. JMIR Med. Inform. **11**, e46477 (2023). https://doi.org/10.2196/46477
5. Zahn, L., et al.: The fault in our sets: a mixed methods analysis of clinical value set errors. medRxiv (2025). https://doi.org/10.1101/2025.02.27.25323054
6. Lukyanchikov, N., Kawamoto, K.: Evaluation of discrepancies among national library of medicine (nlm) value set authority center (vsac) icd-10-cm value sets: case study for diagnoses of common chronic conditions, implications, and potential solutions. AMIA Annu. Symp. Proc. **2023**, 1087–1095 (2024)
7. Chu, L., et al.: SNOMED CT concept hierarchies for computable clinical phenotypes from electronic health record data: comparison of intensional versus extensional value sets. JMIR Med. Inform. (2019). https://doi.org/10.2196/11487

# A Scoring Strategy to Assess AI Prediction Reliability: Validation and Impact on Medical Decision Making

Lorenzo Peracchio[1(✉)], Laura Bergomi[1], Ana Isabel Hernáiz Ferrer[2], Chandra Bortolotto[2,3], Valentina Zuccaro[2,4], Francesco Salinaro[5], Lorenzo Preda[2,3], Riccardo Bellazzi[1], and Giovanna Nicora[1]

[1] Department of Electrical, Computer and Biomedical Engineering, University of Pavia, Pavia, Italy
lorenzo.peracchio01@universitadipavia.it

[2] Department of Clinical, Surgical, Diagnostic and Pediatric Sciences, University of Pavia, Pavia, Italy

[3] Radiology Department, Fondazione IRCCS Policlinico San Matteo, Pavia, Italy

[4] Infectious Diseases Unit, Fondazione IRCCS Policlinico di Pavia, Pavia, Italy

[5] Emergency Medicine Unit and Emergency Medicine Postgraduate Training Program, Department of Internal Medicine, IRCCS Policlinico San Matteo Foundation, University of Pavia, Pavia, Italy

**Abstract.** Trustworthy Artificial Intelligence (AI) is essential for safe deployment in healthcare, where erroneous predictions may have serious clinical consequences. In this work, we propose a predictive reliability approach based on two continuous and complementary scores: a similarity score, measuring how closely a new sample resembles the training distribution, and a local performance score, estimating the model's expected accuracy in the neighborhood of that sample. Together, these scores provide an interpretable assessment of prediction reliability. We evaluated their impact on medical decision-making through a two-stage survey with medical residents from a research hospital in Pavia, Italy. Participants first judged AI predictions based on patient data alone; then, after reliability disclosure, they confirmed or revised their decisions. By comparing responses before and after the disclosure of reliability information, we provide a preliminary analysis of how adding a reliability measure influences the perception and acceptance of AI predictions.

**Keywords:** Human-AI Interaction · Clinical Decision Support · Trust · Uncertainty · Questionnaire · User Study · Survey

## 1 Introduction

Trust is a fundamental prerequisite for the adoption of Artificial Intelligence (AI) and Machine Learning (ML) in clinical practice [1]. Beyond average predictive performance, trustworthy AI requires systems to behave reliably, transparently, and fairly. The formulation of the European AI Act stands as a prominent example of this perspective, as

© The Author(s), under exclusive license to Springer Nature Switzerland AG 2027
P. Andreev et al. (Eds.): AIME 2026, LNAI 16748, pp. 268–273, 2027.
https://doi.org/10.1007/978-3-032-30710-1_33

it explicitly defines the components of a trustworthy system. In clinical settings, reliability is especially important because standard validation metrics describe cohort-level performance but do not indicate whether a prediction can be trusted for an individual patient [2]. Pointwise prediction reliability addresses this need by estimating whether a single prediction produced at deployment is likely to be correct [3]. In prior works, we introduced methods for pointwise reliability assessment [4, 5] grounded in the two key principles proposed by [6]: the Density Principle (DP) evaluates whether a new case resembles the training data, whereas the Local Fit Principle (LFP) assesses whether the model is expected to perform well in the local region of the new case. Building on these principles, our previously developed package RelAI [5] implements the DP through an autoencoder (AE) reconstruction-error threshold strategy, and the LFP through a proxy classifier trained to predict local reliability labels. In its current form RelAI returns a binary decision; while operationally simple, this binary categorization can be too sharp for end-users as it hides differences between clear and borderline cases. In real-world clinical workflows, reliability is better represented as a continuous measure, which can be used to rank cases, support context-dependent thresholds, and align decision policies with local risk tolerance and available resources.

In this work, we propose an extension of RelAI that outputs a continuous reliability score, providing a more informative and usable indicator of the likelihood of a correct prediction on a given case in deployment. Moreover, we assess whether presenting our reliability score influences clinicians' judgments by conducting a survey in which they evaluate the correctness of ML predictions on real-world cases while being presented with the proposed continuous reliability score.

## 2 Materials and Methods

### 2.1 Use Case: An AI System to Predict Hospitalization

To test our approach on a real-world use case, we exploited our previously developed model within the Alfabeto project, an initiative aiming at developing automatic approaches for predicting COVID-19 patients' hospitalization needs, based on clinical information and chest X-ray characteristics. The ML model was trained on data from patients who entered the Emergency Department of the IRCCS San Matteo Hospital in Pavia (Italy) during the I wave of the pandemic (March–May 2020), while test data were collected during the III wave (March–May 2021). More details can be found in [7].

### 2.2 Reliability Score

**Density Principle.** We use the AE reconstruction error to derive a continuous similarity score: after training, we compute the per-sample reconstruction error on the training data to define the empirical reference distribution of errors (ECDF). Then, for any new sample $x$, we compute its reconstruction error $e(x)$ and evaluate its empirical cumulative probability $F(e(x))$ under the training-error ECDF. Finally, we convert it into a DP reliability score using the upper-tail probability.

$$r_{DP}(x) = 1 - F(e(x)) \tag{1}$$

The score describes the proportion of training samples whose reconstruction error is larger than that of $x$, where a high score indicates similarity to the training set, whereas a low one suggests an atypical or potentially out-of-distribution sample.

**Local Fit Principle.** We estimate the LFP as a probability of correctness. First, for each training sample $x$ we compute a correctness label $c = 1\{f(x) = y\}$, where $f$ denotes the original model and $c = 1$ if the prediction matches the ground truth. A proxy classifier $g$ is then trained to predict $c$ from the input features. At inference, we define the LFP reliability as the posterior probability of $g$ for the $c = 1$ class.

$$r_{LFP}(x) = \Pr_g(c = 1 \mid x) \tag{2}$$

The score describes the estimated likelihood that the base model's prediction will be correct for the new sample $x$. High values indicate regions of the feature space where the base model has historically achieved high local accuracy, whereas low ones indicate regions where it is more prone to errors.

### 2.3 Survey Development

The survey aims to evaluate the impact of the reliability score on medical decision-making, involving 70 residents from the IRCCS San Matteo Hospital in Pavia (Italy) specializing in Radiology or Infectious Diseases. The study was designed to collect participants' agreement to AI in two stages: before and after the disclosure of the reliability score. The survey comprised 20 instances, each describing a patient case selected from the III wave of the COVID-19, including 7 True Positive (TP), 7 True Negative (TN), 2 False Positives (FP) and 4 False Negatives (FN). A read-only version of the questionnaire is available at https://ee.kobotoolbox.org/preview/TsWTscqo.

## 3 Results

### 3.1 Reliability Score Validation

To validate the DP, we measured sample-to-training proximity as the average Euclidean distance between each test sample $x$ and its $k$-nearest training neighbors. Mean distance decreased as reliability increased, with the largest distance in the lowest-reliability bin and the smallest for $r_{DP}(x) \geq 0.8$ (Table 1). For the LFP, we trained a Random Forest proxy classifier to predict training correctness labels and used it to assign $r_{LFP}(x)$ scores to test samples. Bin-wise base-model accuracy increased with LFP reliability (Table 1), indicating that the score captures the classifier's local competence.

**Table 1.** DP and LFP scores validation results on the Alfabeto project test set.

| | [0.0–0.2) | [0.2–0.4) | [0.4–0.6) | [0.6–0.8) | [0.8–1.0] |
|---|---|---|---|---|---|
| Distance-to-train (DP) | 2.15 | 1.43 | 1.17 | 1.00 | 0.98 |
| Accuracy (LFP) | / | 0.50 | 0.52 | 0.75 | 0.95 |

### 3.2 Survey Results

Across respondents (26/70), clinicians' accuracy showed a strong monotonic association with reliability category even before score disclosure, supporting the score as an indicator of case-level reliability (Table 2). This ordering persisted after disclosure, but without an overall accuracy improvement.

Decisions were highly stable, with only 4.04% of switches (Table 3). Switching was most frequent in low-reliability cases (6.04%), followed by medium (3.29%) and high reliability (2.56%). Among revisions, shifts from agreement to disagreement were more common than the reverse, especially in low-reliability cases. This directionality suggests that, when clinicians did revise their judgments, the reliability score more often prompted a withdrawal of initial endorsement of the AI than an increased adoption of it, particularly in low-reliability cases. Stratification by prediction outcome showed that high reliability increased agreement for TP cases (+3.8%) and had minimal effect for TN cases (−0.8%). In the medium-reliability group, agreement was unchanged for wrong predictions (FP/FN = 0.0%) and slightly decreased for TP (−1.5%). In the low-reliability group, agreement decreased across all outcomes (TP: −7.7%, TN: −5.8%, FP: −3.8%, FN: −1.3%), indiscating a broad reduction in willingness to endorse AI recommendations rather than selective correction of wrong predictions.

**Table 2.** Clinicians' accuracy on the survey's instances stratified by reliability category.

| Reliability Category | Before Reliability | After Reliability |
|---|---|---|
| Low | 0.654 | 0.637 |
| Medium | 0.802 | 0.791 |
| High | 0.949 | 0.949 |

**Table 3.** Transition matrix of clinicians' agreement with AI after reliability-score disclosure, stratified by reliability category (1: agree, 0: disagree).

| Reliability Category | $0 \rightarrow 0$ | $1 \rightarrow 1$ | $0 \rightarrow 1$ | $1 \rightarrow 0$ | Switches |
|---|---|---|---|---|---|
| Overall | 125 | 374 | 6 | 15 | 21 (4.04%) |
| Low | 89 | 82 | 2 | 9 | 11 (6.04%) |
| Medium | 30 | 146 | 2 | 4 | 6 (3.29%) |
| High | 6 | 146 | 2 | 2 | 4 (2.56%) |

## 4 Discussion and Conclusions

The growing adoption of AI in healthcare requires rigorous assessment of trustworthiness to support safe clinical deployment. In this study, we proposed two continuous reliability scores capturing similarity to the training data and expected local accuracy, and evaluated their impact on decision-making through a two-stage survey with 26 residents from an Italian research hospital. In a real-world scenario, the scores captured both distributional similarity and case-level model accuracy (Table 1).

The survey further showed that the reliability indicator aligned with clinicians' performance: even before score disclosure, accuracy decreased monotonically from high- to low-reliability cases. However, revealing the score had limited behavioral impact, as respondents mostly maintained their initial decisions. When revisions occurred, low reliability prompted reconsideration, sometimes even when the initial decision was correct. This suggests a trade-off: reliability information can encourage scrutiny, but may also lead to a general shift away from AI recommendations rather than selectively correcting erroneous ones. These preliminary findings suggest that reliability may be more useful as a system-level signal for post-deployment monitoring, detection of high-risk subgroups and distribution shifts, and prioritization of cases for audit or model refinement, rather than as a real-time decision aid for end-users. However, this interpretation remains preliminary, as the survey included a limited number of residents, who may differ from senior clinicians in calibration and interaction with decision-support tools. Future work will test alternative score presentations and replicate the study in a larger cohort of senior clinicians to assess whether reliability disclosure can better support selective reliance and improve decision accuracy in realistic clinical workflows.

**Acknowledgments.** We thank all survey participants. This work was supported by PNRR Ricerca DM 118/2023 CUP F13C23000490007, PRIN PNRR 2022 InXAID - Interaction with eXplainable Artificial Intelligence in (medical) Decision-making CUP: H53D23008090001.

**Disclosure of Interests** The authors have no competing interests to declare that are relevant to the content of this article.

## References

1. Mohsin Khan, M., et al.: Towards secure and trusted AI in healthcare: a systematic review of emerging innovations and ethical challenges. Int. J. Med. Inform. **195**, 105780 (2025). https://doi.org/10.1016/j.ijmedinf.2024.105780
2. Banerji, C.R.S., et al.: Clinical AI tools must convey predictive uncertainty for each individual patient. Nat. Med. **29**(12), 2996–2998 (2023). https://doi.org/10.1038/s41591-023-02562-7
3. Kukar, M., Kononenko, I.: Reliable classifications with machine learning. In: Elomaa, T., Mannila, H., Toivonen, H. (eds.) Machine Learning: ECML 2002, pp. 219–231. Springer, Berlin, Heidelberg (2002). https://doi.org/10.1007/3-540-36755-1_19
4. Nicora, G., et al.: Evaluating pointwise reliability of machine learning prediction. J. Biomed. Inform. **127**, 103996 (2022). https://doi.org/10.1016/j.jbi.2022.103996
5. Peracchio, L., et al.: RelAI: an automated approach to judge pointwise ML prediction reliability. Int. J. Med. Inform. **197**, 105857 (2025). https://doi.org/10.1016/j.ijmedinf.2025.105857

6. Saria, S., Subbaswamy, A.: Tutorial: safe and reliable machine learning. arXiv: arXiv, 1904.07204 (2019). https://doi.org/10.48550/arXiv.1904.07204
7. Nicora, G., et al.: Bayesian networks in the management of hospital admissions: a comparison between explainable AI and black box AI during the pandemic. J. Imag. **10**(5), 117 (2024). https://doi.org/10.3390/jimaging10050117

# Vessel-Aware Bilateral Learning for Retina-Based Subclinical Atherosclerosis Screening

Ibrahim Sani(✉), Muhammad Saad, Nafisa Anjum, Ananna Saha, and Salekul Islam

North South University, Dhaka, Bangladesh
{ibrahim.sani,muhammad.saad01,nafisa.anjum12,ananna.saha, salekul.islam}@northsouth.edu

**Abstract.** Early identification of subclinical atherosclerosis is essential for preventing cardiovascular disease, yet conventional screening approaches such as carotid ultrasound are costly and unsuitable for large-scale population screening. Retinal fundus imaging provides a low-cost and non-invasive alternative, as retinal microvascular patterns reflect systemic vascular health. In this work, we propose a vessel-aware gated bilateral learning framework for joint CIMT regression and cardiovascular risk classification using paired left and right retinal fundus images. The proposed approach models inter-eye interactions through a confidence-aware fusion mechanism that adaptively weights bilateral features based on relative reliability, while emphasizing vascular-relevant representations. Experiments conducted on the publicly available Fundus-CIMT-2903 dataset show that the proposed image-only model achieves an AUROC of **0.921** and CIMT error of **0.1169 MAE**, outperforming strong baselines. A late-fusion ensemble with metadata further improves AUROC to **0.936**. These results demonstrate the effectiveness of vessel-aware bilateral retinal modeling for non-invasive cardiovascular risk screening.

**Keywords:** Retinal fundus imaging · Subclinical atherosclerosis · Carotid intima–media thickness · Bilateral learning · Multimodal medical AI

## 1 Introduction

Subclinical atherosclerosis is a precursor to cardiovascular disease, often progressing silently before clinical symptoms appear. Early identification of vascular abnormalities is crucial for effective prevention. Carotid intima–media thickness (CIMT), measured via ultrasound, is a well-established biomarker for subclinical atherosclerosis. However, ultrasound-based screening is resource-intensive and impractical for large-scale use.

Retinal fundus imaging offers a non-invasive, low-cost alternative for vascular assessment, as retinal vessels share similarities with cerebral and coronary

© The Author(s), under exclusive license to Springer Nature Switzerland AG 2027
P. Andreev et al. (Eds.): AIME 2026, LNAI 16748, pp. 274–284, 2027.
https://doi.org/10.1007/978-3-032-30710-1_34

vasculature. The Fundus-CIMT-2903 dataset, recently released by Guo et al. [2], links bilateral retinal imaging with CIMT measurements, providing a valuable resource for screening subclinical atherosclerosis at scale.

Most existing methods rely on single-eye analysis or simplistic bilateral fusion strategies that assume symmetry between the two eyes. However, retinal vascular changes often exhibit inter-eye asymmetry, localized pathology, and image-quality variability, limiting the effectiveness of naive fusion approaches. This highlights the need for principled bilateral modeling that adapts to inter-eye reliability.

In this work, we propose a **vessel-aware gated bilateral learning framework** for joint CIMT regression and cardiovascular risk classification using paired retinal fundus images. The proposed architecture explicitly models left-right retinal interactions through a **confidence-aware fusion mechanism** that adaptively weighs bilateral features based on their relative reliability. This allows the model to focus on the most informative retinal cues while suppressing unreliable or low-quality signals. We further investigate a multimodal extension incorporating demographic metadata via a lightweight ensemble strategy. Experiments on the Fundus-CIMT-2903 dataset show consistent improvements over single-eye, paired-eye, and multimodal baselines. We term our framework vessel-aware as the gating mechanism implicitly prioritizes retinal features correlating with vascular structures. The main contributions are:

- Introducing a **vessel-aware gated bilateral learning framework** that models inter-eye reliability for effective joint prediction of CIMT and cardiovascular risk.
- Performing a comprehensive evaluation on the publicly available Fundus-CIMT-2903 dataset, demonstrating consistent improvements over baselines, and examining the complementary role of demographic metadata via a lightweight ensemble strategy.

## 2 Related Work

**Retinal Imaging for Cardiovascular Risk Prediction.** Retinal fundus imaging has emerged as a promising non-invasive modality for systemic disease analysis, including cardiovascular risk assessment. Poplin *et al.* demonstrated that deep learning models can predict multiple cardiovascular risk factors directly from retinal fundus photographs, highlighting the potential of retinal data for surrogate disease markers [1]. The recently released Fundus-CIMT-2903 dataset provides paired left and right eye images with clinical CIMT measurements and demographic information, enabling systematic study of subclinical atherosclerosis screening using retinal inputs [2]. While this dataset has facilitated baseline investigations, most existing approaches either focus on single-eye analysis or adopt simplistic bilateral aggregation techniques, leaving room for more principled bilateral modeling.

**Bilateral Retinal Learning.** Learning frameworks that explicitly leverage bilateral retinal information are relatively underexplored. Earlier bilateral fusion techniques rely on straightforward concatenation or feature averaging, ignoring inter-eye variability. Yan *et al.* [3] introduced joint bilateral learning, but lacked adaptive reliability weighting. Kendall and Gal [4] highlighted uncertainty modeling in vision systems; our confidence-aware gating aligns with this reliability-aware learning by adaptively weighting bilateral features.

**Multimodal Fusion in Medical Imaging.** Multimodal fusion of retinal images with clinical data can improve prediction [5]; we adopt a lightweight decision-level ensemble to preserve interpretability.

**Architectures and Evaluation Strategies.** We adopt ConvNeXt [6] as our backbone due to its strong representational capacity. The clinical relevance of retinal vascular features is supported by large-scale analyses linking retinal vessel characteristics with cardiovascular outcomes [8]. For imbalanced screening settings, we report AUROC and AUPRC (the latter more informative under imbalance [7]). Recent work by Tohà-Dalmau et al. [9] further supports multimodal retinal imaging for cardiovascular risk prediction, complementing our approach.

## 3 Materials and Dataset

This study is conducted using the publicly available Fundus-CIMT-2903 dataset, introduced by Guo et al. [2] to support research on non-invasive screening of subclinical atherosclerosis. The dataset consists of retinal fundus images acquired from a Chinese population cohort, with each subject associated with carotid ultrasoundderived carotid intima–media thickness (CIMT) measurements and corresponding cardiovascular risk labels.

Each subject is associated with a pair of color fundus images corresponding to the left and right eyes, enabling bilateral retinal analysis. CIMT values are provided as a continuous measure of subclinical atherosclerosis, along with a binary cardiovascular risk label derived from established clinical criteria. In addition to imaging data, demographic metadata, including age and sex, are available and are used in this study to support multimodal modeling experiments.

To ensure a fair and clinically realistic evaluation, we adopt the official group-wise train, validation, and test split provided with the dataset, where subjects are strictly separated across splits. This protocol prevents subject-level information leakage and enables robust assessment of both regression and classification performance under real-world screening conditions (Table 1).

The official group-wise split yields 2,032 subjects for training (70%), 435 for validation (15%), and 436 for testing (15%), ensuring subject-level separation across splits.

**Table 1.** Overview of the Fundus-CIMT-2903 dataset used in this study.

| Attribute | Description |
|---|---|
| Total subjects | 2,903 |
| Population | Chinese cohort |
| Image modality | Color retinal fundus images |
| Images per subject | 2 (left and right eye) |
| Regression target | Carotid intima–media thickness (CIMT) |
| Classification target | Binary cardiovascular risk label |
| Available metadata | Age, sex |
| Evaluation protocol | Subject-level group-wise split |

**Table 2.** Distribution of subjects by CIMT-based cardiovascular risk group.

| Group | Overall | Normal | Thickened |
|---|---|---|---|
| Male | 1,862 (64.1%) | 568 (66.9%) | 1,294 (63.0%) |
| Female | 1,041 (35.9%) | 281 (33.1%) | 760 (37.0%) |
| Total | 2,903 (100%) | 849 (100%) | 2,054 (100%) |

# 4 Methods

## 4.1 Problem Formulation

Given a subject $i$, we are provided with a pair of color retinal fundus images $\{I_i^L, I_i^R\}$ corresponding to the left and right eyes. Each subject is associated with a continuous carotid intima–media thickness (CIMT) value $y_i \in \mathbb{R}$ and a binary cardiovascular risk label $c_i \in \{0, 1\}$, where 0 denotes normal (low-risk) and 1 denotes thickened (high-risk) CIMT.

The objective of this study is to learn a predictive model that jointly performs (i) CIMT regression and (ii) cardiovascular risk classification using paired retinal fundus images. Formally, the model learns a mapping

$$f: \{I_i^L, I_i^R\} \rightarrow (\hat{y}_i, \hat{p}_i),$$

where $\hat{y}_i$ denotes the predicted CIMT value and $\hat{p}_i \in [0, 1]$ denotes the predicted probability that the subject belongs to the thickened (high-risk) group.

## 4.2 Input Representation and Preprocessing

All retinal fundus images are resized to a fixed spatial resolution and normalized using channel-wise mean and standard deviation computed from the training set. To improve model generalization, standard data augmentation techniques are applied during training, including random horizontal flipping, small-angle rotation, and color jittering.

For bilateral modeling, left and right eye images are processed independently through a shared-weight backbone network. This design preserves eye-specific representations while ensuring parameter efficiency and enabling subsequent bilateral feature fusion.

## 4.3 Baseline Models

We compare against diverse baselines: ResNet50, EfficientNet-B0 (CNNs), Swin-Tiny (transformer), ConvNeXt-Tiny (modernized CNN), and XATTN-ConvNeXt (cross-attention). These four architectures cover three design paradigms while respecting dataset size (N=2,903).

Our evaluation encompasses:

- **Single-eye baselines:** Models using only a single retinal fundus image as input to establish a performance floor.
- **Paired-eye baselines:** Independent processing of left and right images combined via simple late-fusion strategies like concatenation or averaging.
- **Multimodal baselines:** Models integrating retinal features with demographic metadata (age and sex) through early or late fusion, utilizing both CNN and transformer-based backbones.

The overall workflow of the proposed VG-CAF framework is shown in Fig. 1.

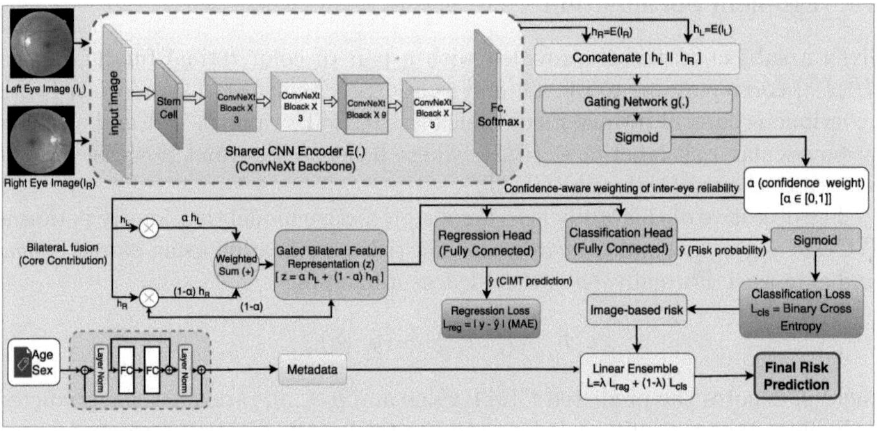


**Fig. 1.** Overall workflow of the proposed Vessel-Aware Gated Bilateral Framework (VG-CAF) for joint CIMT regression and cardiovascular risk classification. Paired retinal fundus images are processed through a shared encoder, followed by confidence-aware gated bilateral fusion. The fused representation is used for multi-task prediction, with an optional decision-level ensemble incorporating demographic metadata.

### 4.4 Proposed Vessel-Aware Gated Bilateral Framework

We propose a vessel-aware gated bilateral learning framework that explicitly models interactions between paired retinal fundus images. The core motivation is to leverage complementary vascular information from both eyes while accounting for inter-eye variability and asymmetric image quality.

Each retinal image is first processed independently using a shared convolutional backbone encoder to extract high-level retinal representations:

$$\mathbf{h}^L = E(I^L), \quad \mathbf{h}^R = E(I^R), \tag{1}$$

where $E(\cdot)$ denotes the shared-weight encoder, and $\mathbf{h}^L$ and $\mathbf{h}^R$ represent features extracted from the left and right eyes, respectively.

To adaptively model the relative reliability of bilateral features, we introduce a confidence-aware gating mechanism. A gating weight $\alpha \in [0, 1]$ is computed as:

$$\alpha = \sigma\big(g([\mathbf{h}^L \| \mathbf{h}^R])\big), \tag{2}$$

where $g(\cdot)$ denotes a lightweight gating network, $[\cdot\|\cdot]$ denotes feature concatenation, and $\sigma(\cdot)$ is the sigmoid activation function.

The bilateral retinal representation is then obtained through gated fusion:

$$\mathbf{z} = \alpha\mathbf{h}^L + (1 - \alpha)\mathbf{h}^R. \tag{3}$$

This fused representation $\mathbf{z}$ emphasizes more informative retinal cues while suppressing unreliable signals, enabling robust bilateral modeling for downstream prediction tasks.

### 4.5 Multimodal Extension with Demographic Metadata

To evaluate the complementary contribution of non-imaging clinical information, we further explore a multimodal extension of the proposed framework by incorporating demographic metadata, including age and sex. Metadata features are encoded using a lightweight fully connected network.

The encoded metadata representation is fused with the bilateral retinal feature representation at the decision level, enabling joint prediction without altering the core image-based learning pipeline. This design allows a direct comparison between image-only and multimodal models, while preserving the interpretability and robustness of retinal-based predictions.

### 4.6 Training Objectives and Implementation Details

The proposed framework is trained using a multi-task learning objective that jointly optimizes CIMT regression and cardiovascular risk classification. The overall training loss is defined as a weighted combination of task-specific losses:

$$\mathcal{L} = \lambda\mathcal{L}_{\text{reg}} + (1 - \lambda)\mathcal{L}_{\text{cls}}, \tag{4}$$

where $\lambda$ controls the relative importance of the two tasks.

For CIMT regression, we employ the mean absolute error (MAE) loss:

$$\mathcal{L}_{\text{reg}} = |y - \hat{y}| \,. \tag{5}$$

For cardiovascular risk classification, we use the binary cross-entropy loss:

$$\mathcal{L}_{\text{cls}} = -\left(c \log \hat{p} + (1-c)\log(1-\hat{p})\right). \tag{6}$$

All models are optimized using a stochastic gradient-based optimizer with early stopping based on validation performance. Hyperparameters are selected using the validation set, and final results are reported on the held-out test set.

Algorithm 1 summarizes the forward pass and training objective of the proposed vessel-aware gated bilateral framework.

**Algorithm 1:** Vessel-Aware Gated Bilateral Multi-Task Learning (VG-CAF)

**Input**: Paired fundus images $(I^L, I^R)$, CIMT target $y$, risk label $c$
**Output**: Predicted CIMT $\hat{y}$, risk probability $\hat{p}$, and loss $\mathcal{L}$

$h^L \leftarrow E(I^L)$ ; `// Shared backbone feature extraction`
$h^R \leftarrow E(I^R)$
$\alpha \leftarrow \sigma(g([h^L \| h^R]))$ ; `// Confidence-aware gating`
$z \leftarrow \alpha h^L + (1-\alpha)h^R$ ; `// Bilateral feature fusion`
$\hat{y} \leftarrow f_{\text{reg}}(z)$ ; `// Regression head`
$\hat{p} \leftarrow f_{\text{cls}}(z)$ ; `// Classification head`
$\mathcal{L}_{\text{reg}} \leftarrow |y - \hat{y}|$ ; `// Regression loss`
$\mathcal{L}_{\text{cls}} \leftarrow -\big(c \log \hat{p} + (1-c)\log(1-\hat{p})\big)$ ; `// Classification loss`
$\mathcal{L} \leftarrow \lambda \mathcal{L}_{\text{reg}} + (1-\lambda)\mathcal{L}_{\text{cls}}$ ; `// Multi-task objective`
**return** $(\hat{y}, \hat{p}), \mathcal{L}$

## 5 Experiments

### 5.1 Experimental Setup

All experiments are conducted on the publicly available Fundus-CIMT-2903 dataset. We follow the official subject-level group-wise split provided with the dataset, ensuring that no subject appears in more than one of the training, validation, or test sets. This protocol prevents information leakage and enables clinically realistic evaluation.

All baseline and proposed models are trained using identical data splits, preprocessing pipelines, and optimization settings to ensure fair comparison. Hyperparameter selection and model selection are performed using the validation set, and final performance is reported on the held-out test set.

### 5.2 Evaluation Metrics

For CIMT regression, model performance is evaluated using mean absolute error (MAE), which provides an interpretable measure of prediction deviation in millimeters and is commonly used in clinical regression tasks.

For cardiovascular risk classification, we report the area under the receiver operating characteristic curve (AUROC) and the area under the precision–recall curve (AUPRC). AUROC measures overall discriminative ability, while AUPRC is particularly informative under class imbalance and reflects performance on high-risk case identification.

### 5.3 Comparison with Baseline Models

Table 3 reports the performance of all baseline and proposed models on the Fundus-CIMT-2903 test set. Overall, our proposed vessel-aware gated bilateral framework (VG-CAF) consistently outperforms strong single-eye, paired-eye, and multimodal baselines across both CIMT regression and cardiovascular risk classification tasks.

To contextualize our findings and validate our claim of state-of-the-art performance, we compare our results with the benchmarks established by Guo et al. [2] on the same dataset. While the baseline ResNet-based architectures in the original study reported a classification AUROC in the range of 0.74–0.80, our proposed VG-CAF-ConvNeXt-Tiny model achieves a substantially higher AUROC of **0.9212**. This significant improvement demonstrates that explicitly modeling bilateral interactions through our confidence-aware gating provides a clear advantage over traditional single-eye or simple fusion approaches used in existing work.

To examine whether left and right retinal images produce consistent predictions, we evaluated single-eye models separately. Using the ResNet50 backbone, the left-eye model achieved a test AUROC of 0.74 (reported in Table 3), while the right-eye model achieved a test AUROC of 0.8170 under identical training conditions. The higher performance of the right-eye model suggests some inter-eye asymmetry in this dataset. This observation motivates the need for an adaptive fusion mechanism that can dynamically weigh bilateral features based on their relative reliability, which is precisely the role of our confidence-aware gating.

Figure 2 illustrates the classification performance of the proposed VG-CAF-ConvNeXt-Tiny model. The ROC curve demonstrates strong discriminative ability, with a steep ascent at low false positive rates indicating effective separation between risk groups. The corresponding confusion matrix confirms the model's robustness, correctly identifying 48 out of 50 high-risk subjects.

Among image-only methods, our model outperforms established CNNs like EfficientNet-B0 and transformer designs like Swin-Tiny. Notably, the cross -attention variant (XATTN-ConvNeXt-Tiny) yields inferior results (0.8520 AUROC) compared to VG-CAF, highlighting that adaptive reliability-based weighting is more effective for bilateral fusion than standard attention mechanisms.

**Table 3.** Performance comparison of baseline and proposed models on the Fundus-CIMT-2903 test set.Higher AUROC and AUPRC indicate better cardiovascular risk classification performance,while lower MAE indicates better CIMT regression accuracy.

| Category | Model | AUROC ↑ | AUPRC ↑ | MAE ↓ |
|---|---|---|---|---|
| Single-Eye | ResNet50 | 0.74 | 0.71 | 0.18 |
| Paired-Eye | ResNet50 (Late Fusion) | 0.80 | 0.78 | 0.16 |
| Multimodal | MM-Early EfficientNet-B0 | 0.90 | 0.89 | 0.12 |
| Multimodal | MM-Early Swin-Tiny | 0.9188 | 0.9221 | 0.1177 |
| Multimodal | CAF-ResNet50 | 0.8900 | 0.8797 | 0.1210 |
| Multimodal | XATTN-ConvNeXt-Tiny | 0.8520 | 0.8055 | 0.1270 |
| Proposed | **VG-CAF-ConvNeXt-Tiny (Ours)** | **0.9212** | **0.9159** | **0.1169** |
| Proposed | **VG-CAF + Metadata (Linear Ensemble)** | **0.9356** | **0.9315** | – |

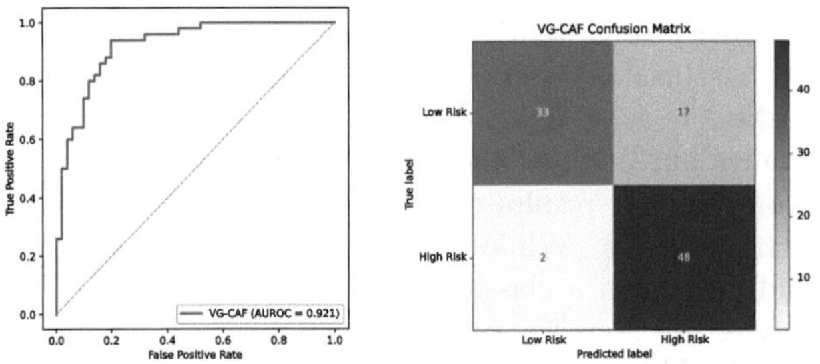


**Fig. 2.** Performance visualization of the proposed VG-CAF-ConvNeXt-Tiny model on the Fundus-CIMT-2903 test set. Left: Receiver operating characteristic (ROC) curve for cardiovascular risk classification (AUROC = 0.921). Right: Confusion matrix at the optimal operating threshold.

Incorporating demographic metadata via a linear ensemble further improves performance to an AUROC of **0.9356**. Even without metadata, our image-only model remains highly competitive, underscoring the strength of vessel-aware bilateral retinal modeling.

### 5.4 Ablation Study

To examine the effect on the proposed confidence-aware gating mechanism, we performed ablation analysis and compared our vessel-aware gated bilateral framework (VG-CAF) with one that removed the gating mechanism and directly fused bilateral features.

*Handling Class Imbalance.* As shown in Table 2, the dataset exhibits class imbalance (normal:thickened ≈ 1:2.4). To mitigate its impact, we employed two strategies. First, we used class-weighted binary cross-entropy loss, assigning higher weight to the minority (normal) class. Second, we report AUPRC alongside

AUROC, as AUPRC is more informative under imbalance. The confusion matrix in Fig. 2 shows 17 false positives out of 50 true negatives (34% FPR). While this reflects a conservative threshold, the operating point can be adjusted during deployment to prioritize either sensitivity or specificity based on clinical requirements. Without class weighting, our model's AUROC dropped to 0.89, confirming that addressing imbalance is beneficial.Beyond class-weighting, future work could explore data-level resampling techniques such as SMOTE to further address class imbalance

*Effect of Gating Mechanism.* As shown in Table 4, removing the confidence-aware gating mechanism leads to a substantial performance drop, confirming its importance for adaptive bilateral weighting.

**Table 4.** Ablation of gating mechanism.

| Configuration | AUROC ↑ | MAE ↓ |
|---|---|---|
| No Gating | 0.873 | 0.1421 |
| VG-CAF | 0.921 | 0.1169 |

## 6 Conclusion

In this paper, we proposed a vessel-aware gated bilateral learning framework for simultaneous CIMT regression and cardiovascular risk classification based on pairs of retinal fundus images. Inter-eye variability and variation of image quality is well addressed by our proposed explicit modeling of the relationship between the left and right eyes. The quantitative experimental results on the Fundus-CIMT-2903 dataset show that VG-CAF significantly outperforms all considered baselines and the established benchmark on this dataset [2], achieving an excellent AUROC of 0.921 for risk classification.

Furthermore, combining demographic metadata using a lightweight ensemble strategy further enhances the classification performance to an AUROC of 0.936. Our framework may lead to better non-invasive cardiovascular risk screening through retinal imaging, and can be directly applied in large health check-up systems as well as clinical practice. In the future, vessel segmentation will be integrated, and validation in other populations will be pursued in order to improve generalizability.

## References

1. Poplin, R., et al.: Prediction of cardiovascular risk factors from retinal fundus photographs via deep learning. Nature Biomed. Eng. **2**(3), 158–164 (2018). https://doi.org/10.1038/s41551-018-0195-0

2. Guo, X., et al.: Fundus-CIMT-2903: a retinal fundus image dataset with carotid intima-media thickness measurements for subclinical atherosclerosis screening. Sci. Data **12**, 2025 (2025). https://doi.org/10.1038/s41597-025-04930-z
3. Yan, Z., et al.: Joint bilateral learning for retinal image analysis. IEEE Trans. Med. Imaging **39**(6), 1852–1863 (2020). https://doi.org/10.1109/TMI.2020.2974250
4. Kendall, A., Gal, Y.: What uncertainties do we need in Bayesian deep learning for computer vision? Adv. Neural Inf. Process. Syst. (NeurIPS), 5574–5584 (2017). https://doi.org/10.5555/3295222.3295337
5. Huang, S.C., et al.: Fusion of medical imaging and electronic health records using deep learning: a systematic review. NPJ Digit. Med.**3**, 136 (2020). https://doi.org/10.1038/s41746-020-00310-9
6. Liu, Z., et al.: A ConvNet for the 2020s. In: Proceedings of the IEEE/CVF Conference on Computer Vision and Pattern Recognition (CVPR), pp. 11976–11986 (2022). https://doi.org/10.1109/CVPR52688.2022.01167
7. Saito, T., Rehmsmeier, M.: The precision-recall plot is more informative than the ROC plot when evaluating binary classifiers on imbalanced datasets. PLoS ONE **10**(3), e0118432 (2015). https://doi.org/10.1371/journal.pone.0118432
8. Cheung, C.Y., et al.: Retinal vascular caliber and risk of cardiovascular disease: a systematic review and meta-analysis. J. Am. Coll. Cardiol. **59**(20), 1780–1791 (2012). https://doi.org/10.1016/j.jacc.2012.03.007
9. Tohà-Dalmau, A., et al.: Machine learning prediction of cardiovascular risk in type 1 diabetes mellitus using radiomic features from multimodal retinal images. Ophthalmol. Sci. **5**(6), 100874 (2025). https://doi.org/10.1016/j.xops.2025.100874

# ECG-SurvHF: Adversarial Transformer Modeling for Heart Failure Risk Prediction

Tadiyos Hailemichael Mamo[1(✉)], Mohammed Hasanuzzaman[1], Hui Wang[1], and Pietro Lio[2]

[1] School of Electronics, Electrical Engineering and Computer Science, Queen's University Belfast, Belfast, Northern Ireland, UK
tmamo01@qub.ac.uk

[2] Department of Computer Science and Technology, University of Cambridge, Cambridge, England, UK

**Abstract.** Heart failure (HF) remains a leading cause of morbidity and mortality, with early-stage risk signals often embedded in subtle and spatially localized ECG deviations that are difficult to capture using conventional modeling approaches. We introduce ECG-SurvHF, a multimodal survival framework for HF risk prediction that integrates 12-lead electrocardiograms (ECGs) with demographic-aware clinical text representations under a unified time-to-event objective. The ECG component employs a transformer-based encoder trained with a focus-guided adversarial reconstruction strategy, where reconstruction residuals are used to dynamically emphasize weak but prognostically informative waveform regions while maintaining stable representation learning. Clinical notes are encoded using a demographic-aware contrastive learning scheme that extends BioClinicalBERT with age- and sex-conditioned supervision, producing context-sensitive textual embeddings without treating demographic attributes as direct predictors. ECG and text representations are aligned in a shared latent space and jointly optimized through a multitask objective combining survival analysis, adversarial reconstruction, and cross-modal alignment. We evaluate ECG-SurvHF on large-scale cohorts derived from MIMIC-IV, including high-risk populations with hypertension and myocardial infarction. Experimental results demonstrate improved discrimination of time-to-event HF risk compared with competitive baselines, highlighting the value of focus-guided adversarial transformer modeling and demographic-aware multimodal integration for clinically meaningful HF risk stratification using routinely collected data.

**Keywords:** Heart failure risk prediction · Electrocardiogram (ECG) analysis · Survival modeling · Multimodal learning

**Supplementary Information** The online version contains supplementary material available at https://doi.org/10.1007/978-3-032-30710-1_35.

© The Author(s), under exclusive license to Springer Nature Switzerland AG 2027
P. Andreev et al. (Eds.): AIME 2026, LNAI 16748, pp. 285–295, 2027.
https://doi.org/10.1007/978-3-032-30710-1_35

# 1 Introduction

Heart failure (HF) is a progressive syndrome characterized by impaired cardiac function and remains a major global health burden. Prevalence continues to rise, with projections estimating more than 11 million affected individuals in the United States by 2050 [3]. Despite therapeutic advances, one-year mortality approaches 20% [15], and many deaths occur suddenly without clear preceding deterioration [16]. These trends highlight the need for proactive, patient-specific risk assessment capable of identifying high-risk individuals before overt decompensation.

Routinely collected clinical data offer an opportunity for earlier HF risk stratification. The 12-lead electrocardiogram (ECG) provides low-cost, high-resolution temporal information about cardiac electrophysiology [7], while electronic health records (EHRs) contain complementary contextual information in clinical narratives. Subtle ECG deviations often acquire prognostic meaning only when interpreted alongside documented comorbidities and disease progression. Joint modeling of ECG signals and clinical text therefore enables more personalized and context-aware risk estimation.

However, effective multimodal risk prediction remains challenging. Traditional models rely on handcrafted features and linear assumptions, limiting their ability to capture complex interactions in high-dimensional physiological and textual data. Although deep learning approaches improve performance, many employ shallow fusion strategies that inadequately model temporal dependencies and cross-modal relationships [19]. Furthermore, demographic heterogeneity and the subtle nature of early-stage electrophysiological changes complicate robust and equitable risk modeling.

We propose ECG-SurvHF, a demographic-aware multimodal survival framework for HF risk prediction. The ECG component uses a transformer-based encoder trained with a focus-guided adversarial reconstruction objective to amplify weak but prognostically relevant waveform deviations while preserving stable representation learning. Clinical notes are encoded using a demographic-aware contrastive strategy that incorporates age and sex context without treating these attributes as direct predictors. ECG and text representations are aligned in a shared latent space and jointly optimized under a multi-task objective combining survival analysis, adversarial reconstruction, and cross-modal alignment.

We evaluate ECG-SurvHF on large-scale MIMIC-IV cohorts, including patients with hypertension and myocardial infarction. Results demonstrate improved discrimination of time-to-event HF risk compared with strong baselines and stable performance across demographic subgroups. Our main contributions are:

1. A dual-decoder transformer architecture for ECG modeling that employs adversarial reconstruction with a focus score-based conditioning mechanism, enhancing sensitivity to subtle ECG deviations relevant to HF risk.
2. A demographic-aware contrastive text encoding strategy that integrates patient context into clinical representations.

3. A unified multimodal survival framework aligning ECG and text representations in a shared latent space and jointly optimizes survival prediction, adversarial reconstruction, and cross-modal alignment for patient-specific risk prediction.
4. Comprehensive evaluation on large real-world cohorts demonstrating improved discrimination and clinical interpretability.

## 2 Related Work

Deep learning has increasingly been applied to survival modeling and ECG-based risk prediction. Classical approaches such as the Cox Proportional Hazards model [6] have been extended through neural variants including DeepSurv [11] and attention-based architectures. Recent hybrid models further improve ECG feature extraction for cardiovascular risk assessment [12]. ECG-SurvHF builds on these developments by introducing an adversarial reconstruction strategy to enhance sensitivity to subtle, early-stage waveform deviations relevant to time-to-event prediction.

Adversarial learning has also been widely used for anomaly detection in time-series data. GANs and their temporal extensions, such as GAN-TAD [14] and TranAD [21], demonstrate the effectiveness of reconstruction-based objectives for highlighting weak or rare patterns. In contrast to generic anomaly detection, ECG-SurvHF adapts adversarial learning specifically for prognostic representation learning within a survival modeling framework.

In clinical informatics, transformer-based language models such as ClinicalBERT [8] and Med-BERT [17] have substantially improved representation learning from electronic health records [10]. Meanwhile, contrastive learning strategies for multimodal alignment [5,9,22] have enabled more robust integration of heterogeneous clinical data. Our work extends these ideas by incorporating demographic-aware contrastive supervision to produce patient-contextualized text embeddings aligned with ECG representations. Additional discussion of related frameworks is provided in Appendix C of the Electronic Supplementary Material (ESM).

## 3 Methodology

We propose ECG-SurvHF, an end-to-end multimodal framework for HF risk prediction that jointly models 12-lead ECG waveforms and clinical notes under a survival objective. The framework consists of three components: (i) a demographic-aware clinical text encoder, (ii) a focus-guided adversarial ECG transformer, and (iii) cross-modal alignment with survival-based fusion. An overview is shown in Fig. 1. Extended implementation details and training procedures are provided in the Appendix D.

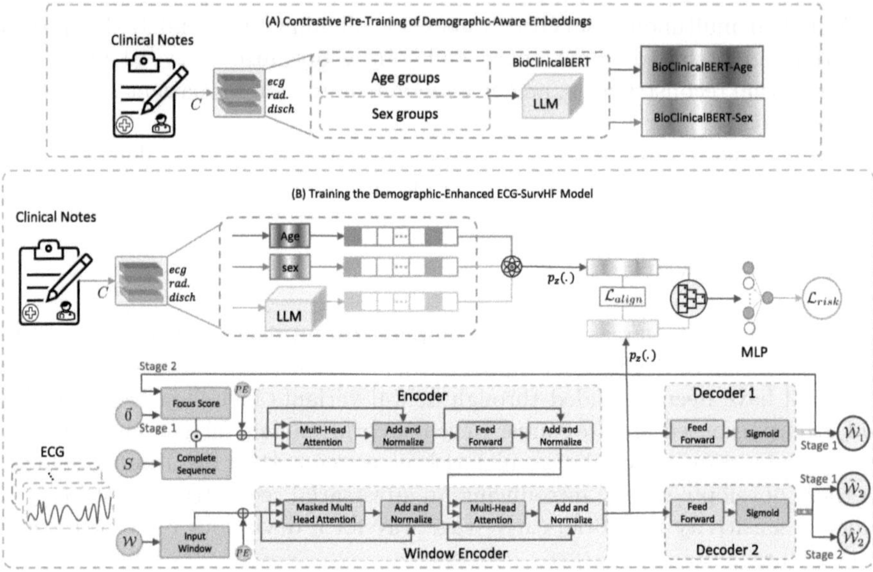


**Fig. 1.** ECG-SurvHF Framework: (A) Pre-training of demographic-aware embeddings for age/sex. (B) Adversarial ECG transformer and cross-modal alignment for HF risk prediction.

## 3.1 Problem Formulation

For each patient $p_i$, we observe ECG signals $\mathcal{S}_i \in \mathbb{R}^{12\times T}$, clinical notes $\mathcal{C}_i$, demographic attributes $d_i$ (age, sex), and survival outcomes $(t_i, \delta_i)$. From $\mathcal{S}_i$, fixed-length windows $\mathcal{W}_i \in \mathbb{R}^{12\times K}$ are sampled for modeling. These window-level representations are integrated through the sequence-level transformer to produce a single patient-level embedding used for survival prediction.

The goal is to learn a nonlinear mapping $f_\theta$ that produces a patient-specific risk score $r_i = f_\theta(z_i)$ from fused multimodal representations $z_i$. Following the Cox proportional hazards formulation [6], the hazard function is:

$$\lambda_i(t) = \lambda_0(t)\exp(r_i), \tag{1}$$

where $\lambda_0(t)$ is the baseline hazard and $r_i$ represents the log-relative risk. Unlike linear Cox models, $f_\theta$ is learned as a deep function over multimodal inputs, enabling nonlinear interactions between physiological and textual features.

## 3.2 Demographic-Aware Clinical Text Encoder

Clinical language varies systematically with patient age and sex, influencing both terminology and prognostic interpretation. Instead of concatenating demographic variables, we incorporate them through supervised contrastive pre-training.

Two specialist BioClinicalBERT encoders are trained using age- and sex-conditioned contrastive objectives, encouraging notes from similar demographic groups to form cohesive representations. A general BioClinicalBERT encoder is retained to preserve global semantics.

At inference, note embeddings from the general, age-aware, and sex-aware encoders are aggregated via learned weights to produce a unified demographic-aware representation $z_{\text{text}}$. (full procedure in Appendix D.1).

### 3.3 Adversarial ECG Transformer

Standard ECG encoders tend to prioritize dominant normal morphology, potentially overlooking weak deviations that precede HF. To improve sensitivity to subtle but prognostically relevant waveform changes, we introduce a focus-guided adversarial transformer (details in Appendix D.2 that couples a shared encoder with dual decoders in a staged training strategy.

*ECG Encoder.* A transformer encoder $E_{\text{ecg}}$ processes ECG windows $W \in \mathbb{R}^{K\times 12}$ (500 Hz sampling) and produces a latent representation $z_{\text{ecg}}$. The ECG signal for each patient is processed as both an input window and a complete sequence within the transformer architecture, yielding a unified patient-level representation for survival prediction. Multi-head self-attention models long-range temporal dependencies across leads, while positional encoding preserves temporal structure. The resulting embedding captures both global morphology and localized waveform dynamics relevant to HF risk.

*Two-Phase Training Strategy.* Training proceeds in two stages using decoders $D_1$ (stability branch) and $D_2$ (deviation branch), as detailed in Appendix D.2.

In Phase 1 (Stable Reconstruction), both decoders learn to reconstruct the input window using the shared latent representation $z_{\text{ecg}}$, minimizing reconstruction errors:

$$\min_{D_i} \|W - \hat{W}_i\|_2, \quad i \in \{1, 2\}, \tag{2}$$

where $\hat{W}_i = D_i(z_{\text{ecg}})$. This phase establishes a stable reconstruction of dominant ECG morphology.

In Phase 2 (Focus-Guided Refinement), a focus score is computed as the element-wise reconstruction error $F = (W - \hat{W}_1)^2$, which preserves temporal and lead-wise structure and highlights regions that are difficult to reconstruct. This deviation map is used to condition the encoder by reweighting its input representation, producing a refined latent representation $z'_{\text{ecg}}$. Decoder $D_2$ then generates a focus-guided reconstruction $\hat{W}'_2$. Instead of a strict min–max formulation, training encourages $D_2$ to emphasize deviations highlighted by $F$ while $D_1$ preserves stable reconstruction. The deviation-sensitive objective is:

$$\min_{D_1} \max_{D_2} \|W - \hat{W}'_2\|_2, \tag{3}$$

which is jointly optimized with the survival and alignment objectives (Sect. 3.5). An epoch-dependent weighting schedule gradually shifts emphasis from stable reconstruction toward deviation-sensitive refinement, improving training stability.

This staged adversarial refinement enhances sensitivity to localized waveform irregularities (e.g., subtle ST–T or QRS deviations) while retaining global morphological coherence. Focus maps derived from $F$ provide an interpretable visualization of waveform regions contributing to the learned representation.

*Inference-Time Sensitivity Control.* At inference, detection sensitivity can be adjusted without retraining by weighting stable and focus-guided reconstructions:

$$\mathcal{L}_{\text{inf}} = \alpha \|W - \hat{W}_1\|_2^2 + \beta \|W - \hat{W}_2'\|_2^2, \quad \alpha + \beta = 1. \tag{4}$$

Higher $\beta$ increases sensitivity to subtle deviations, enabling calibration according to clinical screening or monitoring contexts. Further details on clinical calibration of $\alpha$ and $\beta$ using patient-specific context are provided in Appendix D.4.

### 3.4 Cross-modal Alignment and Fusion

To integrate physiological and contextual information, ECG and clinical text representations are aligned in a shared embedding space prior to fusion. Clinical notes (e.g., ECG reports, discharge summaries, radiology reports) are encoded using the demographic-aware text module described in Sect. 3.2, yielding a patient-level embedding $z_{\text{text}}$. The ECG transformer produces $z_{\text{ecg}}$ from waveform inputs.

Both embeddings are projected into a common latent space: $e_{\text{ecg}} = p_{\text{ecg}}(z_{\text{ecg}})$, $e_{\text{text}} = p_{\text{text}}(z_{\text{text}})$, where $p_{\text{ecg}}$ and $p_{\text{text}}$ are learned projection layers. Alignment is encouraged through a cosine-based objective:

$$\mathcal{L}_{\text{align}} = \frac{1}{N} \sum_{i=1}^{N} \left( 1 - \frac{e_{\text{ecg}}^i \cdot e_{\text{text}}^i}{\|e_{\text{ecg}}^i\| \|e_{\text{text}}^i\|} \right), \tag{5}$$

which promotes semantic consistency between modalities for the same patient while preserving modality-specific structure.

The aligned embeddings are then fused hierarchically: $z_i = \text{Fusion}(e_{\text{ecg}}, e_{\text{text}})$, where fusion operates in three stages (Appendix D.3): (1) modality-specific refinement, (2) cross-modal interaction modeling, and (3) final patient-level integration. This structured fusion strategy allows ECG-derived physiological features and text-derived clinical context to interact while avoiding naive feature concatenation.

### 3.5 Survival Prediction and Training Objectives

The fused patient representation $z_i$ is passed through a lightweight multi-layer perceptron (MLP) to produce a scalar risk score:

$$r_i = f_\theta(z_i) = \text{MLP}(z_i). \tag{6}$$

The score $r_i$ represents the log-relative hazard of HF for patient $i$, where larger values indicate higher predicted risk.

Model training follows the Cox proportional hazards framework [6]. For uncensored patients ($\delta_i = 1$), the partial likelihood loss is:

$$\mathcal{L}_{\text{risk}} = -\frac{1}{N_{\delta=1}} \sum_{i:\delta_i=1} [r_i - \log( \sum_{j:t_j \geq t_i} \exp(r_j))], \tag{7}$$

which encourages correct ranking of patients according to time-to-event. By optimizing this objective, the model learns a nonlinear survival function without requiring explicit estimation of the baseline hazard.

The overall training objective combines complementary components, which comprises the adversarial reconstruction losses ($\mathcal{L}_{D_1}$ and $\mathcal{L}_{D_2}$) from the ECG branch, the cross-modal alignment loss ($\mathcal{L}_{\text{align}}$), and the survival loss ($\mathcal{L}_{\text{risk}}$). The overall training objective is written as a single weighted sum:

$$\mathcal{L}_{\text{total}} = \mathcal{L}_{\text{risk}} + \lambda_1 (\mathcal{L}_{D_1} + \mathcal{L}_{D_2}) + \lambda_2 \mathcal{L}_{\text{align}}, \tag{8}$$

where $\lambda_1, \lambda_2 \in [0,1]$ satisfy $\lambda_1 + \lambda_2 = 1$ and control the contribution of the adversarial decoder objectives and alignment (Appendix F.7), while the survival term $\mathcal{L}_{\text{risk}}$ anchors training. The epoch-dependent schedule is contained in $\mathcal{L}_{D_1}$ and $\mathcal{L}_{D_2}$ (Appendix D.2). This strategy encourages demographically contextualized, deviation-sensitive representations for time-to-event HF risk prediction. The complete training procedure is summarized in Algorithm 1.

## 4 Experimental Setup

We evaluated ECG-SurvHF on high-risk cohorts derived from the MIMIC-IV database [10]. For each patient, the prediction index time was defined by the index ECG used for risk estimation. All clinical notes are restricted to those recorded at or before the index ECG and prior to any HF diagnosis, ensuring no post-event information is included. Time-to-event was then measured from the baseline admission time to the first HF diagnosis, with patients without HF diagnosis treated as right-censored. Additional preprocessing and cohort construction details are provided in Appendix B.

The model was implemented in PyTorch. Training configuration, preprocessing pipelines, and hyperparameter settings are described in Appendix E.

*Evaluation Metric.* Performance was assessed using the concordance index (C-index), the standard metric for survival analysis:

$$\text{C-index} = \frac{\#\ \text{concordant pairs}}{\#\ \text{concordant pairs} + \#\ \text{discordant pairs}}. \tag{9}$$

A pair of patients $(i, j)$ is concordant if the patient with higher predicted risk experiences the event earlier. A value of 1.0 indicates perfect ranking, while 0.5 corresponds to random ordering. Five-fold stratified cross-validation was used; details are provided in Appendix E.

# 5 Results

**Table 1.** Comparison of risk prediction performance across architectures on MIMIC-IV cohorts: Mean C-index (SD) from 5-fold cross-validation.

| Architecture | MIMIC-HYP | MIMIC-MI | MIMIC-HYP-MI |
|---|---|---|---|
| CNN-VAE | 0.5289 (0.0057) | 0.5166 (0.0237) | 0.5125 (0.0026) |
| XResNet1D | 0.5825 (0.0070) | 0.5248 (0.0273) | 0.5474 (0.0074) |
| ECG Dual Attention | 0.5634 (0.0092) | 0.5416 (0.0438) | 0.5309 (0.0025) |
| ECG-SurvHF | **0.7420 (0.0040)** | **0.9640 (0.0081)** | **0.6251 (0.0118)** |

ECG-SurvHF was evaluated on three MIMIC-IV cohorts: hypertension (MIMIC-HYP), myocardial infarction (MIMIC-MI), and their overlap. Performance was measured using the C-index (SD) across five seeds for each of two-fold cross-validation.

## 5.1 Comparison with Baselines

We compared ECG-SurvHF against established ECG modeling approaches: (1) a CNN-based variational autoencoder (CNN-VAE), widely used for ECG representation learning [1,2,13,18]; (2) XResNet1D [20], a strong convolutional baseline for ECG classification and regression; and (3) a recently proposed ECG dual-attention model [4]. As shown in Table 1, ECG-SurvHF consistently achieved the highest discrimination across all cohorts, with particularly strong gains in the MI cohort (C-index 0.9640). Improvements were stable across folds, indicating robust risk ranking performance across heterogeneous patient groups.

## 5.2 Component Analysis

The ablation results (Table 2) show that performance is driven by complementary contributions from multimodal inputs, adversarial ECG modeling, and hierarchical fusion stages. Removing either modality leads to clear degradation, confirming that clinical text provides strong baseline discrimination while ECG contributes additional physiological signal.

**Table 2.** Ablation study of ECG-SurvHF components on MIMIC-IV cohorts.

| Configuration | MIMIC-HYP | MIMIC-MI | MIMIC-HYP-MI |
|---|---|---|---|
| ECG only | 0.6237 (0.0014) | 0.5696 (0.0189) | 0.5730 (0.0090) |
| Text only (general encoder) | 0.6241 (0.0045) | 0.5716 (0.0313) | 0.5742 (0.0067) |
| Text w/o age conditioning | 0.7161 (0.0035) | 0.8940 (0.0569) | 0.5827 (0.0088) |
| Text w/o sex conditioning | 0.7412 (0.0016) | 0.9274 (0.0319) | 0.6106 (0.0106) |
| w/o adversarial refinement | 0.7365 (0.0087) | 0.9060 (0.0407) | 0.6096 (0.0088) |
| Fusion w/o stage 1 | 0.4896 (0.0153) | 0.4571 (0.0962) | 0.5009 (0.0149) |
| Fusion w/o stage 2 | 0.7209 (0.0031) | 0.8852 (0.0620) | 0.5715 (0.0033) |
| Fusion w/o stage 3 | 0.5184 (0.0561) | 0.6847 (0.0613) | 0.4995 (0.0256) |
| Full model | **0.7420 (0.0040)** | **0.9640 (0.0081)** | **0.6251 (0.0118)** |

*Note:* Configurations evaluate removal or modification of key components including demographic conditioning, adversarial refinement, and hierarchical fusion stages.

Adversarial refinement yields consistent improvements across cohorts, indicating its role in enhancing sensitivity to subtle waveform deviations rather than acting as the primary predictive source (Appendix F.5). Fusion ablations further demonstrate that performance depends not only on modality inclusion but also on effective cross-modal interaction, with early-stage alignment being particularly important. Overall, the results indicate that performance gains arise from the combined effect of contextual information, structured ECG representation, and deviation-sensitive refinement.

## 6 Discussion

The results indicate that multimodal integration is the main contributor to performance, with clinical text providing strong contextual signal and ECG adding complementary physiological structure. Demographic-aware contrastive pre-training (Appendix D.1) helps account for variation in clinical language, with subgroup analyses (Appendix Fig. 9) suggesting broadly consistent risk distributions across demographic strata. While adversarial ECG modeling provides consistent improvements, the results indicate that the primary predictive signal is driven by multimodal integration, with clinical text contributing the strongest baseline and ECG offering complementary physiological refinement.

The ECG branch contributes structured waveform representations, while adversarial refinement improves sensitivity to localized deviations (Appendix F.5). Attention and focus visualizations (Fig. 3) provide qualitative transparency into the regions emphasized by the model.

The joint optimization remains stable across loss-weight settings (Appendix F.7), and the dual-decoder design allows adjustment of deviation sensitivity without retraining (Appendix D.4). External evaluation on PTB-XL (Appendix F.9) supports representational robustness across acquisition settings, although external prognostic validation remains to be established.

## 7 Conclusion and Future Work

We introduced ECG-SurvHF, a multimodal survival framework that integrates 12-lead ECG signals and demographic-aware clinical text for heart failure risk prediction. By combining adversarial transformer modeling, demographic-conditioned text embeddings, and joint survival optimization, the framework enhances sensitivity to subtle electrophysiological deviations while maintaining clinically coherent risk stratification. Future work will extend evaluation to multi-center cohorts, incorporate additional modalities such as imaging and laboratory data, and investigate prospective validation to assess real-world clinical utility.

**Disclosure of Interests.** The authors have no competing interests to declare that are relevant to the content of this article.

## References


1. Beetz, M., Banerjee, A., Grau, V.: Multi-domain variational autoencoders for combined modeling of MRI-based biventricular anatomy and ECG-based cardiac electrophysiology. Front. Physiol. **13**, 886723 (2022)
2. Beetz, M., Banerjee, A., Sang, Y., Grau, V.: Combined generation of electrocardiogram and cardiac anatomy models using multi-modal variational autoencoders. In: IEEE International Symposium on Biomedical Imaging (ISBI), pp. 1–4 (2022)
3. Bozkurt, B., et al.: HF stats 2024: heart failure epidemiology and outcomes statistics. J. Cardiac Fail. **31**(1), 66–116 (2025)
4. Chen, C., et al.: Large language model-informed ECG dual attention network for heart failure risk prediction. IEEE Trans. Big Data (2025)
5. Chen, T., Kornblith, S., Norouzi, M., Hinton, G.: A simple framework for contrastive learning of visual representations. In: International Conference on Machine Learning, pp. 1597–1607 (2020)
6. Cox, D.R.: Regression models and life-tables. J. Roy. Stat. Soc. B **34**(2), 187–220 (1972)
7. Crawford, M.H., et al.: Acc/aha guidelines for ambulatory electrocardiography: executive summary and recommendations. Circulation **100**(8), 886–893 (1999)
8. Huang, K., Altosaar, J., Ranganath, R.: Clinicalbert: modeling clinical notes and predicting hospital readmission. In: Proceedings of the ACM Conference on Health, Inference, and Learning (2020)
9. Huang, S.C., Shen, L., Lungren, M.P., Yeung, S.: Gloria: a multimodal global-local representation learning framework for label-efficient medical image recognition. In: Proceedings of the IEEE/CVF International Conference on Computer Vision, pp. 3942–3951 (2021)
10. Johnson, A.E.W., et al.: MIMIC-IV, a freely accessible electronic health record dataset. Sci. Data **10**(1), 1 (2023)
11. Katzman, J.L., et al.: Deepsurv: personalized treatment recommender system using a cox proportional hazards deep neural network. BMC Med. Res. Methodol. **18**(1), 24 (2018)
12. Kim, D., et al.: A novel hybrid CNN-transformer model for arrhythmia detection without r-peak identification using stockwell transform. Sci. Rep., **15** (2025) arrhythmia detection without r-peak identification using stockwell transform. Scientific Reports 15 (2025)

13. Li, L., Camps, J., Banerjee, A., et al.: Deep computational model for the inference of ventricular activation properties. In: Statistical Atlases and Computational Models of the Heart, pp. 369–380 (2022)
14. Mamo, T.H., Shao, J., Cobbinah, B.M.: Gan-tad: a graph-based adversarial network for time series anomaly detection. Inf. Sci. **733**, 122973 (2026)
15. Meta-analysis global group in chronic heart failure (MAGGIC): the survival of patients with heart failure with preserved or reduced left ventricular ejection fraction: an individual patient data meta-analysis. Eur. Heart J., **33**(14), 1750–1757 (2011)
16. Muhammad, A.N., et al.: Trends in cardiac arrest among heart failure patients aged 25 and older in the united states: Insights from the CDC wonder database. Am. J. Cardiol. **245**, 38–41 (2025)
17. Rasmy, L., Xiang, Y., Xie, Z., Tao, C., Zhi, D.: Med-BERT: pretrained contextualized embeddings on large-scale structured electronic health records for disease prediction. NPJ Digit. Med., **4**(1), 86 (2021)
18. Sang, Y., Beetz, M., Grau, V.: Generation of 12-lead electrocardiogram with subject-specific, image-derived characteristics using a conditional variational autoencoder. In: IEEE International Symposium on Biomedical Imaging (ISBI), pp. 1–5 (2022)
19. Stahlschmidt, S.R., Ulfenborg, B., Synnergren, J.: Multimodal deep learning for biomedical data fusion: a review. Briefings Bioinf., **23**(2) (2022)
20. Strodthoff, N., Wagner, P., Schaeffter, T., Samek, W.: Deep learning for ECG analysis: benchmarks and insights from PTB-xl. CoRR abs/2004.13701 (2020)
21. Tuli, S., Casale, G., Jennings, N.R.: Tranad: deep transformer networks for anomaly detection in multivariate time series data. Proc. VLDB Endowment **15**(6), 1201–1214 (2022)
22. Zang, C., Wang, F.: Scehr: supervised contrastive learning for clinical risk prediction using electronic health records. In: IEEE International Conference on Healthcare Informatics, pp. 1–11 (2022)

# Vision Transformer–Enhanced Voxel-Wise Regression for Neuromuscular Adaptation

Satyar Foroughi(✉), Sergi Garcia-Retortillo, Song Wang, and Rui Xie

University of Central Florida, Orlando, FL, USA
{satyar,sergi.garciaretortillo,song.wang,rui.xie}@ucf.edu

**Abstract.** Wearable biomedical sensing based on surface electromyography (sEMG) enables the modeling of inter-muscular coordination networks, offering critical insights into neuromuscular adaptation while posing challenges for traditional inference due to high dimensionality in small-sample physiological studies. We address this by representing cross-frequency sEMG signals as 3D tensors and proposing a **Vi**sion **T**ransformer–enhanced **V**oxel-wise **T**ensor **R**egression (ViT-VTR) framework. This approach estimates spatially varying coefficient maps for population-level effects (fatigue and aging), while utilizing a ViT to extract and map latent individual signatures to voxel-level deviations. Our model significantly outperforms traditional and neural baselines in reconstruction fidelity. Crucially, the learned coefficient maps offer interpretable physiological insights, capturing the systematic breakdown of muscular synergy during exhaustive exercise and aging.

**Keywords:** Image tensor response regression · Electromyography · Inter-muscular coordination · Vision Transformer · Coordinate MLP · Representation learning

## 1 Introduction

The neuromuscular system coordinates various muscle groups to perform fundamental movements and adapt to physiological stressors like fatigue and aging. Understanding these patterns is central to biomechanics, injury prevention, and rehabilitation [6]. Inter-muscular coordination functions as a complex, multi-scale network where muscle fibers synchronize across frequency bands [3]. Surface electromyography (sEMG) is a noninvasive wearable biomedical sensing technology that measures muscle electrical activity across frequency bands reflecting motor unit recruitment and neural drive. Cross-frequency EMG correlations capture this synchronization and represent the motor system's internal state. Modeling cross-frequency EMG data is challenging because intensive physiological studies often yield highly complex data from limited participant pools [5]. Traditional methods struggle with non-linear, spatially varying structure and individual heterogeneity [7].

In this paper, we propose **Vi**sion **T**ransformer–enhanced **V**oxel-wise **T**ensor **R**egression (ViT-VTR) for modeling EMG coordination maps using image-based

© The Author(s), under exclusive license to Springer Nature Switzerland AG 2027
P. Andreev et al. (Eds.): AIME 2026, LNAI 16748, pp. 296–300, 2027.
https://doi.org/10.1007/978-3-032-30710-1_36

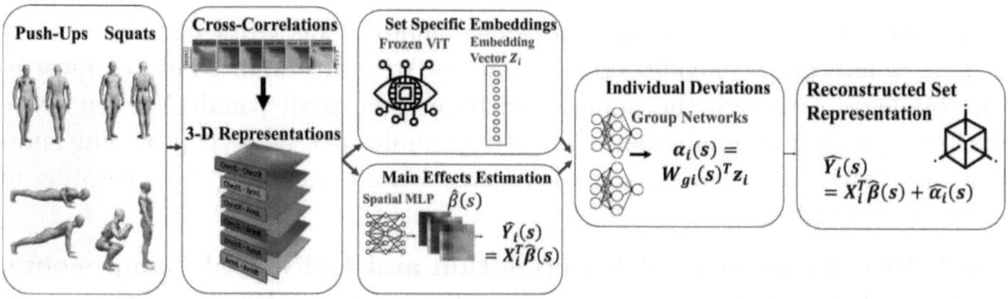


**Fig. 1.** Overview of the ViT-VTR framework for voxel-wise modeling of EMG coordination tensors. Global main effects are estimated via a coordinate-based MLP. A Vision Transformer encoder extracts observation-level latent representations, which are mapped to voxel-specific deviations through group-specific coordinate networks.

tensor response regression with deep neural networks. Specifically, we represent spatial coordination as 3D tensor structures, incorporate a Vision Transformer (ViT) to model subject heterogeneity, and employ voxel-wise regression to capture spatially varying coefficients. Treating individual voxels as effective samples mitigates the limitations of small sample sizes. A key innovation of our work is integrating a pre-trained Vision Transformer to extract individual signatures, which are then mapped to local voxel-level deviations via group-specific networks. This separates population main effects (fatigue/aging) from subject-specific adaptations. We validate this approach on data from two distinct studies: the evolution of inter-muscular networks during push-ups [4], and coordination dynamics comparing young and older adults during squatting exercises [2].

## 2 Methodology

**Inter-Muscular Reorganization Studies: Push-Up and Squat Protocols.** We use two protocols targeting neuromuscular adaptation under exhaustion. The first dataset captures upper-body fatigue [4]. Eight healthy subjects performed three sets of push-ups to volitional exhaustion (five-minute rest intervals). sEMG was recorded bilaterally from the pectoralis major and triceps brachii to observe inter-muscular network reorganization approaching failure. The second dataset examines biological aging during lower-body movement [2]. Two cohorts, 35 young (ages 20–30) and 9 older adults (ages 60–70), performed a single set of squats to exhaustion. Bilateral sEMG from the vastus lateralis and erector spinae provides insight into how leg-back synergy degrades or compensates with age.

**Construction of EMG Coordination Stacks.** Let $u_m(t)$ denote the sEMG signal for muscle $m$. For each observation, we band-limit $u_m(t)$ into $B$ frequency bands. For each muscle pair $(m_a, m_b)$, we compute a $B \times B$ cross-frequency coupling surface. Stacking these $B \times B$ association matrices over the $P$ unique muscle-pair combinations yields a 3D tensor stack $Y_i \in \mathbb{R}^{B \times B \times P}$ for observation $i$.

We interpret $Y_i$ as a volumetric image indexed by voxel coordinate $s = (x, y, z)$, where $(x, y)$ encodes cross-frequency structure and $z$ indexes muscle-pair topology. Although the number of subjects is small (small $N$), the dense voxel grid yields a large number of effective samples per subject, providing sufficient information for stable voxel-wise regression and enabling deep learning in small-cohort studies.

**Voxel-Wise Regression with Population and Individual Components.** Let $X_i \in \mathbb{R}^J$ be a design vector describing the covariates for observation $i$, and let $Y_i(s)$ denote the voxel intensity at coordinate $s$. Following image response regression [7], ViT-VTR decomposes each voxel into a population-level component and an observation-specific deviation:

$$Y_i(s) = X_i^\top \beta(s) + \alpha_i(s) + \epsilon_i(s), \tag{1}$$

where $\beta(s) = [\beta_1(s), \ldots, \beta_J(s)]^\top$ is a spatially varying coefficient field, $\alpha_i(s)$ is an observation-specific signature field, and $\epsilon_i(s)$ is random errors.

To model the main effects via a coordinate MLP, we approximate the coefficient field $\beta(s)$ with a neural function that takes the normalized coordinate $s$ as input, and outputs $\hat{\beta}(s) \in \mathbb{R}^J$, the estimated population-level main effect at voxel $s$. This provides a smooth, nonparametric estimate without explicit smoothing penalties.

To model individualized heterogeneity $\alpha_i(s)$, we introduce a latent signature $z_i$ extracted from the full coordination stack:

$$z_i = E(Y_i) \in \mathbb{R}^d, \tag{2}$$

where $E(\cdot)$ denotes a fixed or trainable encoder based on a Vision Transformer backbone. The latent code $z_i$ captures the global coordination structure of observation $i$. We project $z_i$ back to the voxel domain through a coordinate-based weight field. For observation $i$ in group $g_i$ (e.g., protocol or study), we define $\alpha_i(s) = W_{g_i}(s)^\top z_i$, where $W_g(\cdot)$ is a group-specific coordinate MLP that outputs a $d$-dimensional weight vector at spatial location $s$.

Each group-specific network $W_g(\cdot)$ is trained with an $\ell_1$ loss to predict the residual $Y_i(s) - X_i^\top \hat{\beta}(s)$ from the latent signature $z_i$. The reconstructed signal is given by $\hat{Y}_i(s) = X_i^\top \hat{\beta}(s) + \hat{\alpha}_i(s)$, which combines the population-level main effect and the individualized deviation.

A schematic overview of the full framework is provided in Fig. 1.

## 3 Results

**Data Representation and Training Details.** Across both protocols, each exercise set is represented as a 3D coordination stack with $B = 10$ frequency bands and $P = 6$ muscle-pair channels, yielding $Y_i \in \mathbb{R}^{10\times10\times6}$. The combined analysis includes $N = 68$ total observations.

For modeling systematic condition effects, we instantiate $X_i \in \mathbb{R}^J$ using $J = 5$ one-hot indicators corresponding to the five experimental conditions in our pooled dataset: three fatigue sets from the push-up protocol and two age cohorts from the squat protocol. This yields condition-specific maps $\hat{\beta}_j(s)$ as population coordination templates. For the latent encoder $E(\cdot)$, we use a frozen OpenCLIP Vision Transformer backbone [1]. We tile the six slices into a $2 \times 3$ mosaic, resize to $224 \times 224$, and replicate channels to match the ViT input. The resulting embedding dimension is $d = 512$, so $z_i \in \mathbb{R}^{512}$.

We use two group-specific maps $W_g(\cdot)$ for push-ups and squats. The spatial MLP for $\beta(\cdot)$ and the $W_g(\cdot)$ networks are trained with a mean absolute error objective over all voxels and observations, using 500 epochs and five random initializations; reported neural results are averaged over these initializations.

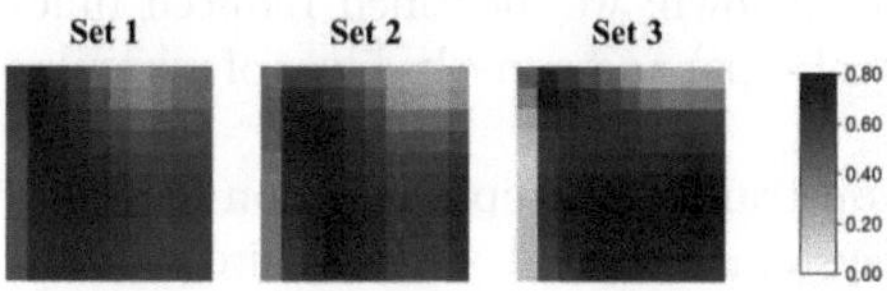


**Fig. 2.** Push-up main-effect maps for right pectoralis vs left triceps across fatigue progression. From left to right: $\beta_1$ (Set 1), $\beta_2$ (Set 2), $\beta_3$ (Set 3).

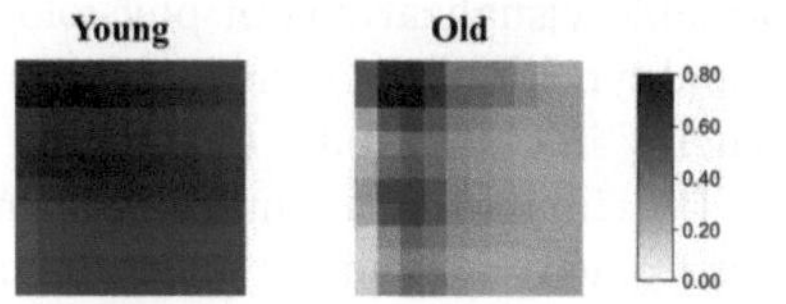


**Fig. 3.** Squat main-effect maps for right vastus lateralis vs left erector spinae by cohort. Left: $\beta_4$ (young); right: $\beta_5$ (older).

**Reconstruction Accuracy.** We compare the proposed method against IRRNN [7] and two mass-univariate baselines fit voxel-wise using the same $X_i$. We report our results in Table 1. Metrics reported are Pearson correlation ($r$), cosine similarity, structural similarity index measure (SSIM), Peak signal-to-noise ratio (PSNR), and Mean Absolute Error (MAE). Results for ViT-enhanced and IRRNN are averaged over five initializations.

**Table 1.** Quantitative comparison of reconstruction performance

| Method | Pearson ($r$) | Cosine Sim. | SSIM | PSNR (dB) | MAE |
|---|---|---|---|---|---|
| ViT-VTR | **0.9910** | **0.9987** | **0.9554** | **32.5581** | **0.0172** |
| IRRNN [7] | 0.9820 | 0.9970 | 0.9252 | 29.6339 | 0.0238 |
| OLS | 0.6714 | 0.9167 | 0.3288 | 14.8161 | 0.1576 |
| Ridge ($\lambda = 10$) | 0.6714 | 0.9167 | 0.2215 | 11.7259 | 0.2301 |

The learned main effects $\hat{\beta}(s)$ provide condition-specific coordination templates. Figure 2 shows an example muscle-pair map in the push-up protocol across the three fatigue sets. The intensity pattern diminishes across sets, consistent with reduced cross-frequency synchronization as subjects approach exhaustion. Figure 3 shows an example in the squat protocol. The older cohort exhibits markedly attenuated coordination intensity over the frequency grid, consistent with an age-associated reduction in inter-muscular coupling.

## 4 Conclusion

We introduced a novel framework integrating voxel-wise image response regression with Vision Transformers to analyze neuromuscular coordination. Treating cross-frequency coordination as 3D stacks overcomes the high-dimensionality and small sample sizes typical of physiological datasets. Using a frozen OpenCLIP ViT backbone, our approach effectively distills complex muscular interactions into stable, latent individual signatures.

Across upper-body fatigue and lower-body aging studies, our ViT-enhanced model significantly outperforms traditional and neural baselines. Beyond superior reconstruction accuracy, the learned population-level main effects offer interpretable visualizations of physiological breakdown: we identified reduced functional synchronization near exhaustion (push-ups) and a marked loss of muscular synergy in older adults (squats).

By eliminating manual smoothness constraints via representation learning, this framework robustly maps the motor system's internal state. Future research will explore these individual coordination signatures as clinical and athletic biomarkers for neuromuscular health and rehabilitation.

**Disclosure of Interests.** The authors have no competing interests to declare.

## References

1. Cherti, M., et al.: Reproducible scaling laws for contrastive language-image learning. In: 2023 IEEE/CVF Conference on Computer Vision and Pattern Recognition (CVPR), pp. 2818–2829. IEEE (2023). https://doi.org/10.1109/cvpr52729.2023.00276
2. Garcia-Retortillo, S., et al.: Age-related breakdown in networks of inter-muscular coordination. GeroScience **47**(2), 1615–1639 (2025). https://doi.org/10.1007/s11357-024-01331-9
3. Garcia-Retortillo, S., Ivanov, P.C.: Inter-muscular networks of synchronous muscle fiber activation. Front. Netw. Physiol. **2** (2022). https://doi.org/10.3389/fnetp.2022.1059793
4. Garcia-Retortillo, S., Romero-Gómez, C., Ivanov, P.C.: Network of muscle fibers activation facilitates inter-muscular coordination, adapts to fatigue and reflects muscle function. Commun. Biol. **6**(1), 891 (2023). https://doi.org/10.1038/s42003-023-05204-3
5. Konietschke, F., Schwab, K., Pauly, M.: Small sample sizes: a big data problem in high-dimensional data analysis. Stat. Methods Med. Res. **30**(3), 687–701 (2021). https://doi.org/10.1177/0962280220970228. pMID: 33228480
6. Ting, L.H., et al.: Neuromechanical principles underlying movement modularity and their implications for rehabilitation. Neuron **86**(1), 38–54 (2015)
7. Zhang, D., Li, L., Sripada, C., Kang, J.: Image response regression via deep neural networks. J. R. Stat. Soc. Ser. B Stat Methodol. **85**(5), 1589–1614 (2023)

# Late-Fusion of 2D Ultrasound and IVF Cycle Data for Predicting Clinical Pregnancy Outcomes

May Levin[1(✉)], Mo Vali[2(✉)], Saaliha Vali[3], Pietro Lio[1], Staci Meredith Weiss[1,4], and Meen-Yau Thum[5]

[1] Department of Computer Science and Technology, University of Cambridge, Cambridge CB3 0FD, UK
ml2229@cam.ac.uk

[2] Cavendish Laboratory, Department of Physics, University of Cambridge, Cambridge CB3 0US, UK
mmv487@cam.ac.uk

[3] Hillingdon Hospitals NHS Foundation Trust, Uxbridge, UK

[4] School of Psychology, University of Roehampton, London, UK

[5] The Lister Fertility Clinic, part of HCA Healthcare, London, UK

**Abstract.** In vitro fertilisation (IVF) treatment involves regular assessments of ultrasound scans and blood tests. However, this information is underutilised for estimating the likelihood of clinical pregnancy outcome. We propose a pipeline which combines 2D transvaginal ultrasound (TVUS) scans with cycle, hormonal and embryo-related variables to predict clinical pregnancy outcomes throughout IVF treatment. We analyse a retrospective cohort from a UK-based clinic comprising 505 patients and 1,455 TVUS images. We develop two unimodal classification models to predict clinical pregnancy: a tabular model using IVF cycle parameters (CatBoost), and a TVUS ensemble model using 2D ultrasound scans. We then develop multimodal late-fusion models which combine tabular and image predictions, including logistic-stacking base fusion and a rule-gated late-fusion policy. Additionally, we provide post-hoc interpretability to identify IVF cycle data and image regions important for clinical pregnancy prediction (SHAP). Under patient-grouped 5-fold cross-validation, pooled record-level AUROC was 0.771 for the tabular model and 0.680 for the TVUS ensemble. Late fusion improved discrimination, with base fusion achieving AUROC 0.809 and the final rule-gated fusion achieving AUROC 0.811. Integrating routine ultrasound scans with IVF cycle data therefore provides a route to utilising multimodal information collected in IVF clinics to support better informed decision-making during IVF treatment.

**Keywords:** IVF · Pregnancy Prediction · Fusion Models · Post-hoc Interpretability

M. Levin and M. Vali—Equal contribution.

© The Author(s), under exclusive license to Springer Nature Switzerland AG 2027
P. Andreev et al. (Eds.): AIME 2026, LNAI 16748, pp. 301–311, 2027.
https://doi.org/10.1007/978-3-032-30710-1_37

# 1 Introduction

Infertility affects approximately 17.5% of the adult population, and many couples pursue assisted reproduction methods such as in vitro fertilisation (IVF) in an effort to aid in conception [12]. IVF care is data-rich: patients undergo regular transvaginal ultrasound (TVUS) scan monitoring, blood tests, and detailed embryology assessments [13]. However, these data are often stored and interpreted in separate workflows. As a result, clinicians may lack a holistic estimate of the likelihood of a successful clinical pregnancy outcome which integrates all available information. This leaves patients and clinicians making high-stakes decisions under uncertainty across ovarian stimulation protocol, timing of follicular and embryo transfer, and embryo selection.

There is growing interest in predicting IVF outcomes to support patient counselling, inform protocol selection, and improve resource allocation. However, much of the existing work focuses on structured cycle variables alone or on single-modality pipelines, limiting use of the range in routine IVF data.

TVUS is a core component of IVF monitoring and provides a direct view of endometrial characteristics relevant to implantation. Unlike many laboratory variables, ultrasound captures morphological and spatial information that may reflect uterine and ovarian physiology in ways that are not fully captured in tabular records. This motivates evaluating whether routine TVUS can add predictive signal beyond structured IVF cycle variables. In turn, IVF cycle features such as age, embryo features, number of oocytes collected, in combination with ultrasound imaging, might capture additional signal relevant to stimulation protocol efficacy, implantation and pregnancy outcomes. However, integrating heterogeneous modalities in IVF is non-trivial: data arrive at different timepoints, imaging quality varies and is subject to ultrasound sonographer (operator) bias, and naive fusion can obscure how each modality contributes to prediction of IVF success. Interpretability is therefore important for clinical use into which features and regions of the uterus drive model predictions of a successful IVF outcome.

In this work, we evaluate whether combining routine 2D TVUS images with structured cycle, hormone, and embryology variables improves clinical pregnancy prediction in a real-world, retrospective IVF cohort. We benchmark tabular-only and image-only baselines, and introduce an interpretable late-fusion approach that in some cases reclassifies both of these baselines, and clarifies the contribution of each modality.

# 2 Related Work

## 2.1 Prediction of IVF Outcomes from Structured Tabular Data

IVF tabular data include predictors such as female age, ovarian reserve markers (e.g., AMH, AFC, basal FSH), infertility duration and aetiology, stimulation protocol details, and embryology variables. Large-scale retrospective analyses have shown that tree-based models can achieve strong performance while providing ranked feature importance to support clinical interpretation [10]. Bereczki et al. demonstrated that an XGBoost-based model using pre-procedural variables (e.g., age, AMH, BMI, gonadotropin dosing, and semen parameters) can support early treatment triage [1]. Other studies have deployed web-based risk calculators to encourage real-world adoption [4]. Despite these advances, tabular cycle and patient factors alone may not capture the full physiological state during treatment and can miss time-varying signals, motivating our approach: to incorporate additional routine data sources, specifically ultrasound imaging, collected frequently throughout the IVF cycle.

### 2.2 Imaging-Based Prediction in IVF

Deep learning has been widely explored in embryo assessment, especially with time-lapse data. CNN-based approaches have reported strong performance in predicting IVF live birth outcomes from embryo image sequences [3]. Ultrasound, by contrast, is ubiquitous across IVF clinics, but is typically applied to inform intermittent clinical decision-making, rather than for predicting treatment outcome. Emerging research has started to quantify ultrasound-derived predictors, combining ultrasound with radiomics for instance, outperforming clinical-only and radiomics-only models, or using functional signals from TVUS recordings [2]. However, compared with embryo time-lapse research, ultrasound-based outcome prediction remains fragmented across endpoints and patient types, motivating ultrasound-based modelling.

### 2.3 Multimodal Fusion for Clinical Prediction

Multimodal clinical AI is commonly grouped into several strategies including (i) early fusion, whereby inputs or features are concatenated before the model has been trained, (ii) joint/intermediate fusion, where modality-specific representations are learned, and then fused, and (iii) late fusion, which combines separate outputs from unimodal models [5]. Medical images can be affected by data bias, missing data, and limited sample size [11]. The effectiveness of early vs intermediate vs late fusion can depend on whether modalities are complementary and often requires careful modelling choices [9]. In IVF, these multimodal considerations are particularly relevant since structured variables (age, AMH, stimulation details, embryology) are often strong predictors, while 2D images may provide more subtle signals and can vary in acquisition and anatomical context. To our knowledge, there is limited published work evaluating fusion models for IVF cycle outcome prediction that integrate routine TVUS images with structured cycle variables.

### 2.4 Explainability in IVF Prediction

The opacity of AI models is a major barrier to their adoption particularly in clinical settings, where accountability and understanding results are essential for care [8]. One of the most widely used techniques to understand model outputs is SHAP (SHapley Additive exPlanations), which assigns each feature (age or oocytes for instance) an importance value representing its fair contribution to the difference between the model's prediction and a baseline [6]. In a broader medical context, SHAP has been used extensively, particularly for explaining EHR-based risk prediction models [7], however there is very limited work on using SHAP in an IVF context.

## 3 Methods

### 3.1 Cohort and Outcomes

A retrospective patient study is performed with 1,455 2D TVUS images and IVF data from 505 patients undergoing fresh and frozen embryo transfer (ET) cycles at a single UK-based IVF clinic after being filtered for extensive missing data. IVF data included clinical pregnancy outcome (confirmed via ultrasound), age, endometrial thickness, oocytes collected, embryo culture and grading, and several other patient-level variables. Clinical pregnancy outcome (ultrasound-confirmed) was available for all records (640 positive, 815 negative).

### 3.2 Data Preprocessing

Tabular data such as IVF cycle data (age, number of oocytes, embryo grading etc.) were encoded and normalised to values between 0 and 1. For text-based data such as embryo stage, a linear scale from 1 to 6 was used to encode entries ranging from 'cells' and 'morula' to 'early', 'expanded', 'full' and 'hatching blastocyst'. These values were then normalised to 0–1.

TVUS images were collected in DICOM format and contained sonographer-applied caliper annotations associated with endometrial thickness. After cropping, these images were then passed through an automated caliper removal stage, using a simple U-Net which was trained to remove caliper annotations. These scans were then resized to (256,256,3) and used as model inputs. All metadata was removed from DICOM files before processing.

To prevent data leakage, we used patient-level partitioning within a grouped 5-fold cross-validation framework, such that all records from a given patient were assigned exclusively to one fold partition at a time. Primary evaluation was performed at the record level. To assess whether repeated records from the same patient or treatment cycle affected performance, we also computed patient- and cycle-level metrics by averaging out-of-fold probabilities within each unit before calculating AUROC and accuracy.

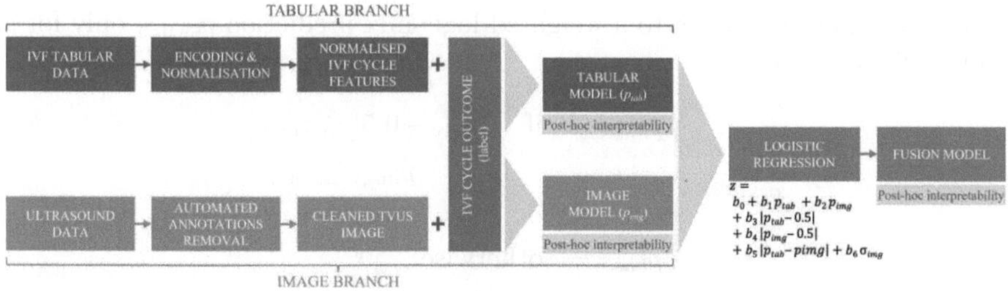


**Fig. 1. Overview of the multimodal IVF prediction pipeline**. TVUS scans are preprocessed with caliper removal, while IVF cycle data are encoded and normalised. Tabular and TVUS branches are fused, followed by post-hoc interpretability.

### 3.3 Model Architecture

**Tabular Model.** The final tabular branch used a CatBoost classifier trained under patient-grouped 5-fold cross-validation. Hyperparameters were selected via fold-wise search on the training folds only, and the best configuration was then refit per fold and evaluated on the held-out fold. As tabular baselines, we also benchmarked Random Forest and gradient-boosted tree models (e.g., XGBoost-style learners).

**Image Model.** The image branch is a 2D image classifier trained on preprocessed TVUS frames resized to 256×256. For fusion experiments, we use a small heterogeneous ensemble (ConvNeXt-Small, Swin-T, ResNet-50) chosen using training-fold OOF predictions only. For sample $i$, the fused image probability is the mean $p_{\text{img},i} = \frac{1}{M}\sum_{m=1}^{M} p_{\text{img},i}^{(m)}$ (with $M = 3$), and the standard deviation across members is used as a proxy for ensemble uncertainty (disagreement), $\sigma_{\text{img},i} = \text{std}(\{p_{\text{img},i}^{(m)}\}_{m=1}^{M})$.

**Late-Fusion Baselines.** We evaluated weighted logit mixing and logistic stacking as late-fusion strategies. The reported base-fusion model is the logistic-stacking output:

$$p_{\text{base}} = \sigma(b_0 + b_1 p_{\text{tab}} + b_2 p_{\text{img}} + b_3 |p_{\text{tab}} - p_{\text{img}}| + b_4 \sigma_{\text{img}}),$$

where $p_{\text{tab}}$ and $p_{\text{img}}$ denote tabular and TVUS ensemble probabilities, and $\sigma_{\text{img}}$ denotes image-ensemble uncertainty. Base fusion in the results table refers to $p_{\text{base}}$. Weighted logit mixing was also evaluated and used as the switch prediction in the rule-gated model:

$$p_{\text{mix}} = \sigma(\alpha \,\text{logit}(p_{\text{tab}}) + (1 - \alpha)\,\text{logit}(p_{\text{img}})), \qquad \alpha \in [0, 1].$$

**Rule-Gated Late Fusion (Final Model).** Our final multimodal model uses a rule-gated late-fusion policy. The default prediction is the base logistic-stacking output $p_{\text{base}}$, and we switch to a weighted logit-mix prediction $p_{\text{switch}}$ only for a small hard-case subset:

$$p_{\text{rule}} = \begin{cases} p_{\text{switch}}, & \text{if } \ |p_{\text{tab}} - 0.5| \le \tau_{\text{unc}}, \\ & \qquad |p_{\text{tab}} - p_{\text{img}}| \ge \tau_{\text{gap}}, \\ & \qquad \qquad \sigma_{\text{img}} \le \tau_{\sigma} \\ p_{\text{base}}, & \text{otherwise.} \end{cases}$$

$$p_{\text{switch}} = \sigma(\alpha_{\text{sw}} \, \text{logit}(p_{\text{tab}}) + (1 - \alpha_{\text{sw}}) \, \text{logit}(p_{\text{img}}))\,.$$

Gate parameters were selected on training-fold predictions and locked before held-out evaluation: $\alpha_{\text{sw}} = 0.4$, $\tau_{\text{unc}} = 0.15$, $\tau_{\text{gap}} = 0.25$, and $\tau_{\sigma} = 0.12$.

### 3.4 Calibration and Interpretability

Calibration was performed within each fold by fitting a probability calibrator (none/Platt scaling/isotonic regression) on training-fold predictions only and applied to the held-out fold, ensuring no cross-fold leakage (Fig. 2).

**Table 1.** Performance under patient-grouped 5-fold cross-validation. Patient- and cycle-level metrics aggregate out-of-fold probabilities within each unit.

| Model | Rec. AUC | Rec. ACC | Pat. AUC | Pat. ACC | Cyc. AUC | Cyc. ACC |
|---|---|---|---|---|---|---|
| Tabular-only | 0.771 | 0.685 | 0.768 | 0.673 | 0.765 | 0.663 |
| TVUS-only | 0.680 | 0.598 | 0.718 | 0.610 | 0.699 | 0.589 |
| Base fusion | 0.809 | 0.713 | **0.810** | **0.723** | 0.809 | **0.718** |
| Rule-gated fusion | **0.811** | **0.715** | **0.810** | **0.723** | **0.809** | 0.716 |

For the tabular branch, SHAP attribution was used to identify influential structured predictors. For the image branch, SHAP-based attribution maps were used to inspect salient regions in TVUS scans driving predictions. For the fusion policy, we report switched coverage and analyze the conditions under which switching occurs (confidence, disagreement, and uncertainty).

## 4 Results

All results are reported under patient-grouped 5-fold cross-validation, ensuring that all records from a given patient were exclusive to a single held-out fold; performance is reported at record, patient, and cycle level.

### 4.1 Overall Performance

Table 1 summarises discrimination (AUROC) and accuracy (ACC) for the final tabular, image, and multimodal models under patient-grouped 5-fold cross-validation. Fusion improves discrimination over both unimodal models, with rule-gated fusion achieving the highest AUROC. Rule-gated switching occurred in 66 records (4.5%), and base fusion accounted for most of the multimodal gain. We interpret the gate as a targeted hard-case refinement rather than a large independent source of improvement. Patient- and cycle-level aggregation preserved the multimodal gain.

Additional pooled record-level baselines were lower than the final fusion models, including Random Forest (AUROC 0.740), XGBoost/LightGBM (0.719), ResNet-50 (0.651), Swin-T (0.669), and ConvNeXt-Small (0.663). Figure 2 shows ROC, calibration, and incremental fusion performance. The TVUS branch shows weaker discrimination than the tabular and fusion branches, while both fusion models achieve the highest AUROC with broadly similar calibration.

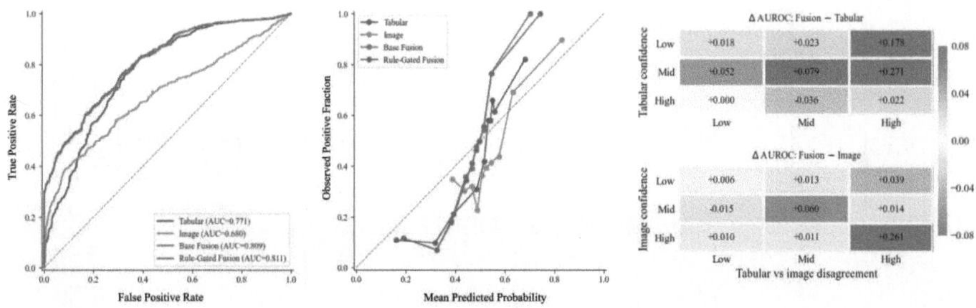


**Fig. 2. ROC, calibration and incremental fusion model performance under patient-grouped 5-fold cross-validation.** (Left) Comparison of tabular model (CatBoost), TVUS ensemble, base fusion, and rule-gated fusion. (Middle) Calibration curves showing reliability curves for the same models, with $y = x$ indicating perfect calibration. (Right) Incremental AUROC for fusion over tabular (upper) and TVUS ensemble (lower) models. Fusion improves discrimination relative to either unimodal branch with broadly similar calibration, and outperforms both tabular and image models when they disagree most.

Figure 2 (right panel) shows that fusion gains were largest when tabular and TVUS predictions disagreed, supporting late fusion for cases where single-modality predictions were uncertain or conflicting.

As shown in Table 2, base fusion significantly improved AUROC over the tabular branch ($\Delta$AUROC = 0.037), while the additional gain from rule-gated fusion over base fusion was small and statistically uncertain ($\Delta$AUROC = 0.003).

We next evaluate how often fusion reclassifies unimodal predictions. Upward corrections (Not pregnant → Pregnant) were more reliable than downward corrections (Pregnant → Not pregnant). For rule-gated fusion, upward corrections

**Table 2.** Paired bootstrap AUROC differences. Confidence intervals were estimated with 10,000 resamples.

| Comparison | $\Delta$AUROC | 95% CI | $p$ |
|---|---|---|---|
| Base fusion vs. Tabular-only | 0.037 | 0.014–0.062 | 0.001 |
| Rule-gated fusion vs. Base fusion | 0.003 | −0.002–0.010 | 0.469 |
| Rule-gated fusion vs. Tabular-only | 0.040 | 0.015–0.067 | $< 0.001$ |

were correct in 73.9% of tabular comparisons and 86.1% of TVUS comparisons, while downward corrections were correct in 53.7% and 66.7%, respectively. This suggests that fusion is more useful for identifying additional high-likelihood cases than as a reliable rule-out signal.

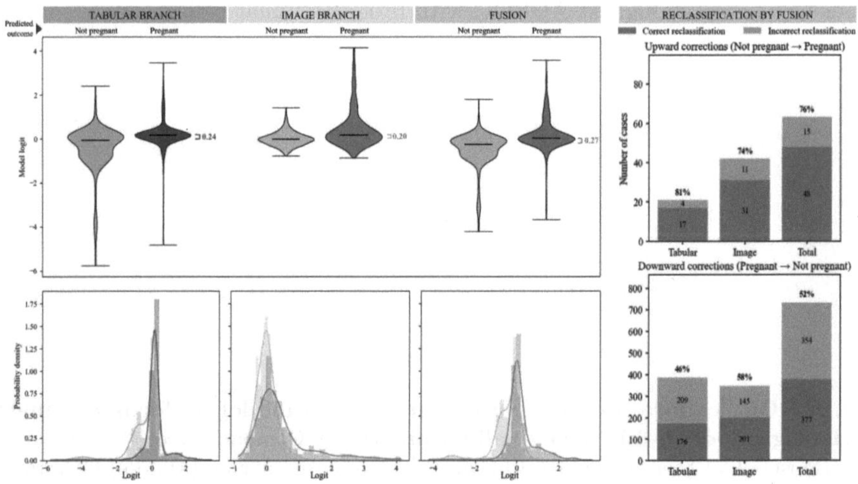


**Fig. 3.** Distribution of logits and directional reclassification by fusion model. (Upper left panel) Plots showing median and extremal logit values by model and true outcome class. (Bottom left panel) Probability density of logits by true outcome class. (Right panel) Directional reclassification relative to unimodal models, showing that upward corrections are more reliable than downward corrections.

Figure 3 compares logit distributions by true outcome class and summarizes directional reclassification by the fusion model. The fusion model shows greater separation between the true outcome medians than either unimodal branch. This aligns with Fig. 2, where the image branch exhibits weaker discrimination. Consistently, the density plots show greater overlap between classes for the image model relative to the tabular and fusion models.

Figure 4 shows that the tabular branch placed high attribution on embryo-development and ovarian-response variables, while image attributions often

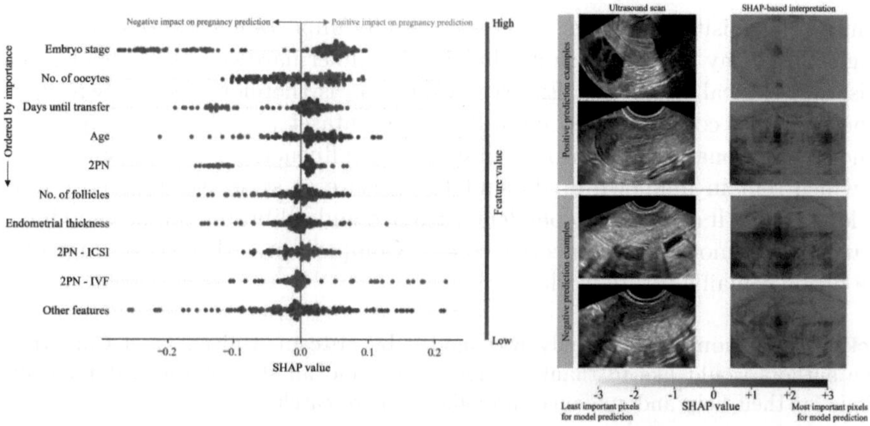


**Fig. 4. Post-hoc interpretability by model type using SHAP**. SHAP analysis showing feature importance values for tabular branch. Tabular branch shows embryo stage, oocytes and age are most important for prediction of IVF pregnancy outcome, while image attributions highlight regions near the endometrium.

localised around the endometrial region. In many cases, the model uses pixels related to the endometrial tissue in predicting the likelihood of a successful IVF cycle outcome. This is in line with current IVF practice which uses endometrial thickness as a key parameter in assessing the readiness for embryo transfer. Because several IVF variables are clinically correlated, SHAP values should be interpreted as showing which features the model used for prediction, rather than as independent physiological effects.

# 5 Conclusion

Our work develops a methodology for utilising more modalities available in routine IVF care for IVF embryo transfer outcome prediction, in an end-to-end approach, from raw data collection through to prediction and post-hoc interpretability.

This is a first step in using AI-aided pipelines to review initial cycle treatment response for patients with recurrent ovarian or implantation failure, and in turn design data-driven protocols personalised around prior cycle data or ultrasound monitoring of ovarian stimulation. We hope this work can also empower patients with tailored information beyond just age in assessing their likelihood of IVF cycle success.

## 5.1 Limitations

This dataset is from a single IVF clinic based in London, UK. Although patient-grouped cross-validation prevents the same patient from appearing in both training and test folds, it does not test how well the model would generalise to other clinics or acquisition settings. This is especially important because data from a single clinic may reflect the same clinicians, scanner hardware, treatment protocols, and clinical workflows. External validation is therefore needed before this type of model could be used clinically. This dataset also does not capture all genetic, hormonal, and environmental factors influencing IVF outcomes, some of which remain unknown or difficult to measure at scale. We focused on late fusion because it allowed independently trained and calibrated tabular and image branches in a modest retrospective cohort. Comparison with early or intermediate fusion remains future work.

**Acknowledgments.** This study was funded by ai@cam, University of Cambridge. The authors would like to thank Nichola Evans and all staff at the Lister Fertility Clinic for their help and guidance throughout the research.

**Data Availability Statement.** Clinical images and IVF records cannot be publicly released due to patient confidentiality. Code and derived analysis materials may be shared on reasonable request, subject to data-sharing agreements.

**Disclosure of Interests.** The authors have no competing interests to declare that are relevant to the content of this article.

## References

1. Bereczki, K.G., et al.: Machine learning-based prediction of IVF outcomes: the central role of female preprocedural factors. Biomedicines **13**(11), 2768 (2025)
2. Cheng, A., et al.: Prediction of in-vitro fertilization outcome by ultrasound strain analysis and machine learning: a multi-center study. Ultrasound J. **18**(1), 18257 (2026)
3. Huang, B., et al.: Using deep learning to predict the outcome of live birth from more than 10,000 embryo data. BMC Pregnancy Childbirth **22**(1), 36 (2022)
4. Huang, S., et al.: Machine learning-based preliminary screening tool for clinical pregnancy prediction: towards management of IVF/ICSI stages. Ann. Med. **57**(1) (2025)
5. Huang, S.C., Pareek, A., Seyyedi, S., Banerjee, I., Lungren, M.P.: Fusion of medical imaging and electronic health records using deep learning: a systematic review and implementation guidelines. NPJ Digit. Med. **3**, 136 (2020)
6. Lundberg, S.M., Lee, S.I.: A unified approach to interpreting model predictions. In: Advances in Neural Information Processing Systems (2017)
7. Lundberg, S.M.: Explainable machine-learning predictions for the prevention of hypoxaemia during surgery. Nat. Biomed. Eng. **2**(10), 749–760 (2018)
8. Rudin, C.: Stop explaining black box machine learning models for high stakes decisions and use interpretable models instead. Nat. Mach. Intell. **1**(5), 206–215 (2019)
9. Simon, B.D., Ozyoruk, K.B., Gelikman, D.G., Harmon, S.A., Türkbey, B.: The future of multimodal artificial intelligence models for integrating imaging and clinical metadata: a narrative review. Diagn. Interv. Radiol. **31**(4), 303–312 (2025)
10. Wang, C.W., Kuo, C.Y., Chen, C.H., Hsieh, Y.H., Su, E.C.Y.: Predicting clinical pregnancy using clinical features and machine learning algorithms in in vitro fertilization. PLoS ONE **17**(6), e0267554 (2022)

11. Warner, E., et al.: Multimodal machine learning in image-based and clinical biomedicine: survey and prospects. Int. J. Comput. Vision **132**, 3753–3769 (2024)
12. World Health Organization: 1 in 6 people globally affected by infertility: WHO (Apr 2023). https://www.who.int/news/item/04-04-2023-1-in-6-people-globally-affected-by-infertility, official press release
13. Zhang, Q., Liang, X., Chen, Z.: A review of artificial intelligence applications in in vitro fertilization. J. Assist. Reprod. Genet. **42**(1), 3–14 (2025)

# A Benchmark Study for Reporting Feasibility in AI-Based Infant Hearing Screening: Exploring the Limits of Passive Sensing

Lorenzo Corso[1(✉)], Samuele Pe[1], Anisa Visram[2], Iain Jackson[2], Michael Stone[2], Kevin Munro[2,3], Enea Parimbelli[1,4], Giovanna Nicora[1], and Arianna Dagliati[1]

[1] Department of Computer, Electrical and Biomedical Engineering, University of Pavia, Pavia 27100, Italy
lorenzo.corso01@universitadipavia.it

[2] Manchester Centre for Audiology and Deafness, School of Health Sciences, University of Manchester, Manchester, United Kingdom

[3] Manchester Academic Health Science Centre, Manchester University Hospitals NHS Foundation Trust, Manchester, United Kingdom

[4] Telfer School of Management, University of Ottawa, Ottawa, Canada

**Abstract.** Assessing hearing in infants with a developmental age of 3–7 months remains a clinical challenge. Too mature for neonatal reflexes, yet too immature for visual reinforcement, this demographic relies on Behavioural Observation Audiometry (BOA), a subjective method with high inter-observer variability. This preliminary study investigated whether State-of-the-Art (SOTA) machine learning could automate a modified BOA protocol, distinguishing auditory responses in a passive listening task.

We analysed facial video recordings from 46 infants (mean age 4.68 months; central 95% range: 3.68–6.44). The protocol used a central "attention-holding" visual stimulus and loudspeakers at $\pm 45°$. Using OpenFace 2.0, we extracted 38 facial, gaze, and pose channels over 12 s windows ($-2$ s pre-stimulus to $+10$ s post-stimulus). We benchmarked eight time-series architectures—ranging from Logistic Regression to the MOMENT foundation model—to classify "Stimulus" (80.25%) vs. "Control/Silence" (19.75%).

Despite subject-independent validation and augmentation, no model exceeded chance-level performance (Balanced Accuracy 0.50–0.60). UMAP projections revealed a complete topological overlap between stimulus and control frames, both in raw feature space and learned embedding space. Unlike our previous success with older infants (7–24 months), these findings suggest automated facial analysis during this specific passive listening paradigm may be unlikely to serve as an effective screening method for this demographic. We attribute this to insufficient stimulus salience and high inter-subject variability—both in response timing and idiosyncratic baseline movements—which obscure the transient response signal.

Future work must prioritise protocol adaptations to enhance response clarity, supporting a reframing from supervised classification toward anomaly detection and clinician-validated models.

**Keywords:** Action Units · Negative findings · Audiology · Computer Vision · BAMBINO Project

© The Author(s), under exclusive license to Springer Nature Switzerland AG 2027
P. Andreev et al. (Eds.): AIME 2026, LNAI 16748, pp. 312–322, 2027.
https://doi.org/10.1007/978-3-032-30710-1_38

# 1 Introduction

Early detection of hearing loss is critical for preventing developmental delays in speech and cognition [1, 2]. While Universal Newborn Hearing Screening (UNHS) effectively identifies issues in neonates [3], and Visual Reinforcement Audiometry (VRA) is the standard for infants with a developmental age of 7 months or older, a diagnostic "blind spot" exists for infants with a developmental age of 3–7 months. Ideally, an automated tool for this demographic would serve as a rapid screening device, identifying infants who fail to respond for referral to definitive diagnostic testing.

Infants in this developmental window present a unique assessment challenge. They have largely outgrown the primitive startle reflexes used in neonatal testing but have not yet developed the neck muscle control or cognitive association skills required for VRA. Consequently, clinicians rely on Behavioural Observation Audiometry (BOA). In BOA, experienced audiologists present suprathreshold sounds, often broadband in nature, and observe the infant for subtle, reflexive changes in behaviour—such as eye widening, a pause in sucking, or a slight head turn [4, 5]. While usually effective in expert hands, BOA is inherently subjective, making standardisation difficult.

Recent advances in Computer Vision (CV) offer a potential solution by quantifying subtle facial behaviours. Artificial Intelligence (AI) has been successfully applied to detect neonatal pain [6] and screen for developmental markers [7]. In our previous work [8], we successfully automated hearing screening for older infants (7–24 months) using VRA data, where head turns are distinct and reinforced.

This study explored whether this success extends to the more challenging 3–7 month demographic, benchmarking State-of-the-Art (SOTA) time-series models—from statistical baselines to Foundation Models—on behavioural responses to sound in a passive BOA-like paradigm. By reporting these negative findings, we mitigate positive publication bias [9] and delimit the boundaries of current sensing capabilities.

# 2 Materials and Methods

## 2.1 Participants and Clinical Protocol

**Cohort.** We analysed data from 46 healthy infants (mean age 4.68 months; central 95% range: 3.68–6.44) recruited as part of the BAMBINO project (details available at: https://sites.manchester.ac.uk/bambino/) at the University of Manchester. Infants with risk factors for hearing loss (e.g., Neonatal Intensive Care Unit stay >48h, family history) were excluded to ensure a normative sample.

**Experimental Setup.** The study was conducted in a sound-treated booth.

- *Positioning*: Infants were seated on a caregiver's lap, facing a monitor at 1 m. Caregivers were provided with a surgical mask to wear during the session to prevent their face from appearing in the videos.
- *Visual Stream*: To ensure the infant's face remained visible to the camera, a central monitor displayed colourful shapes continuously. This served to hold the infant's attention in a frontal position.

- *Audio Stimuli*: Stimuli consisted of 4-s sounds presented at 70 dB sound pressure level (SPL) via loudspeakers positioned at $\pm 45^\circ$ azimuth, grouped into four macro-categories: (i) a 1 kHz warble tone, (ii) 1 kHz narrowband noise, (iii) 1 kHz filtered samples of speech and music (covering generic, personalised, and caregiver-selected options), and (iv) 'other' generic/personalised sounds. The absence of sound (500 ms silent intervals) defined the control condition.
- *Passive Paradigm*: Unlike VRA, no visual reward was provided upon hearing the sound. The focus was on capturing naturalistic, reflexive responses.
- *Data Acquisition*: High-definition video was recorded at 25 fps using a Sony HDR-CX625 positioned below the monitor. Each infant contributed ~20 trials, randomly interleaving Stimulus (Class 1, ~80.25%) and Control (Class 0, ~19.75%) conditions.

## 2.2 Pipeline

**Data Preprocessing.** We utilised OpenFace 2.0 [10] to extract high-dimensional behavioural data. For each frame, we obtained 38 channels, comprising Action Units (AUs) representing facial muscle movements, gaze direction, and head pose.

For each trial we extracted a 12 s window ($-2$ s pre-stimulus to $+10$ s post-stimulus); only the post-stimulus segment (0 s to $+10$ s) was fed to the classifiers. To maintain high data integrity, we implemented an automated quality control filter: any trial where more than 50% of the frames yielded an OpenFace confidence score below 50%, typically due to physical occlusion or extreme head angles, was excluded from analysis.

**Benchmarking Framework.** To rigorously assess feasibility, we evaluated a spectrum of architectures ranging from interpretable baselines to state-of-the-art foundation models. Two CNN baselines (CNN 1D & 2D) from our prior work [8] are also reported, without augmentation, to preserve comparability with that study:

- *Baseline* (Logistic Regression): We extracted 17 statistical, temporal, and complexity descriptors per channel (e.g., mean, skew, zero-crossing rate) using custom NumPy and SciPy routines, resulting in ~650 total features per trial.
- *Time-Series Classifiers*: We benchmarked three distinct approaches: MiniRocket [11], a fast transform using random convolutional kernels coupled with XGBoost; InceptionTime [12], a deep ensemble of CNNs serving as the current standard benchmark; and FiLM-CNN [13], a custom CNN conditioned on demographic covariates (age, sex) to adapt to developmental differences.
- *Image Encoding*: ResNet-18 (GASF) transformed time-series data into 2D images using Gramian Angular Fields, enabling the use of a pre-trained ImageNet backbone [14, 15].
- *Foundation Model*: We leveraged MOMENT [16], a Large Time-Series Model based on the Transformer architecture. We utilised its pre-trained backbone to extract embeddings, hypothesising that training on massive datasets enables the detection of subtle signal changes that smaller models might miss.

A schematic overview of this processing pipeline is presented in Fig. 1.

**Validation Strategy.** To ensure generalisability, we employed a Subject-Independent Hold-out strategy. Infants were strictly separated between training and test sets to prevent data leakage (i.e., no infant appeared in both). We report balanced accuracy, AUROC, and specificity to account for the ~80:20 class imbalance.

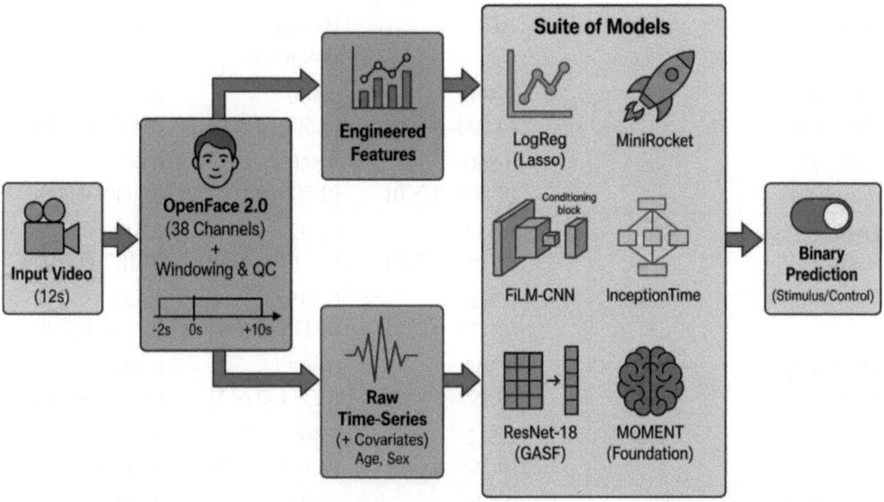


**Fig. 1.** *Overview of the automated screening pipeline.* Facial signals extracted via OpenFace 2.0 are windowed (−2 s to +10 s) and quality-controlled; only the 10-s post-stimulus segment (0–10 s) is used as classifier input. The data is then processed via two parallel representations—hand-crafted statistical, temporal, and complexity descriptors (custom NumPy/SciPy implementation) and raw multivariate time-series (with demographic covariates)—before being fed into a suite of 8 diverse machine learning architectures to predict the presence of an acoustic stimulus.

## 3 Results

### 3.1 Classification Performance

Table 1 summarises the performance of all 22 experimental configurations. To address class imbalance, we applied a randomised augmentation pipeline to the minority class. The primitives included jittering ($\sigma = 0.05$), scaling (0.8–1.2×), time-warping (max warp 0.2), and random shifting (±1 s), with a protective constraint applied to the first 0.6 s of positive trials to preserve stimulus onset dynamics. Three configurations showed modest above-chance AUC — LogReg with augmentation (0.568), ResNet-GASF with augmentation (0.642), and MOMENT+TabPFN without augmentation (0.591); notably, adding augmentation to MOMENT+TabPFN reduced its AUC to 0.514, indicating that the apparent gains do not generalise across configurations. Bootstrap 95% CIs for all three crossed 0.50 and corresponding Balanced Accuracies remained ≤0.60, indicating that the apparent signal is not statistically robust across subjects.

**Table 1.** *Classification performance on the held-out test set* (95% CI on 200 bootstrap sampling with 70% extractions each time). The 'Augmented' column indicates whether the model was trained using data augmentation. Despite rigorous training, with hyperparameter optimisation, optimal threshold selected based on validation set performance on the best validation model, learning rate scheduler, and early stopping, no model significantly exceeds chance (Balanced Accuracy ≈ 0.50).

| Model | Augmented | AUC | Balanced Accuracy | Specificity |
|---|---|---|---|---|
| *CNN 1D (baseline)* | No | 0.500 [0.500–0.500] | 0.500 [0.500–0.500] | 0.000 [0.000–0.000] |
| *CNN 2D (baseline)* | No | 0.500 [0.500–0.500] | 0.500 [0.500–0.500] | 0.000 [0.000–0.000] |
| *LogReg (Lasso)* | No | 0.534 [0.367–0.709] | 0.532 [0.417–0.660] | 0.419 [0.187–0.667] |
| | Yes | 0.568 [0.427–0.722] | 0.595 [0.470–0.699] | 0.528 [0.316–0.739] |
| *MiniRocket (XGB)* | No | 0.307 [0.193–0.417] | 0.497 [0.374–0.617] | 0.780 [0.588–0.950] |
| | Yes | 0.512 [0.368–0.660] | 0.490 [0.389–0.619] | 0.701 [0.533–0.889] |
| *FiLM-CNN* | No | 0.536 [0.354–0.663] | 0.502 [0.413–0.603] | 0.195 [0.048–0.376] |
| | Yes | 0.465 [0.305–0.629] | 0.495 [0.408–0.587] | 0.200 [0.038–0.358] |
| *InceptionTime* | No | 0.472 [0.320–0.673] | 0.468 [0.338–0.598] | 0.634 [0.400–0.883] |
| | Yes | 0.532 [0.400–0.658] | 0.515 [0.402–0.640] | 0.300 [0.111–0.534] |
| *ResNet (GASF)* | No | 0.480 [0.342–0.628] | 0.448 [0.320–0.562] | 0.550 [0.312–0.750] |
| | Yes | 0.642 [0.499–0.776] | 0.576 [0.475–0.699] | 0.398 [0.182–0.609] |
| *MOMENT (MLP)* | No | 0.454 [0.275–0.597] | 0.500 [0.500–0.500] | 0.000 [0.000–0.000] |
| | Yes | 0.544 [0.382–0.695] | 0.516 [0.382–0.633] | 0.345 [0.105–0.591] |
| *MOMENT (HistGB)* | No | 0.485 [0.312–0.658] | 0.536 [0.415–0.668] | 0.333 [0.133–0.534] |

(*continued*)

**Established Baselines (CNN 1D and 2D).** Despite achieving >80% accuracy and F1 on older infants in prior work, both CNN baselines collapsed to majority-class prediction

**Table 1.** *(continued)*

| Model | Augmented | AUC | Balanced Accuracy | Specificity |
|---|---|---|---|---|
| | Yes | 0.540 [0.369–0.705] | 0.543 [0.429–0.653] | 0.374 [0.158–0.600] |
| *MOMENT (LogReg)* | No | 0.526 [0.375–0.677] | 0.532 [0.405–0.657] | 0.554 [0.316–0.750] |
| | Yes | 0.506 [0.363–0.645] | 0.470 [0.373–0.566] | 0.773 [0.571–0.941] |
| *MOMENT (PCA + TabPFN)* | No | 0.557 [0.421–0.708] | 0.546 [0.432–0.673] | 0.358 [0.158–0.572] |
| | Yes | 0.526 [0.394–0.680] | 0.532 [0.418–0.662] | 0.335 [0.118–0.546] |
| *MOMENT (TabPFN)* | No | 0.591 [0.442–0.727] | 0.556 [0.461–0.671] | 0.251 [0.071–0.462] |
| | Yes | 0.514 [0.379–0.673] | 0.500 [0.401–0.621] | 0.215 [0.050–0.438] |

here (BA = 0.500, Specificity = 0.000) despite extensive hyperparameter optimisation. The raw waveform and spectrogram representations that worked for older infants do not capture the more nuanced behaviours of this younger demographic.

**General Performance and Feasibility.** Across the entire architectural spectrum, predictive performance plateaued near random chance, with Balanced Accuracy scores largely confined to the 0.50–0.60 range. This suggests that, for this specific cohort and experimental setup, the behavioural signal is either extremely subtle or heavily obscured by noise.

**Model Complexity.** Furthermore, we observed that increased model complexity did not correlate with better performance.

- *The Logistic Regression (Lasso) baseline*, when trained with augmentation, achieved one of the highest Balanced Accuracies (0.595) and a competitive AUROC (0.568). This indicates that simple, interpretable statistical features (e.g., variance, entropy) may be more robust than deep learned representations in this low-signal-to-noise regime.
- *The MOMENT foundation model*, despite its pre-training on massive time-series datasets, failed to provide a decisive breakthrough. While the MOMENT + TabPFN configuration reached an AUROC of 0.591, it did not significantly outperform the simpler linear baseline.
- The only deep architecture to show a notable improvement in AUROC was the *ResNet* (GASF) model, achieving a test AUROC of 0.642 following augmented training. This suggests that transforming the time-series into a 2D image domain might offer a slight advantage over sequence modelling.

## 3.2 Manifold Visualisation

To better investigate the possible reasons for classification failure, we mapped the data at two distinct stages using Uniform Manifold Approximation and Projection (UMAP).

First, we mapped the raw, pre-processed time-series features into a 2D space prior to any learning. As shown in Fig. 2a, the Stimulus and Control classes exhibit a complete topological overlap. This initial structure confirms that there is no obvious separability in the raw behavioural data; responses are not characterised by simple, high magnitude triggers distinct from baseline movement.

Next, we visualised the learned embeddings from our best-performing deep architecture, the ResNet-18 (GASF). If the model had successfully extracted discriminative latent features, we would expect to see the emergence of distinct class-based clusters.

Figure 2b reveals that while the ResNet latent space shows a slight tendency towards clustering compared to the raw data, this topological structure did not translate into significant classification performance. The Stimulus and Control classes remain overlapped, suggesting that the observed clusters are likely driven by subject-specific features (e.g., individual movement patterns) rather than class separability. This persistence of inseparability suggests that the limitation is informational—the signal is simply not present in the video feed with sufficient magnitude—rather than a failure of model capacity.

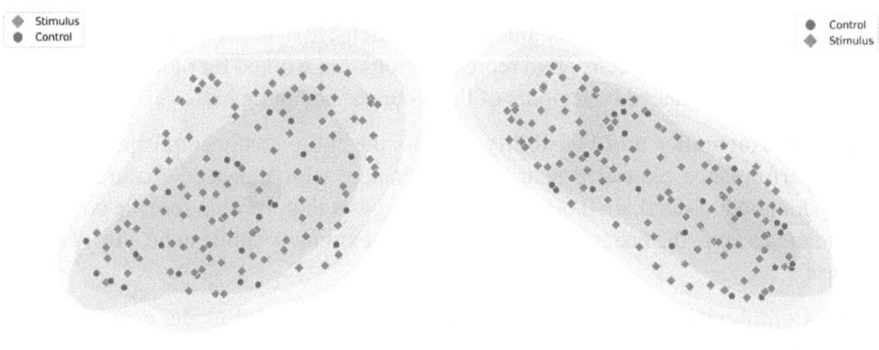


*(a)* *(b)*

**Fig. 2.** *Manifold visualisation of behavioural features using UMAP on the held-out test set.* (a) Projection of raw, pre-processed time-series features prior to model training. The complete overlap between Stimulus (Orange) and Control (Blue) classes indicates a lack of separability in the input space. (b) Projection of the learned latent embeddings from the best-performing deep architecture, ResNet-18 (GASF). While the latent space exhibits a slight increased structural clustering compared to the raw input, the Stimulus and Control classes remain topologically indistinguishable. This indicates that the model learned to extract some features (likely subject-specific) but failed to find a decision boundary that separates auditory responses from baseline movement. *UMAP parameters*: n_neighbors = 30, min_dist = 0.1, metric = Euclidean, random_state = 42.

## 4 Discussion

This study investigated the feasibility of automated hearing screening for infants with a developmental age of 3–7 months. Our previous work achieved high accuracy with older infants (developmental age of 7–24 months) under VRA, where reinforced head turns produce a strong, time-locked signal. The current results show that a passive listening paradigm in younger infants does not yield a comparable signal: no SOTA time-series model exceeded chance-level performance. In the remainder of this section, we interpret this negative result along three axes—model behaviour, protocol geometry, and response biology—and use these interpretations to motivate a reformulation of the task as anomaly detection.

Model behaviour itself is informative. The CNN 1D and 2D baselines collapsed to majority-class prediction, and deep 1D architectures such as InceptionTime did not substantively outperform simpler alternatives. The strongest configurations were the L1-regularised Logistic Regression on extracted features, the 2D ResNet-GASF, and the MOMENT + TabPFN pipeline. Although three models exceeded chance on point estimates, their 95% bootstrap confidence intervals all crossed 0.50, so we do not interpret these as evidence of a robust learnable signal. The pattern—statistical and 2D texture-based encodings marginally outperforming deep 1D sequence models—is consistent with a signal that, when present, manifests as a brief non-stationary excursion (e.g., a momentary spike in variance or entropy) rather than a structured, time-locked head turn with consistent morphology.

Turning to protocol factors, we attribute the difficulty of this task primarily to the specific constraints of the passive protocol used for this age group. First, the high level of attentional engagement elicited by the central stimulus likely played a key role [17]. Research shows that infants aged 3–7 months display markedly reduced peripheral localisation when sustaining attention on a complex central visual target, a phenomenon known as the competition effect. In our setup, the central video featuring moving colourful shapes, while necessary to maintain visibility of the infant's face, also acted as a powerful visual anchor. As a result, visual salience may have overridden auditory orienting responses: although the infant likely perceived the sound, they may have inhibited the oculomotor head-turn reflex to maintain fixation on the engaging visual stimulus. To mitigate this in future automated screenings, protocols should consider momentarily reducing the visual salience (e.g., replacing the video with a static, neutral image) immediately prior to stimulus onset to 'release' the infant's attention and facilitate a reflexive response.

A second protocol factor is speaker geometry. The geometric configuration of the BAMBINO protocol differs significantly from the VRA setup used in our previous work. VRA typically employs speakers at 90°, eliciting a large, distinct head profile turn. In contrast, this study used speakers at ±45°. Biomechanically, a 45° turn is subtle and difficult to distinguish from natural postural instability in a 2D frontal feed. While 90° turns, standard in VRA, generate clearer motion signals, they are developmentally challenging for 3–7-month-olds who lack independent sitting balance. Supportive seating (e.g., a baby chair) could enable a safe 90° layout, maximising head-turn magnitude and the resulting Signal-to-Noise Ratio (SNR).

Biologically, the absence of reinforcement, incompatible with this age group, is expected to produce rapid habituation. In VRA, turning is rewarded and the response is sustained; in a passive paradigm the response remains purely reflexive. An infant may respond to the first one or two trials, but subsequent stimuli likely elicit no observable behavioural change, rendering most "Stimulus" trials behaviourally indistinguishable from "Control" trials. We consider this not a contradiction of our design but a principal finding of the benchmark: under fixed binary labels, habituation injects structured label noise that is invisible to any supervised learner, regardless of capacity. The topological collapse observed in Fig. 2—in both raw feature space and deep embedding space—is the signature one would predict under this hypothesis.

This interpretation motivates a reformulation of the task as *anomaly detection*. Rather than learning a decision boundary between uniformly-labelled Stimulus and Control trials, one can model each infant's baseline behavioural manifold $M_i$ from pre-stimulus windows and silent controls, then score post-stimulus windows by their deviation from $M_i$. Candidate instantiations include one-class SVMs on extracted features, reconstruction-error scoring with subject-conditioned autoencoders, and self-supervised contrastive encoders trained on baseline segments. Three properties make this formulation well-matched to the present setting: (i) it is habituation-tolerant, since early-trial excursions remain detectable without requiring a consistent response across the session; (ii) it absorbs inter-subject variability by conditioning on $M_i$ rather than on a population-level boundary; and (iii) it converts the output from a binary prediction into a continuous novelty score that a clinician can threshold, aligning with BOA's native decision logic. Validating this framework on the BAMBINO cohort, together with stimulus schedules designed to counteract habituation (e.g., varying acoustic content across trials), is the natural next study.

## 5 Conclusion

We provide a rigorous benchmark for AI-based hearing screening in the 3–7 month diagnostic blind spot. Under the passive listening protocol studied here, the behavioural response to suprathreshold sound is too subtle to be reliably separated from baseline movement by current SOTA computer vision models. The persistence of topologically overlapping clusters from raw features through deep embeddings indicates that this is not an algorithmic failure but an informational limit of the current sensing paradigm.

Two conclusions follow. First, progress in this demographic depends more on protocol engineering—reducing central visual competition, exploiting 90° speaker geometry with supportive seating, and counteracting habituation with varied stimuli—than on further scaling of model capacity. Second, the supervised binary formulation is itself a limiting assumption: trial-wise habituation induces label noise that no classifier can overcome, whereas an anomaly-detection formulation over subject-specific baseline manifolds might be both biologically and statistically better matched to the task. Consequently, identifying these methodological limits establishes a clear baseline to guide the future development of AI-assisted BOA systems.

**Acknowledgments.** The authors thank the BAMBINO project team and all participating families. Project information is available at https://sites.manchester.ac.uk/bambino/. Lorenzo Corso and

Samuele Pe are enrolled in the National PhD Program in Artificial Intelligence (XL cycle for LC, XXXIX cycle for SP) – Health and Life Sciences, organised by Università Campus Bio-Medico di Roma.

**Disclosure of Interests** The authors have no competing interests to declare that are relevant to the content of this article.

## References

1. Yoshinaga-Itano, C., et al.: Language of early-and later-identified children with hearing loss. Pediatrics. **102**(5), 1161–1171 (1998). https://doi.org/10.1542/peds.102.5.1161
2. Moeller, M.P.: Early intervention and language development in children who are deaf and hard of hearing. Pediatrics. **106**(3), e43 (2000). https://doi.org/10.1542/peds.106.3.e43
3. Thompson, D.C., et al.: Universal newborn hearing screening: summary of evidence. JAMA. **286**(16), 2000–2010 (2001). https://doi.org/10.1001/jama.286.16.2000
4. Madell, J.R., Flexer, C. (eds.): Pediatric Audiology: Diagnosis, Technology, and Management. Thieme (2014)
5. Ewing, I.R., Ewing, A.W.G.: The ascertainment of deafness in infancy and early childhood. J. Laryngol. Otol. **59**(9), 309–333 (1944). https://doi.org/10.1017/S0022215100007465
6. Zamzmi, G., et al.: A review of automated pain assessment in infants: features, classification tasks, and databases. IEEE Rev. Biomed. Eng. **11**, 77–96 (2018). https://doi.org/10.1109/RBME.2017.2777907
7. Egger, H.L., et al.: Automatic emotion and attention analysis of young children at home: a ResearchKit autism feasibility study. Npj Digit. Med. **1**(1), 20 (2018). https://doi.org/10.1038/s41746-018-0024-6
8. Pe, S., et al.: Hearing impairment assessment in infants through explainable computer vision analysis of facial features. In: Proceedings of the 1st Workshop on Artificial Intelligence for Biomedical Data (AIBio) 2025 Held in conjunction with the 28th European Conference on Artificial Intelligence (ECAI), Bologna, Italy (2025) (in press)
9. Mlinarić, A., et al.: Dealing with the positive publication bias: why you should really publish your negative results. Biochem. Med. **27**(3), 030201 (2017). https://doi.org/10.11613/BM.2017.030201
10. Baltrusaitis, T., et al.: OpenFace 2.0: facial behavior analysis toolkit. In: 2018 13th IEEE International Conference on Automatic Face & Gesture Recognition (FG 2018), pp. 59–66 (2018). https://doi.org/10.1109/FG.2018.00019
11. Dempster, A., et al.: MINIROCKET: a very fast (almost) deterministic transform for time series classification. In: Proceedings of the 27th ACM SIGKDD Conference on Knowledge Discovery & Data Mining, pp. 248–257 (2021). https://doi.org/10.1145/3447548.3467231
12. Fawaz, H.I., et al.: InceptionTime: finding AlexNet for time series classification. Data Min. Knowl. Discov. **34**(6), 1936–1962 (2020). https://doi.org/10.1007/s10618-020-00710-y
13. Perez, E., et al.: FiLM: visual reasoning with a general conditioning layer. arXiv:1709.07871. (2017). https://doi.org/10.48550/arXiv.1709.07871
14. Wang, Z., Oates, T.: Imaging time-series to improve classification and imputation. In: Proceedings of the 24th International Conference on Artificial Intelligence, in IJCAI'15, pp. 3939–3945. AAAI Press, Buenos Aires, Argentina (2015)
15. Garibo-i-Orts, Ò., et al.: Gramian angular fields for leveraging pretrained computer vision models with anomalous diffusion trajectories. Phys. Rev. E. **107**(3), 034138 (2023). https://doi.org/10.1103/PhysRevE.107.034138

16. Goswami, M., et al.: MOMENT: a family of open time-series foundation models. arXiv: 2402.03885. (2024). https://doi.org/10.48550/arXiv.2402.03885
17. Richards, J.E.: Peripheral stimulus localization by infants: attention, age, and individual differences in heart rate variability. J. Exp. Psychol. Hum. Percept. Perform. **23**(3), 667–680 (1997). https://doi.org/10.1037/0096-1523.23.3.667

# ExpertoRhythm: Morphology-Aware Learning for Waveform Reconstruction and Cuffless Blood Pressure Estimation from Single-Channel PPG

Amir Arjomand(✉), Kenneth B. Kent, and Georgiy Krylov

University of New Brunswick, Fredericton, Canada
{a.arjomand,ken,georgiy.krylov}@unb.ca

**Abstract.** Continuous cuffless blood pressure (BP) monitoring from photoplethysmography (PPG) has strong potential for wearable health and telemonitoring, but accurate estimation remains difficult because PPG-to-BP mapping must preserve subtle waveform morphology and pressure-range-dependent dynamics. We introduce *ExpertoRhythm*, an attention-enhanced 1D U-Net that reconstructs the arterial blood pressure (ABP) waveform from a single-channel PPG signal and derives systolic and diastolic BP directly from the reconstructed waveform. The central contribution is a composite morphology-aware learning objective that integrates range-weighted SmoothL1 reconstruction with a window-range regularizer to emphasize high-dynamic BP segments and reduce amplitude under/over-shoot. On the UCI cuff-less BP dataset with 942 subjects, ExpertoRhythm achieves 2.46/1.46 mmHg MAE for systolic/diastolic BP (SBP/DBP), while obtaining a 30.4% average relative error reduction over pure MSE across waveform reconstruction and BP estimation metrics. Clinical-style evaluation further demonstrates low bias and strong agreement across the BP range, including high-pressure windows up to 200 mmHg, satisfying AAMI criteria and achieving BHS Grade A. These results suggest that morphology-aware waveform reconstruction from a single PPG channel can provide an accurate and practical pathway toward continuous cuffless BP monitoring in wearable and remote-care settings.

**Keywords:** Cuffless blood pressure · PPG · ABP waveform reconstruction · 1D U-Net · channel attention · morphology-aware loss · SmoothL1 · amplitude regularization · composite loss · SBP/DBP

## 1 Introduction

Blood pressure (BP) is a key marker of cardiovascular risk, but cuff-based measurements are inconvenient to take frequently and do not provide continuous trends. This has accelerated interest in *cuffless* BP estimation using wearable-friendly sensors, especially photoplethysmography (PPG), which is inexpensive

© The Author(s), under exclusive license to Springer Nature Switzerland AG 2027
P. Andreev et al. (Eds.): AIME 2026, LNAI 16748, pp. 323–333, 2027.
https://doi.org/10.1007/978-3-032-30710-1_39

and already embedded in many consumer devices. A widely used deep-learning strategy is to reconstruct the arterial blood pressure (ABP) waveform from PPG and then derive systolic/diastolic values from the reconstructed waveform, retaining more hemodynamic detail than direct scalar regression [5,14].

However, a practical mismatch remains between how these models are trained and how BP is ultimately read out. Most PPG→ABP methods optimize pointwise waveform losses (MSE/MAE/SmoothL1), which improve average sample fidelity, but systolic/diastolic values are governed by localized morphology, here defined as peak/trough amplitudes and the immediate shape around those turning points. Consequently, small errors in these regions can yield noticeable BP error even when overall waveform error is low, making our loss a better surrogate by emphasizing these morphology critical points.

We address this gap with ExpertoRhythm, a channel-prior convolutional attention (CPCA) enhanced 1D U-Net for PPG→ABP reconstruction [3,11] and composite training loss functions. ExpertoRhythm is trained with a composite loss that (i) range-weights a robust SmoothL1 loss to emphasize high-dynamic windows and (ii) applies a window-range regularizer to penalize amplitude under/over-shoot. On the UCI cuff-less BP dataset (942 subjects; 10 s at 125 Hz), controlled ablations show consistent improvements over standard pointwise objectives, achieving SBP/DBP MAE of 2.46/1.46 mmHg while including high-pressure windows up to SBP 200 mmHg and meeting established medical evaluation standards (AAMI and BHS).

*Contributions*

- We propose a morphology-aware training objective for PPG→ABP reconstruction that combines range-weighted SmoothL1 with a window-range amplitude regularizer to improve waveform-derived SBP/DBP.
- We provide controlled ablations over both objective terms and model capacity, quantifying their effects on waveform fidelity and BP accuracy.
- We present a 4-layers CPCA 1D U-Net model and report standards-style evaluation demonstrating strong agreement under AAMI/BHS criteria.

## 2 Background and Related Work

*Baselines and Fair-Comparison Protocol.* We benchmark our morphology-aware enhanced-CPCA 1D U-Net (ExpertoRhythm) against a focused, representative set of state-of-the-art PPG-to-ABP reconstruction methods that cover the dominant paradigms in the literature: convolutional encoder–decoder architectures (PPG2ABP [14], ABP-Net [5]), transformer-based models (our prior TransfoRhythm [2]), and recent morphology-aware or hybrid-objective approaches (De Palma *et al.* [6]).

These baselines were chosen because they (i) operate exclusively on single-channel PPG, (ii) target continuous waveform reconstruction for clinical

SBP/DBP extraction, and (iii) are the most widely cited and directly comparable works under resource-constrained deployment scenarios.

For fair and reproducible comparison, we use the performance numbers **as originally reported** in each paper and adopt the identical evaluation protocol (MAE on the waveform, absolute SBP/DBP errors, etc.) and test-set definitions described by the authors. Where public test splits or preprocessing details are available, we follow them exactly. This approach eliminates confounding factors from data partitioning or metric variations and isolates performance gains to architectural and objective choices.

# 3 Method

## 3.1 Regression Architecture and I/O

We reconstruct ABP from PPG using a 1D U-Net encoder–decoder with skip connections for time-series translation [20,24]. The network follows a 4-level multi-scale design as illustrated in Fig. 1. Concretely, with base width $C$=72, encoder widths are $\{C, 2C, 4C, 8C\}$ with bottleneck $16C$, and the decoder mirrors this with skip concatenation.

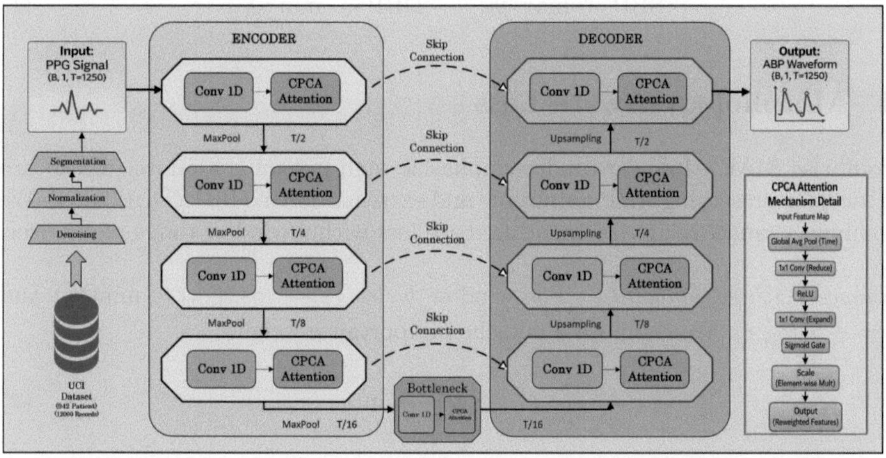


**Fig. 1.** CPCA-enhanced 1D U-Net for PPG→ABP regression (4-level encoder–decoder with skip connections and CPCA blocks).

- **Encoder:** progressively downsamples temporal resolution using MaxPool1D(2) to learn hierarchical representations.
- **Bottleneck:** operates at the lowest resolution, aggregating long-range context across the full window into a compact representation that guides the decoder.

- **Decoder:** upsamples using nearest-neighbor interpolation and concatenates corresponding encoder features (skip connections) to recover fine-grained detail.

Each encoder and decoder stage uses the same lightweight block:

- **Convolutional block:** two Conv1D layers (kernel size 3) with ReLU and batch normalization [16].
- **CPCA attention:** appended at the end of each block to adaptively reweight channels using a squeeze-and-excitation style mechanism [3,10,23].

All convolutions use same-length padding, preserving temporal resolution within each scale and ensuring alignment for skip concatenation. Model capacity is controlled by the base number of channels in the first stage; we evaluate multiple widths in an ablation study in the Results section. Inputs are provided in channel-first form as $X \in \mathbb{R}^{B\times 1\times T}$, and the network outputs a time-aligned ABP estimate $\hat{Y} \in \mathbb{R}^{B\times 1\times T}$ for each window.Here, $B$ is the batch size, $T$ is the window length (samples), and $t$ indexes time. For window-level reporting, SBP/DBP are computed from the predicted waveform extrema, consistent with prior PPG→ABP reconstruction work [3,4,14]:

$$\widehat{\mathrm{SBP}} = \max_{t\in[1,T]} \hat{y}_t, \qquad \widehat{\mathrm{DBP}} = \min_{t\in[1,T]} \hat{y}_t. \tag{1}$$

## 4 Morphology-Aware Loss

Pointwise MAE/MSE can under-emphasize high-dynamic windows, which are critical for preserving ABP amplitude and extrema-derived SBP/DBP [4,14]. We combine a range-weighted SmoothL1 base loss with a window-range regularizer.

*Range-Weighted SmoothL1.* For window $b$, let $r_b = \max(Y_b) - \min(Y_b)$ and $\bar{r} = \frac{1}{B}\sum_{j=1}^{B} r_j$. We compute a detached importance weight

$$w_b = \frac{r_b}{\bar{r}+\epsilon}, \qquad w_b \leftarrow \min(w_b, w_{\max}), \tag{2}$$

and minimize

$$\mathcal{L}_{\text{base}} = \frac{1}{B}\sum_{b=1}^{B} w_b\,\mathrm{SmoothL1}_{\beta}(\hat{Y}_b, Y_b), \tag{3}$$

where $\mathrm{SmoothL1}_{\beta}(\hat{Y}_b, Y_b)$ [13] denotes the mean over time samples in the window. Here $\epsilon$ ensures numerical stability (e.g., $r_b{\approx}0$), and $w_{\max} \in [3,5]$ prevents rare high-range windows from dominating updates.

*Units.* Losses are computed on min–max normalized ABP, while metrics are reported in mmHg after inverse scaling; thus $\delta$ is in normalized units (mmHg equivalent: $\delta\,(y_{\max} - y_{\min})$).

*Range Regularizer.* To preserve within-window amplitude, after trimming $\tau$ samples at both ends we define $\Delta R_b = (\max \hat{y}_b - \min \hat{y}_b) - (\max y_b - \min y_b)$ (over the trimmed interval) and penalize under/over-shoot beyond margin $\delta$ via a smooth gate:

$$\mathcal{L}_{\text{AR}} = \frac{1}{B}\sum_{b=1}^{B}\Big(\sigma(s(-\Delta R_b - \delta))\,\text{ReLU}(-\Delta R_b)^2 + \sigma(s(\Delta R_b - \delta))\,\text{ReLU}(\Delta R_b)^2\Big), \tag{4}$$

where $\sigma(z) = 1/(1+e^{-z})$ and $s > 0$ controls gate steepness.

*Overall.*

$$\mathcal{L} = \mathcal{L}_{\text{base}} + \lambda_{\text{AR}}\mathcal{L}_{\text{AR}}. \tag{5}$$

*Hyperparameters.* Unless stated otherwise, we set SmoothL1 $\beta = 1.0$, $\epsilon = 10^{-6}$, $w_{\max} = 5$, and trim $\tau = 10$ samples per side; the range regularizer uses $\delta = 0.01$ and gate slope $s = 10$. [1]

## 5 Data and Training Protocol

We use the widely used UCI dataset, derived from the MIMIC Waveform Database [8,15,21]. It contains synchronized PPG and invasive ABP sampled at 125 Hz (12,000 records from 942 subjects), segmented into 10 s windows ($T$=1250).

Records are stored contiguously per subject; to prevent leakage, we split at the subject level by treating each subject's block as indivisible. We keep a fixed 25% held-out test split(random seed) and run 5-fold cross-validation on the remaining 75% for model selection(per fold: 60% train, 15% validation, 25% test); after choosing hyperparameters, we retrain on the full 75% and evaluate once on the test set.

Preprocessing includes edge trimming and a 4th-order Butterworth bandpass (0.1–30 Hz) with zero-phase filtering. We apply global min–max normalization separately for PPG and ABP; extrema are computed on each fold's training split and applied to its validation data, and for the final model computed on the full 75% pool and reused for the test set.

Models are implemented in PyTorch and trained on an RTX 3060 using batch size $B$=256 and Adam (lr $10^{-3}$, weight decay $10^{-5}$) for up to 150 epochs with early stopping on validation SBP/DBP MAE (patience 10) and ReduceLROnPlateau (factor 0.5). We set $\lambda_{\text{AR}}$=0.6, $w_{\max}$=5, and $\epsilon$=$10^{-6}$.

## 6 Results

### 6.1 Ablation Study

We ablate two axes: model capacity (base width $C$) and objective design (morphology-aware loss). We first sweep $C$ under a fixed protocol, then fix the chosen width for loss ablations to isolate objective effects. All runs share identical splits, preprocessing, optimization, and metrics.

*Architecture Ablation (Table 1).* We vary only the base channel width $C$. Increasing capacity from $C$=32 (prior work [3]) to $C$=72 clearly reduces SBP/DBP MAE, while $C$=86 yields only marginal gains at much higher cost. We therefore use $C$=72 for the best accuracy and size trade-off.

**Table 1.** Channel-width with MSE loss ablation

| Base channels ($C$) | Params (M) | Model size (MB) | SBP/DBP MAE (mmHg) |
|---|---|---|---|
| 32 | 2.58 | 9.54 | 4.92/2.97 |
| 48 | 5.63 | 21.46 | 4.41/3.09 |
| 72 | 12.66 | 48.31 | **3.86/2.38** |
| 86 | 18.06 | **68.89** | 3.78/2.26 |

*Loss Ablation (Table 2).* On fixed architecture ($C$ = 72), range-weighted SmoothL1 ($\mathcal{L}_{\text{base}}$) outperforms MSE on waveform and BP errors. Adding $\mathcal{L}_{\text{AR}}$ gives further gains, peaking at $\lambda_{\text{AR}}$ = 0.6; higher values cause slight over-regularization.

**Table 2.** Loss ablation. $\mathcal{L}_{\text{base}}$: range-weighted SmoothL1; $\mathcal{L}_{\text{AR}}$: range regularizer. Wave: MAE/RMSE; SBP/DBP from ABP extrema (mmHg). Improvement is the average relative error reduction versus pure MSE across Wave MAE, Wave RMSE, SBP MAE, and DBP MAE.

| Loss setting | $\lambda_{\text{AR}}$ | Wave (MAE/RMSE) | SBP MAE | DBP MAE | Improvement vs. MSE |
|---|---|---|---|---|---|
| MSE (`MSELoss`) | 0.0 | 4.68 / 6.97 | 3.86 | 2.38 | – |
| $\mathcal{L}_{\text{base}}$ | 0.0 | 4.37 / 6.69 | 3.51 | 2.19 | +6.9% |
| $\mathcal{L}_{\text{base}} + \lambda_{\text{AR}}\mathcal{L}_{\text{AR}}$ | 0.2 | 4.09 / 6.51 | 3.17 | 1.95 | +13.8% |
| $\mathcal{L}_{\text{base}} + \lambda_{\text{AR}}\mathcal{L}_{\text{AR}}$ | 0.4 | 3.67 / 6.27 | 2.78 | 1.70 | +22.0% |
| $\mathcal{L}_{\text{base}} + \lambda_{\text{AR}}\mathcal{L}_{\text{AR}}$ | **0.6** | **3.13 / 6.02** | **2.46** | **1.46** | **+30.4%** |
| $\mathcal{L}_{\text{base}} + \lambda_{\text{AR}}\mathcal{L}_{\text{AR}}$ | 0.8 | 3.16 / 6.05 | 2.52 | 1.48 | +29.6% |

### 6.2 Metrics and Clinical Result

Across the held-out test set, the proposed model achieves low waveform reconstruction error and strong clinical agreement when BP values are extracted from predicted ABP extrema. The errors derived from extrema are small and near-unbiased: SBP MAE is 2.46 mmHg (mean error −0.37 mmHg, SD 4.38 mmHg) and DBP MAE is 1.46 mmHg (mean error −0.07 mmHg, SD 3.63 mmHg), with error histograms tightly centered around zero (Fig. 3). Predicted-versus-true scatter plots further confirm strong agreement with the identity line, with high correlation for both DBP ($R = 0.949$, MAE 1.46 mmHg) and SBP ($R = 0.965$, MAE 2.46 mmHg) over $n$ = 27,260 windows (Fig. 2a, Fig. 2b). Bland–Altman analysis shows near-zero bias and tight limits of agreement for both SBP and DBP, with no evident proportional bias across the pressure range (Fig. 4) . Finally, using established medical standards (AAMI and BHS), our evaluation (Table 4) meets AAMI mean/SD requirements for both SBP and DBP and achieves BHS Grade A for both pressures. Errors are near-unbiased with variability within AAMI limits, and the BHS threshold criteria are satisfied across the standard tolerance bands.

### 6.3 Comparison to State-of-the-Art

Table 3 compares representative cuffless BP methods while highlighting key comparability factors. ExpertoRhythm achieves 2.46/1.46 mmHg SBP/DBP MAE using a single raw PPG channel, improving over widely used UCI baselines such as Dual-DS-U-Net [14] and ResNet34 [19] and remaining competitive with recent sequence models [7]. Several strong results rely on richer representations (e.g., PPG+STFT [25]) or additional derived inputs (PPG/VPG/APG [18]), whereas our gains are achieved under a minimal sensing constraint by optimizing for peak-sensitive morphology via a composite loss. Notably, U-Net+BiLSTM [18] reports SBP/DBP errors close to ours, but it is evaluated on a substantially smaller subset (150 records versus 12,000), which can materially affect difficulty and comparability. The MIMIC-III entries also suggest that accuracy depends strongly on modality and preprocessing (e.g., ECG+PPG or engineered features [22]), motivating PPG-only methods that better preserve waveform structure.

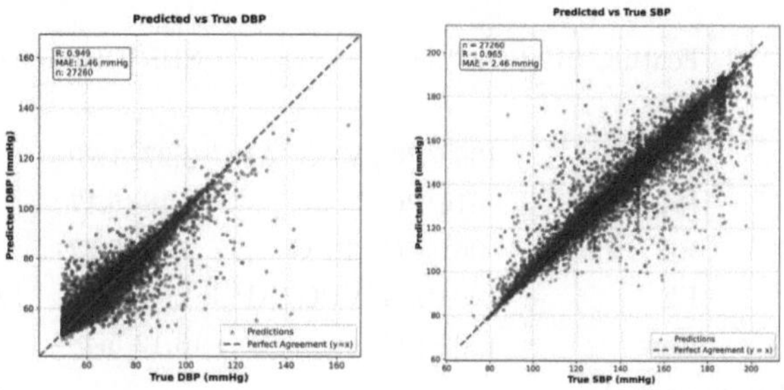


**(a)** DBP **(b)** SBP

**Fig. 2.** Predicted versus reference blood pressure on the test set. The dashed line indicates the identity line.

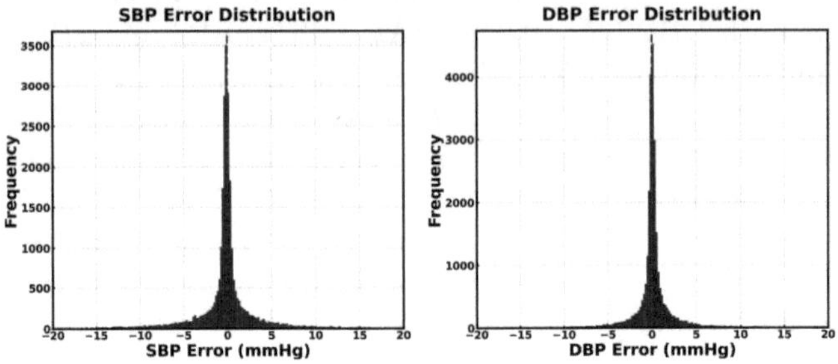


**Fig. 3.** Error distributions for SBP and DBP on the test set.

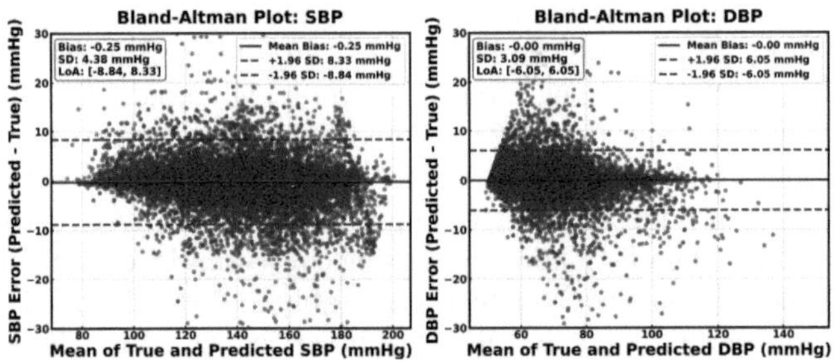


**Fig. 4.** Bland–Altman plots for SBP/DBP. Solid: mean bias; dashed: 95% LoA (mean $\pm 1.96$ SD).

**Table 3.** Comparison of cuffless BP estimation models. ND = not disclosed.

| Model | Feature | #Patients | Input | SBP | DBP | Records | Comp. Loss |
|---|---|---|---|---|---|---|---|
| **MIMIC-III** | | | | | | | |
| ABP-Net [5] | Raw | 106 | PPG/VPG/APG | 3.27 | 1.90 | ND | Yes |
| ArterialNet [12] | Raw | 61 | PPG | 4.18 | 5.17 | ND | Yes |
| Ensemble_NN [22] | FE | 96 | ECG+PPG | 3.74 | 2.22 | ND | Yes |
| MLR [17] | FE | 109 | PPG/VPG/APG | 4.59 | 2.47 | 12000 | No |
| Residual U-Net [6] | Raw | 120 | PPG | 13.12 | 5.48 | ND | Yes |
| **UCI(MIMIC-II extension)** | | | | | | | |
| Dual-DS-U-Net [14] | Raw | 942 | PPG | 5.73 | 3.45 | 12000 | No |
| Transformer [7] | Raw | 942 | PPG | 2.97 | 1.60 | 12000 | No |
| LSTM autoenc. [9] | Raw | 942 | PPG | 4.05 | 2.41 | 5289 | No |
| MCAFNet [25] | Freq | 942 | PPG+STFT | 2.48 | 1.29 | ND | No |
| ResNet34 [19] | Raw | 942 | PPG | 5.98 | 3.24 | 12000 | No |
| U-Net+BiLSTM [18] | Raw | ND | PPG/VPG/APG | 2.48 | 1.42 | 150 | Yes |
| ExpertoRhythm (ours) | Raw | 942 | PPG | 2.46 | 1.46 | 12000 | Yes |

**Table 4.** Clinical evaluation under AAMI and BHS.

| Metric | SBP | | | DBP | | |
|---|---|---|---|---|---|---|
| | Val. | Crit. | Res. | Val. | Crit. | Res. |
| **AAMI** | | | | | | |
| ME (mmHg) | -0.36 | $\leq 5$ | PASS | -0.07 | $\leq 5$ | PASS |
| SD (mmHg) | 4.38 | $\leq 8$ | PASS | 3.63 | $\leq 8$ | PASS |
| AAMI overall | **PASS** | | | **PASS** | | |
| **BHS** | | | | | | |
| $\leq \pm 5$ (%) | 87.2 | $\geq 60$ | A | 93.3 | $\geq 60$ | A |
| $\leq \pm 10$ (%) | 94.6 | $\geq 85$ | A | 97.6 | $\geq 85$ | A |
| $\leq \pm 15$ (%) | 96.9 | $\geq 95$ | A | 98.9 | $\geq 95$ | A |
| BHS grade | **A** | | | **A** | | |

## 7 Discussion and Conclusion

The results highlight two practical drivers of performance: model capacity and objective alignment. The channel-width sweep (Table 1) shows that increasing width improves SBP/DBP accuracy up to a moderate setting, after which gains saturate. Holding architecture fixed, the loss ablation (Table 2) demonstrates that the proposed morphology-aware objective consistently reduces SBP/DBP error by improving amplitude precise waveform reconstruction, rather than relying on architectural scaling alone. Further analyses support clinical credibility under established medical evaluation standards (Table 4). Overall, ExpertoRhythm shows that the waveform can be recovered from a single PPG channel when the training objective is designed to preserve it, achieving strong accuracy and meeting clinical grade criteria. A remaining limitation is deployability: wearable use requires low-latency, energy-efficient edge inference. Future work will report efficiency metrics (latency, memory, compute/energy proxies) and study deployment-oriented optimization, including quantization and hybrid mixtures-of-experts for dynamic compute. Also we will validate ExpertoRhythm on MIMIC-III, MIMIC-IV, and wearable-acquired PPG datasets to assess cross-dataset generalizability using consistent subject-level protocols.

**Acknowledgements.** Funding for this research was provided by ResearchNB through the Academic Start-up Fund, formerly the Talent Recruitment Fund program (TRF_2025_005). The authors gratefully acknowledge this support.

**Data Availability Statement.** The source code used in this study is available at: https://github.com/amirarjmand93/aime2026_loss_function.

## References

1. Smoothl1loss — pytorch documentation. https://docs.pytorch.org/docs/stable/generated/torch.nn.SmoothL1Loss.html. Accessed 29 Jan 2026
2. Arjomand, A., Boudesh, A., Bayatmakou, F., Kent, K.B., Mohammadi, A.: Transforhythm: a transformer architecture conductive to blood pressure estimation via solo ppg signal capturing (2024). arXiv:2404.15352
3. Arjomand, A., Kent, K.B., Krylov, G.: Lightweight 1d unet-cpca regression model for energy-efficient blood pressure estimation from raw PPG signals. In: Proceedings of the 36th International Workshop on Rapid System Prototyping (RSP '25). Taipei, Taiwan (2025). https://doi.org/10.1145/3768617.3770734
4. Athaya, T., Choi, S.: An estimation method of continuous non-invasive arterial blood pressure waveform using photoplethysmography: a U-Net architecture-based approach. Sensors **21**(5), 1867 (2021). https://doi.org/10.3390/s21051867
5. Cheng, J., et al.: Prediction of arterial blood pressure waveforms from photoplethysmogram signals via fully convolutional neural networks. Comput. Biol. Med. **138**, 104877 (2021). https://doi.org/10.1016/j.compbiomed.2021.104877
6. De Palma, L., Andria, G., Attivissimo, F., Lanzolla, A.M.L., Di Nisio, A.: Enhancing ABP estimation through comprehensive ppg signal analysis and advanced loss function optimization. Measurement 118210 (2025)
7. Fan, C., Wei, Y., Qiu, M., Haghi, M., TaheriNejad, N.: Dual-path cuffless PPG-based blood pressure estimation using conformer and swin transformer. IEEE J. Biomed. Health Inform. **29**(12), 8695–8702 (2025)
8. Goldberger, A.L., et al.: Physiobank, physiotoolkit, and physionet: components of a new research resource for complex physiologic signals. Circulation **101**(23), e215–e220 (2000). https://doi.org/10.1161/01.CIR.101.23.e215
9. Harfiya, L.N., Chang, C.C., Li, Y.H.: Continuous blood pressure estimation using exclusively photoplethysmography by LSTM-based signal-to-signal translation. Sensors **21**(9), 2952 (2021)
10. Hu, J., Shen, L., Sun, G.: Squeeze-and-excitation networks. In: Proceedings of the IEEE Conference on Computer Vision and Pattern Recognition (CVPR), pp. 7132–7141 (2018)
11. Huang, H., Chen, Z., Zou, Y., et al.: Channel prior convolutional attention for medical image segmentation. Comput. Biol. Med. **178**, 108784 (2024)
12. Huang, S., Jafari, R., Mortazavi, B.J.: ArterialNet: reconstructing arterial blood pressure waveform with wearable pulsatile signals, a cohort-aware approach. IEEE Open J. Eng. Med. Biol. (2025)
13. Huber, P.J.: Robust estimation of a location parameter. Ann. Math. Stat. **35**(1), 73–101 (1964). https://doi.org/10.1214/aoms/1177703732
14. Ibtehaz, N., Rahman, M.S.: PPG2ABP: translating photoplethysmogram (PPG) signals to arterial blood pressure (ABP) waveforms using fully convolutional neural networks (2020). arXiv:2005.01669
15. Kachuee, M., Kiani, M.M., Mohammadzade, H., Shabany, M.: Cuff-less high-accuracy calibration-free blood pressure estimation using pulse transit time. In: IEEE International Symposium on Circuits and Systems (ISCAS), pp. 1006–1009. IEEE (2015)
16. Kiranyaz, S.: 1D convolutional neural networks and applications: a survey. Mech. Syst. Signal Process. **151**, 107398 (2021)
17. Lin, W.H., et al.: Towards accurate estimation of cuffless and continuous blood pressure using multi-order derivative and multivariate photoplethysmogram features. Biomed. Signal Process. Control **63**, 102198 (2021)

18. Pan, J., et al.: Robust modelling of arterial blood pressure reconstruction from photoplethysmography. Sci. Rep. **14**(1), 30333 (2024). https://doi.org/10.1038/s41598-024-82026-1
19. Qin, C., Li, Y., Liu, C., Ma, X.: Cuff-less blood pressure prediction based on photoplethysmography and modified resnet. Bioengineering **10**(4), 400 (2023)
20. Ronneberger, O., Fischer, P., Brox, T.: U-Net: convolutional networks for biomedical image segmentation. In: Medical Image Computing and Computer-Assisted Intervention (MICCAI), pp. 234–241. Springer (2015)
21. Saeed, M., et al.: Multiparameter intelligent monitoring in intensive care II (mimic-II): a public-access ICU database. Crit. Care Med. **39**(5), 952–960 (2011)
22. Shen, Z., et al.: Uncertainty quantification of cuffless blood pressure estimation based on parameterized model evidential ensemble learning. Biomed. Signal Process. Control **92**, 106104 (2024). https://doi.org/10.1016/j.bspc.2024.106104
23. Si, Y., et al.: SCSA: exploring the synergistic effects between spatial and channel attention. Neurocomputing **634**, 129866 (2025)
24. Stoller, D., Ewert, S., Dixon, S.: Wave-U-Net: a multi-scale neural network for end-to-end audio source separation (2018). arXiv:1806.03185 arXiv preprint
25. Tian, Z., Liu, A., Chen, J., Wang, D., Chen, X.: Ppg-based continuous arterial blood pressure estimation via multi-scale cross attention fusion. Biomed. Signal Process. Control **113**, 108833 (2026). https://doi.org/10.1016/j.bspc.2025.108833

# Phenotypic Profile of Subclinical Alcohol Use Disorder and Liver Cancer in Type 2 Diabetes

Melissa Larbi[1(✉)], Edouard Audit[1], Joel Chavas[2], Simplice Donfack[1,3], and Vincent Mallet[4]

[1] Université Paris-Saclay, UVSQ, CNRS, CEA, Maison de la Simulation, 91191 Gif-sur-Yvette, France
melissa.larbi0207@gmail.com
[2] Université Paris-Saclay, CEA, Neurospin, 91191 Gif-sur-Yvette, France
[3] IDRIS, 91403 Orsay, France
[4] Université Paris Cité, AP-HP.Centre Université Paris Centre, Groupe Hospitalier Cochin Port Royal, DMU Cancérologie et spécialités médico-chirurgicales, Service d'Hépatologie, Paris, France

**Abstract.** Hepatocellular carcinoma (HCC) incidence is rising alongside the global type 2 diabetes (T2D) pandemic, with alcohol use disorder (AUD) as a major risk factor. However, a substantial population with undiagnosed subclinical AUD (sAUD) remains overlooked in current estimates. Using XGBoost and One-Class SVM, we identified hidden sAUD populations whose clinical profiles resemble those of diagnosed AUD patients, suggesting that the alcohol-related burden of HCC in T2D patients may be underestimated by 10–30%. Beyond prevalence, the two identified populations exhibit distinct phenotypes reflecting different pathways to HCC. XGBoost-identified sAUD patients are primarily characterized by advanced liver disease and cirrhosis, a common HCC precursor, while One-Class SVM identifies a subgroup concentrated around metabolic syndrome risk factors, a particularly relevant target for prevention and monitoring. Finally, gender-stratified analyses reveal sex-specific detection biases, with models performing substantially better in men than in women. We examine the sources of these biases and propose methodological strategies to mitigate them.

**Keywords:** XGBoost · One-Class SVM · Bias mitigation · subclinical alcohol detection · type 2 diabetes · hepatocellular carcinoma · phenotypic characterization

## 1 Introduction

The global rise in type 2 diabetes (T2D), obesity, and alcohol consumption contributes to the increasing incidence of hepatocellular carcinoma (HCC), the third leading cause of cancer-related deaths. Alcohol use disorder (AUD) is a major

© The Author(s), under exclusive license to Springer Nature Switzerland AG 2027
P. Andreev et al. (Eds.): AIME 2026, LNAI 16748, pp. 334–339, 2027.
https://doi.org/10.1007/978-3-032-30710-1_40

contributor [2], yet a significant proportion of AUD cases remain underdiagnosed, hidden within non-AUD cohorts. This group, known as subclinical AUD (sAUD), shares clinical profiles similar to diagnosed AUD patients and exhibits high HCC prevalence. Identifying sAUD early is crucial for timely intervention and more accurate quantification of alcohol-related HCC risk. In a previous work [1], we identified an sAUD population within a nationwide cohort of 2.8 million T2D patients, suggesting that alcohol-related HCC burden could be up to 30% higher than current estimates. The present study builds on this work, focusing on improving sAUD detection by reducing gender bias and characterizing the clinical profiles of the identified sAUD populations.

**Dataset and Methodology Overview.** This study uses data from the French National Hospital Discharge database, covering 2,755,292 anonymized T2D patients followed from 2011 to 2020. Among them, 0.59% developed HCC recorded from 2013 onward. The analysis focuses on 21 variables per patient, with the target variable being alcohol use disorder (AUD). Of the cohort, 7.3% were diagnosed with AUD, while 92.7% were non-AUD, with subclinical AUD (sAUD) hidden within the non-AUD group. To capture complementary perspectives on sAUD detection, we used both unsupervised (One-Class SVM) and supervised (XGBoost) models. The One-Class SVM (SVM) was trained solely on AUD patients to define an AUD boundary, while XGBoost(XGB) was trained on both AUD and non-AUD data. Both models were optimized via bootstrap sampling ($B = 6$) and hyperparameter tuning to maximize AUC. After training, models were applied to the non-AUD population providing a score (probability for XGB, distance for SVM) for each patient. A threshold was then selected to define the sAUD subgroup based on minimizing the Wasserstein distance (WD) between the sAUD and AUD age distribution at HCC onset (AHO). An overview of the used models and their performances is provided in Table 1.

## 2 Gender Differences in Models' Performance

To evaluate the baseline models named $\text{XGB}_{m0}$ and $\text{SVM}_{m0}$ across demographic subgroups, we examined their performance separately for men and women.

For $\text{XGB}_{m0}$, the TPR was lower for women (0.48) compared to men (0.66), missing nearly half of female AUD cases. $\text{SVM}_{m0}$ showed high sensitivity for both sexes but with low specificity, especially in women. Stratification by sex $\text{XGB}_{m0}$ identified more sAUD men (0.44%) than women (0.04%), while $\text{SVM}_{m0}$ detected more sAUD in women (0.47%) than men (0.11%), with higher HCC prevalence in men (83.4%) than in women (9.8%).

The AHO analysis shows better alignment between sAUD and AUD in men, while poor alignment is seen in women as showen in Fig. 1. These results underscore pronounced gender-related disparities in model performance, highlighting the need for targeted strategies to improve sAUD detection in women.

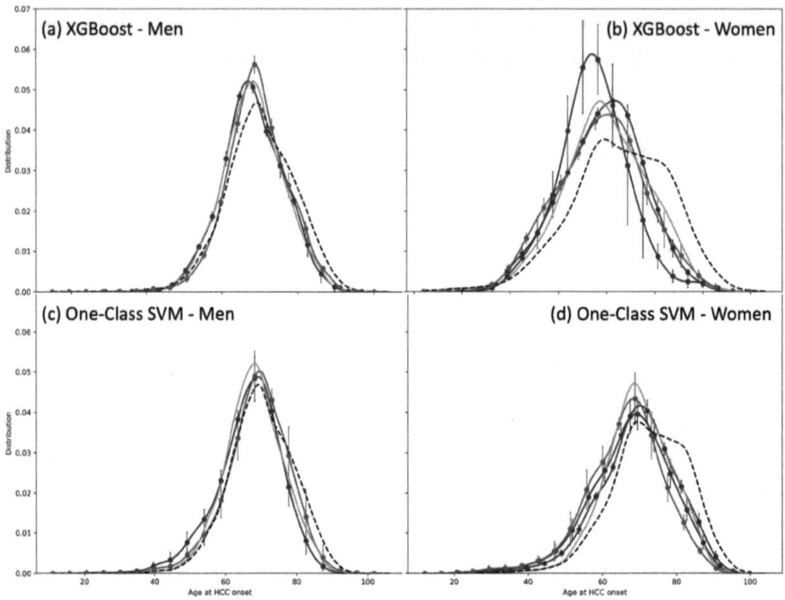


**Fig. 1.** Model variants across algorithms and sex. Each panel shows the full population in black, AUD in yellow, sAUD populations identified by the model variants: m0 in blue, m0_wa in purple and the gender-specific models in red. (Color figure online)

## 3 Strategies to Address Gender Performance Gaps

This section explores strategies to refine the models and better align sAUD and AUD populations in AHO distributions, especially in female patients.

**Sex Adapted Threshold**: In this approach, we retain the trained $m0$ models but adopt a sex-specific thresholds, re-estimating them separately for males and females to better align the sAUD and AUD AHO distributions. For men, the adapted models perform similarly to the original ones due to the larger male data volume. However, for women, the adapted models ($\text{XGB}_{m0\_wa}$ and $\text{SVM}_{m0\_wa}$) show improved identification of female sAUD cases and better alignment of AHO distributions. With $\text{XGB}_{m0\_wa}$, the proportion of identified female sAUD cases increased (0.10% vs 0.04% with $\text{XGB}_{m0}$), along with a higher HCC prevalence (20.2% vs 17.1%). The alignment with true female AUD cases also improved, as shown in Fig. 1 and by reduction in WD from 2.88 to 0.69. A similar improvement was observed with $\text{SVM}_{m0\_wa}$, which identified nearly five times more female sAUD cases (2.46% vs 0.47%) and showed better alignment of HCC density distributions, with a reduction in WD from 2.18 to 1.11.

**Gender-Specific Models**: To further reduce sex-related biases, separate XGB and SVM models were trained exclusively on male or female patients.

XGB gender-specific models maintained overall classification performance while significantly improving the alignment with true AUD populations. The unified model showed good alignment for men (WD=0.37), but poor alignment for women (WD= 2.88). Gender-specific models improved this (1.19 for men, 1.23 for women), offering better sex-specific disease patterns. The $\text{XGB}_{men}$ model identified more at-risk men (1.01%) with a lower HCC prevalence (19.38%), indicating broader risk detection. The $\text{XGB}_{women}$ model increased identification rates (0.10% vs. 0.04%) while maintaining a clinically plausible HCC prevalence (21.29%). For SVM, gender-specific training showed mixed results. While it improved classification balance, alignment improvements were inconsistent. For men, $\text{SVM}_{men}$ showed moderate alignment with true AUD AHO (WD=1.76), better than the baseline (1.93). For women, however, the model $\text{SVM}_{women}$ had the worst alignment (WD=3.58), despite identifying 0.22% of female cases with HCC prevalence of 21.90%. This suggests challenges in capturing female-specific disease patterns due to the limited number of female AUD cases (20%).

Overall, gender-specific XGB outperformed SVM in sex-specific AUD modeling, achieving better fairness, distributional consistency, and clinically meaningful results. For men, the best model was $\text{XGB}_{m0}$, while for women, adapted models improved performance, with $\text{XGB}_{m0\_wa}$ leading, followed by $\text{SVM}_{m0\_wa}$ and $\text{XGB}_{women}$. These findings underscore the importance of gender-tailored models in effectively identifying sAUD.

**Table 1.** Overview of the models used for sAUD identification across genders

| Model | Gender | % sAUD over non-AUD | sAUD's HCC prevalence (%) | Wasserstein Distance | Description |
|---|---|---|---|---|---|
| $\text{XGB}_{m0}$ | Men | 0.44±0.21 | 23.60±4.50 | 0.35±0.15 | trained on both sexes' data; threshold |
| | Women | 0.04±0.02 | 17.05±5.50 | 2.88±1.05 | |
| $\text{SVM}_{m0}$ | Men | 0.11±0.09 | 83.41±10.08 | 1.93±0.99 | selected on the full dataset. |
| | Women | 0.47±0.21 | 9.77±2.76 | 2.18±1.24 | |
| $\text{XGB}_{m0\_wa}$ | Women | 0.10±0.02 | 20.17±5.62 | 0.69±0.15 | trained on the full dataset with |
| $\text{SVM}_{m0\_wa}$ | | 2.46±2.22 | 7.11±6.17 | 1.11±0.46 | an adapted threshold for female sAUD. |
| $\text{XGB}_{men}$ | Men | 1.01±0.11 | 19.38±0.40 | 1.19±0.38 | trained and threshold selected |
| $\text{SVM}_{men}$ | | 0.59±0.10 | 26.07±10.93 | 1.76±1.37 | on the men data only |
| $\text{XGB}_{women}$ | Women | 0.10±0.01 | 21.29 ±2.90 | 1.23±0.5 | trained and threshold selected |
| $\text{SVM}_{women}$ | | 0.22±0.08 | 21.90±2.65 | 3.58±1.98 | on the women data only |

## 4 Clinical Profiles of Identified sAUD Populations

To better assess the clinical profiles of sAUD populations identified by each model, we analyzed the prevalence of key comorbidities and risk factors across model variants (Table 1). This helps determine if the models capture clinically coherent subgroups and how closely these profiles resemble the known AUD.

XGB models predominantly identified patients with advanced liver disease, with extremely high cirrhosis prevalence and elevated rates of viral hepatitis and other liver conditions. This suggests detection of late-stage, undiagnosed AUD, consistent with the high HCC prevalence observed. In contrast, SVM models captured a distinct subgroup characterized by metabolic and cardiovascular comorbidities, including very high rates of obesity, hyperlipidemia, hypertension, and smoking, indicating a metabolically driven sAUD phenotype. Additional differences in smoking and non-liver risk factors further reinforce this distinction. Despite these contrasts, all models preserved socioeconomic patterns similar to true AUD populations, with slight concentration in more deprived groups.

Overall, these results highlight two complementary sAUD phenotypes: a liver-disease-driven profile by XGB and a metabolic-risk-driven profile by SVM (Fig. 2).

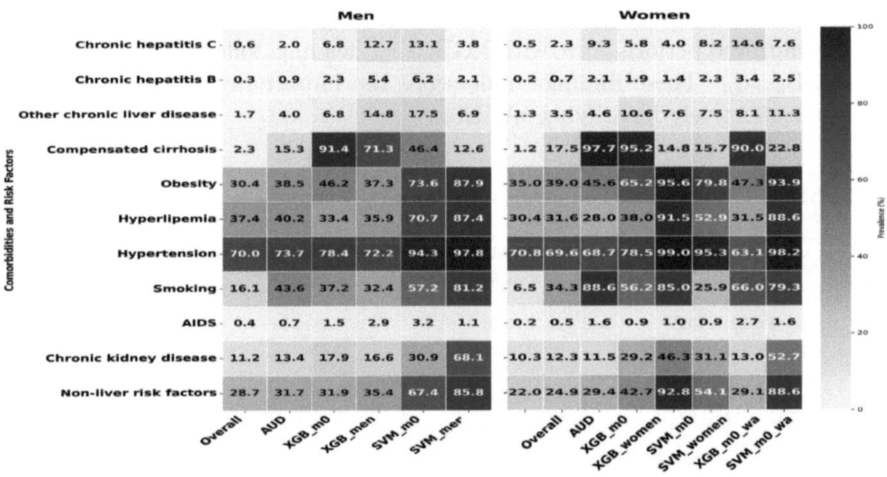


**Fig. 2.** Prevalence of key comorbidities and risk factors across models and sex.

## 5 Conclusions

This study shows that machine learning models can effectively identify subclinical AUD (sAUD) in T2D patients, revealing hidden alcohol-related risk that may increase the HCC burden by 10–30%. The analysis highlights strong sex-related differences in alcohol-related behaviors and clinical consequences, with models performing better in men, while female profiles are less well captured without sex-specific adaptations.

The study also shows that the sAUD population is heterogeneous, with two distinct clinical phenotypes: one linked to advanced liver disease and the other to metabolic syndrome. XGB and SVM capture these phenotypes differently, offering complementary insights into the underlying risk structures of HCC.

A more comprehensive evaluation of alcohol-related HCC burden could benefit from integrating both phenotypes. Further clinical research is needed to explore their relevance for patient monitoring, prevention, and epidemiology.

## References

1. Larbi, M., et al.: AI-Driven identification of subclinical alcohol use disorder in type 2 diabetes patients. In: International Conference on Artificial Intelligence in Medicine, pp. 218-223. Springer, Cham (2025)
2. Mallet, V., et al.: Burden of liver disease progression in hospitalized patients with type 2 diabetes mellitus. J. Hepatology **76**(2), 265–274 (2022)

# Gradient-Based Counterfactual Optimization for Kidney Transplant Allocation Using Gumbel-Softmax Relaxation

Syed Asil Ali Naqvi[1(✉)], Karthik Tennankore[2], Amanda Vinson[2], George Worthen[2], and Syed Sibte Raza Abidi[1]

[1] NICHE Research Group, Dalhousie University, Halifax, Nova Scotia, Canada
a.naqvi@dal.ca

[2] Division of Nephrology, Department of Medicine, Dalhousie University, Halifax, Nova Scotia, Canada

**Abstract.** Kidney transplantation (KT) remains the optimal treatment for end-stage renal disease, yet severe organ scarcity necessitates maximally efficient donor-recipient matching (DRM) strategies. Current allocation systems rely on rule-based scoring mechanisms that cannot predict individualized treatment effects (ITE) for specific donor-recipient combinations. Moreover, transplant registries exhibit substantial systematic biases from allocation policies that introduce confounding, which standard machine learning models tend to reproduce rather than correct. This paper addresses the challenge of transforming counterfactual treatment estimation into counterfactual treatment optimization for DRM in KT. Building on our Confounding-Adjusted Model (CAM) for predicting outcomes of alternative donor-recipient pairings, this work introduces a specialized search strategy to identify optimal matches from a high-dimensional treatment space. We leverage gradient-based optimization combined with Logit masking and Gumbel-Softmax relaxation techniques to efficiently identify the optimal counterfactual recipients for a given donor ensuring that the recommendations satisfy clinical donor-recipient compatibility criterion. Applied to a comprehensive dataset of 186,000 kidney transplants from the Scientific Registry of Transplant Recipients (2000–2023), our framework demonstrates substantial improvements over baseline prediction models with nearest-neighbor retrieval validation revealing that our counterfactual optimization corresponds to 394 additional days of observed post-transplant survival ($p < 0.001$).

**Keywords:** Machine Learning · Causal Inference · Counterfactual Optimization · Kidney Transplantation

## 1 Introduction

Kidney transplantation remains the optimal treatment for kidney failure, yet organ scarcity, (acknowledging that there are approximately 90,000 patients awaiting a transplant but only 25,000 kidneys available annually in the United States), demands maximally efficient donor-recipient matching (DRM) strategies [1, 2]. Current DRM systems rely primarily on rule-based scoring mechanisms such as the Kidney Donor Profile

© The Author(s), under exclusive license to Springer Nature Switzerland AG 2027
P. Andreev et al. (Eds.): AIME 2026, LNAI 16748, pp. 340–350, 2027.
https://doi.org/10.1007/978-3-032-30710-1_41

Index (KDPI) and Expected Post-Transplant Survival (EPTS), which stratify risk based on population-level associations but cannot predict individualized treatment effect (ITE) for specific donor-recipient combinations [3, 4].

Transplant registries exhibit substantial systematic biases arising from allocation policies that preferentially match high-quality organs with low-risk recipients ("best-to-best") while directing marginal organs to older, sicker patients [5–7]. These policy-driven patterns create confounding that standard ML models tend to reproduce rather than correct, leading to recommendations that appear optimal based on historical correlations but fail to maximize true biological utility [8–10].

In our previous work [11], we established a novel CAM learning pipeline reframing DRM as an ITE problem where donor organs are the units and recipients represent high-dimensional treatments. The CAM enables reliable counterfactual prediction, estimating what would happen under alternative donor-recipient pairings. For example, it might predict that matching Donor A with Recipient B would yield 1,800 days of post-transplant survival, while matching Donor A with Recipient C would yield 1,500 days. However, in the absence of an explicit recipient set (i.e., the waitlist), the CAM does not determine which recipient has a longer survival after receiving a kidney from Donor A. This gap between counterfactual estimation and counterfactual optimization represents the central challenge addressed in this work.

In binary treatment settings (e.g., drug vs. placebo), optimization is straightforward – compare two potential outcomes and select the larger. However, in our DRM setting, this problem is compounded by two fundamental challenges: (1) the treatment space is high-dimensional and discrete (recipient features such as blood type, age groups), making exhaustive evaluation computationally infeasible; and (2) clinical constraints (e.g., ABO blood type compatibility) must be strictly enforced throughout the optimization process. To the best of our knowledge, no existing counterfactual optimization methods can handle high-dimensional discrete treatment spaces with hard constraints.

In this paper, we present a counterfactual optimization framework to efficiently identify optimal donor-recipient matches from a learned causal model while satisfying all clinical compatibility constraints. The intent is to enable clinicians introspect counterfactual outcomes for any given donor and recipient pair to identify which recipients will most benefit from receiving a given donor kidney.

Given the high-dimensional and discrete nature of the recipient feature space exhaustive evaluation of all possible recipient profiles is computationally infeasible, necessitating an efficient search strategy. We introduce a gradient-based search strategy that leverages a learned CAM to explore the recipient space and rank counterfactual candidates by directly optimizing predicted survival outcomes, while enforcing biological compatibility constraints (Fig. 1). Our search strategy follows a gradient ascent optimization technique which iteratively updates the input space of a pre-trained neural network to maximize a specific objective function, such as a predicted outcome. However gradient ascent requires a differentiable (continuous) search space which is a problem in our case because recipient features are all discrete. To solve this, we use Gumbel-Softmax (GS) relaxation to transform that discrete, high-dimensional space into a continuous, differentiable approximation [12]. This allows gradient ascent to successfully navigate and optimize those high-dimensional recipient characteristics.

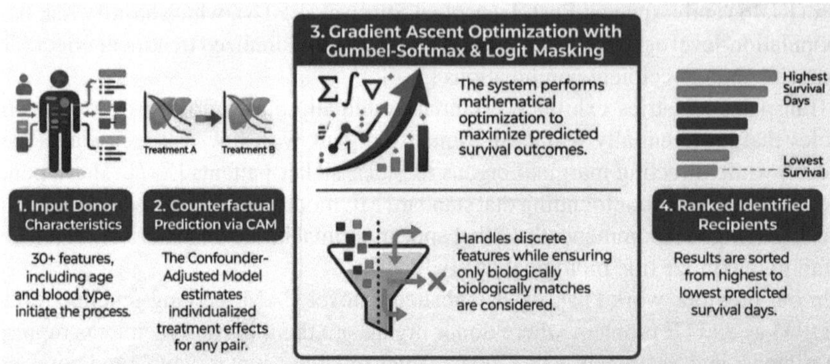


**Fig. 1.** Illustration of our counterfactual optimization approach.

Since this optimization can find any recipient that maximizes the survival outcome, a lot of biologically incompatible recipients can be found. To address that we incorporate a logit masking technique which ensures all generated recommendations satisfy biological compatibility requirement [13].

The remainder of this paper is organized as follows: Sect. 2 reviews related work on counterfactual treatment generation and optimization. Section 3 formalizes the optimization problem and establishes the challenge of discrete feature spaces. Section 4 details our GS methodology and constraint enforcement mechanisms. Section 5 presents the large-scale application to KT data, including implementation details, comprehensive evaluation. and in-depth case study analysis with clinical interpretation. Section 6 concludes with a discussion highlighting contributions, limitations and future directions.

## 2 Related Work

This section reviews key approaches to counterfactual optimization in an ITE problem. Early work on counterfactual optimization focused primarily on binary treatments where treatment with better outcome is selected [14–17]. Categorical treatments with multiple discrete options extend binary treatment methods to handle multiple treatment arms. Schwab et al. [18] introduced Perfect Match, a neural network framework that learns treatment-invariant representations and predicts outcomes for each treatment, selecting the one with the most favorable prediction.

When treatment is continuous (e.g., drug dosage, exercise duration, pollution levels), the problem becomes one of estimating dose-response functions and selecting optimal doses. This optimization problem is more challenging than the discrete case because we must search over a continuous space. Kallus et al. [19] proposed policy learning methods that parameterize treatment policies and optimize them using numerical methods such as L-BFGS. Similarly, SCIGAN [20] uses generative adversarial networks to estimate dose-response curves and applies SLSQP for optimization. However, these approaches are limited to low-dimensional continuous treatments and do not generalize well to constrained settings. A promising recent direction combines deep learning with constrained optimization for treatment selection. Schweisthal et al. [21] trains a policy neural network that predicts optimal dosage combinations by solving a constrained optimization problem using gradient descent-ascent. The optimization maximizes the estimated dose-response. Extending to high-dimensional treatments, where the treatment is characterized by dozens of interacting variables, requires fundamentally different optimization strategies, as the search space grows exponentially and current methods struggle with discrete categorical features. Gradient-based optimization approach provides an effective workaround for counterfactual optimization when treatment is continuous, high-dimensional and effectively handling constraints.

# 3 Problem Formulation

## 3.1 Data

This study used data from the Scientific Registry of Transplant Recipients (SRTR). The SRTR data system includes data on all donor, wait-listed candidates, and transplant recipients in the US, submitted by the members of the Organ Procurement and Transplantation Network (OPTN). The Health Resources and Services Administration (HRSA), U.S. Department of Health and Human Services provides oversight to the activities of the OPTN and SRTR contractors. The data reported here have been supplied by the Hennepin Healthcare Research Institute (HHRI) as the contractor for the Scientific Registry of Transplant Recipients (SRTR). The interpretation and reporting of these data are the responsibility of the author(s) and in no way should be seen as an official policy of or interpretation by the SRTR or the U.S. Government.

We used historical KT donor and recipient data (2000–2023) comprising 186,000 transplant instances. We also generated semi-synthetic data according to the approach detailed in our previous work [11]. The feature space is divided into two distinct categories:

- Donor Characteristics: This set comprises over 30 features, including demographics (age, sex, race), physiological metrics (BMI, blood pressure), organ quality indicators (e.g., serum creatinine), medical history, and critical biological markers such as ABO blood type and viral status
- Recipient Characteristics: Similarly defined by over 30 features, this set includes demographics, clinical status (dialysis vintage, panel reactive antibodies), functional scores, and comorbidities like diabetes or cardiovascular disease

The primary outcome measure is post-transplant graft survival time in days.

Following established preprocessing protocols from clinical literature, we discretized continuous variables into clinically meaningful categories and applied one-hot encoding. While optimizing over continuous features is mathematically efficient, our dataset contains numerous inherent categorical features that cannot be authentically transformed into a continuous space without losing their fundamental meaning. Conversely, converting continuous variables into discrete binary categories is not only possible but beneficial; it creates a uniform, high-dimensional space suitable for gradient-based optimization. This approach allows the model to maintain clinical interpretability by respecting the categorical boundaries, such as specific age brackets or lab result thresholds, familiar to medical practitioners.

### 3.2 Mathematical Framework

In our previous work [11], we adopted an organ-centric perspective where each available donor organ must be optimally allocated among potential recipients on the waitlist. For donor organ $\boldsymbol{o} \in \mathcal{O}$ and recipient $\boldsymbol{r} \in \mathcal{R}$, the CAM $\mu$ provides:

$$\mu(\boldsymbol{o}, \boldsymbol{r}) \rightarrow \hat{y},$$

where $\hat{y}$ represents predicted post-transplant survival (days). Given donor **o**, our objective is to identify the recipient profile **r*** that maximizes predicted outcomes:

$$\boldsymbol{r}^* = \underset{r \in \mathcal{R}}{\arg\max}\ \mu(\boldsymbol{o}, \boldsymbol{r})$$

## 4 Methodology

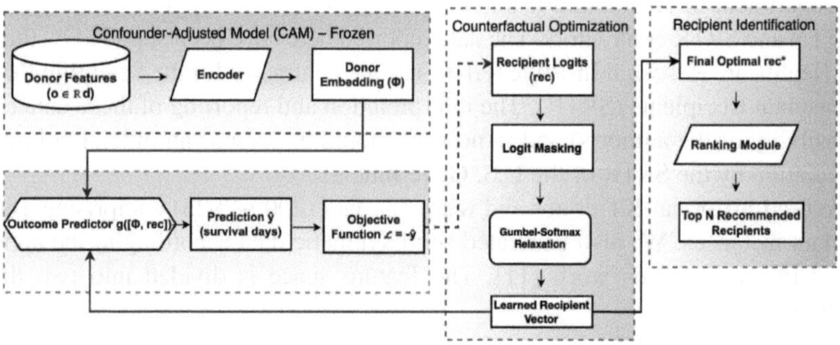


**Fig. 2.** Methodology schematic for gradient based optimization.

A fundamental challenge arises because the recipient profile is represented as a high-dimensional sparse binary (one-hot encoded) vector. Gradient-based optimization requires computing ∂μ/∂r, which assumes that the input space is continuous and differentiable. However, one-hot encoded features are discrete and can only take values of 0 or 1. Changing a categorical feature (e.g., blood type A to B) requires switching one indicator from 0 to 1 and another from 1 to 0, constituting a discontinuous jump rather than an infinitesimal perturbation. Because no infinitesimal variation of exists in this discrete space, gradients with respect to are undefined, making direct gradient ascent infeasible [12]. In addition, DRM in KT is governed by hard biological constraints, such as ABO incompatibility, that cannot be violated at any stage of the optimization process. We address these requirements through GS relaxation combined with logit masking [12, 13]. Figure 2 provides a methodology of the optimization pipeline.

### 4.1 Enforcing Clinical Constraints via Logit Masking

The optimization process requires safeguards to ensure that only clinically viable donor-recipient matches are explored. Without constraints, the algorithm could converge toward biologically impossible combinations, such as assigning a Type A kidney to a Type O recipient. To prevent this, the methodology employs logit masking, a technique applied directly to the learnable parameters before probability conversion [13].

The process begins with the initialization of learnable logits $\Phi$ for each feature that representing the characteristics of a potential recipient. For a given donor, the algorithm identifies incompatible recipient blood types using standard clinical rules based on ABO compatibility matrices. A logit mask is then applied by assigning negative infinity ($-\infty$) to logits corresponding to incompatible categories. This structural modification prevents the optimization algorithm from exploring or selecting invalid matching options. During each forward pass, the algorithm identifies indices corresponding to incompatible blood types and assigns very large negative values to their associated logits. The masked logit values ensure that incompatible blood types receive zero probability, effectively restricting the optimization to clinically feasible combinations. This approach was chosen over post-hoc filtering because allowing exploration of infeasible regions causes gradients to converge toward invalid local maxima. By masking incompatible logits prior to the Softmax step, the optimization landscape is constrained, forcing the gradient to navigate exclusively within the clinically feasible manifold and ensuring computational resources focus on refining valid candidates.

### 4.2 Gumbel-Softmax Relaxation

The masked logits (learnable parameters after constraint enforcement) are transformed to probabilities via GS where the masked logits are passed through a Softmax function. Because incompatible logits are set to $-\infty$, the exponential of negative infinity becomes zero, guaranteeing that the probability of sampling an incompatible match is exactly zero. This mathematical property ensures clinical constraints are maintained throughout optimization.

Instead of selecting a single discrete category, which would break differentiability and prevent gradient-based optimization, the method samples a continuous relaxed vector using the GS trick. The relaxed sample is computed by adding Gumbel noise to the logits and dividing by a temperature parameter $\tau$ before applying Softmax. The temperature parameter controls the degree of relaxation: as $\tau$ approaches zero, the relaxed sample approaches a discrete one-hot vector, while higher temperatures produce smoother distributions. This continuous relaxation preserves differentiability while approximating discrete categorical sampling.

### 4.3 The Optimization Approach

The optimization procedure follows an iterative gradient ascent loop for each donor organ in the test set. At each step t, the algorithm executes a three-phase process combining the techniques described in the previous sections.

The forward pass begins by applying logit masking to enforce clinical constraints. The algorithm then generates a synthetic recipient vector using GS sampling with the masked logits. This synthetic recipient, combined with frozen donor features, is fed into the outcome predictor to estimate post-transplant survival. We linearly anneal $\tau$ from 1.0 to 0.1 over optimization to balance exploration (high $\tau$) early and exploitation (low $\tau$) late. This schedule empirically converged reliably across diverse donor profiles.

The backward pass computes gradients of the loss with respect to the recipient logits and updates these logits using the Adam optimizer. This loop repeats iteratively until the logits converge to a recipient profile that maximizes the predicted post-transplant survival outcome.

Optimization terminates after 2000 iterations. Empirically, 95% of cases converged within 1500 iterations. The optimization output is a list of 10 synthetic feature vector representing the ideal candidate for the specific donor organ ranked by their predicted days of survival. The algorithm in Fig. 3. below shows the step-by-step optimization process.

**Algorithm 1:** Counterfactual Recipient Profile Optimization

**Input** : Donor feature vector $\mathbf{x}_{donor}$, Pre-trained Counterfactual Model $\mu(\cdot)$, Recipient Feature Groups $\mathcal{G}$, ABO Compatibility Matrix $\mathbf{C}$
**Output:** Optimal Recipient Feature Vector $\mathbf{x}^*_{rec}$, Predicted Survival $\hat{y}^*$

**1. Initialization:**
**foreach** *categorical group* $g \in \mathcal{G}$ **do**
    Initialize learnable logits $\Phi_g \sim \mathcal{N}(0, 0.01)$;
**2. Constraint Setup:**
Extract donor blood type from $\mathbf{x}_{donor}$;
Identify compatible recipient indices $I_{compat}$ based on $\mathbf{C}$;
**3. Optimization Loop:**
**for** $t \leftarrow 1$ **to** $T_{steps}$ **do**
    *(a) Forward Pass:*
    /* Apply Logit Masking for ABO constraints */
    Let $\Phi_{ABO}$ be the logits for the blood-type group;
    **foreach** $j \notin I_{compat}$ **do** $\Phi_{ABO}[j] \leftarrow -\infty$ ;
    /* Gumbel-Softmax Relaxation */
    Sample $\epsilon \sim \text{Gumbel}(0, 1)$;
    Generate continuous recipient vector:;
    $\hat{\mathbf{x}}_{rec} \leftarrow \text{Concat}_{g \in \mathcal{G}} \left( \frac{\exp((\Phi_g + \epsilon)/\tau)}{\sum \exp((\Phi_g + \epsilon)/\tau)} \right)$;
    *(b) Prediction:*
    $\hat{y} \leftarrow \mu(\mathbf{x}_{donor}, \hat{\mathbf{x}}_{rec})$;
    *(c) Backward Pass:*
    $\mathcal{L} \leftarrow -\hat{y}$ ; /* Maximize survival */
    Compute gradients $\nabla_\Phi \mathcal{L}$;
    Update logits $\Phi \leftarrow \Phi - \eta \nabla_\Phi \mathcal{L}$;
**4. Final Selection:**
$\mathbf{x}^*_{rec} \leftarrow \text{argmax}(\Phi)$ ; /* Convert logits to discrete profile */
$\hat{y}^* \leftarrow \mu(\mathbf{x}_{donor}, \mathbf{x}^*_{rec})$;
**return** $\mathbf{x}^*_{rec}, \hat{y}^*$

**Fig. 3.** Algorithm showing detailed optimization process.

## 5 Results and Discussion

Our evaluation seeks to quantify two distinct contributions: (1) the accuracy of the CAM in estimating counterfactual outcomes of DRM, and (2) the clinical utility of the gradient-based optimization in identifying superior matches. Before optimization can occur, the system must accurately predict outcomes for unseen donor-recipient pairs.

### 5.1 Counterfactual Estimation

Adhering to the methodology established in our previous work [11], we evaluate the CAM alongside a simple baseline deep neural network (DNN) prediction model (described in our previous work [11]). Table 1 presents these results across both semi-synthetic (counterfactual accuracy) and real-world (factual prediction) scenarios the held-out test set ($N_{test} = 37{,}200$). Performance is evaluated using normalized root mean squared error (*n-RMSE*) and mean absolute error in days (*MAE*). As shown in Table 1, the CAM significantly outperforms the baseline DNN across both semi-synthetic and real-world datasets (paired t-test, $p < 0.001$).

**Table 1.** Performance comparison of the CAM versus a baseline DNN for counterfactual and factual prediction accuracy.

| | Semi-Synthetic n-RMSE | Real n-RMSE | MAE |
|---|---|---|---|
| CAM | 0.46 (0.08) | 0.912 (0.07) | 1030 (20) |
| DNN | 0.69 (0.1) | 1.05 (0.12) | 1168 (22) |

## 5.2 Counterfactual Optimization

Clinical utility was validated via *k*-nearest neighbor retrieval within the joint donor-recipient manifold. For each donor, we generated an optimal recipient profile using both our CAM and baseline DNN model. Since these optimized matches are counterfactual, we retrieved the closest historical transplants based on Euclidean distance, utilizing their average observed survival as the ground-truth proxy (Table 2).

**Table 2.** Nearest Neighbor Retrieval Validation Results

| Metric | Baseline Prediction | Counterfactual (Ours) |
|---|---|---|
| Average Proxy Survival | 2324 days | 2718 days |
| Improvement | | +394 days |
| Win Rate | | 85.47% |
| Statistical Significance for Paired t-test | | $p < 0.001$ |

The counterfactual model's recommendations corresponded to historical matches with an average of 394 additional days of observed survival ($p < 0.001$), confirming that confounding-adjusted optimization translates to genuine clinical benefit. In 85.47% of pairwise comparisons, our model identified neighbors with superior actual outcomes, demonstrating systematic improvement over correlation-based prediction.

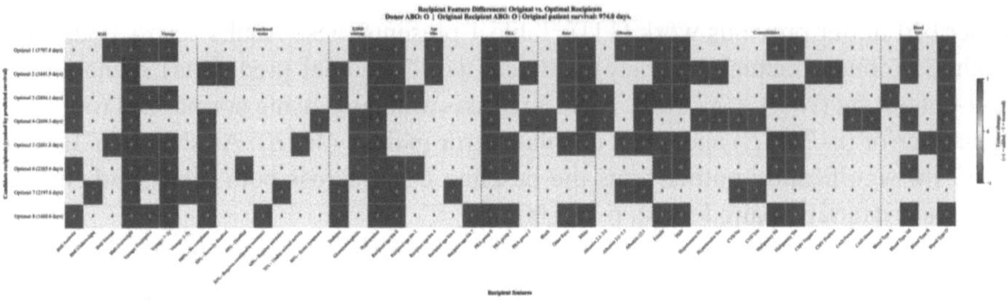

**Fig. 4.** Counterfactual recipient profiles where orange cells denote feature deviations from the historical match; blue cells indicate agreement.

To provide clinically grounded insight into the framework's decision-making, we examine a near-exemplary historical allocation: an 18-year-old donor (KDPI = 8%) matched to a 24-year-old Type O recipient (EPTS = 11%, 100% functional status, no diabetes, dialysis vintage 2.92 years). A model merely encoding historical policy would rigidly reproduce near-identical candidates. Instead, Fig. 4 shows our framework surfaces a broader set of high-utility recipients – with the top-ranked counterfactual yielding 3,707 predicted days versus 974 days for the original recipient – including those in slightly older age bins with comparable physiological resilience and recipients with marginally lower functional scores offset by strong overall health profiles. This demonstrates that our framework contributes to DRM by identifying ranked, clinically defensible alternatives that challenge policy-induced allocation biases rather than replicating them.

# 6 Conclusion

This research addresses the gap between counterfactual estimation and optimization in DRM for KT. We propose a gradient-based optimization framework that integrates GS relaxation with logit masking to efficiently navigate high-dimensional treatment spaces while strictly enforcing clinical compatibility constraints. While existing methods can estimate outcomes under alternative treatments, they do not provide a mechanism for identifying the optimal treatment within a constrained feasible set, particularly when the treatment space is high-dimensional and discrete. Our primary contribution is enabling counterfactual optimization in such settings, transforming causal estimation into actionable decision-making. Clinically, we demonstrate that counterfactual optimization can identify superior donor-recipient matches that challenge policy-driven allocation patterns, with nearest-neighbor validation confirming meaningful improvements in observed post-transplant survival.

While developed for kidney transplantation, this framework generalizes to other organ allocation problems (liver, lung, heart) and broader clinical decision-making scenarios involving high-dimensional treatments under compatibility constraints. However, the current framework optimizes solely for graft survival; therefore, its outputs should be considered clinical decision support rather than a replacement for clinician judgment. Human oversight remains essential, particularly in cases where predicted survival differences fall within margins of statistical uncertainty. In practice, clinical decision-making involves multiple competing objectives, including equity and urgency. Future work should extend this framework to a multi-objective optimization setting to better balance these priorities.

## References

1. Cron, D.C., Patzer, R.E., Adler, J.T.: Supply, demand, and a growing US kidney transplant waiting list. JAMA Netw. Open. **8**(3), e251675 (2025)
2. Rabb, H., Lee, K., Parikh, C.R.: Beyond kidney dialysis and transplantation: what's on the horizon? J. Clin. Invest. **132**(7) (2022)
3. Montgomery, J.R., Berger, J.C., Warren, D.S., James, N.T., Montgomery, R.A., Segev, D.L.: Outcomes of ABO-incompatible kidney transplantation in the United States. Transplantation. **93**(6), 603–609 (2012)
4. Yeung, M.Y., Coates, P.T., Li, P.K.-T.: Kidney organ allocation system: how to be fair. Semin. Nephrol. **42**(4), 151274 (2022)
5. Senanayake, S., et al.: Deceased donor kidney allocation: an economic evaluation of contemporary longevity matching practices. BMC Health Serv. Res. **20**(1) (2020)
6. Israni, A.K., et al.: New national allocation policy for deceased donor kidneys in the United States and possible effect on patient outcomes. J. Am. Soc. Nephrol. **25**(8), 1842–1848 (2014)
7. Lee, D., Kanellis, J., Mulley, W.R.: Allocation of deceased donor kidneys: a review of international practices. Nephrology. **24**(6), 591–598 (2019)
8. Ghosh, S., Yu K., Arabshahi, F., Batmanghelich, K.: Tackling Shortcut Learning in Deep Neural Networks: An Iterative Approach with Interpretable Models (2023)
9. Zhu, Y., Li, J., Bian, Y., Zheng, Z., Chen, L.: One Fits All: Learning Fair Graph Neural Networks for Various Sensitive Attributes (2025)
10. Wei Koh, P., Liang, P.: Understanding Black-Box Predictions via Influence Functions (2017)
11. Naqvi, S.A.A., Tennankore, K., Abidi, S.S.R.: A Counterfactual Analysis Framework based on Uncertainty Guided Contrastive Learning for Donor-Recipient Matching in Organ Transplantation. (2026) Available at SSRN: https://ssrn.com/abstract=6250498
12. Jang, E., Gu, S., Poole, B.: Categorical Reparameterization with Gumbel-Softmax (2017)
13. Hou, Y., Liang, X., Zhang, J., Yang, Q., Yang, A., Wang, N.: Exploring the use of invalid action masking in reinforcement learning: a comparative study of on-policy and off-policy algorithms in real-time strategy games. Appl. Sci. **13**(14), 8283 (2023)
14. Schrod, S., et al.: BITES: balanced individual treatment effect for survival data. Bioinformatics. **38**, I60–I67 (2022)
15. Shah, A., Ahuja, K., Shanmugam, K., Wei, D., Varshney, K.R., Dhurandhar, A.: Treatment effect estimation using invariant risk minimization. In: ICASSP, IEEE International Conference on Acoustics, Speech and Signal Processing-Proceedings, vol. 2021, pp. 5005–5009 (2021)
16. Manski, C.F.: Statistical treatment rules for heterogeneous populations. Econometrica. **72**(4), 1221–1246 (2004)
17. Künzel, S.R., Sekhon, J.S., Bickel, P.J., Yu, B.: Metalearners for estimating heterogeneous treatment effects using machine learning. Proc. Natl. Acad. Sci. USA. **116**(10), 4156–4165 (2019)
18. Schwab, P., Linhardt, L., Karlen, W.: Perfect Match: A Simple Method for Learning Representations for Counterfactual Inference with Neural Networks (2019)
19. Kallus, N., Zhou, A.: Policy evaluation and optimization with continuous treatments. In: International Conference on Artificial Intelligence and Statistics, AISTATS 2018, vol. 84, pp. 1243–1251 (2018)

20. Bica, I., Jordon, J., van der Schaar, M.: Estimating the effects of continuous-valued interventions using generative adversarial networks. Adv. Neural Inf. Process. Syst. **2020**. Decem, no. NeurIPS (2020)
21. Schweisthal, J., Frauen, D., Melnychuk, V., Feuerriegel, S.: Reliable Off-Policy Learning for Dosage Combinations (2023)

# How Do LLMs Handle Conflict in Healthcare? Hierarchy, Collaboration Defaults, and Autonomy

Saba Ghanbari Haez, Claudio Giuliano, Renan Lirio De Souza, and Mauro Dragoni(✉)

Digital Health and Wellbeing Research Center, Fondazione Bruno Kessler, Trento, Italy
{sghanbarihaez,giuliano,rliriodesouza,dragoni}@fbk.eu

**Abstract.** This study examines how Large Language Models advise users during healthcare conflicts where power differences matter (e.g., patient vs. clinician, junior vs. senior staff). We introduce a Thomas–Kilmann–grounded benchmark of 150 short healthcare conflict vignettes constructed from author-defined role, hierarchy, and option-style rules, with LLM-assisted drafting followed by validation and revision. Each vignette is paired with five response options representing common conflict styles: accommodate, assert, compromise, collaborate, and avoid. We evaluate multiple leading LLM families in both single-turn (stateless) and history-conditioned settings, and compare their choices with a small human-judgment study. Across models, recommendations concentrate heavily on collaboration, with assertion a distant second and very little accommodation or avoidance. Models show hierarchy-sensitive shifts in assertiveness, while remaining strongly collaboration-dominant overall. Human choices are more varied, suggesting LLMs may over-default to one "best" conflict approach. These findings motivate conflict-aware evaluation and calibration to better support autonomy in healthcare advice.

**Keywords:** Conflict Resolution · Large Language Models · Bias

## 1 Introduction

In recent years, the use of Large Language Models (LLMs) as conversational advisors in the context of health and well-being has increased significantly, whether the users are patients or expert clinicians. For example, patients use them to ask about their symptoms and possible treatments, clinicians, on the other hand, consult them for second opinions, and healthcare institutions apply them in triage, documentation, and decision support [5,7,12,17]. However, a less-studied critical area is when LLMs are used to provide recommendations in cases of a clash of interests or views between individuals/groups. Inspired by [22], we use *conflict* to refer to these situations. Following [1], conflict is an expressed struggle between interdependent parties with perceived incompatible goals or

© The Author(s), under exclusive license to Springer Nature Switzerland AG 2027
P. Andreev et al. (Eds.): AIME 2026, LNAI 16748, pp. 351–362, 2027.
https://doi.org/10.1007/978-3-032-30710-1_42

constraints. Conflict and resolution strategies are central to organizational communication and collective decision-making [9,18,24], and are common in health and well-being (e.g., safety vs. workload, honesty vs. hope, or institutional rules vs. clinical judgment). How such conflicts are handled affects clinical outcomes, relationship quality, and professional well-being [6,19]. Conflicts are closely tied to autonomy: advice that encourages deference (conformity) can constrain self-determination, while advice that supports reasoned push back (assertion) can strengthen it. Compromise and collaboration can enable shared decision-making, but may also dilute autonomy under power asymmetries by discouraging clear refusals or independent choices. This makes healthcare conflicts a useful lens for assessing how LLM advice may support or restrict autonomy [16,29].

Existing evaluations of medical LLMs focus mainly on factual accuracy, guideline adherence, and safety filters, while less is known about model behavior in *interpersonal* or *role-based* conflicts. To our knowledge, no structured benchmark targets healthcare conflict styles while comparing how LLM families distribute advice across conformity, assertion, compromise, collaboration, and avoidance. We address this gap with a Thomas–Kilmann–grounded, conflict-based evaluation: author-defined roles and option rules guide LLM-assisted scenario drafting, followed by validation and revision. Each vignette is paired with five response options reflecting Thomas–Kilmann conflict modes [14,15, 26–28]: conform/accommodate, assert/compete, compromise, collaborate, and avoid/defer. Models select the single best option for the focal actor. Building on our prior scenario-based work on autonomy-relevant response patterns in LLM advice, we focus here on healthcare conflicts and extend the evaluation from broad autonomy dilemmas to clinically situated hierarchy and conflict-resolution scenarios.

Our contributions are: (1) a healthcare conflict-style benchmark with author-guided, LLM-assisted structured options; (2) an analysis of how model choices shift under power asymmetries; (3) an examination of autonomy-relevant reasoning in justifications; and (4) a human evaluation ($n = 9$) that benchmarks model choices against human distributions.

## 2 Related Work

While LLMs are increasingly embedded in clinical workflows, recent meta-analyses show that evaluation remains fragmented and often centered on narrow technical metrics rather than the social and situational realities of care [4,5]. Benchmarks likewise emphasize factual correctness, safety, and guideline adherence in complex clinical interactions [2,8]. Prior work argues these criteria are insufficient: LLMs should also be assessed on communication quality, expression of uncertainty, and potential for harm, since impact depends on how advice is framed and interpreted in real settings [13,25]. Scenario-based evaluations similarly show that apparently neutral prompts can reveal systematic LLM biases, supporting the need for structured, socially situated benchmarks beyond factual accuracy alone [10]. Empirical evidence further shows that strong standalone model capability does not necessarily translate into better human decision-making: controlled studies report limited or inconsistent benefits when lay users or clinicians consult LLMs during medical reasoning, highlighting interaction effects and reliance dynamics [3,11]. Robustness studies also find that models can be overly swayed by medical text that looks authoritative (such as clinical notes), which matters in hierarchical settings where institutional language is often treated as especially credible [21]. From a psychological perspective, conflict and its resolution are established interpersonal and organizational processes shaped by goals, relationships, and power asymmetries, with canonical conflict-handling modes widely used in healthcare research [20,23]. However, despite extensive work on medical LLM accuracy and safety, there is little structured evaluation of how LLMs *advise* users in role-based conflicts (e.g., junior vs. senior, patient vs. clinician), or whether model recommendations systematically privilege deference, assertion, compromise, collaboration, or avoidance under hierarchy. Our work addresses this gap by benchmarking multiple model families on healthcare conflict vignettes with options mapped to canonical conflict modes, explicitly testing hierarchy effects and history-conditioned (informed) versus stateless (non-informed) model behavior.

## 3 Methodology

We use a scenario-based evaluation of healthcare conflict: each role-specific vignette includes five response options mapped to canonical conflict styles, and models select the single best option. We analyze how choices and justifications vary by model family, hierarchy (lower vs. higher role), and protocol (independent vs. access to prior answers).

### 3.1 Scenario Creation and Conflict-Style Options

We construct $N = 150$ short healthcare conflict vignettes spanning clinical and organizational tensions (e.g., patient–clinician disagreement, junior–senior escalation, clinician–policy constraints). The corpus is balanced by hierarchy: questions 1–75 place the focal actor in a higher-power role (e.g., attending physician, supervisor, institution), and questions 76–150 place the focal actor in a lower-power role (e.g., patient, junior staff). The focal role denotes the advice recipient and decision-maker, not a persona assigned to the LLM; other actors mentioned in the vignette form the conflict context. All vignettes are fictional research scenarios and are not based on real patient records or clinician-provided cases.

Each vignette is paired with one single-sentence option per style, adapted from the Thomas–Kilmann [14,15] conflict mode framework: **conform/accommodate (A)**, **assert/compete (B)**, **compromise (C)**, **collaborate (D)**, and **avoid/defer (E)**. We use Thomas–Kilmann as a compact analytic scaffold rather than a clinical gold standard: it maps naturally to forced-choice conflict-style options while allowing transparent comparison of whether LLM advice favors deference, assertion, compromise, collaboration, or avoidance. Options are written to maintain style purity, similar length, and neutral tone across scenarios. A representative example vignette with its focal role and A–E response options is shown in Fig. 1. The benchmark was developed through an author-guided, LLM-assisted pipeline: we first defined the role, hierarchy, conflict-style, and option-format rules, used GPT-5.2 to draft scenarios and A–E options under these constraints, and then validated, repaired, normalized, and reviewed the items for clinical plausibility, role consistency, neutral wording, and conflict-style purity. We audited redundancy with pairwise character-trigram cosine similarity across all 150 vignettes (median = 0.332, 95th percentile = 0.447, max = 0.668) and found no near-duplicates using a conservative 0.88 threshold (no clusters > 1). We also applied an LLM-as-judge check with GPT-5.2-Pro to verify that each vignette and its A–E options followed the intended conflict logic and style constraints; it was used to flag unclear or inconsistent items, not to assign preferred answers. Because GPT-5.2-Pro is also evaluated, this validation step may introduce some construction bias; however, it did not assign preferred answers, and the main patterns appear across multiple model families. The released benchmark and code are available in our public repository.[1]

**Example scenario (ID 4).**
**Focal role:** Attending physician
**Scenario:** After a postoperative bleed, I discover the intern mistakenly doubled the anticoagulant dose and urges me to chart it as "expected." The patient's family demands an explanation, and hospital policy requires timely documentation. What do I do next right now?
**Options:**
**A)** I use the intern's "expected" wording in the note and tell the family bleeding is a known risk, keeping details minimal.
**B)** I document that the anticoagulant was overdosed, inform the family directly about the mistake, and file the required incident report immediately.
**C)** I document the bleed and a possible dosing discrepancy without calling it an error, and I tell the family a medication concern is being reviewed.
**D)** I meet with the intern to agree on a factual chart entry and a shared explanation for the family, then we document and report together.
**E)** I postpone the family conversation and my formal note, ask the intern not to finalize documentation, and step away until I decide later.

**Fig. 1.** Example vignette with focal role, scenario text, and five response options (A–E).

### 3.2 Models and Inference Protocols

We evaluate instruction-tuned LLMs available through OpenRouter[2] spanning multiple model families: OpenAI (`gpt-4.1`, `gpt-5.2`, `gpt-5.2-pro`), Anthropic (`claude-3.5-sonnet`, `claude-sonnet-4.5`), Alibaba/Qwen (`qwen3-max-thin-`

[1] https://github.com/Saba-Gh-H/Healthcare-Conflict-Resolution-Benchmark.
[2] https://openrouter.ai/.

king), Meta (llama-3.2-3b-instruct), and DeepSeek (deepseek-v3.2). For each model and scenario, we run two protocols with identical prompts at temperature 0: **non-informed** (stateless single-turn calls; the model sees only the current vignette and response options) and **informed** (history-conditioned sequential calls; for question $t$, the model also sees its own prior question–answer pairs $1, \ldots, t-1$ and is instructed to remain consistent when appropriate). The prompt template was identical across protocols except for history: non-informed calls included only the current vignette and A–E options, while informed calls additionally included the model's own previous question–answer pairs. Full prompts and parsing scripts are in the public repository. In addition, for the non-informed setting, we run three temperature conditions ($T \in \{0, 0.8, 1.5\}$), chosen to span low, medium, and high sampling noise to test the robustness of option distributions. The three temperatures represent deterministic, moderate-randomness, and high-randomness settings for testing sampling robustness. We log the selected option, the one-sentence justification, and the raw response for analysis.

### 3.3 Analysis and Human Evaluation

We compare option frequencies (A–E) across models, protocols (non-informed vs. informed), and hierarchy (Q1–Q75 vs. Q76–Q150), and we examine justifications for autonomy-relevant framing (e.g., deference to authority vs. self-determination, rule/policy vs. relational emphasis, and confidence/hedging). To compare option frequencies with real users, we collected responses from 9 members of a digital-health research unit who were familiar with healthcare contexts but were not necessarily clinicians or domain experts. We quantify results using option counts/percentages, hierarchy differences, temperature mean/min–max ranges, intra-rater agreement, Fleiss' $\kappa$, human-majority agreement, and model–human distribution distance. Accordingly, we treat these responses as an exploratory human baseline rather than a representative sample of patients, clinicians, or other conflict stakeholders. We developed a custom web interface and adopted an "anchor and partition" approach to ensure a balanced distribution across the 150 vignettes. Each participant initially answers a fixed set of 18 anchor vignettes, which serve as the baseline for cross-participant comparisons. After that, the system assigns a subset of 10 additional questions (partition), selected using a greedy depth-first algorithm. This method prioritizes questions with the fewest recorded responses, thereby ensuring a balanced distribution and meeting a target of at least 3 classifications per vignette. Finally, the session concludes by re-presenting 2 randomly selected anchor vignettes that the participant previously answered to assess user consistency.

## 4 Results

In this section, we summarize how models distribute their conflict-style choices (A–E) across settings and roles, and relate these patterns to human judgments using anchor and randomly assigned questions with repeat-item consistency checks.

### 4.1 Non-informed (stateless) Responses

In the non-informed setting, each scenario is answered independently without access to prior responses. Table 1 reports how often each option was selected. Across models, option D (collaborate) dominates, indicating a strong default toward joint problem-solving and relationship-preserving advice in healthcare conflicts. Option B (assert/compete) is typically the second most common choice, suggesting occasional autonomy- or safety-driven push back, but far less often than collaboration. Options A (conform/accommodate) and E (avoid/defer) are rare, which may reflect instruction-tuned safety norms and the broad applicability of collaborative wording across scenarios. The near absence of A in some models (e.g., GPT-5.2 and GPT-5.2-Pro) further suggests reluctance to recommend simple compliance.

### 4.2 Informed (History-Conditioned) Responses

In the informed setting, each model answers with access to its own prior question–answer history and is instructed to remain consistent when appropriate. Table 2 reports option counts for models that completed this protocol. Providing history often increases concentration on a single style, consistent with path dependence: early choices tend to be reinforced. DeepSeek-V3.2, GPT-4.1, GPT-5.2, GPT-5.2-Pro, and Llama-3.2-3B become strongly D-heavy, suggesting that the consistency instruction amplifies the collaboration default. In contrast, Claude-3.5-Sonnet shifts from D toward B (and some E), suggesting that some models use history to justify a change in stance rather than simply repeating it. Persistently rare A and E likely reflect the option/prompt design (and the "single best option" instruction) that favors broadly applicable collaboration over accommodation or avoidance.

**Table 1.** Non-informed counts (out of 150). Cells report: count (percentage).

| Option | claude35sonnet | claudesonnet45 | deepseekv32 | gpt41 | gpt52 | gpt5pro | llama323binstruct | qwen3maxthinking |
|---|---|---|---|---|---|---|---|---|
| A | 4 (2.7%) | 2 (1.3%) | 2 (1.3%) | 2 (1.3%) | 0 (0.0%) | 0 (0.0%) | 1 (0.7%) | 1 (0.7%) |
| B | 15 (10.0%) | 23 (15.3%) | 19 (12.7%) | 26 (17.3%) | 11 (7.3%) | 15 (10.0%) | 26 (17.3%) | 20 (13.3%) |
| C | 2 (1.3%) | 2 (1.3%) | 6 (4.0%) | 10 (6.7%) | 3 (2.0%) | 3 (2.0%) | 12 (8.0%) | 7 (4.7%) |
| D | 129 (86.0%) | 121 (80.7%) | 121 (80.7%) | 111 (74.0%) | 135 (90.0%) | 131 (87.3%) | 111 (74.0%) | 121 (80.7%) |
| E | 0 (0.0%) | 2 (1.3%) | 2 (1.3%) | 1 (0.7%) | 1 (0.7%) | 1 (0.7%) | 0 (0.0%) | 1 (0.7%) |
| Total | 150 | 150 | 150 | 150 | 150 | 150 | 150 | 150 |

*Note.* Colors denote response option; darker intensity indicates larger counts within each option row.

**Table 2.** Informed counts. Cells report: count (percentage).

| Option | claude35sonnet | claudesonnet45 | deepseekv32 | gpt41 | gpt52 | gpt5pro (inf.) | llama323binstruct | qwen3maxthinking |
|---|---|---|---|---|---|---|---|---|
| A | 5 (3.3%) | 0 (0.0%) | 0 (0.0%) | 0 (0.0%) | 0 (0.0%) | 0 (0.0%) | 0 (0.0%) | 0 (0.0%) |
| B | 69 (46.0%) | 38 (25.3%) | 3 (2.0%) | 2 (1.3%) | 9 (6.1%) | 16 (10.7%) | 1 (0.7%) | 27 (18.0%) |
| C | 1 (0.7%) | 4 (2.7%) | 0 (0.0%) | 1 (0.7%) | 1 (0.7%) | 2 (1.3%) | 0 (0.0%) | 3 (2.0%) |
| D | 62 (41.3%) | 107 (71.3%) | 147 (98.0%) | 147 (98.0%) | 138 (93.2%) | 132 (88.0%) | 149 (99.3%) | 120 (80.0%) |
| E | 13 (8.7%) | 1 (0.7%) | 0 (0.0%) | 0 (0.0%) | 0 (0.0%) | 0 (0.0%) | 0 (0.0%) | 0 (0.0%) |
| Total | 150 | 150 | 150 | 150 | 148 | 150 | 150 | 150 |

*Note.* gpt52 has 2 missing outputs overall (total 148).

## 4.3 Hierarchy Effect (Higher vs. Lower Role)

We split scenarios into questions 1–75, where the decision-maker is higher in the hierarchy, and questions 76–150, where the decision-maker is lower in the hierarchy. Table 3 reports the non-informed hierarchy split, and Table 4 reports the informed hierarchy split. Across both conditions, models remain dominated by option D, the collaborative response, in both hierarchy groups. In the non-informed condition, hierarchy-related differences are modest. In the informed condition, several models select option B, the assertive response, more often for lower-power focal actors than for higher-power focal actors, especially Claude and Qwen, while other models show smaller or mixed shifts. DeepSeek remains strongly collaboration-dominant in both groups, suggesting that access to prior answers can amplify or dampen hierarchy sensitivity depending on the model. One possible explanation is healthcare-specific: lower-power actors such as patients, junior clinicians, nurses, and caregivers are often at risk of being overridden by authority, so LLMs may treat assertive responses as autonomy- or safety-protective when the focal actor has less power. This pattern has mixed ethical implications: encouraging lower-power actors to be assertive may strengthen autonomy and voice, but it can also understate the risks of challenging authority; encouraging collaboration may support relationships and shared decision-making, but in strongly unequal settings it may weaken accountability.

**Table 3.** Non-informed counts by hierarchy. Cells report: count (percentage).

| Option | claude35sonnet | claudesonnet45 | deepseekv32 | gpt41 | gpt52 | gpt5pro | llama323binstruct | qwen3maxthinking |
|---|---|---|---|---|---|---|---|---|
| **Higher hierarchy (Q1–Q75)** | | | | | | | | |
| A | 1 (1.3%) | 1 (1.3%) | 0 (0.0%) | 0 (0.0%) | 0 (0.0%) | 0 (0.0%) | 1 (1.3%) | 0 (0.0%) |
| B | 3 (4.0%) | 8 (10.7%) | 7 (9.3%) | 13 (17.3%) | 5 (6.7%) | 7 (9.3%) | 13 (17.3%) | 7 (9.3%) |
| C | 2 (2.7%) | 2 (2.7%) | 3 (4.0%) | 6 (8.0%) | 2 (2.7%) | 2 (2.7%) | 4 (5.3%) | 4 (5.3%) |
| D | 69 (92.0%) | 64 (85.3%) | 65 (86.7%) | 56 (74.7%) | 68 (90.7%) | 66 (88.0%) | 57 (76.0%) | 64 (85.3%) |
| E | 0 (0.0%) | 0 (0.0%) | 0 (0.0%) | 0 (0.0%) | 0 (0.0%) | 0 (0.0%) | 0 (0.0%) | 0 (0.0%) |
| **Lower hierarchy (Q76–Q150)** | | | | | | | | |
| A | 3 (4.0%) | 1 (1.3%) | 2 (2.7%) | 2 (2.7%) | 0 (0.0%) | 0 (0.0%) | 0 (0.0%) | 1 (1.3%) |
| B | 12 (16.0%) | 15 (20.0%) | 12 (16.0%) | 13 (17.3%) | 6 (8.0%) | 8 (10.7%) | 13 (17.3%) | 13 (17.3%) |
| C | 0 (0.0%) | 0 (0.0%) | 3 (4.0%) | 4 (5.3%) | 1 (1.3%) | 1 (1.3%) | 8 (10.7%) | 3 (4.0%) |
| D | 60 (80.0%) | 57 (76.0%) | 56 (74.7%) | 55 (73.3%) | 67 (89.3%) | 65 (86.7%) | 54 (72.0%) | 57 (76.0%) |
| E | 0 (0.0%) | 2 (2.7%) | 2 (2.7%) | 1 (1.3%) | 1 (1.3%) | 1 (1.3%) | 0 (0.0%) | 1 (1.3%) |

**Table 4.** Informed counts by hierarchy. Cells report: count (percentage).

| Option | claude35sonnet | claudesonnet45 | deepseekv32 | gpt41 | gpt52 | gpt5pro (inf.) | llama323binstruct | qwen3maxthinking |
|---|---|---|---|---|---|---|---|---|
| **Higher hierarchy (Q1–Q75)** | | | | | | | | |
| A | 0 (0.0%) | 0 (0.0%) | 0 (0.0%) | 0 (0.0%) | 0 (0.0%) | 0 (0.0%) | 0 (0.0%) | 0 (0.0%) |
| B | 30 (40.0%) | 14 (18.7%) | 3 (4.0%) | 2 (2.7%) | 1 (1.3%) | 5 (6.7%) | 1 (1.3%) | 9 (12.0%) |
| C | 1 (1.3%) | 3 (4.0%) | 0 (0.0%) | 1 (1.3%) | 1 (1.3%) | 1 (1.3%) | 0 (0.0%) | 3 (4.0%) |
| D | 44 (58.7%) | 58 (77.3%) | 72 (96.0%) | 72 (96.0%) | 71 (94.7%) | 69 (92.0%) | 74 (98.7%) | 63 (84.0%) |
| E | 0 (0.0%) | 0 (0.0%) | 0 (0.0%) | 0 (0.0%) | 0 (0.0%) | 0 (0.0%) | 0 (0.0%) | 0 (0.0%) |
| **Lower hierarchy (Q76–Q150)** | | | | | | | | |
| A | 5 (6.7%) | 0 (0.0%) | 0 (0.0%) | 0 (0.0%) | 0 (0.0%) | 0 (0.0%) | 0 (0.0%) | 0 (0.0%) |
| B | 39 (52.0%) | 24 (32.0%) | 0 (0.0%) | 0 (0.0%) | 8 (11.0%) | 11 (14.7%) | 0 (0.0%) | 18 (24.0%) |
| C | 0 (0.0%) | 1 (1.3%) | 0 (0.0%) | 0 (0.0%) | 0 (0.0%) | 1 (1.3%) | 0 (0.0%) | 0 (0.0%) |
| D | 18 (24.0%) | 49 (65.3%) | 75 (100.0%) | 75 (100.0%) | 67 (91.8%) | 63 (84.0%) | 75 (100.0%) | 57 (76.0%) |
| E | 13 (17.3%) | 1 (1.3%) | 0 (0.0%) | 0 (0.0%) | 0 (0.0%) | 0 (0.0%) | 0 (0.0%) | 0 (0.0%) |

### 4.4 Temperature Sensitivity

Our main non-informed results use greedy decoding ($T = 0$; Table 1), which is effectively deterministic and thus yields a single stable option distribution per model. To assess robustness under stochastic decoding, we reran the same protocol at higher temperatures and summarize multiple runs using the mean count with the min–max range in parentheses, reporting the effective number of valid responses in the Total row (Tables 5–6).

At $T = 0.8$ (3 runs; Table 5), the qualitative pattern remains unchanged from $T = 0$: all models still favor **D**, while **A** and **E** remain rare. Run-to-run variability is small for most models but larger for `llama323binstruct` (e.g., **B**: 26–45; **D**: 95–112). At $T = 1.5$ (5 runs; Table 6), dispersion into **B**/**C** and run-to-run ranges increase, again most noticeably for `llama323binstruct`, which also has the lowest mean valid responses (Total = 147.6, min = 138); other models remain close to 150 with narrower ranges.

**Table 5.** Non-informed counts at temperature 0.8 (3 runs). Cells report: mean count (min–max) across runs.

| Option | claude35sonnet | claudesonnet45 | deepseekv32 | gpt41 | gpt52 | gpt5pro | llama323binstruct | qwen3maxthinking |
|---|---|---|---|---|---|---|---|---|
| **Temperature 0.8 (3 runs: mean (min–max))** | | | | | | | | |
| A | 4.7(4–5) | 2 | 1.7(1–2) | 2 | 0 | 0 | 1.3(1–2) | 1 |
| B | 14.7(14–15) | 23.7(23–24) | 15.0(12–17) | 28.0(27–29) | 12.7(11–15) | 14.7(14–16) | 32.3(26–45) | 19.7(19–20) |
| C | 2.0(0–3) | 2 | 7.3(5–10) | 11.0(10–12) | 2.7(2–3) | 3.0(2–4) | 10.0(7–12) | 8.7(8–9) |
| D | 128.3(127–129) | 120.3(120–121) | 125 | 108.0(106–110) | 133.0(132–134) | 131.0(130–133) | 106.0(95–112) | 117.3(113–120) |
| E | 0.3(0–1) | 2 | 1 | 1 | 1.3(1–2) | 1.3(1–2) | 0.3(0–1) | 1 |
| Total | 150 | 150 | 150 | 150 | 149.7(149–150) | 150 | 150 | 147.7(143–150) |

**Hierarchy Under Temperature.** Using the hierarchy ordering (Q1–75 = higher-power roles; Q76–150 = lower-power roles), raising temperature to $T = 0.8$ preserves the main qualitative pattern: option **D**, the collaborative response, remains dominant for all models in both hierarchy groups. However, across the three runs, several models assign relatively more mass to option **B**, the assertive response, in the lower-power group than in the higher-power group,

**Table 6.** Non-informed counts at temperature 1.5 (5 runs). Cells report: mean count (min–max) across runs.

| Option | claude35sonnet | claudesonnet45 | deepseekv32 | gpt41 | gpt52 | gpt5pro | llama323binstruct | qwen3maxthinking |
|---|---|---|---|---|---|---|---|---|
| **Temperature** 1.5 **(5 runs: mean (min–max))** | | | | | | | | |
| A | 3.8(3–4) | 1.8(1–2) | 1.4(0–3) | 1.6(1–2) | 0 | 0 | 0.8(0–1) | 1 |
| B | 17.0(15–19) | 23.0(22–24) | 17.2(13–21) | 28.0(26–30) | 13.2(12–14) | 14.8(13–16) | 26.8(25–32) | 19.0(18–20) |
| C | 2.6(1–5) | 2 | 10.0(7–13) | 10.8(10–11) | 3.2(2–4) | 2.6(2–3) | 12.6(11–17) | 10.2(9–11) |
| D | 125.4(121–128) | 121.2(121–122) | 119.8(113–126) | 108.6(107–111) | 131.0(128–132) | 131.2(130–134) | 106.6(85–113) | 118.8(117–120) |
| E | 1.2(1–2) | 2 | 1.4(1–2) | 1 | 1.2(1–2) | 1.2(1–2) | 0.8(0–4) | 1 |
| Total | 150 | 150 | 149.8(149–150) | 150 | 148.6(147–149) | 149.8(149–150) | 147.6(138–150) | 150 |

while differences for **C** remain smaller and more variable. Run-to-run variability is modest for most models, with the largest instability again appearing for `llama323binstruct`. Across the five $T = 1.5$ runs, the same hierarchy pattern largely persists. Collaboration remains the dominant style in both groups, but higher temperature increases dispersion into **B**/**C** and produces more occasional **A**/**E** selections. The Higher–Lower differences for **B** are often negative, indicating that assertive choices occur more frequently in lower-power scenarios for several models, although the size of this effect varies by model and run. This pattern has mixed ethical implications: encouraging lower-power actors to be assertive may strengthen autonomy and voice, but it can also understate the risks of challenging authority; encouraging collaboration may support relationships and shared decision-making, but in strongly unequal settings it may weaken accountability.

### 4.5 Human Evaluation and LLM Comparison

We collected multiple-choice judgments (options A–E) from 9 members of a digital-health research unit who were familiar with healthcare contexts but were not necessarily clinicians or domain experts. Anchor questions were answered by all participants, while the remaining items were sampled at random until each question received at least 3 independent human answers. We report *coverage* using the number of *unique raters* per question and aggregate one vote per participant per question for option distributions. Reliability was assessed with repeated anchor items (10% per participant; 2/20), yielding intra-rater exact-match agreement of $15/18 = 0.833$. Inter-rater agreement on anchors was low (Fleiss' $\kappa = 0.061$, 95% bootstrap CI [0.004, 0.103]). As a robustness check, excluding raters with repeat agreement $< 0.5$ removed none (9/9 retained), leaving the human option distribution unchanged. For LLM baselines, we apply the same A–E choices and compare models to humans via option-distribution shifts and agreement with the human majority on sufficiently covered questions. Overall, humans show a broader spread across options, whereas LLMs are strongly concentrated on option D, indicating a narrower default strategy. Four models tied for highest human-majority agreement on anchor items (10/18 = 55.6%): `qwen3maxthinking`, `gpt5pro`, `claude35sonnet`, and `gpt52`. Among them, `qwen3maxthinking` was closest by option-distribution similarity, so we treat it as the closest overall to the human anchor distribution; this comparison is exploratory because the human sample is small. Table 7 summarizes human reliability and anchor option distributions.

**Table 7.** Human reliability and anchor distributions. Top: intra-rater agreement and Fleiss' $\kappa$; bottom: option distributions for humans vs. LLMs (count, row %).

| | #pairs | #match | rate |
|---|---|---|---|
| Anchor repeats (10%) | 18 | 15 | 0.833 |

| | |
|---|---|
| Fleiss' $\kappa$ | 0.061 |
| 95% CI | [0.004, 0.103] |

| | A | B | C | D | E | Total |
|---|---|---|---|---|---|---|
| Humans (anchors) | 23 ( 12.8% ) | 26 ( 14.4% ) | 45 ( 25.0% ) | 68 ( 37.8% ) | 18 ( 10.0% ) | 180 |
| LLMs (anchors) | 0 ( 0.0% ) | 24 ( 16.7% ) | 1 ( 0.7% ) | 118 ( 81.9% ) | 1 ( 0.7% ) | 144 |

## 5 Conclusion

We introduced a Thomas–Kilmann–grounded benchmark of 150 healthcare conflict vignettes and found a robust *collaboration* default across instruction-tuned LLMs, with *assertion* as a secondary pattern and near-zero *conformity* and *avoidance*. Models show modest hierarchy-sensitive shifts, with more assertive advice for lower-power roles, while collaboration remains dominant overall. Human judgments were reliable on repeated anchor checks and showed a broader spread across options than LLMs, indicating greater sensitivity to situational trade-offs and highlighting autonomy-relevant gaps when models collapse to a narrow conflict style. Together, these results suggest that current medical LLM advice may be less flexible than human judgment in conflict settings, especially under hierarchy. Future work will scale and diversify human studies beyond our small forced-choice sample ($n = 9$), collect brief human justifications and confidence ratings, and move from fictional single-turn research vignettes to higher-fidelity, multi-turn clinical interactions. We will also test interventions to reduce over-concentration on a single style (e.g., prompting or preference tuning) and evaluate robustness across institutions, cultures, and real-world power dynamics, while considering how prompt phrasing, option design, and model alignment tendencies may shape model responses.

## References

1. Adler, R.B., Rosenfeld, L.B., Towne, N., Scott, M.: Interplay: The Process of Interpersonal Communication. Oxford University Press (2007)
2. Arora, R.K., Wei, et al.: HealthBench: evaluating large language models towards improved human health. arXiv preprint arXiv:2505.08775 (2025)
3. Bean, A.M., et al.: Reliability of LLMs as medical assistants for the general public: a randomized preregistered study. Nat. Med., 1–7 (2026)

4. Bedi, S., Liu, et al.: Testing and evaluation of health care applications of large language models: a systematic review. Jama **333**(4), 319–328 (2025)
5. Busch, F., Hoffmann, et al.: Current applications and challenges in large language models for patient care: a systematic review. Commun. Med. **5**(1), 26 (2025)
6. Clarke, S., Oakley, et al.: Misaligned hope and conviction in health care. Bioethics **39**(3), 232–239 (2025)
7. Consolandi, M., Magnolini, S., Dragoni, M.: Risk communication in healthcare: the management of misunderstandings. J. Med. Syst. **50**(1), 15 (2026). https://doi.org/10.1007/s10916-026-02347-8
8. Fast, D., Adams, et al.: Autonomous medical evaluation for guideline adherence of large language models. NPJ Digit. Med. **7**(1), 358 (2024)
9. Gaba, V., Joseph, J.: Content and process: organizational conflict and decision making. Front. Psychol. **14**, 1227966 (2023)
10. Ghanbari Haez, S., Dragoni, M.: Neutral is not unbiased: evaluating implicit and intersectional identity bias in LLMs through structured narrative scenarios. In: Findings of the Association for Computational Linguistics: EMNLP 2025, pp. 15060–15088 (2025). https://doi.org/10.18653/v1/2025.findings-emnlp.814
11. Goh, E., Gallo, R., Hom, et al.: Large language model influence on diagnostic reasoning: a randomized clinical trial. JAMA Netw. Open **7**(10), e2440969 (2024)
12. Gómez, C., Yin, et al.: How large language model-powered conversational agents influence decision making in domestic medical triage contexts. Front. Comput. Sci. **6**, 1427463 (2024)
13. Haltaufderheide, J., Ranisch, R.: The ethics of ChatGPT in medicine and healthcare: a systematic review on large language models. NPJ Digit. Med. **7**(1), 184 (2024). https://doi.org/10.1038/s41746-024-01157-x
14. Kilmann, R.H., Thomas, K.W.: Interpersonal conflict-handling behavior as reflections of Jungian personality dimensions. Psychol. Rep. **37**(3), 971–980 (1975)
15. Kilmann, R.H., Thomas, K.W.: Developing a forced-choice measure of conflict-handling behavior: the "mode" instrument. Educ. Psychol. Measur. **37**(2), 309–325 (1977)
16. Kim, M.S., Lee, et al.: Large language models for pre-mediation counseling in medical disputes: a comparative evaluation against human experts. Healthc. Inform. Res. **31**(2), 200–208 (2025)
17. Maity, S., Saikia, M.J.: Large language models in healthcare and medical applications: a review. Bioengineering **12**(6), 631 (2025)
18. Majer, J.M., Barth, et al.: Resolving conflicts between people and over time in the transformation toward sustainability: a framework of interdependent conflicts. Front. Psychol. **12**, 623757 (2021)
19. Miaoulis, G., Jr., Manev, I.M.: Personal and organizational responsibility in the delivery of healthcare services: breaking the code of silence. Health Serv. Insights **18**, 11786329251356096 (2025)
20. Nikitara, M., Dimalibot, et al.: Conflict management in nursing: analyzing styles, strategies, and influencing factors: a systematic review. Nurs. Rep. **14**(4), 4173–4192 (2024)
21. Omar, M., et al.: Mapping the susceptibility of large language models to medical misinformation across clinical notes and social media: a cross-sectional benchmarking analysis. Lancet Digit. Health **8**(1) (2026)
22. Rice, S.: Non-violent conflict management: conflict resolution, dealing with anger, and negotiation and mediation. California Social Work Education Center, California State University (2000)

23. Scherer, K.A., Büdenbender, et al.: Power asymmetry and embarrassment in shared decision-making: predicting participation preference and decisional conflict. BMC Med. Inform. Decis. Making **25**, 120 (2025)
24. Somaraju, A.V., Griffin, D.J., et al.: The dynamic nature of interpersonal conflict and psychological strain in extreme work settings. J. Occup. Health Psychol. **27**(1), 53 (2022)
25. Tam, T.Y.C., Sivarajkumar, et al.: A framework for human evaluation of large language models in healthcare derived from literature review. NPJ Digit. Med. **7**(1), 258 (2024)
26. Thomas, K.W.: Conflict and conflict management: reflections and update. J. Organ. Behav., 265–274 (1992)
27. Thomas, K.W.: Thomas-Kilmann conflict mode. TKI Profile Interpretive Rep. **1**(11), 1–11 (2008)
28. Thomas, K.W., Kilmann, R.H.: Comparison of four instruments measuring conflict behavior. Psychol. Rep. **42**(3_suppl), 1139–1145 (1978)
29. Wu, W., Xu, et al.: Assessing and mitigating medical knowledge drift and conflicts in large language models. arXiv preprint arXiv:2505.07968 (2025)

# Evaluating Static and Dynamic Approaches for Assessing Trustworthiness in Medical Risk Factor Forecasting


Ana Krstevska[1(✉)], Rianne M. Schouten[2], Soroush Ghandi[2], Mykola Pechenizkiy[2], and Mitja Luštrek[1]

[1] Jožef Stefan Institute and Jožef Stefan International Postgraduate School, Ljubljana, Slovenia
{ana.krstevska,mitja.lustrek}@ijs.si

[2] Eindhoven University of Technology, Eindhoven, The Netherlands
{r.m.schouten,s.ghandi,m.pechenizkiy}@tue.nl



**Abstract.** The adoption of machine-learning models in clinical practice requires not only accurate predictions but also an understanding of their trustworthiness. We study predictive trustworthiness in forecasting cardiovascular risk factors from childhood and adolescence to later ages using real-world medical data. We compare two approaches for identifying unreliable predictions: a dynamic approach based on predictive uncertainty from a probabilistic heteroscedastic regression model and a static approach that identifies interpretable subgroups with consistently high prediction error. We further evaluate whether combining both approaches improves performance, and gather feedback from domain experts on practical utility. Across multiple risk factors, both approaches perform similarly, with a slight advantage for the static approach (F1 score 0.58 vs 0.56). We combine them into a conservative strategy that improves detection of unreliable predictions at the cost of rejecting reliable ones, and a permissive one that does the opposite. Domain experts favored the conservative strategy, and said that predictive uncertainty is particularly useful for refining patient dialogue.



**Keywords:** Trustworthy AI · Medical Risk Factor Forecasting · Exceptional Model Mining · Probabilistic Modeling · Experimental Evaluation


## 1 Introduction

When a Machine Learning (ML) model is used in a medical context, it is important to know when its predictions can be trusted. If critical decisions depend on the model, the users demand a high accuracy, and if a sufficiently accurate model cannot be built, no model will be used. However, if the information that the user obtains from the model has a measure of certainty added to it, this gives valuable information about when to trust the model and when to lean more on their own expertise.


© The Author(s), under exclusive license to Springer Nature Switzerland AG 2027


P. Andreev et al. (Eds.): AIME 2026, LNAI 16748, pp. 363–367, 2027.
https://doi.org/10.1007/978-3-032-30710-1_43

In this paper, we address the forecasting of cardiovascular risk factors from childhood or adolescence (input age) to later ages (output age), where they begin to significantly affect the health risk. This is an important problem because tools for risk assessment of children and adolescents are lacking, even though young age is a critical period for formation of health behaviors.

Prediction uncertainty can arise both from inherent variability in the data (aleatoric uncertainty) and from limited knowledge due to finite training data (epistemic uncertainty). To capture both, we use a probabilistic heteroscedastic regression model [4] that outputs both the mean and standard deviation for each prediction. As a complementary static approach, we apply Exceptional Model Mining (EMM) [1,3], which identifies interpretable subgroups where prediction error is consistently high. These two approaches were chosen because they capture different but complementary aspects of trustworthiness. We compare how well these two approaches identify predictions that should be rejected, and combine them into more conservative and more permissive decision strategies. In addition, we perform a small qualitative assessment with domain experts to explore the practical usefulness of these methods.

To obtain a sufficiently rich and diverse dataset for forecasting cardiovascular risk factors, we constructed a single merged dataset by combining multiple longitudinal sources, harmonizing differing risk factor coverages and applying synthetic data generation to fill in missing features [2]. Training and validation samples were then created by forming all available younger-to-older age pairs per individual, resulting in a varying number of instances per subject depending on available measurements. Model training used both real and synthetic data, while evaluation was restricted to real records with input ages 6–18 and output ages 18–55. The training and validation sets contained 48101 and 11621 records, respectively, with each individual assigned to only one split, and evaluation used 4778 real records.

## 2 Approaches for Assessing Trustworthiness

### 2.1 Dynamic Trustworthiness with Probabilistic Modeling

To perform a principled assessment of when model predictions can be trusted, we follow the methodology proposed in [4] and adopt a probabilistic regression model. First, we implement a feed-forward neural network with two fully connected hidden layers with 512 and 128 neurons. Rectified Linear Unit (ReLU) activations are used throughout the network, and dropout with a rate of 0.2 is applied to reduce overfitting. Optimization was performed using the Adam optimizer, and early stopping was employed based on validation performance. We then introduce an additional output head to predict the log-variance alongside the mean. The log-variance is trained to be large when the mean is far from the ground truth, and small otherwise. We adapt the loss function following the faithful heteroscedastic formulation [4] to ensure that the uncertainty estimation does not influence the mean prediction updates, i.e., it is not inflated to avoid the penalty for poor mean prediction. As a result, our model outputs both a mean prediction $\hat{y}$ and a log-variance $s = \log(\sigma^2)$. We convert the latter into standard deviations $\sigma = e^{0.5s}$, which serve as explicit measures of predictive uncertainty.

### 2.2 Static Trustworthiness with Interpretable Subgroups

We investigate static trustworthiness using EMM [1,3], a pattern mining framework that identifies interpretable subgroups of instances where model performance is exceptionally good or poor compared to the whole dataset. A subgroup is defined by a description $S$, typically a conjunction of conditions on input features, and consists of all records covered by that description [1]. For our evaluation, we use six descriptive attributes: input age, output age, body mass index (BMI), physical activity (PA), fitness score, and diet score.

The goal is to discover subgroups with exceptional behavior with respect to prediction error. We therefore define the target attribute as the absolute prediction error, $\ell_{\text{err}} = |\hat{y} - y|$, where $\hat{y}$ is the predicted value and $y$ is the true value. To quantify exceptionality, we use the mean gain quality measure $\varphi^a_M(S) = n^a|m_S - m_0|$, with $a = 0$, meaning subgroup size is not explicitly weighted. Here, $m_S$ is the mean value of $\ell_{\text{err}}$ in subgroup $S$, and $m_0$ is the mean over the full test dataset. We additionally enforce a minimum subgroup size of $n > 0.1N$, where $N = 4778$ is the size of the entire test dataset.

To search for the top-$q$ exceptional subgroups, we use beam search [1], a level-wise search algorithm that iteratively refines promising subgroup descriptions. We set the search depth to $d = 2$, beam width to $w = 20$, and return the top $q = 5$ subgroups.

## 3 Evaluation

### 3.1 Quantitative Evaluation

**Experimental Design.** We evaluate the static and dynamic approach for assessing trustworthiness from Subsects. 2.1 and 2.2. All analyses were performed separately for four model outputs: BMI, systolic blood pressure (SBP), low-density lipoprotein cholesterol (LDL), and PA.

For each risk factor, every instance is assigned three binary labels (accepted or rejected), corresponding to the static approach, dynamic approach, and ground truth. In the static approach, instances belonging to the q = 5 exceptional subgroups are identified as untrustworthy, yielding a rejection rate defined as the proportion of such instances.

The dynamic approach assesses trustworthiness at the instance level using the predicted standard deviation. As no "natural" rejection threshold exists, the threshold is set per risk factor to match the rejection rate of the static approach by rejecting instances with the highest standard deviations.

Furthermore, we define a ground-truth notion of untrustworthy predictions based on actual model performance. For each risk factor, predictions with the largest absolute error were rejected, using the same rejection rate as in the static and dynamic approaches.

We further examine whether combining the static and dynamic criteria improves performance. Two strategies are considered: a conservative strategy, where a prediction is rejected if either approach rejects it, and a permissive strategy, where a prediction is rejected only if both approaches reject it. Performance across all approaches is evaluated using precision, recall and F1 score.

**Table 1.** Average metrics for four risk factors

| Method | Accept | | | Reject | | | Macro average | | |
|---|---|---|---|---|---|---|---|---|---|
| | Precision | Recall | F1 | Precision | Recall | F1 | Precision | Recall | F1 |
| Static | 0.83 | 0.83 | 0.83 | 0.32 | 0.32 | 0.32 | 0.58 | 0.58 | 0.58 |
| Dynamic | 0.82 | 0.82 | 0.82 | 0.30 | 0.30 | 0.30 | 0.56 | 0.56 | 0.56 |
| Conservative | 0.84 | 0.72 | 0.77 | 0.29 | 0.46 | 0.36 | 0.57 | 0.59 | 0.56 |
| Permissive | 0.82 | 0.94 | 0.87 | 0.37 | 0.16 | 0.22 | 0.59 | 0.55 | 0.55 |

**Experimental Results.** This section presents a comparison of the static and dynamic approaches. The numeric performance metrics averaged over all the risk factors are shown in Table 1.

A direct comparison of the static and dynamic approaches shows that the static approach slightly outperforms the dynamic approach. This is true on average and for individual risk factors except BMI. The reason could be that the static approach has direct access to the actual error, whereas the dynamic approach uses standard deviation as a confidence measure, which is only indirectly related to the error. This advantage apparently outweighs the disadvantage of not being able to reject individual instances but only subgroups.

The low F1 score for the reject class can be attributed to class imbalance (mean rejection rate of 19.6%) and limitations in uncertainty estimation. Evaluation of uncertainty estimation showed a fairly strong Spearman correlation of 0.46 between absolute error and predicted standard deviation for BMI, but weaker correlations for the other risk factors, explaining the superior performance of the dynamic approach for BMI. Reliability diagrams indicated some underconfidence, with predicted standard deviations being too high, consistent with qualitative feedback from domain experts in Subsect. 3.2.

We conducted additional experiments to evaluate whether combining the static and dynamic approaches into conservative or permissive strategies improves performance over the standalone approaches. As expected, the conservative strategy increases reject recall but reduces accept recall, while precision remains largely unchanged. In contrast, the permissive strategy increases accept recall but substantially lowers reject recall, with slightly higher precision. The preferred strategy therefore depends on the clinical objective, balancing the detection of unreliable predictions against the preservation of reliable ones.

### 3.2 Qualitative Evaluation

To investigate the practical usability of our methods, we interviewed three health experts. All of them were presented with an example consisting of six independent variables used in forecasting, the forecast BMI, the confidence interval (dynamic approach) and an example of an unreliable subgroup (static approach). They found confidence intervals useful for expressing uncertainty but considered them too wide to inspire trust. Unreliable subgroups were also viewed as useful, although some defining variables were not clinically meaningful, suggesting that users should have input in how such subgroups are described. In promoting a healthy lifestyle, the experts preferred avoiding unreliable predictions even at the cost of discarding some reliable ones to prevent misinformation, although the priorities could be different in different use cases.

## 4 Conclusion

Our analyses show that both the static and dynamic approaches provide useful insights into trustworthiness in long-term cardiovascular risk forecasting, with comparable performance and a slight overall advantage for the static approach in both performance and interpretability. Combining both methods allows either more conservative or more permissive decision strategies depending on the clinical goal. Future work should evaluate generalizability across additional datasets, investigate the impact of temporal distribution shifts, and conduct a more extensive user study. Overall, this work highlights the importance of research on trustworthy AI for supporting clinical decision-making.

**Acknowledgments.** This work was carried out as part of the SmartCHANGE project (grant agreement No 101080965). The datasets were provided by University of Ljubljana, KU Leuven, University of Porto, VUMC, the Helena study group and University of Turku. We furthermore acknowledge the domain experts who provided valuable qualitative feedback: Maroje Sorić, Tuija Tammelin and Syed-Abdul Shabbir.

**Disclosure of Interests.** The authors have no competing interests to declare that are relevant to the content of this article.

**Declaration of AI Assistance Technologies during Manuscript Preparation.** The author(s) used AI assistance from Gemini/ChatGPT for refinement, correction, editing or formatting the manuscript to improve clarity of language (cf. class 1).

## References

1. Duivesteijn, W., Feelders, A., Knobbe, A.: Exceptional model mining. Data Min. Knowl. Disc. **30**(1), 47–98 (2016)
2. Reščič, N., et al.: SmartCHANGE risk prediction tool: next-generation risk assessment for children and youth. In: Proceedings of the IS (2025)
3. Schouten, R.M.: Exceptional model mining for hierarchical data. Ph.D. thesis, Eindhoven University of Technology (2025)
4. Stirn, A., Wessels, H., Schertzer, M., Pereira, L., Sanjana, N., Knowles, D.: Faithful heteroscedastic regression with neural networks. In: Proceedings of the AISTATS (2022)

# Can LLMs Accurately Score Medical Diagnoses and Clinical Reasoning?

Amy Rouillard[1(✉)], Sitwala Mundia[2], Linda Camara[2], Ziyaad Dangor[3], Michael Cameron Gramanie[3], Ismail Kalla[4], Shabir A. Madhi[3], Kajal Morar[3], Marlvin T. Ncube[3], Haroon Saloojee[5], and Bruce A. Bassett[1,2,6]

[1] Wits MIND Institute, University of the Witwatersrand, Johannesburg, South Africa
{amy.rouillard,bruce.bassett1}@wits.ac.za
[2] Grai Labs, Cape Town, South Africa
[3] South African Medical Research Council Vaccines and Infectious Diseases Analytics Research Unit, Faculty of Health Sciences, University of the Witwatersrand, Johannesburg, South Africa
[4] Department of Internal Medicine, Faculty of Health Sciences, Charlotte Maxeke Johannesburg Academic Hospital, University of the Witwatersrand, Johannesburg, South Africa
[5] Department of Paediatrics and Child Health, Faculty of Health Sciences, University of the Witwatersrand, Johannesburg, South Africa
[6] School of Computer Science and Applied Mathematics, University of the Witwatersrand, Johannesburg, South Africa

**Abstract.** Evaluating medical AI systems using expert clinician panels is costly and slow, motivating the use of large language models (LLMs) as alternative adjudicators. Here, we evaluate an LLM Jury, composed of three frontier AI models, for scoring 3333 diagnoses on 300 real-world low- and middle-income country (LMIC) hospital cases. Both LLM- and clinician-generated diagnoses are scored against expert panel diagnoses across four dimensions: diagnosis, differential diagnosis, clinical reasoning, and negative treatment risk. The LLM Jury scores are compared with expert and independent re-scoring panel scores, assessing error metrics, inter-rater agreement, severe risk errors, and the effect of post hoc calibration using isotonic regression. In our data, we find that: (i) the uncalibrated LLM Jury scores preserve ordinal agreement with the expert clinician panel scores, but are systematically lower; (ii) the probability of severe risk errors is lower for the LLM Jury than the human expert re-score panels; (iii) the LLM Jury combined with LLM diagnoses can be used to identify diagnoses at high risk of error, enabling targeted expert review and improved panel efficiency; (iv) the calibrated LLM Jury rankings of diagnosing agents show excellent agreement with primary expert panel rankings. Together, these results provide evidence that a calibrated, multi-model LLM jury is a trustworthy and reliable proxy for expert clinician evaluation in medical AI benchmarking. Confirming these findings in other clinical settings is an important direction for future work.

© The Author(s), under exclusive license to Springer Nature Switzerland AG 2027
P. Andreev et al. (Eds.): AIME 2026, LNAI 16748, pp. 368–377, 2027.
https://doi.org/10.1007/978-3-032-30710-1_44

**Keywords:** Large language models (LLMs) · LLM-as-a-judge · Medical AI evaluation

# 1 Introduction

Healthcare applications of generative Artificial Intelligence (AI) demand rigorous model evaluation to ensure safety and accuracy. Traditionally, expert clinicians review AI-generated answers, but this approach is labour-intensive, inconsistent, and not easily scalable [1,3,10]. Evaluating a number of AI models rigorously across a large number of cases with human panels is simply not feasible. Researchers have instead explored using LLMs as evaluators, an approach often termed "LLM-as-a-Judge", to provide efficient and reproducible assessments of medical AI outputs [5,7,8,10]. Early results suggest that strong LLM-based judges can approximate human judgment closely [4,11]. Such findings indicate that LLM evaluators could serve as a scalable proxy for human review in medicine, where obtaining consistent expert feedback is often costly and slow.

However, relying on a single LLM as the sole "judge" has notable limitations. Studies have documented that individual LLM evaluators, which mimic a single human, may exhibit systematic biases [11] and hence may be less robust than a jury of multiple experts. Even state-of-the-art LLM judges do not uniformly agree with human experts across all medical criteria. In a recent healthcare quality assessment (QA) study, the best-performing LLM judge achieved expert-level agreement on only 4 of 11 evaluation criteria, with some models proving overly harsh while others were overly lenient [10]. Such variability underscores that single-LLM judgments can be unreliable in nuanced clinical contexts. More robust evaluation frameworks are valuable in harnessing LLMs' scalability without inheriting a lone model's biases or blind spots.

Our work assesses a frontier-level LLM Jury for evaluating medical diagnoses and reasoning with expert-level rigour in an LMIC context. While prior studies have tested multi-LLM evaluators in general domains and even shown modest gains in specialised medical settings [6,9,10], the approach has not yet been fully validated. We fill this gap by systematically assessing how an LLM Jury can reproduce expert physician panel scoring on medical tasks. We analyse scoring errors, inter-rater agreement, severe risk errors, and diagnosing agent rankings, and discuss post-hoc calibration. These results provided evidence that a suitable LLM Jury can serve as a trustworthy surrogate for human evaluation in medicine.

# 2 Data, Panels and LLM Jury

**Datasets** used in the work were collected as part of the VALID study [2] that evaluated the multimodal diagnostic performance of LLMs on a South African public health hospital cohort. During the study, a team of medical officers captured 539 complete medical cases together with primary, secondary, and differential diagnoses made by the treating physicians, which we refer to collectively as the *ward diagnoses*. This multimodal dataset comprises admission records, structured clinical reports, laboratory test results, and medical imaging data, including computerised tomography (CT), magnetic resonance imaging (MRI) and X-rays. The dataset is not publicly available, making it suitable for independent evaluation of LLMs.

**Primary panel diagnoses** are diagnoses made by expert panels of two internal medicine physicians or two paediatricians. These panels reviewed 300 speciality-relevant cases: members examined cases independently in advance, then met to provide a consensus primary, secondary, and differential diagnoses, document clinical reasoning, and record binary agreement with ward diagnoses (examples in [2]). **Primary panel scores** are evaluations provided by these panels. In total, they scored 30 ward and 300 LLM diagnoses, one per case, against their own expert diagnoses. This yielded four Likert-scale scores (1–5): diagnosis (Dx), differential diagnosis (DDx), clinical reasoning (Reasoning), and negative treatment risk. Higher scores are better except for negative treatment risk, which we replace with a patient safety (Safety) score, defined as 6 minus the negative treatment risk. The clinical reasoning of the treating doctors was not available; therefore, the clinical reasoning score is omitted for ward diagnoses.

**The LLM Jury** was formed from three leading LLM models: Anthropic's Claude Opus 4.1 (2025-08-05), Google's Gemini 2.5 Pro (2025-06-17) and OpenAI's o3 (2025-04-16). These reasoning AI models were chosen from different labs to enhance diversity and were identically prompted to provide each of the four scores (Dx, DDx, Reasoning, negative treatment risk) on the same 1–5 scale as the human panels. In total, each LLM Jury model evaluated 3333 diagnoses: 300 ward diagnoses associated with the cases reviewed by the primary panels, and 3033 LLM diagnoses made by a variety of models. In the prompt, the primary panel's diagnoses and clinical reasoning were supplied as ground truth. The final LLM Jury scores are computed as the mean of the three LLM Jury model scores. We do not round these values, preserving the granularity and reflecting uncertainty from inter-jury-model disagreement.

The **re-score panels**, a second set of expert panels, re-scored a random duplicate sample of 30 LLM diagnoses to assess inter-panel agreement. Re-score panels were not provided with the full case details, only the AI model predictions and the primary panel's diagnoses and clinical reasoning as ground truth, exactly mirroring the data provided to the LLM Jury. For efficiency, the primary panels scored diagnoses immediately after recording their diagnoses and clinical reasoning, and therefore were aware of the full case details. However, because scoring was anchored to concordance with the panel's own diagnoses and reasoning using predefined criteria, this context was unlikely to systematically bias the assigned scores, although this should be explored in future work.

## 3 Summary Statistics: Panels vs LLM Jury Scores

Analysis of the score differences between the primary panels and the LLM Jury models (see Table 1 Offset) indicates that all LLM Jury models systematically gave lower scores than the panel's scores. Figure 1 shows confusion matrices allowing comparison of the scores given by the primary panel (y-axis) to the scores given by the LLM Jury models and the re-score panel (x-axis) for each case. These plots further demonstrate the consistent strictness of the LLM Jury models (most data lie above the diagonals). In particular, the LLM Jury rarely gives the highest score, 5. The ordinal consistency is, however, generally preserved. In contrast to the LLM Jury models, the human re-score panels (Fig. 1d) had more random, symmetric disagreement with the panels, with lower correlations and a higher exact-match percentage.

**Table 1.** Offset and RMSE for each evaluator relative to primary panels. Offset is defined as an evaluator's score minus the primary panel's score, averaged over the 330 (30) cases scored by the primary panels (re-score panels). A positive offset indicates that the evaluator's scores are, on average, lower than the primary panels' scores. Bold indicates the lowest values across evaluators. For all scores, the LLM Jury has lower RMSE than the re-score panels, though a larger offset.

| Metric | Model | Dx | DDx | Reasoning | Safety |
|---|---|---|---|---|---|
| Offset | Opus 4.1 | 1.00 | 1.30 | 1.10 | 1.00 |
| | Gemini 2.5 Pro | 0.94 | 1.30 | 1.10 | 1.10 |
| | o3 | 0.72 | 1.20 | 0.86 | 0.66 |
| | LLM Jury | 0.89 | 1.30 | 0.99 | 0.93 |
| | Re-score Panel | **0.40** | **0.37** | **0.67** | **0.10** |
| RMSE | Opus 4.1 | 1.50 | 1.80 | 1.50 | 1.80 |
| | Gemini 2.5 Pro | 1.50 | 1.80 | 1.80 | 2.00 |
| | o3 | **1.30** | 1.80 | **1.40** | **1.60** |
| | LLM Jury | 1.40 | **1.70** | 1.50 | 1.70 |
| | Re-score Panel | 1.50 | 1.80 | 1.60 | 1.90 |

## 4 Panel-LLM Jury Inter-rater Agreement

To evaluate the consistency of the judgments provided by the LLM Jury and re-score panels relative to the primary panels, we calculate two complementary inter-rater agreement metrics: Spearman's $\rho$, defined as the Pearson correlation coefficient between rank variables, is a non-parametric measure of agreement of orderings and is insensitive to calibration errors. And, quadratic weighted Cohen's $\kappa$, which quantifies absolute agreement and allows for weighting of ordinal differences. Table 2 shows that there is fair to moderate agreement between the LLM Jury and the primary panels, with consistently better agreement than between re-score and the primary panels. We note that the diagnoses evaluated by the re-score panels represent a small subset of those evaluated by the LLM Jury, and the observed differences are not all statistically significant. Across all

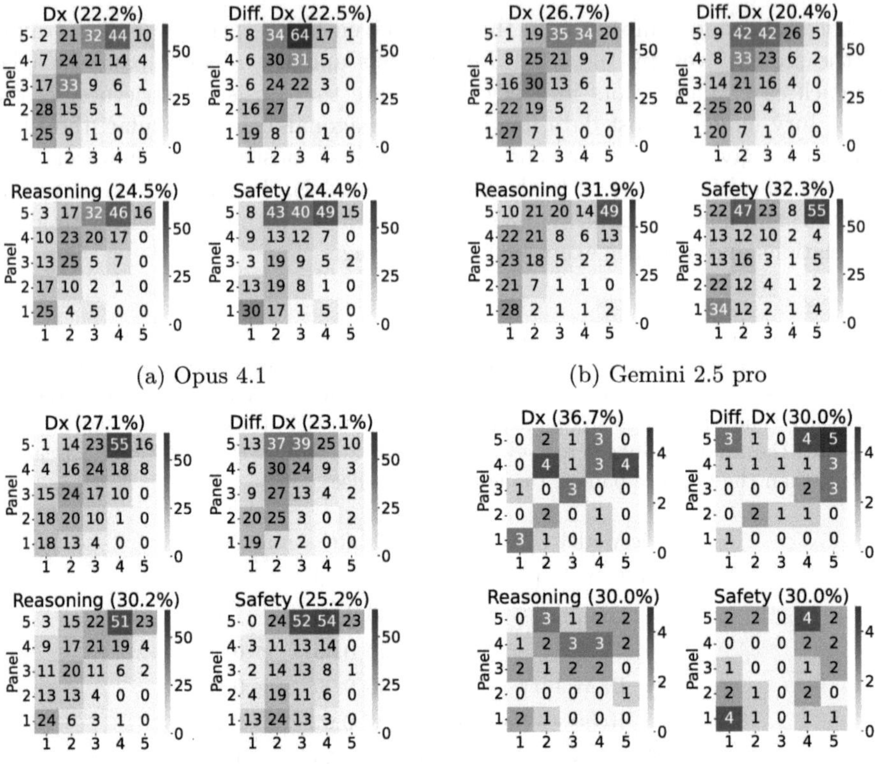


(a) Opus 4.1 (b) Gemini 2.5 pro

(c) o3 (d) Re-score Panels

**Fig. 1.** Confusion matrices showing the concordance between the primary panels and (a)–(c) the LLM Jury models and (d) the re-score panels, for each score. The percentage of exact matches is shown in brackets. The LLM Jury models (a)–(c) systematically assign stricter scores compared to the primary panels, while the re-score panels (d) differ symmetrically from the primary panels.

scores, there is a strong positive association between metrics. However, Spearman's $\rho$ is marginally higher than Cohen's $\kappa$, indicating greater ordinal alignment than absolute agreement, consistent with Fig. 1. Across all LLM Jury models and all metrics, inter-rater agreement is highest for the diagnosis score and lowest for the differential diagnosis score.

## 5 Severe Risk Errors: LLM Jury vs Human Evaluators

While the LLM Jury scores are systematically lower than the primary panel's, this does not exclude the possibility of the LLM Jury misclassifying a subset of dangerous misdiagnoses as harmless. To assess this risk, we define the *severe error rate* as the proportion of potentially harmful diagnoses (primary panel's patient safety score $\leq 2$) that also received a patient safety score from an LLM

**Table 2.** For each score, Spearman's $\rho$ and Cohen's $\kappa$ between the primary panels and all other evaluators (LLM Jury and re-score panels). Bold indicates the highest values across all evaluators. Across all scores, all jury models align more closely with the primary panels than the re-score panels do, giving strong evidence for LLM Jury consistency.

| Metric | Model | Dx | DDx | Reasoning | Safety |
|---|---|---|---|---|---|
| $\rho$ | Opus 4.1 | 0.652 | 0.463 | 0.639 | 0.501 |
| | Gemini 2.5 Pro | 0.640 | 0.494 | 0.590 | 0.450 |
| | o3 | 0.638 | 0.442 | 0.628 | 0.482 |
| | LLM Jury | **0.679** | **0.523** | **0.656** | **0.523** |
| | Re-score Panel | 0.398 | 0.113 | 0.309 | 0.286 |
| $\kappa$ | Opus 4.1 | 0.476 | 0.268 | 0.467 | 0.365 |
| | Gemini 2.5 Pro | 0.487 | **0.293** | 0.423 | 0.329 |
| | o3 | **0.541** | 0.285 | **0.514** | **0.399** |
| | LLM Jury | 0.438 | 0.220 | 0.402 | 0.325 |
| | Re-score Panel | 0.411 | 0.151 | 0.309 | 0.320 |

Jury model or re-score panel of at least 3 points higher (i.e. diagnoses with strong disagreement with the primary panel on potential harm). This corresponds to the error rate for the binary classification of 'patient risk', which can be computed from Fig. 1. Table 3 shows the severe error rates for the LLM Jury models (approx 5%), which are significantly lower than the severe error rate estimated for the re-score panels (16.7%). In a beta–binomial model with a flat prior, the posterior probability that the severe error rate in the LLM Jury is lower than in the re-score panel is $\simeq 96.3\%$. These estimates provide further confidence in the quality of the LLM Jury.

The LLM Jury model scores are highly correlated. As a result, the LLM Jury does not achieve a lower severe error rate than the individual LLM Jury models. Given the limited number of cases, we cannot infer any underlying failure modes. Despite this, a qualitative examination of individual cases can provide useful insights. For instance, in a case diagnosed as pneumonia/myasthenia gravis, the LLM Jury was lenient despite the model hallucinating a 'large pleural effusion' excluded by the CT scan. Opus 4.1's reasoning relied on the panel's clinical reasoning that omitted the negative CT finding, while o3 dismissed the hallucination as clinically insignificant, despite the potential that a falsely identified large effusion could trigger an unnecessary thoracentesis, introducing procedural risks like iatrogenic pneumothorax. Interestingly, the re-score panel also gave a low negative treatment risk, agreeing with the LLM Jury scores.

## 6 LLM Jury Scores for Incorrect Diagnosis Detection

A novel test of the LLM Jury is its ability to identify cases in which the ward diagnoses were likely incorrect. In this study, 54% of cases reviewed by the panels

**Table 3.** Observed severe error rates relative to primary panels' scores. The probability that the re-score panels have a higher severe error rate than the LLM Jury models ($\mathbf{P}_{\text{severe}}$) is approximately 96.3%.

| | Opus 4.1 | Gemini 2.5 Pro | o3 | LLM Jury | Re-score Panels | $\mathrm{P}_{\text{severe}}$ |
|---|---|---|---|---|---|---|
| Rate | 5.3% | 7.4% | 3.2% | 5.3% | 16.7% | 96.3% |

were selected because all tested AI models scored poorly with the ward diagnoses as ground truth. Specifically, these cases were chosen for primary panel review based on the ranked patient safety scores. During review, the primary panel indicated whether they agreed or disagreed with the ward diagnoses, as mentioned in Sect. 2. The probability of primary panel disagreement with the ward diagnosis as a function of the average patient safety score, as scored by the LLM Jury using the ward diagnosis as ground truth, is shown in Fig. 2. There is a clear negative correlation between the patient safety score and the likelihood of panel disagreement, $P(\text{Disagreement})$. Panel disagreement with the ward diagnosis provides joint evidence for the quality of the AI diagnoses and the LLM Jury scoring.

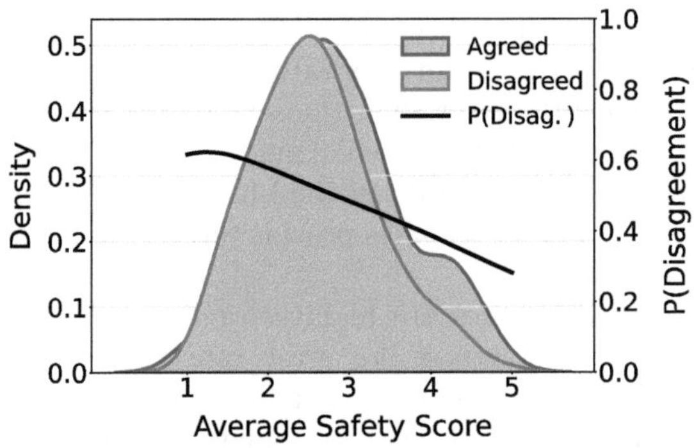


**Fig. 2.** Patient safety score as a predictor of primary panel disagreement with ward diagnoses. Shaded regions show kernel density estimates (KDE) of LLM Jury patient safety scores, using ward diagnoses as ground truth, subdivided into cases where primary panels agreed (blue; $n = 163$) or disagreed (orange; $n = 137$) with the ward. The empirical probability of disagreement, $P(\text{Disagreement})$ (right axis, purple), is linearly correlated with the LLM Jury patient safety score. (Color figure online)

## 7 Calibrating LLM Jury Scores to Panels' Scores

Previously, we observed that LLM Jury models' scores are lower than the expert panels'. To improve agreement with the primary panels, we perform a post-hoc calibration of LLM Jury scores using isotonic regression for each LLM Jury model and each score to calibrate the predicted scores to the primary panels' scores. Isotonic regression is well-suited for calibration here because it preserves the Likert-scale ordering. The LLM Jury score prediction is then taken as the mean over the calibrated LLM Jury model scores. After calibration, there is a statistically significant improvement in offset and RMSE across all scores, while there is no statistically significant change to Spearman's $\rho$ (Table 4). Cohen's $\kappa$ improved for all scores except patient safety, for which the improvement was not statistically significant. Metrics are computed across a 5-fold cross-validation to avoid over-fitting.

**Table 4.** LLM Jury performance after calibration. Offset, RMSE, Spearman's $\rho$, and Cohen's $\kappa$ for the calibrated LLM Jury relative to panel scores are reported, with parentheses indicating pre–post differences and * denoting statistical significance. For offset and RMSE, negative differences indicate improvement, whereas for Spearman's $\rho$ and Cohen's $\kappa$, positive differences indicate improvement. Statistical significance is defined as an absolute change exceeding 2× the combined standard error (SE), estimated via bootstrap sampling ($n = 1000$). Metrics are averaged over 330 case diagnoses reviewed by the primary panels, and all show either statistically significant improvement or no statistically significant change.

| Metric | Dx | DDx | Reasoning | Safety |
|---|---|---|---|---|
| Offset | 0.00 (−0.89)* | 0.00 (−1.27)* | 0.00 (−1.00)* | 0.00 (−0.93)* |
| RMSE | 1.00 (−0.37)* | 1.14 (−0.58)* | 1.05 (−0.46)* | 1.33 (−0.34)* |
| $\rho$ | 0.67 (−0.01) | 0.50 (−0.02) | 0.63 (−0.02) | 0.51 (−0.01) |
| $\kappa$ | 0.54 (+0.10)* | 0.39 (+0.17)* | 0.50 (+0.10)* | 0.36 (+0.03) |

## 8 LLM Jury Model Rankings Align with Expert Panels

The diagnoses evaluated by the primary panels spanned a variety of models, including the LLM Jury models themselves and models from other providers. Figure 3 shows the anonymised rankings of 8 diagnosing agents, labelled $M_i$, based on a 'universal quality score', $S_3$, assigned by the primary panels. The $S_3$ score was computed as a weighted sum of the diagnosis, differential diagnosis, and patient safety scores, weighted 40:20:40, respectively. Across all scores, we found no evidence of scoring bias toward LLM diagnoses from the same provider. LLM Jury models generally ranked their own outputs similarly to how other jury models ranked them. Mixed-effects regression controlling for case-level variability and LLM Jury model effects showed that same-provider evaluations differed by at most 0.041 points on average, with confidence intervals overlapping zero for all LLM Jury models. These effects were also small relative to inter-case variability, with same-provider effects ($\leq 0.041$) substantially smaller than case-level variance ($\geq 0.32$). Each case contributed between 9 and 30 same-provider observations, with a mean of 27.3, providing adequate within-case replication for estimating case-level random effects.

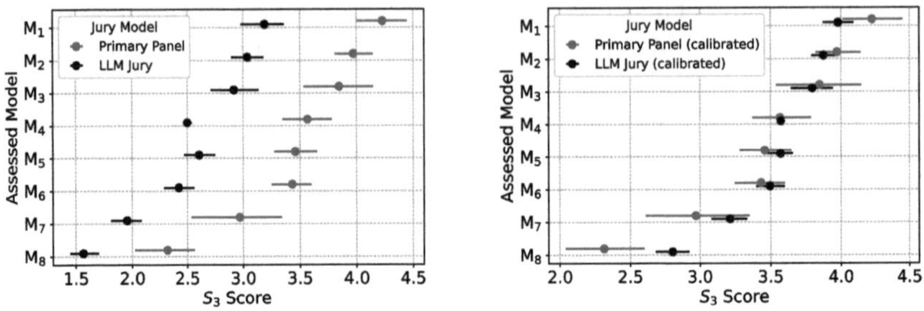


(a) Before calibration

(b) After calibration

**Fig. 3.** Mean $S_3$ score for 8 anonymised diagnosing agents ($M_i$) as scored by the primary panel and the LLM Jury, (a) before and (b) after calibration, with 68% confidence intervals computed using bootstrap sampling ($n = 1000$). Diagnosing agents are ranked according to the primary panels. After calibration, there is improved absolute agreement between the LLM Jury and the primary panels.

# 9 Conclusion

In this study, we provide a detailed assessment of a state-of-the-art LLM Jury for evaluating clinical case diagnoses and clinical reasoning. We discuss complementary approaches to assess accuracy, consistency, and reliability, including agreement with expert panels and rates of severe safety errors. We examine ranking consistency, potential bias toward same-provider LLM diagnoses, and the ability of LLM Jury models to identify incorrect ward diagnoses. We also present post hoc calibration of LLM Jury scores to better align with primary panels and assess the impact on errors, inter-rater agreement, and ranking agreement.

Together, these analyses provide a holistic, multi-dimensional evaluation of LLMs for scoring medical diagnoses. In our data, the LLM Jury assigns lower scores than primary panels but preserves ordinal agreement. Post hoc calibration using isotonic regression improves LLM Jury performance, and we find no evidence of preferential scoring of same-provider diagnoses. Combining the LLM Jury with AI-generated diagnoses enables identification of cases at high risk of ward diagnostic error, allowing targeted expert review and improved efficiency. Finally, in our study, the probability of severe safety errors is significantly lower for LLM Jury models than for human evaluators, a finding that should be tested in other settings. Together, these results provide evidence that an LLM Jury can reliably assess diagnostic accuracy, safety, and clinical reasoning.

**Acknowledgments.** This study was funded by the Gates Foundation under Grant INV-081034. We thank Jess Rees for valuable discussions.

**Disclosure of Interests.** The authors have no competing interests to declare.

**Declaration of AI Assistance.** The authors used ChatGPT for the formatting of LaTeX tables. After using this technology, the authors reviewed the results and take full responsibility for the contents of the manuscript.

## References


1. Arora, R.K., et al.: Healthbench: evaluating large language models towards improved human health. arXiv preprint arXiv:2505.08775 (2025)
2. Bassett, B.A., et al.: Evaluating multimodal LLMs for inpatient diagnosis: real-world performance, safety, and cost across ten frontier models. arXiv preprint arXiv:2604.16980 (2026)
3. Bedi, S., et al.: Holistic evaluation of large language models for medical tasks with MedHELM. Nat. Med. 1–9 (2026)
4. Chiang, C.H., Lee, H.Y.: Can large language models be an alternative to human evaluations? In: Proceedings of the 61st Annual Meeting of the Association for Computational Linguistics (Volume 1: Long Papers), pp. 15607–15631 (2023)
5. Croxford, E., et al.: Automating evaluation of AI text generation in healthcare with a large language model (LLM)-as-a-judge. medRxiv (2025). https://doi.org/10.1101/2025.04.22.25326219
6. Croxford, E., et al.: Evaluating clinical AI summaries with large language models as judges. NPJ Digit. Med. **8**(1), 640 (2025)
7. Genovese, A., et al.: Artificial authority: the promise and perils of LLM judges in healthcare. Bioengineering **13**(1) (2026). https://doi.org/10.3390/bioengineering13010108
8. Li, D., et al.: From Generation to Judgment: Opportunities and Challenges of LLM-as-a-Judge (2025)
9. Reese, M.L., Zeneli, M., Ng, M., Haimes, J., Damien, A., Stade, E.: Using LLM-as-a-Judge/Jury to Advance Scalable, Clinically-Validated Safety Evaluations of Model Responses to Users Demonstrating Psychosis. arXiv preprint arXiv:2604.02359 (2026)
10. Williams, G., Rutunda, S., Nzabakira, F., Mateen, B.A.: Human Evaluators vs. LLM-as-a-Judge: Toward Scalable, Real-Time Evaluation of GenAI in Global Health. medRxiv (2025). https://doi.org/10.1101/2025.10.27.25338910
11. Zheng, L., et al.: Judging LLM-as-a-judge with MT-bench and chatbot arena. In: Advances in Neural Information Processing Systems (NeurIPS), Datasets and Benchmarks Track (2023)

# Causal Models with Tiny Data: The Case of Rural People Living with Dementia

Ranveer Singh[1(✉)], Saurabh Mathur[2], Kavimayil P. Komarasamy[1], Ameet Soni[3], Cliff Whetung[4], Wayne Warry[4], Kristen Jacklin[4], Melissa Blind[4], and Sriraam Natarajan[1]

[1] The University of Texas at Dallas, Richardson, TX 75080, USA
ranveer.singh@utdallas.edu
[2] Technische Universität Darmstadt, Darmstadt, Germany
[3] Swarthmore College, Swarthmore, PA 19081, USA
[4] University of Minnesota Medical School, Duluth Campus, Duluth, MN 55812, USA

**Abstract.** Causal modeling for specialized populations like non-urban dementia patients is critical for developing targeted interventions, yet reliable causal models are unavailable. Moreover, the inherent scarcity of data makes automatic causal discovery challenging. We study several approaches for building causal graphs under this data-scarce setting: expert elicitation, Large Language Model (LLM) generation, a data-driven method, and a hybrid method that refines expert and LLM-elicited graphs using data. Through direct structural comparison, our analysis reveals areas of agreement between the graphs, but also contradictions in different tendencies impacting the directionality and inclusion of socioeconomic and clinical factors. Additionally, we show that tiny data sets can be used to empirically validate conditional independencies encoded in these candidate causal graphs, concluding that causal modeling for specialized populations requires reconciling expert and LLM-generated causal discovery with tiny datasets.

**Keywords:** Life-Space Assessment · Causal Discovery · Data Scarce Domains · Large Language Models

## 1 Causal Modeling for Life-Space Assessment

Dementia is a progressive decline in cognitive functions. It can negatively impact the medical, social, functional, and psychological well-being of a patient, ranging from memory loss to depression to social withdrawal [2]. As the average life expectancy and aging population increase, dementia diagnoses will rise as well. Therefore, it is necessary to conduct more comprehensive studies to understand dementia and improve clinical outcomes. Persons Living with Dementia (PLWD)

---

We acknowledge support from NIH awards R01NS133142 and 1R21AG072566.
R. Singh and S. Mathur—Equal Contribution.

© The Author(s), under exclusive license to Springer Nature Switzerland AG 2027
P. Andreev et al. (Eds.): AIME 2026, LNAI 16748, pp. 378–383, 2027.
https://doi.org/10.1007/978-3-032-30710-1_45

can be studied by assessing their life-space mobility. It captures a person's physical and social environment, movement, and daily activities [1,8]. A decrease in life-space is associated with various measures of declining health in older adults, including cognitive decline [9].

Life-space mobility is primarily measured through a written survey called the Life-Space Assessment (LSA), which quantifies an older adult's geographic area in environmental zones and captures the rate at which they travel throughout the day [7]. For PLWD, LSA can be a useful tool to chart a patient's progress or mental decline [9]. However, LSAs have primarily focused on urban populations, limiting the applicability of LSAs to rural or Indigenous settings, where dementia risk is higher [10]. Therefore, LSA should be adapted for these settings, for example, by redefining environmental zones for rural and Indigenous contexts.

While life-space is an effective indicator of quality of life, developing interventions to improve outcomes requires causally modeling its relationship with relevant demographic and environmental variables. Causal models are often expressed as graphs, consisting of nodes representing the variables of interest, and directed edges between nodes representing cause-effect relationships [5]. Causal graphs concisely represent qualitative causal knowledge about a domain. In the absence of such domain knowledge, they might be learned from data.

Data-driven causal discovery methods exploit patterns in large amounts of high-dimensional data, along with assumptions about the underlying causal dynamics, to induce causal graphs. However, the paucity of data about understudied populations makes data-driven causal discovery challenging [3]. In low-data settings, a hybrid approach is adopted; smaller datasets are used to refine graphs derived from incomplete domain knowledge obtained from either domain experts or from LLMs [4], owing to their ability to capture correlations over causal facts from their vast training corpora [11]. Each of these approaches depends on good initial causal graphs, which are difficult to come by in understudied domains.

We aim to analyze the plausibility and mutual compatibility of the graphs obtained by these methods in terms of the empirical validity of their inferences. Specifically, we empirically evaluate the statistical independence statements inferred from each graph. Alongside qualitatively analyzing the similarities and differences across the graphs, the analysis furthers the goal of creating more comprehensive causal graphs by combining the expert knowledge, approximate knowledge from LLMs, and tiny data.

## 2 Qualitative and Quantitative Evaluation

We answer the following research questions:

**(Q1)** Is there any consensus in causal relations identified by experts and LLMs?

**(Q2)** Are the graphs obtained from experts and LLMs compatible with the statistical patterns present in the tiny dataset?

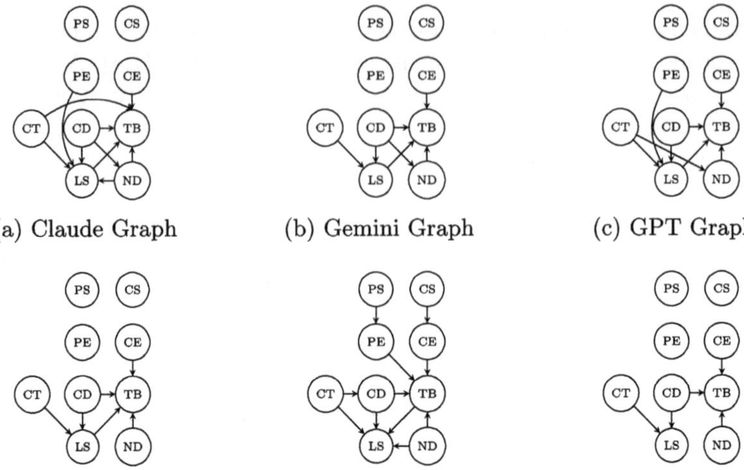


(a) Claude Graph (b) Gemini Graph (c) GPT Graph

(d) LLMs Consensus (e) Expert Graph (f) Overall Consensus

**Fig. 1.** The causal graphs for the Life-space Domain. (**a-c**) shows the causal graphs provided by the different LLMs, (**d**) shows the consensus (common causal relationships) across the different LLMs, (**e**) shows the expert causal graph, and (**f**) shows the consensus between the LLMs and the experts.

*Dataset.* To answer these questions, we constructed a dataset from LSAs of **20** patients conducted in **rural** and **Indigenous** communities in northern Minnesota, USA, and Ontario, Canada. We extracted nine boolean features from the LSA, demographic data for patients and caregivers, and the daily diaries completed by the caregiver over the course of a month. The features include the life-space score (LS), sex of the patient (PS) and caregiver (CS), education of the patient (PE) and caregiver (CE), and their community type (CT). We also consider the number of non-routine days (ND) and challenging days (CD) for the patient, as well as the total burden on the caregiver (TB). Continuous variables were binarized using expert-provided or sample mean-based thresholds[1]

*Methods.* For these variables, we consider 4 types of causal graph construction methods: Expert elicitation, LLM-generation, data-driven discovery, and Hybrid subtractive refinement. We obtain candidate causal graphs from multiple experts' consensus and 3 LLMs – Claude (4.5 Sonnet), Gemini (3 Thinking), and ChatGPT (GPT 5.2). To construct the graphs using the LLMs, they were prompted five times each with the variables and their description, and asked to come up with causal relationships as well as their corresponding weight[1]. The graphs were then pooled to form a single graph by adding causal edges in decreasing order of their average weight, excluding any edges introducing a cycle or having an average weight below a threshold. Additionally, we considered a hybrid subtractive refinement method [4] that refines the above graphs

[1] The thresholds, prompts, and their responses are provided in the supplementary.

by deleting edges to optimize the Minimal Description Length score. Finally, we implemented the purely data-based baseline using the Fast Causal Inference (FCI) algorithm [6].

*Results.* To answer **(Q1)**, we compare the graphs structurally using consensus sets (relations common to all graphs) and conflict sets (disagreements between candidate graphs). Figure 1 shows that the **LLMs agree on six direct causal relationships with each other**: Non-routine days (ND), community type (CT), education of caregiver (CE), and life-space score (LS) are direct causes of total burden (TB); challenging days (CD), and community type (CT) are direct causes of life-space score (LS). While experts agree with the LLMs on five of these six relationships, *they invert the final edge*, placing the causal direction from TB to LS. This disparity suggests a fundamental difference in modeling perspectives: *the experts appear to be more interested in the patient's outcomes*, treating the life-space score (LS) as the final sink node, while the LLMs consistently identify the caregiver's total burden (TB) as the ultimate sink variable. This disparity might also point to the bidirectional nature of the relationship, requiring a disaggregation across time. Further, the LLMs exclude socio-economic factors such as sex and education, which the experts identify as significant causal drivers.

**Table 1.** Empirically validating candidate graphs. For each model, we summarize (i) Total: number of conditional independencies (CI) implied by graph structure (via d-separation), (ii) Precision: fraction of CI statements entailed by the model that were compatible with the data, and (iii) False positive rate (FPR): fraction of CI statements incompatible with the data that were entailed by the model. CIs were empirically tested using the G-test at a significance threshold of $\alpha = 0.05$ and a conditioning set of size at most one.

| Model | Total | Precision | FPR |
|---|---|---|---|
| Expert | 113 | 0.73 | 0.53 |
| GPT | 45 | 0.67 | 0.48 |
| Claude | 45 | 0.73 | 0.39 |
| Gemini | 23 | 0.70 | 0.33 |
| LLM Consesus | 31 | 0.68 | 0.48 |
| Overall Consesus | 39 | 0.72 | 0.52 |

To answer **(Q2)**, we examine the results of the refinement procedure. The number of edges deleted during this process serves as a measure of compatibility between the causal models and the dataset. Refinement eliminated nearly all edges, leaving fewer than three in the final graphs. Further, while the data-driven baseline did not identify any causal edges, it did identify 3 undirected associations: caregiver's sex with patient's sex, caregiver's education with community type, and challenging days with total burden. These results indicate high incompatibility between the tiny dataset and the LLMs' and the experts' graphs.

Next, we analyze the nature of this incompatibility by empirically evaluating the conditional independence (CI) relations entailed by each graph. We treat each network as a model that predicts whether variables $X$ and $Y$ are independent given a variable $Z$. We evaluate these predictions against data-driven labels using the G-test. Since incorrectly assuming independence is more detrimental to causal inference than failing to identify it, we quantify each graph's divergence from data-driven CIs using False Positive Rate (FPR) and Precision metrics. Table 1 summarizes the results. Clearly, the expert graph entails more CIs than the LLM graphs. As a result, it has a higher or equal precision, but a higher FPR than the LLM graphs. On the other hand, the LLM graphs entail fewer independencies overall, but still entail independencies incompatible with data. Of these, Claude's graph has a lower FPR and the same precision as the expert graph, but entails less than half the number of independencies.

Neither the LLM-generated graphs nor the expert-constructed graphs are compatible with the data. However, they are incompatible in different ways, illustrating the differences between expert and LLM-based causal models.

## 3 Discussion

We considered the problem of causally modeling the life-space mobility of people living with dementia in non-urban environments. The domain's understudied nature and the resulting data paucity make this a challenging problem. We considered two additional sources of causal knowledge: domain experts and LLMs. While data-driven causal discovery and refinement of expert and LLM-elicited causal graphs proved unsuccessful, the tiny dataset allowed us to compare the two types of graphs. The graph structures reveal distinct underlying assumptions. Experts prioritized patient-centric outcomes and integrated socio-economic factors like sex and education into the causal structure. In contrast, the LLMs focused on the total burden and ignored the socio-economic factors. Our analysis of the differences among sources of causal knowledge – domain experts, LLMs, and tiny datasets – provides a foundation for hybrid causal models. Understanding the interplay between expert-led and LLM-driven discovery remains essential for developing robust clinical decision-support systems.

## References

1. Baker, P.S., Bodner, E.V., Allman, R.M.: Measuring life-space mobility in community-dwelling older adults. J. Am. Geriatr. Soc. **51**(11), 1610–1614 (2003)
2. Geldmacher, D.S., Whitehouse, P.J.: Evaluation of dementia. N. Engl. J. Med. **335**(5), 330–336 (1996)
3. Hasan, U., Hossain, E., Gani, M.O.: A survey on causal discovery methods for IID and time series data. TMLR (2023)
4. Mathur, S., Singh, R., et al.: LLM-guided causal Bayesian network construction for pediatric patients on ECMO. In: Bellazzi, R., Juarez Herrero, J.M., Sacchi, L., Zupan, B. (eds.) AIME 2025. LNCS, vol. 15735, pp. 255–260. Springer, Cham (2025). https://doi.org/10.1007/978-3-031-95841-0_48

5. Pearl, J.: Causality. Cambridge University Press, Cambridge (2009)
6. Spirtes, P.: An anytime algorithm for causal inference. In: AISTATS, pp. 278–285. PMLR (2001)
7. Stalvey, B.T., Owsley, C., et al.: The life space questionnaire: a measure of the extent of mobility of older adults. J. Appl. Gerontol. **18**(4) (1999)
8. Taylor, J.K., Buchan, I.E., Van Der Veer, S.N.: Assessing life-space mobility for a more holistic view on wellbeing in geriatric research and clinical practice. Aging Clin. Exp. Res. **31**(4), 439–445 (2019)
9. Ullrich, P., Eckert, T., et al.: Life-space mobility in older persons with cognitive impairment after discharge from geriatric rehabilitation. Arch. Gerontol. Geriatr. **81**, 192–200 (2019)
10. Xie, Z., Hu, J., et al.: Rural-urban differences in modifiable dementia risk factors among us populations aged 45 years or older. J Alzheimers Dis. Rep. **9** (2025)
11. Zečević, M., Willig, M., Dhami, D.S., Kersting, K.: Causal parrots: large language models may talk causality but are not causal. TMLR (2023)

# Assessing Mental Health Therapeutic Capacity in AI Agents

Piergiorgio Maruotti[1], Mattia Rampazzo[1], Sergio Muñoz[2], Mauro Dragoni[1], and Patrizio Bellan[1](✉)

[1] Digital Health and Wellbeing Research Center, Fondazione Bruno Kessler, Trento, Italy
{maruotti,rampazzo,dragoni,pbellan}@fbk.eu
[2] Universidad Politécnica de Madrid, Madrid, Spain
sergio.munoz@upm.es

**Abstract.** Large Language Models (LLMs) have been widely investigated for conversational support in mental health. However, their therapeutic reliability in empathy and perspective-taking remains uncertain. We aim to fill this gap by introducing a comprehensive evaluation of the Pool of Experts framework, a multi-agent approach that enables role-specific identities without retraining the underlying model. Beyond its effectiveness, this framework provides a controlled test-bed to study whether personality framing induces measurable behavioral variation across roles and tasks. We systematically assess the Pool of Experts capability in empathy and theory-of-mind-oriented benchmarks through question-answering tasks, evaluating accuracy via strict and relaxed match against gold answers, and compare structured multi-agent orchestration with less structured conditions. Results demonstrate three main findings. First, architectural orchestration with deliberative aggregation consistently improves performance: a Final Decision Maker agent improves accuracy by up to 4.1% points compared with individual experts. This aggregation mechanism also provides superior error recovery compared to majority voting. Second, such improvements generalize robustly across model families without requiring larger parameter scales. Compact and large-scale architectures achieve comparable benefits. Third, process-oriented frameworks yield the strongest gains, while theory-of-mind tasks benefit more reliably from structured orchestration than empathy tasks. This suggests perspective-taking is currently more tractable for optimization than affective alignment. These findings support structured multi-agent orchestration as a reliable way to improve socio-cognitive behaviors in mental-health-oriented LLM systems.

**Keywords:** Agent Personality Framing · Mental Health · Empathy · Theory of Mind · Multi-Agent Systems

© The Author(s), under exclusive license to Springer Nature Switzerland AG 2027
P. Andreev et al. (Eds.): AIME 2026, LNAI 16748, pp. 384–394, 2027.
https://doi.org/10.1007/978-3-032-30710-1_46

## 1 Introduction

The rapid growth of Large Language Models (LLMs) has enabled the development of persona agents capable of adopting structured roles and simulating psychological perspectives [11,22]. These systems are increasingly deployed in domains such as digital health, coaching, education, and therapeutic support, where they must interact with human reasoning and emotional attunement [28]. A concrete deployment scenario is provided by ChatFAQ within the TREC-Mamma project, a Trentino-based application designed to support pregnant women through accessible digital information services. In this setting, our Pool of Experts (PoE) architecture has been integrated into the conversational pipeline, where specialized agents support query assessment, response validation, and the generation of contextually appropriate outputs. PoE is also being adapted for additional applied pipelines, indicating the practical relevance of evaluating such systems beyond controlled experimental benchmarks. As these applications expand, evaluating empathic capacity and perspective-taking has become critical. Traditional evaluations of empathy and theory of mind in LLMs have predominantly focused on single-agent architectures [6], leaving the ability of multi-agent systems grounded in psychological frameworks to demonstrate these capacities largely unexplored [8].

Multi-agent systems offer a promising alternative by simulating collaborative processes [35]. Among these approaches, the Pool of Experts (PoE) architecture represents a distinctive approach in which agent prompts incorporating personality profiles are generated by a dedicated LLM-wise agent based on psychological and user-design science frameworks [1]. A central feature of PoE is that these profiles grounded in identity are not handcrafted but produced systematically for specialized roles, including project managers, expert agents, and final decision makers. However, the comparative effectiveness of different theoretical frameworks in guiding these agents has not been systematically evaluated.

This study evaluates whether multi-agent systems grounded in psychological frameworks can reliably demonstrate empathic capacity and adopt human perspectives, by organizing selected frameworks into distinct structural types: interpretative or role-based (User-Centered Design, Freudian Psychoanalysis); process-oriented (Dual Process Theory, Cognitive Load Theory); dynamic or motivational (Flow Theory); and minimally specified baseline conditions. The proposed PoE-based agents were evaluated for accuracy on question-answering tasks across six datasets: three in the empathy domain and three in the theory of mind domain. Therefore, we focus on the following research questions (RQs):

- **RQ1**: Which psychological frameworks perform best across empathy and theory of mind tasks for different agent roles and datasets?
- **RQ2**: How do different framework types compare in terms of empathic capacity and perspective-taking abilities?
- **RQ3**: Does the system generalize across different LLM models of different scales?

The original contributions of this work are threefold. First, we provide the first systematic evaluation of the Pool of Experts framework on socio-cognitive benchmarks targeting empathy and theory of mind, covering six datasets across both domains. Second, we introduce a controlled experimental design that disentangles the effect of psychological framework choice from architectural orchestration, comparing deliberative aggregation via a Final Decision Maker, majority voting, and single-agent baselines across five LLMs of varying scale and three model families. Third, we demonstrate that structured multi-agent orchestration yields consistent improvements over individual expert agents and unstructured conditions, with gains that generalize across model families independently of parameter count. The remainder of the paper is structured as follows. Section 2 provides an overview of the relevant literature on agent personality and multi-agent systems. Section 3 presents the PoE framework. In Sect. 4, we detail the datasets, evaluation metrics, and experimental setup. Section 5 presents the results and discusses the main findings organized by research question. Finally, Sect. 6 presents the conclusions and outlines potential avenues for future research.

## 2 Related Work

We review two complementary streams of research: *agent personalization*, which studies how psychologically grounded personas shape LLM behavior, and *multi-agent systems*, which investigates how coordination and aggregation shape collective intelligence.

*Agent Personality.* Conversational agents have long leveraged psychological frameworks (most prominently the Big Five) to induce consistent interaction styles and enable personalization [24,30]. In applied domains such as healthcare, persona-based design can improve perceived empathy, trust, and task outcomes [12,14]. Prompt- and data-driven approaches have also been proposed to improve contextual awareness and diversify dialogue behaviors in LLMs [17,25]. Recent work scales persona diversity and evaluates trait stability under synthetic personas, including persona-aligned datasets and analyses of Big Five and social-identity effects on downstream behavior [10,16]. These studies typically focus on a single framework or a narrow set of tasks. Personality- and identity-grounded prompting provides further evidence of *propagated* influence. Big Five traits and upstream profile definitions can induce stable patterns and shape downstream agents [7,16], including effects on task selection over time [20]. Together, these results motivate our use of psychologically grounded identities as a controllable inductive bias for both expert roles and the coordinator. Beyond trait prompting, recent studies investigate how LLMs can *define* profiles and generate persona-consistent content [7], and how automatically generated expert roles can improve diversity and factual accuracy in multi-agent reasoning [13,18].

*Multi-agent Systems.* Prior work in multi-agent systems shows that a single coordinator can substantially shape group behavior, including debate-style judges, proactive controllers, and hierarchical leaders that align plans and fuse peer outputs [15,27,36]. Control-loop and multi-expert pipelines show that monitoring and synthesis can redirect other agents' reasoning [2,18,19], while simple ensembles illustrate protocol-level aggregation. By contrast, we steer the identity of the aggregator agent: our `Final Decision Maker` (FDM) agent is described with (or without) psychologically grounded traits, and we compare it to voting baselines to isolate how identity conditions aggregation and group-level outcomes.

## 3 The Pool of Experts Framework

The **PoE** framework, first introduced in [1], addresses complex queries by integrating multiple specialized viewpoints, similarly to how interdisciplinary teams support human decision-making. PoE implements this idea by coordinating a set of LLM-based agents, each assigned a distinct role and guided by an explicit profile that shapes how it interprets and reasons about the query and communicates its conclusions. Here, an *agent* is an autonomous entity instantiated from an LLM and guided by a personality description injected into the system prompt.

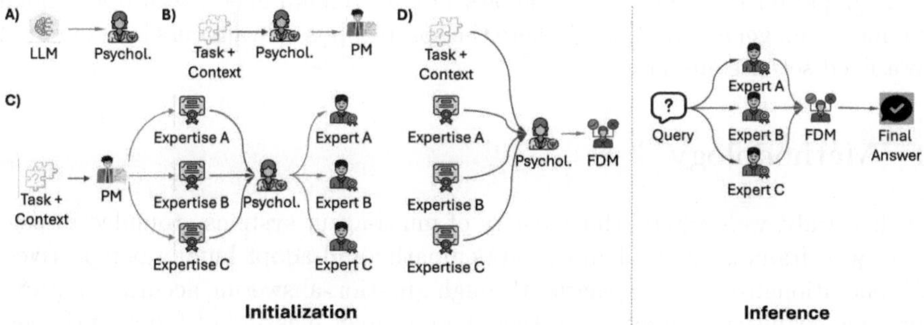


**Fig. 1.** The figure, taken from [1], shows an overview of the PoE framework. The pipeline is divided in two phases: (i) initialization where roles are defined and experts are instantiated and (ii) inference where experts work on a query and FDM provides the final answer.

Behavioral diversity is not achieved through model fine-tuning, but induced through prompt-based personality framings. Concretely, each agent is associated with a textual personality description generated under the guidance of a chosen description framework taken from psychological (or user-design) theory, which is injected into the prompt before inference. The profile acts as an inductive bias that can influence the agent's reasoning and communication style. In this work, we investigate whether specific profile-description frameworks consistently support better accuracy across question-answering tasks in empathy and theory-of-mind domains, and whether personality-driven variation within a single task yields significant differences in performance.

PoE comprises two stages: *initialization* and *inference* (see Fig. 1). During initialization, the framework configures a set of role-specialized agents, each shaped by a tailored profile mirroring interdisciplinary decision-making teams. Initialization begins with a **Psychologist Agent (PA)** (Fig. 1-A), which generates profile descriptions for all subsequent agents by conditioning each description on the agent's functional role, the task instruction, and the problem domain. The first agent generated by the PA is the **Project Manager (PM)** (Fig. 1-B), which serves as system orchestrator: it analyzes the task and identifies the domains of expertise required of the **Expert Agents (EAs)** (Fig. 1-C), who collaborate on the problem. Note that the number of EAs may vary, as PoE dynamically recruits agents based on task demands, though the architectural dynamics related to expert selection fall outside the scope of this paper.

Finally, a **Final Decision Maker (FDM)** (see Fig. 1-D) is instantiated to integrate the EAs' outputs and produce the final response. The FDM is an LLM agent drawn from the same backbone as the experts, prompted to review all expert responses, identify convergences and disagreements, and synthesize a single coherent answer. Rather than relying on simple averaging or majority voting the FDM operates through prompted deliberation: its output is emergent from the underlying LLM conditioned on expert responses, rather than a deterministic aggregation rule. This design allows PoE to remain effective in open-ended settings (e.g., generative Q&A) where the space of possible answers is not limited to a fixed set of candidates.

## 4 Methodology

In this study, we evaluate the capacity of multi-agent systems grounded in psychological frameworks to demonstrate empathy and adopt human perspectives. We operationalize these capacities through question-answering accuracy, a proxy for socio-cognitive competence rather than a direct measure of therapeutic performance. To this end, we systematically vary three experimental dimensions: (i) the description framework assigned to the agents; (ii) the backbone LLM; and, (iii) the task dataset. Each combination is compared against a baseline condition consisting of standard single-call LLM inference without identity framing.

Psychological identity descriptions were organized by theoretical architecture: interpretative or role-based (User-Centered Design [21] *UCD*, User Design Persona [3] *UDP* and Freudian Psychoanalysis [5] *FP*), process-oriented (Dual-Process Theory [31] *DPT*, Cognitive Load Theory [29] *CLT*), dynamic or motivational (Flow Theory [4] *FT*), and unstructured baselines (no-description and no-personality). For each framework, we instantiate the full PoE multi-agent system across all selected models and tasks.

We evaluated five LLMs drawn from three major model families selected to reflect variation in architectural design, parameter scale and accessibility. From the Gemma family, we included gemma-3-12b-it and gemma-3-27b-it. From the LLaMA family, we evaluated llama-3.3-70b-instruct and llama-4-scout. In addition, we included nova-micro-v1 as a compact, cost-efficient baseline model.

All experiments were conducted via the OpenRouter API[1] using fixed decoding parameters and deterministic random seeds to ensure reproducibility and consistency across runs.

To evaluate language model capabilities on empathy and Theory of Mind (ToM), we selected three datasets per domain and built reproducible evaluation subsets via stratified sampling with fixed random seeds. For empathy, we used *EDOS* [32], annotated with 32 fine-grained emotions; *IEMPATHIZE* [9], labeled by empathy direction (seeking, providing, none); and *EmpatheticDialogues* [23], a corpus of nearly 25K conversations across 32 emotion categories. For ToM, we used *Hi-ToM* [33], with Sally-Anne-style stories targeting different ToM reasoning levels; *ToMATO* [26], covering multiple mental-state dimensions; and *OpenToM* [34], probing ToM through narrative questions on location tracking, multi-hop inference, and attitude attribution. Due to computational constraints, subsets were built via stratified sampling: *EDOS* and *EmpatheticDialogues* with 10 dialogues per emotion label (32 labels), *IEMPATHIZE* with 40 sentences per class. *Hi-ToM* was stratified by question order, story length, and deceptive communication (30 subgroups, 5 samples each); *ToMATO* by ToM order, mental-state category, and false-belief condition (20 subgroups); *OpenToM* by question type, ToM order, and answer granularity.

We evaluated question-answering performance against gold answers using two complementary metrics. First, *strict match* counted a prediction as correct only when it exactly matched the gold answer. Second, *relaxed match* counted a prediction as correct when the system returned either the correct option label (e.g., "[a]") or the corresponding option content (e.g., "seeking"), or both (e.g., "[a] seeking").

## 5 Results and Discussion

In Sect. 1, we outlined three key research questions. Here, we report the results of the analyses in Table 1 and discuss the findings.

The primary focus of the first question (**RQ1**) was to investigate which psychological frameworks perform best across empathy and ToM tasks. The results show that the effects of the identity description framework exist but are compact. Overall, averaging strict-match in the FDM condition across models and datasets, *no-descr* is the strongest condition (0.528), followed by *CLT* (0.514) and *DPT* (0.513). The spread between best and worst framework in FDM is small (about 2.7% points), indicating that framework choice matters, but less than orchestration choices.

Role effects do exist and are systematic. Compared with the average of the EAs, FDM always provides slight improvements, without exception. MV also improves over EAs, but FDM remains the strongest integrator on average. We run Mann-Whitney-U-statistic tests to compare FDM, MV, and baseline. The results confirm a statistical mean difference between the two aggregation methods and baseline, but no statistical difference between the two methods.

[1] https://openrouter.ai/.

**Table 1.** Strict-match accuracy by model, identity description framework, and dataset across FDM, MV, and Expert Agents mean. Bold values indicate the best performance for each model-dataset pair across all frameworks and roles. Baseline (Base) scores are reported in Exp column. In this condition, FDM and MV are not applicable.

| Model | Desc.f. | EDOS | | | IEMPATHIZE | | | EmpDialog | | | HiToM | | | OpenToM | | | ToMATO | | |
|---|---|---|---|---|---|---|---|---|---|---|---|---|---|---|---|---|---|---|---|
| | | FDM | MV | Exp | FDM | MV | Exp | FDM | MV | Exp | FDM | MV | Exp | FDM | MV | Exp | FDM | MV | Exp |
| nova-micro-v1 | CLT | 0.40 | 0.38 | 0.33 | 0.60 | 0.59 | 0.59 | 0.39 | 0.37 | 0.36 | 0.51 | 0.45 | 0.40 | 0.44 | 0.43 | 0.40 | 0.49 | 0.49 | 0.48 |
| | DPT | **0.42** | 0.41 | 0.36 | 0.61 | 0.60 | 0.60 | 0.38 | 0.38 | 0.37 | **0.53** | 0.51 | 0.43 | 0.45 | 0.46 | 0.41 | **0.51** | 0.49 | 0.49 |
| | FT | 0.40 | 0.40 | 0.34 | 0.62 | 0.61 | 0.55 | 0.36 | 0.36 | 0.35 | 0.48 | 0.50 | 0.40 | 0.44 | **0.50** | 0.45 | 0.49 | 0.50 | 0.49 |
| | FP | 0.38 | 0.38 | 0.35 | 0.66 | 0.64 | 0.62 | 0.37 | 0.37 | 0.36 | 0.48 | 0.49 | 0.41 | 0.45 | 0.46 | 0.46 | 0.49 | 0.50 | 0.49 |
| | UDP | 0.41 | 0.39 | 0.34 | 0.64 | 0.65 | 0.61 | 0.38 | 0.38 | 0.36 | 0.52 | 0.47 | 0.41 | 0.43 | 0.42 | 0.40 | 0.48 | 0.47 | 0.47 |
| | UCD | 0.41 | 0.39 | 0.36 | 0.65 | 0.64 | 0.60 | 0.38 | 0.38 | 0.35 | 0.45 | 0.46 | 0.41 | 0.42 | 0.42 | 0.42 | 0.50 | 0.49 | 0.50 |
| | no-descr | **0.42** | **0.42** | 0.38 | 0.67 | **0.68** | 0.64 | 0.40 | **0.42** | 0.39 | 0.48 | 0.45 | 0.39 | 0.45 | 0.41 | 0.40 | 0.50 | **0.51** | 0.49 |
| | no-pers | 0.39 | 0.38 | 0.35 | 0.61 | 0.58 | 0.61 | 0.39 | 0.39 | 0.37 | 0.45 | 0.49 | 0.39 | 0.43 | 0.44 | 0.42 | 0.46 | 0.50 | 0.47 |
| | baseline | - | - | 0.36 | - | - | 0.43 | - | - | 0.00 | - | - | 0.00 | - | - | 0.00 | - | - | 0.01 |
| gemma-3-12b-it | CLT | 0.45 | 0.43 | 0.38 | 0.67 | 0.66 | 0.64 | **0.47** | 0.45 | 0.43 | 0.56 | 0.57 | 0.53 | 0.47 | 0.48 | 0.48 | 0.65 | 0.66 | 0.66 |
| | DPT | 0.48 | 0.44 | 0.39 | **0.68** | 0.64 | 0.63 | 0.44 | 0.43 | 0.42 | 0.57 | 0.60 | 0.55 | 0.43 | 0.45 | 0.46 | 0.64 | 0.65 | 0.64 |
| | FT | 0.42 | 0.45 | 0.38 | 0.62 | 0.63 | 0.63 | 0.45 | 0.45 | 0.44 | 0.61 | **0.63** | 0.55 | 0.49 | **0.50** | 0.47 | 0.68 | 0.67 | 0.65 |
| | FP | 0.32 | 0.32 | 0.27 | 0.61 | 0.59 | 0.61 | 0.44 | 0.44 | 0.42 | 0.59 | 0.60 | 0.54 | 0.45 | 0.45 | 0.46 | 0.66 | 0.63 | 0.63 |
| | UDP | 0.42 | 0.44 | 0.38 | 0.64 | 0.66 | 0.66 | **0.47** | 0.44 | 0.41 | 0.56 | 0.59 | 0.55 | 0.43 | 0.45 | 0.45 | 0.68 | 0.67 | 0.65 |
| | UCD | 0.45 | 0.44 | 0.40 | 0.63 | 0.63 | 0.62 | 0.43 | 0.44 | 0.44 | 0.55 | 0.59 | 0.53 | 0.43 | 0.45 | 0.46 | 0.67 | 0.66 | 0.66 |
| | no-descr | **0.49** | **0.49** | 0.45 | 0.66 | 0.67 | 0.65 | 0.44 | 0.44 | 0.44 | 0.57 | 0.59 | 0.53 | 0.47 | 0.49 | 0.48 | 0.68 | **0.69** | 0.64 |
| | no-pers | 0.44 | 0.43 | 0.38 | 0.66 | 0.66 | 0.65 | 0.46 | 0.45 | 0.43 | 0.59 | 0.59 | 0.53 | 0.46 | 0.43 | 0.44 | 0.67 | 0.65 | 0.64 |
| | baseline | - | - | 0.44 | - | - | 0.66 | - | - | 0.42 | - | - | 0.00 | - | - | 0.00 | - | - | 0.67 |
| gemma-3-27b-it | CLT | 0.44 | 0.42 | 0.38 | 0.66 | 0.63 | 0.63 | 0.45 | 0.45 | 0.43 | 0.08 | 0.05 | 0.08 | 0.52 | 0.54 | 0.53 | 0.65 | 0.65 | 0.66 |
| | DPT | 0.41 | 0.42 | 0.37 | 0.60 | 0.62 | 0.62 | 0.44 | 0.44 | 0.42 | 0.05 | 0.03 | 0.07 | 0.54 | **0.56** | 0.52 | 0.67 | 0.68 | 0.67 |
| | FT | 0.40 | 0.42 | 0.37 | 0.66 | 0.66 | 0.65 | **0.47** | 0.46 | 0.44 | 0.08 | 0.09 | 0.09 | 0.54 | 0.54 | 0.52 | **0.69** | 0.67 | 0.67 |
| | FP | 0.32 | 0.33 | 0.30 | 0.64 | 0.63 | 0.63 | 0.41 | 0.40 | 0.38 | **0.12** | 0.06 | 0.08 | 0.52 | 0.54 | 0.52 | 0.67 | **0.69** | 0.67 |
| | UDP | 0.39 | 0.41 | 0.37 | 0.66 | 0.69 | 0.67 | 0.44 | 0.45 | 0.41 | 0.09 | 0.05 | 0.08 | 0.53 | 0.54 | 0.53 | 0.67 | **0.69** | 0.68 |
| | UCD | 0.42 | 0.43 | 0.40 | 0.65 | 0.68 | 0.66 | 0.43 | 0.43 | 0.42 | 0.09 | 0.05 | 0.08 | 0.54 | **0.56** | 0.53 | 0.68 | 0.68 | 0.68 |
| | no-descr | **0.47** | 0.45 | 0.43 | 0.67 | 0.69 | 0.66 | 0.46 | 0.46 | 0.44 | 0.09 | 0.03 | 0.07 | 0.51 | 0.53 | 0.54 | 0.68 | 0.67 | 0.68 |
| | no-pers | 0.43 | 0.43 | 0.40 | 0.62 | 0.65 | 0.63 | 0.45 | 0.46 | 0.43 | 0.06 | 0.04 | 0.06 | 0.54 | 0.53 | 0.53 | 0.67 | **0.69** | 0.67 |
| | baseline | - | - | 0.42 | - | - | **0.74** | - | - | 0.21 | - | - | 0.00 | - | - | 0.00 | - | - | 0.20 |
| llama-3.3-70b | CLT | 0.47 | 0.46 | 0.45 | 0.67 | 0.68 | 0.67 | 0.44 | 0.45 | 0.44 | 0.68 | 0.68 | 0.66 | 0.53 | 0.54 | 0.53 | 0.75 | 0.76 | 0.76 |
| | DPT | 0.47 | 0.46 | 0.44 | 0.66 | 0.67 | 0.66 | 0.45 | 0.46 | 0.45 | 0.67 | 0.68 | 0.67 | **0.56** | 0.52 | 0.53 | 0.74 | 0.76 | 0.75 |
| | FT | 0.47 | 0.47 | 0.45 | 0.68 | 0.67 | 0.67 | 0.46 | 0.44 | 0.44 | 0.65 | 0.69 | 0.67 | 0.53 | 0.51 | 0.52 | 0.77 | **0.79** | 0.76 |
| | FP | 0.46 | 0.45 | 0.45 | 0.67 | 0.68 | 0.65 | 0.44 | 0.45 | 0.44 | 0.65 | 0.67 | 0.67 | 0.52 | 0.55 | 0.53 | 0.73 | 0.75 | 0.74 |
| | UDP | 0.46 | 0.45 | 0.44 | 0.70 | 0.69 | 0.69 | 0.46 | 0.46 | 0.45 | **0.70** | 0.69 | 0.68 | 0.50 | 0.51 | 0.52 | 0.75 | 0.75 | 0.75 |
| | UCD | 0.47 | 0.46 | 0.44 | 0.68 | 0.68 | 0.67 | 0.44 | 0.45 | 0.44 | 0.68 | **0.70** | 0.67 | **0.56** | 0.55 | 0.54 | 0.75 | 0.75 | 0.75 |
| | no-descr | **0.48** | **0.48** | 0.46 | 0.69 | 0.69 | 0.69 | 0.46 | **0.47** | 0.46 | 0.67 | 0.69 | 0.67 | 0.52 | 0.50 | 0.52 | 0.75 | 0.75 | 0.74 |
| | no-pers | 0.47 | 0.47 | 0.45 | 0.67 | 0.67 | 0.66 | 0.45 | 0.46 | 0.44 | 0.69 | 0.68 | 0.67 | 0.55 | 0.52 | 0.54 | 0.73 | 0.76 | 0.76 |
| | baseline | - | - | 0.45 | - | - | **0.71** | - | - | 0.00 | - | - | 0.00 | - | - | 0.00 | - | - | 0.76 |
| llama-4-scout | CLT | 0.43 | 0.43 | 0.42 | 0.66 | 0.66 | 0.65 | **0.46** | 0.45 | 0.43 | 0.19 | 0.21 | 0.20 | 0.54 | 0.52 | 0.51 | 0.71 | 0.73 | 0.69 |
| | DPT | **0.47** | **0.47** | 0.44 | 0.67 | 0.66 | 0.66 | **0.46** | 0.43 | 0.43 | 0.14 | 0.11 | 0.14 | 0.52 | 0.53 | 0.52 | 0.74 | **0.75** | 0.72 |
| | FT | **0.47** | 0.44 | 0.44 | 0.66 | 0.63 | 0.64 | 0.44 | 0.43 | 0.42 | 0.11 | 0.16 | 0.15 | 0.49 | 0.50 | 0.50 | 0.72 | 0.72 | 0.71 |
| | FP | 0.46 | 0.43 | 0.43 | 0.65 | 0.67 | 0.66 | **0.46** | 0.45 | 0.43 | 0.17 | 0.15 | 0.14 | 0.50 | 0.53 | 0.51 | 0.72 | 0.73 | 0.70 |
| | UDP | 0.45 | 0.43 | 0.42 | 0.66 | 0.64 | 0.65 | 0.44 | 0.43 | 0.42 | 0.08 | 0.09 | 0.12 | 0.54 | 0.53 | 0.52 | 0.68 | 0.70 | 0.71 |
| | UCD | **0.47** | 0.44 | 0.43 | 0.65 | 0.66 | 0.65 | 0.45 | **0.46** | 0.43 | 0.19 | 0.21 | 0.19 | 0.54 | 0.53 | 0.53 | 0.71 | 0.71 | 0.70 |
| | no-descr | 0.44 | 0.44 | 0.41 | **0.68** | 0.67 | 0.67 | 0.43 | 0.44 | 0.44 | **0.31** | 0.23 | 0.25 | **0.58** | 0.57 | 0.55 | 0.71 | 0.72 | 0.68 |
| | no-pers | 0.46 | 0.44 | 0.43 | 0.65 | 0.63 | 0.65 | 0.44 | 0.44 | 0.43 | 0.13 | 0.13 | 0.15 | 0.50 | 0.50 | 0.50 | 0.69 | 0.71 | 0.68 |
| | baseline | - | - | 0.33 | - | - | 0.47 | - | - | 0.00 | - | - | 0.00 | - | - | 0.00 | - | - | 0.17 |

We analyzed the errors of the two aggregation strategies. Both aggregation strategies provide a clear net corrective effect over individual expert outputs. MV corrects 792 expert errors while introducing 266 new errors, yielding a net benefit of +526 cases. FDM achieves the highest absolute recovery: it corrects 1467 errors but introduces 854 new ones, for a higher net benefit of +613 (+16.5% relative to MV). Hence, the FDM is more accurate and preferable when maximizing error recovery, whereas MV is preferable in settings where robustness and low-risk aggregation are prioritized.

The second research question (**RQ2**) addressed how different framework types compare in terms of empathic capacity and perspective-taking abilities. The marked discrepancy between performance in ToM and empathy datasets reveals a structural asymmetry in current LLM capabilities. While one empathy dataset achieved comparable performance, two out of three remained below 50% accuracy, suggesting persistent challenges in affective alignment. A clear domain asymmetry emerges. In the FDM condition, *no-description* is strongest in empathy, whereas *Flow Theory* is strongest in ToM. This suggests that dynamic/motivational formulations are better aligned with perspective-taking tasks.

Overall, the evidence indicates that the current framework engineering improves both capacities, but perspective-taking is currently easier to optimize than affective alignment. Furthermore, all identity description frameworks benefit from an improvement due to the presence of the Final Decision Maker, confirming its utility. Moreover, two of the top three frameworks describe Process Constructs (Dual Process Theory, Cognitive Load Theory), while from the third to the fifth positions, it emerges that frameworks denoting role-based frames (Freudian Psychoanalysis, User Design Persona, User Centered Design) obtained comparable scores. At the bottom, close together, are frameworks that lack a structured description. This ranking pattern in which process-oriented frameworks (DPT, CLT) consistently occupy the top positions, followed by role-based frameworks (FP, UDP, UCD), with unstructured conditions at the bottom suggests that persona conditioning is useful but not sufficient alone. From an application perspective, the fact that perspective-taking can be stronger than affective alignment in several settings indicates that empathy remains a key bottleneck for clinically credible deployment.

The third research question (**RQ3**) examined whether the system generalizes across LLMs of different scales. The results indicate cross-model competitiveness but non-monotonic scaling. In FDM, average strict-match is highest for *llama-3.3-70b-instruct*, followed by *gemma-3-12b-it*, *llama-4-scout*, *nova-micro-v1*, and *gemma-3-27b-it*. Thus, a larger parameter count does not guarantee better performance. No positive correlation was found between model parameter scale and performance, suggesting that architectural configuration and alignment strategies may play a more significant role than parameter count.

Finally, strict match remains intentionally conservative. In the same experimental outputs, relaxed match increases by about 5%, while preserving the main ranking patterns. Overall, these results move the concept of a virtual psychologist from an intuitive prompting strategy to an empirically grounded system design, showing that robust socio-cognitive behavior depends on coordination mechanisms more than on richer identity framing alone.

To ensure transparency and reproducibility, we provide the complete analysis pipeline, code, and detailed results in the paper repository[2].

## 6 Conclusions

This study examined whether a multi-agent setup with psychologically inspired descriptions improves performance on empathy and ToM benchmarks. Regard-

[2] Available at: https://github.com/patriziobellan86/AIME2026.

ing RQ1, identity framework effects are task-dependent and generally modest: richer descriptions do not consistently help, and the no-description condition is often competitive, with the spread between best and worst framework remaining within 2.7% points. Across all settings, adding a Final Decision Maker improves over both individual expert agents and majority voting, with a net error recovery advantage of 16.5% relative to majority voting, supporting explicit deliberative integration as the primary driver of performance gains over persona framing alone. Regarding RQ2, gains are more robust in ToM than in empathy, where performance remains below 50% in two out of three datasets, suggesting that affective alignment remains a key bottleneck for clinically credible deployment. Regarding RQ3, llama-3.3-70b-instruct and gemma-3-12b-it are among the strongest systems, but we do not observe a monotonic scale effect, indicating that architectural configuration matters more than parameter count.

Overall, no single identity description framework dominates across all tasks, and improvements are more sensitive to aggregation strategy than to framework choice alone. The approach generalizes across model families but does not provide a consistent size-driven advantage. These findings suggest that future progress will likely come from tighter task–framework calibration and stronger aggregation design, rather than from model scale or generic persona prompting.

**Acknowledgments.** This research has been partially funded by the AMOR project (TSI-063100-2022-0002), supported by the Spanish Ministry of Economic Affairs and Digital Transformation and the European Union - NextGeneration EU, within the UNICO I+D Cloud Program. Author Sergio Muñoz would like to thank ETSI de Telecomunicación and Universidad Politécnica de Madrid for the mobility grant obtained under *Programa Propio.*

**Disclosure of Interests.** The authors have no competing interests to declare that are relevant to the content of this article.

## References

1. Bellan, P., Haez, S.G., Sanna, L., Magnolini, S., Dragoni, M.: Leveraging multi-agent systems for domain-pertinence query classification in informative chatbots. In: Bellazzi, R., Juarez Herrero, J.M., Sacchi, L., Zupan, B. (eds.) AIME, pp. 44–54 (2025)
2. Chai, Z., et al.: An expert is worth one token: Synergizing multiple expert LLMs as generalist via expert token routing. In: Proceedings of the 62nd Annual Meeting of the ACL (Volume 1: Long Papers) (2024)
3. Cooper, A., Saffo, P.: The Inmates are Running the Asylum. Sams Publishing, Indianapolis, IN, USA (1999)
4. Csikszentmihalyi, M.: Beyond Boredom and Anxiety. Jossey-Bass Behavioral Science Series, Jossey-Bass Publishers, San Francisco, CA, USA (1975)
5. Freud, S., Brill, A.: The Interpretation of Dreams. Classics of World Literature, Wordsworth Editions, Ware, UK (1997)
6. Gandhi, K., Fränken, J.P., Gerstenberg, T., Goodman, N.: Understanding social reasoning in language models with language models. In: Advances in Neural Information Processing Systems, vol. 36, pp. 13518–13529 (2023)

7. Ge, T., Chan, X., Wang, X., Yu, D., Mi, H., Yu, D.: Scaling synthetic data creation with 1,000,000,000 personas. arXiv (2024)
8. Gurney, N., Pynadath, D.V., Ustun, V.: Spontaneous theory of mind for artificial intelligence. In: Kurosu, M., Hashizume, A. (eds.) HCII 2024. LNCS, vol. 14684, pp. 60–75. Springer, Cham (2024). https://doi.org/10.1007/978-3-031-60405-8_5
9. Hosseini, M., Caragea, C.: It takes two to empathize: one to seek and one to provide. In: Proceedings of the AAAI Conference on Artificial Intelligence, pp. 13018–13026 (2021)
10. Hu, T., Collier, N.: Quantifying the persona effect in LLM simulations. In: Proceedings of the 62nd Annual Meeting of the Association for Computational Linguistics (Volume 1: Long Papers), pp. 10289–10307 (2024)
11. Huang, J.t., et al.: Apathetic or empathetic? Evaluating LLMs' emotional alignments with humans. In: Advances in Neural Information Processing Systems, vol. 37, pp. 97053–97087 (2024)
12. Hwang, Y., Shin, D., Baek, S., Suh, B., Lee, J.: Applying the persona of user's family member and the doctor to the conversational agents for healthcare (2021)
13. Jandaghi, P., et al.: Faithful persona-based conversational dataset generation with LLMs. In: Proceedings of the 6th Workshop on NLP4ConvAI 2024, pp. 114–139 (2024)
14. Kocaballi, A.B., et al.: The personalization of conversational agents in health care: systematic review. J. Med. Internet Res. **21**(11) (2019)
15. Liang, T., et al.: Encouraging divergent thinking in LLMs through multi-agent debate. In: Proceedings of the 2024 Conference on EMNLP, pp. 17889–17904 (2024)
16. Liu, A., Diab, M., Fried, D.: Evaluating large language model biases in persona-steered generation. In: Findings of the Association for Computational Linguistics: ACL 2024, pp. 9832–9850 (2024)
17. Liu, J., Symons, C., Vatsavai, R.R.: Persona-based conversational AI: state of the art and challenges (2022)
18. Long, D.X., et al.: Multi-expert prompting improves reliability, safety and usefulness of LLMs. In: Proceedings of the 2024 Conference on Empirical Methods in NLP (2024)
19. Nascimento, N., et al.: Self-adaptive LLMs-based multiagent systems. In: 2023 IEEE International Conference on Autonomic Computing and Self-Organizing Systems Companion (ACSOS-C), pp. 104–109. IEEE (2023)
20. Newsham, L., Prince, D.: Personality-driven decision-making in LLM-based autonomous agents. In: Proceedings of the 24th International Conference on Autonomous Agents and Multiagent Systems (AAMAS 2025), Detroit, Michigan, USA (2025)
21. Norman, D.A., Draper, S.W.: User Centered System Design: New Perspectives on Human-computer Interaction. Lawrence Erlbaum Associates, Hillsdale, NJ, USA (1986)
22. Ozgun, M.C., Pei, J., Hindriks, K., Donatelli, L., Liu, Q.,Wang, J.: Trustworthy AI psychotherapy: multi-agent LLM workflow for counseling and explainable mental disorder diagnosis. In: Proceedings of the 34th ACM International Conference on Information and Knowledge Management, pp. 2263–2272 (2025)
23. Rashkin, H., Smith, E.M., Li, M., Boureau, Y.L.: Towards empathetic open-domain conversation models: a new benchmark and dataset. In: Proceedings of the 57th Annual Meeting of the Association for Computational Linguistics, pp. 5370–5381. Association for Computational Linguistics, Florence, Italy (2019)
24. Roccas, S., Sagiv, et al.: The big five personality factors and personal values. Personal. Soc. Psychol. Bull. **28**(6), 789–801 (2002)

25. Serapio-García, G., et al.: Personality traits in large language models (2023)
26. Shinoda, K., et al.: ToMATO: verbalizing the mental states of role-playing LLMs for benchmarking theory of mind. In: AAAI-25, pp. 1520–1528 (2025)
27. Singh, A.V., et al.: Hierarchical multi-agent reinforcement learning for cyber network defense. In: AAMAS. Detroit, Michigan, USA (2025). Extended Abstract
28. Sorin, V., et al.: Large language models and empathy: systematic review. J. Med. Internet Res. **26**, e52597 (2024)
29. Sweller, J.: Cognitive load during problem solving: effects on learning. Cogn. Sci. **12**(2), 257–285 (1988)
30. Völkel, S.T.: Conversational agents with personality. Ph.D. thesis, LMU Munich (2022)
31. Wason, P., Evans, J.: Dual processes in reasoning? Cognition **3**(2), 141–154 (1974)
32. Welivita, A., Xie, Y., Pu, P.: A large-scale dataset for empathetic response generation. In: Proceedings of the 2021 Conference on Empirical Methods in Natural Language Processing, EMNLP 2021, pp. 1251–1264
33. Wu, Y., He, Y., Jia, Y., Mihalcea, R., Chen, Y., Deng, N.: Hi-ToM: a benchmark for evaluating higher-order theory of mind reasoning in large language models. In: Findings of the Association for Computational Linguistics: EMNLP 2023. pp. 10691–10706 (2023)
34. Xu, H., Zhao, R., Zhu, L., Du, J., He, Y.: OpenToM: a comprehensive benchmark for evaluating theory-of-mind reasoning capabilities of large language models. In: Proceedings of the 62nd Annual Meeting of the Association for Computational Linguistics, pp. 8593–8623 (2024)
35. Xu, Y., Hu, J., Zhao, Z., Duan, Z., Sun, X., Yang, X.: MultiAgentESC: a LLM-based multiagent collaboration framework for emotional support conversation. In: Proceedings of the 2025 Conference on Empirical Methods in Natural Language Processing, pp. 4665–4681 (2025)
36. Zhang, W., et al.: AgentOrchestra: a hierarchical multi-agent framework for general-purpose task solving. arXiv preprint arXiv:2506.12508 (2025)

# Comparative Analysis of U-Net and YOLO Architectures for the Computer-Aided Pathological Diagnosis of Hirschsprung's Disease

Eve Wang[1](✉), Karl Grenier[2], Peter Savadjiev[3], and Dan Poenaru[4]

[1] Faculty of Medicine and Health Sciences, McGill University, Montréal, QC, Canada
yixuan.wang5@mail.mcgill.com
[2] Department of Pathology, The Montreal Children's Hospital, Montréal, QC, Canada
[3] Radiology, Larner College of Medicine, University of Vermont, Burlington, VT, USA
[4] Harvey E. Beardmore Division of Pediatric Surgery, The Montréal Children's Hospital, Montréal, QC, Canada

**Abstract.** Definitive diagnosis of Hirschsprung's Disease (HD) requires time-consuming manual screening for aganglionosis. While computer vision offers a solution, the comparative efficacy of pixel-wise segmentation versus object detection for this specific pathology has yet to be established. This study compares two deep learning frameworks to assist the diagnosis of HD: U-Net, which performs semantic segmentation to produce precise pixel-level boundaries of ganglion cells, and You Only Look Once (YOLO), an object detection model designed to identify and draw bounding boxes around cells in real time. Our dataset consisted of 54 whole slide images that were tiled into 397,731 overlapping 128x128 pixel patches, split into training (70%), validation (15%), and testing (15%) sets. Performance was evaluated based on diagnostic sensitivity, specificity, and balanced accuracy of identifying individual ganglia. Evaluation of 61,184 tiles ($n = 22$ patients) demonstrated that, although U-Net sensitivity was nominally higher (82.9% vs. 79.1%), the difference was not statistically significant ($p = 0.097$). However, YOLO26 achieved significantly superior specificity (96.1% vs. 93.9%; $p < 0.001$) and a 34% reduction in latency. Both models achieved 100% patient-level sensitivity. These findings suggest that the high specificity and speed of object detection architectures make them uniquely suited for high-throughput clinical screening in HD, providing a robust, real-time alternative to pixel-wise segmentation.

**Keywords:** Computer Vision · Computational Pathology · Semantic Segmentation · Object Detection · Computer-Aided Diagnosis

## 1 Introduction

Hirschsprung's Disease (HD) is a rare congenital disorder characterized by the absence of distal colon ganglion cells, leading to chronic obstruction and is potentially fatal if left untreated [1]. The current gold standard for diagnosing HD involves the histopathological examination of rectal biopsy specimens [2]. The diagnostic process ultimately

© The Author(s), under exclusive license to Springer Nature Switzerland AG 2027
P. Andreev et al. (Eds.): AIME 2026, LNAI 16748, pp. 395–399, 2027.
https://doi.org/10.1007/978-3-032-30710-1_47

becomes a laborious search task, in which the pathologist must identify the presence of even one ganglion cell to rule out the disease. While artificial intelligence (AI) offers a potential solution, the optimal architectural paradigm for this task remains an open research question.

Currently, semantic segmentation architectures (e.g., U-Net [3]) are commonly used in HD computational pathology [4, 5]. While they offer precise morphological boundaries, they are computationally expensive and require rigorous pixel-level annotations [6]. Conversely, object detection architectures like You Only Look Once (YOLO) [7] generate bounding boxes rather than pixel maps and are rarely applied to computational pathology. These models are significantly faster and require less granular annotation but may lack the feature resolution necessary to distinguish subtle cell physiologies.

This paper presents a comparative analysis of these two approaches for the assistive diagnosis of HD. By benchmarking a U-Net-based segmentation model against a YOLO-based detection model, we aim to determine whether the rigorous pixel-wise analysis of segmentation is required for clinical accuracy or if the rapid inference of object detection is sufficient for effective screening.

## 2 Methods

### 2.1 Dataset Preparation

The dataset consisted of 54 digitized HPS-stained slides from children ages 0–10 years collected at the Montreal Children's Hospital between 2015 and 2022. All whole slide images (WSIs) were anonymized and annotated for ganglion cells by a pediatric pathologist using QuPath [8], with region-of-interest converted to bounding boxes. The WSIs were tiled into 397,731 overlapping patches of 128x128 pixels, split into training (70%), validation (15%), and testing (15%) sets (Fig. 1). To address class imbalance, we downsampled the majority class, oversampled the minority class, and applied data augmentation techniques including rotation, flipping, and colour jittering.

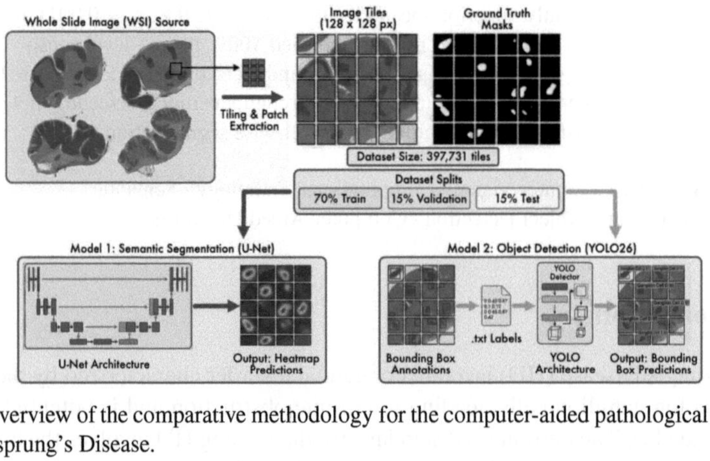


**Fig. 1.** Overview of the comparative methodology for the computer-aided pathological diagnosis of Hirschsprung's Disease.

### 2.2 Model Training and Evaluation

Two distinct model architectures were implemented: U-Net with an EfficientNet-B3 backbone (pre-trained on ImageNet) from the segmentation_models.pytoch library [9], and a YOLO26 model from the Ultralytics library [10] (Fig. 1). Training was conducted on an NVIDIA RTX 5000 GPU.

The U-Net was optimized using AdamW with a scheduler, an initial learning rate of 1e-4, and a batch size of 32. The model was trained for 100 epochs. The loss was minimized using a combination of Dice Loss and Focal Loss. The YOLO26 was trained for 100 epochs using the AdamW optimizer with a learning rate scheduler, starting with an initial rate of 1e-4 and a batch size of 32. The loss was minimized using its standard multi-part loss function.

Performance was evaluated using balanced accuracy, sensitivity, and specificity per tile. To ensure comparable metrics, bounding boxes were generated from U-Net predictions. The inference time per tile was also recorded.

## 3 Results

### 3.1 Tile-Level Performance

Both architectures were evaluated on a standardized test set of 61,184 tiles. Quantitative results are summarized in Table 1.

In terms of diagnostic sensitivity, the U-Net achieved 82.9%, nominally higher than the YOLO26 at 79.1%. However, statistical analysis revealed that this difference was not significant ($p = 0.097$; McNemar's Test at $\alpha = 0.05$), suggesting comparable performance in identifying true positive ganglion cells. Conversely, the YOLO26 demonstrated a statistically significant advantage in specificity (96.1% vs. 93.9%; $p < 0.001$), effectively reducing the false-positive rate by 36% relative to the U-Net. This increased precision contributed to a comparable balanced accuracy between the two models. Regarding computational efficiency, the YOLO26 achieved a mean inference latency of 7.64 ms per tile, representing a 33.97% reduction compared to the U-Net (11.57 ms).

Figure 2 illustrates the predictive outputs across a spectrum of histological complexities, ranging from larger ganglion cells (Fig. 2A) to smaller and partially truncated cases (Fig. 2B). Both models appear to successfully locate the target cell, with the U-Net producing pixel-level masks and the YOLO26 generating bounding boxes.

### 3.2 Patient-Level Diagnostic Feasibility

Model predictions were aggregated at the patient level ($n = 22$). Both the U-Net and YOLO26 achieved 100% patient-level sensitivity, correctly identifying all 5 positive Hirschsprung's cases. However, at a single-tile detection threshold, patient-level specificity was low for both models. The U-Net correctly identified 0/17 negative cases (0%), while the YOLO26 correctly identified 2/17 negative cases (11.7%).

**Table 1.** Summary of the quantitative performance metrics for the U-Net and YOLO26

| Metric | EfficientNet-B3-U-Net | YOLO26 |
|---|---|---|
| Sensitivity | 82.91% | 79.08% |
| Specificity | 93.85% | 96.11% |
| Balanced Accuracy | 88.38% | 87.60% |
| Inference Time (ms/tile) | 11.57 | 7.64 |
| Throughput (tiles/s) | ~86 | ~130 |

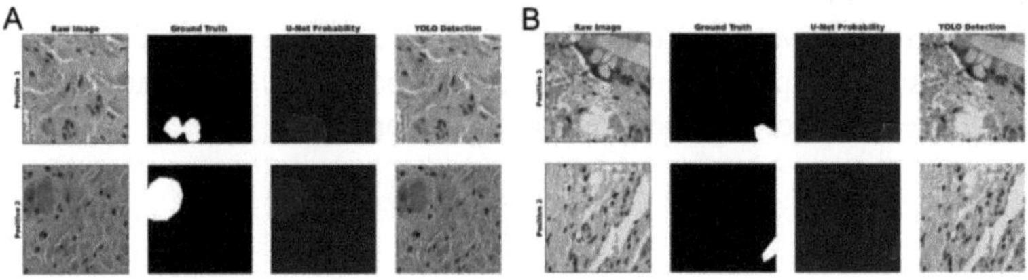


**Fig. 2.** Visualization of predictions. **A.** Larger ganglion cells. **B.** More difficult edge cases.

## 4 Discussion

The diagnosis of HD remains a significant challenge due to the labor-intensive nature of identifying ganglion cells. This study establishes a baseline for assisted diagnosis by comparing the U-Net against YOLO. Unlike typical histopathological diagnoses, HD is a diagnosis of exclusion, making computer vision tools ideal for this workflow as they can maintain constant scrutiny over large datasets.

Existing literature by Duci et al. [4] and Oda et al. [5] has demonstrated the efficacy of U-Net architectures for HD, reporting accuracies and sensitivities of 92.3% and 85.3%, respectively. While our U-Net achieved comparable performance, our work highlights a critical oversight in current research: the trade-off between architectural complexity and clinical utility. We investigated YOLO, a high-speed model previously unexplored in HD, and found its feature-extraction capabilities robust, aligning with nucleus segmentation results observed in other tissues [11].

While the U-Net showed a higher absolute sensitivity, the difference was not statistically significant. YOLO26 demonstrated a statistically significant advantage in specificity and a 34% reduction in inference latency, suggesting that YOLO26 is a viable candidate for rapid clinical triage. Our patient-level analysis further underscores this potential. While both architectures achieved 100% sensitivity, YOLO26 demonstrated better clinical reliability by correctly identifying a subset of negative patients that the U-Net misclassified. In a diagnosis of exclusion, YOLO's ability to reduce the false-positive burden while maintaining perfect sensitivity is important, as it narrows the search space without compromising diagnostic safety.

Several limitations remain. Our dataset remains small, and reliance on single-institution data limits generalizability. Furthermore, converting U-Net maps to bounding boxes for comparison may have penalized U-Net's latency without capturing its full morphological diagnostic value. Future work will focus on expanding the patient cohort through multi-institutional data to refine the data pipeline and auditing misclassifications. We will also benchmark these models against human pathologists to quantify the actual time efficiency of AI-assisted screening versus manual diagnosis.

## 5 Conclusion

Comparing U-Net and YOLO26 for ganglion cell detection, we found no statistically significant sensitivity differences. However, YOLO26 offered significantly higher specificity and 34% lower latency. Given that both models achieved 100% patient-level sensitivity, YOLO26 emerges as the optimal candidate for real-time clinical triage without compromising diagnostic safety.

**Acknowledgments.** This research received no specific grant from any funding agency.

## References

1. Das, K., Mohanty, S.: Hirschsprung disease-current diagnosis and management. Indian J. Pediatr. **84**, 618–623 (2017)
2. Vervloet, G., et al.: Rectal biopsy for Hirschsprung's disease: a multicentre study involving biopsy technique, pathology and complications. Children (Basel). **10** (2023)
3. Ronneberger, O., Fischer, P., Brox, T.: U-Net: Convolutional Networks for Biomedical Image Segmentation. (2015)
4. Duci, M., et al.: Enhancing diagnosis of Hirschsprung's disease using deep learning from histological sections of post pull-through specimens: preliminary results. Pediatr. Surg. Int. **40**, 12 (2023)
5. Oda, H., et al.: Automated ganglion cell detection using fully convolutional networks and evaluation under different training losses. Int. J. Comput. Assist. Radiol. Surg. **13**(Supplement 1), S104–S105 (2018)
6. Lin, T.-Y., et al.: Microsoft COCO: common objects in context. In: Computer Vision–ECCV 2014, pp. 740–755. Springer International Publishing (2014)
7. Redmon, J., Divvala, S., Girshick, R., Farhadi, A.: You Only Look Once: Unified, Real-Time Object Detection. (2016)
8. Bankhead, P., et al.: QuPath: open source software for digital pathology image analysis. Sci. Rep. **7**, 16878 (2017)
9. Iakubovskii, P.: Segmentation models pytorch. GitHub. (2019)
10. Jocher, G., Qiu, J.: Ultralytics YOLO26. (2026)
11. Rong, R., et al.: A deep learning approach for histology-based nucleus segmentation and tumor microenvironment characterization. Mod. Pathol. **36**, 100196 (2023)

# A Case-Based Framework for Explaining AI-Driven Bruise Detection Model Behavior Using Structured Data

Dharmi Desai(✉), Mehrdad Ghyabi, David Lattanzi, Katherine Scafide, and Janusz Wojtusiak

George Mason University, Fairfax, VA 22030, USA
{ddesai8,mghyabi,dlattanz,kscafide,jwojtusi}@gmu.edu

**Abstract.** Object-detection models can perform well on medical images, but their behavior across cases is often unclear. Explanations for object detectors often rely on heatmaps or latent embeddings that are difficult to validate or communicate to clinical experts. We present a model-agnostic, structured-data case-based explanation framework that retrieves context-matched similar and dissimilar cases to enable transparent comparisons of a bruise detector's behavior. The presented method is developed and applied in the context of models for detecting bruises on forensic medical images. 15,513 bruise images were analyzed using a YOLOv5-based detector to generate bounding boxes and confidence scores. For each test image, references were restricted to comparable acquisition conditions (e.g., bruise location, lighting), and matched within a context neighborhood defined by demographic and imaging-specific variables. Similarity was computed from injury features, model outputs, and structured explanation summaries, and $k = 5$ similar and $k = 5$ dissimilar cases were retrieved. Because no standard criteria exist to evaluate retrieved explanation sets, we introduce five retrieval-quality metrics and a weighted composite score assessing context control, injury separation, behavioral contrast, and cohesion. Composite retrieval quality was nearly identical across distance metrics (Euclidean, Cosine, Manhattan, Mahalanobis; 0.50–0.51), indicating that the framework is robust to the choice of distance definition. Composite quality differed by skin tone (Light 0.505, Medium 0.494, Dark 0.493). Post-hoc tests showed differences for Light vs. Dark ($p = 0.02$) and Light vs. Medium ($p = 0.02$), but not Medium vs. Dark ($p = 0.72$). Overall, the proposed framework enables interpretable case comparisons without latent embeddings and supports quantitative evaluation of explanation quality.

**Keywords:** case-based explanation · object detection · bruise detection

## 1 Introduction

While AI-based models can outperform humans in many prediction and detection tasks, their internal decision processes are often difficult to interpret and trust. Explanation has therefore become an important component of model evaluation and deployment.

© The Author(s), under exclusive license to Springer Nature Switzerland AG 2027
P. Andreev et al. (Eds.): AIME 2026, LNAI 16748, pp. 400–411, 2027.
https://doi.org/10.1007/978-3-032-30710-1_48

Common approaches for vision models include saliency and attribution methods that highlight important image regions [1]. Case-based reasoning (CBR) offers a complementary way by explaining predictions through comparison with prior examples [2, 3], a form of reasoning routinely used by clinicians when interpreting new cases.

Recent work has explored CBR for machine learning explainability [4, 5]. However, many image-based explanation approaches use learned latent embeddings to define similarity, but these embeddings compress complex features into opaque dimensions, making it difficult to justify *why* two cases are judged similar. Methods like CEILS use latent representations to generate counterfactual explanations, but they do not make those dimensions interpretable for similarity reasoning [6]. To address this limitation, a structured-data retrieval framework that forms similar and dissimilar case sets using observable context variables, injury descriptors, and explanation-derived behavior summaries rather than latent representations is proposed. The presented method is developed and applied in the context of models for detecting bruises on forensic medical images. The approach is evaluated using a You Only Look Once version 5 (YOLOv5)-based object detector retrained on forensic images, which outputs bounding boxes and confidence scores for a single class [7, 10].

For each query image, the explanation consists of two sets: similar and dissimilar bruises. In this way, the explanation presents prior examples alongside the model's prediction to support transparent, case-based comparison. Because bruise appearance is strongly influenced by imaging conditions, injury-only similarity can be confounded by context [8, 9]. Therefore, context is matched first and then injuries are compared within that matched neighborhood so that differences reflect injury characteristics and model behavior rather than acquisition conditions. Similarity is computed from structured imaging and injury metadata together with SHAP-derived summaries, including a Center Focus Score (CFS), which quantifies how strongly attribution concentrates near the bruise center, and Semantic Region Scores (SRS), which summarize attribution inside, bordering, and outside the bruise region.

Because expert review was not feasible within the scope of this study, the evaluation was done indirectly by using quantitative criteria that reflect properties expected of controlled case-based explanations: context control, injury separation, behavioral/explanation contrast, and cohesion of the similar set. Building on this idea, this paper contributes (1) a structured case-based explanation framework for object detection that retrieves context-matched similar and dissimilar cases using observable context, injury, and SHAP-derived features without latent embeddings; (2) a demonstration on a YOLO-based bruise detector retrained on forensic images; and (3) quantitative metrics to assess whether retrieval outputs meet the framework's design goals, including subgroup evaluation by skin tone.

## 2 Methods

### 2.1 Dataset and Model Development

This study draws on a bruise image dataset previously collected by Scafide et al. [8], containing approximately 32,000 images captured under both natural (white) light and alternate light source (ALS) conditions, along with structured metadata describing subject demographics, imaging conditions, and injury characteristics. This analysis included images with full-consensus bounding-box annotations and complete values for required cohort variables, resulting in 15,513 images (Table 1). Annotation procedures, model development, and training details follow our prior work [12, 14]. Images were split into training, validation, and test sets at the image level. The training counts reported in Table 1 include the validation subset, which was used only for model selection and not for retrieval or evaluation, preventing information leakage into the test set. For each image, the YOLOv5 detector produced bounding boxes and associated confidence scores [11], which were stored in a structured data frame and linked to case metadata. Skin tone was measured using the Individual Typology Angle (ITA) scale [12].

**Table 1.** Test and train set distribution by ITA skin type, gender, and age group.

| Category | Subjects n (%) | | Injuries n (%) | | Images n (%) | |
|---|---|---|---|---|---|---|
| | Test | Train | Test | Train | Test | Train |
| **Skin Tone** | | | | | | |
| Very Light | 20 (14.7) | 21 (14.7) | 21 (13.9) | 23 (13.0) | 270 (15.7) | 2,149 (15.6) |
| Light | 26 (19.1) | 26 (18.2) | 32 (21.2) | 35 (19.8) | 370 (21.5) | 3,119 (22.6) |
| Intermediate | 24 (17.6) | 24 (16.8) | 27 (17.9) | 32 (18.1) | 347 (20.2) | 2,516 (18.2) |
| Tan | 24 (17.6) | 26 (18.2) | 27 (17.9) | 33 (18.6) | 277 (16.1) | 2,406 (17.4) |
| Brown | 22 (16.2) | 25 (17.5) | 23 (15.2) | 28 (15.8) | 274 (16.0) | 2,195 (15.9) |
| Dark | 20 (14.7) | 21 (14.7) | 21 (13.9) | 26 (14.7) | 179 (10.4) | 1,411 (10.2) |
| **Gender** | | | | | | |
| Male | 39 (28.7) | 41 (28.7) | 41 (27.2) | 48 (27.1) | 445 (25.9) | 3,727 (27.0) |
| Female | 97 (71.3) | 102 (71.3) | 110 (72.8) | 129 (72.9) | 1,272 (74.1) | 10,069 (73.0) |
| **Age group (years)** | | | | | | |
| 18–25 | 106 (77.9) | 111 (77.6) | 112 (74.2) | 129 (72.9) | 1,315 (76.6) | 10,673 (77.4) |
| 26–35 | 17 (12.5) | 19 (13.3) | 24 (15.9) | 30 (16.9) | 252 (14.7) | 1,954 (14.2) |
| 36–45 | 9 (6.6) | 9 (6.3) | 11 (7.3) | 11 (6.2) | 93 (5.4) | 744 (5.4) |
| 46–55 | 4 (2.9) | 4 (2.8) | 4 (2.6) | 7 (4.0) | 57 (3.3) | 425 (3.1) |
| **Total** | **136 (100)** | **143 (100)** | **151 (100)** | **177 (100)** | **1,717 (100)** | **13,796 (100)** |

## 2.2 Feature Sets for Similarity Computation

Structured features were cleaned and encoded for comparability (z-score standardization for continuous variables; one-hot encoding for categorical variables), and non-bruise images were excluded. Similarity was defined in two spaces: a context space capturing subject and imaging comparability, and an injury space capturing bruise characteristics and model behavior. This two-stage design first matches cases on acquisition context (subject characteristics and imaging settings) and then ranks them by injury-level similarity. Algorithm 1 summarizes the overall retrieval procedure. For each test image, the explanation output consisted of the $k = 5$ most similar and $k = 5$ most dissimilar cases retrieved from the training set based on injury similarity within the context-matched neighborhood.

**Context Feature Space.** Context variables included demographics and imaging conditions used to define the candidate pool. Demographic features included age, gender, race, body mass index (BMI), and skin tone. Imaging features included anatomical location (upper vs. lower arm), ALS wavelength, and filter type. Each image case $i$ was represented by a context vector $x_c(i)$, and context similarity was used only to define a neighborhood of reference cases comparable to the query case.

**Injury Feature Space.** Injury features captured bruise characteristics, model outputs, and explanation summaries within the context-matched neighborhood. These included bruise age, size, visibility score (BVS), CIELAB color measures [12], region-specific skinfold thickness, and model behavior features (IoU and confidence). Explanation features included CFS and SRS for regions inside, bordering, and outside predicted boxes at 20%, 40%, 60%, and 80% thresholds. Each case $i$ was represented by an injury feature vector $x_i(i)$ constructed from these injury variables. Because available injury features differed by anatomical location, the injury vector $x_i(i)$ was defined using the subset of injury features applicable to the query image (upper-arm features for upper-arm cases and lower-arm features for lower-arm cases). Injury similarity was computed only after context matching and used to rank cases within the neighborhood.

**Algorithm 1.** Proposed case retrieval framework.

**Input:** *Query case q, reference set R, context vectors* $x_c$*, injury vectors* $x_i$*, distance metric d, percentile p=10%, k=5, model behavior features B={IoU, Conf, CFS, SRS}*
**Output:** *Similar set S(q), dissimilar set D(q), CP, CT, IS, BC, SC, CompositeScore*

| | |
|---|---|
| 1. Compute $R' \leftarrow R$ | • Compute candidate reference pool $R'$ by matching imaging conditions and excluding cases from the same subject as $q$. |
| 2. **for** each $j \in R'$ **compute** $d_c(q, j) \leftarrow d(x_c(q), x_c(j))$ | • Loop over each candidate reference case j (training set) in the pool. Compute context distance for each candidate. |
| **end for** | • End context loop. |
| 3. Set $\tau_c \leftarrow$ *p-th* percentile of $\{d_c(q, j)\}$ and define $C(q) = \{j : d_c(q, j) \le \tau_c\}$ | • Define context neighborhood & keep closest p%. |
| 4. **for** each $j \in C(q)$ **compute** $d_i(q, j) \leftarrow d(x_i(q), x_i(j))$ | • Within context neighborhood, compute injury/behavior distance. |
| **end for** | • End injury loop. |
| 5. Rank $C(q)$ by $d_i(q, j)$; select $S(q) \leftarrow$ top $k$ and $D(q) \leftarrow$ bottom $k$ | • Similar vs. dissimilar examples. |
| 6. $CP \leftarrow \lvert \text{mean}_S d_c - \text{mean}_D d_c \rvert$ <br> $CT \leftarrow \frac{1}{2}(\text{mean}_S d_c + \text{mean}_D d_c)$ <br> $IS \leftarrow \text{mean}_D d_i - \text{mean}_S d_i$ | • Compute retreival metrics |
| 7. **for** each $b \in B$ **do** $\Delta_b \leftarrow \lvert \text{mean}_D(b(j) - b(q)) \rvert - \lvert \text{mean}_S(b(j) - b(q)) \rvert$ | • Per-feature contrast between dissimilar & similar sets. |
| **end for** | • End contrast loop. |
| 8. $BC \leftarrow \text{mean}(\{\Delta b\})$ | • Overall behavior/explanation contrast. |
| 9. $SC \leftarrow \text{mean}_B(\text{std}(\{b(j) : j \in S(q)\}))$ | • Within-set variability of behavior/explanation features in $S(q)$. |
| 10. $Composite \leftarrow (0.30)\,CP + (0.15)\,CT + (0.25)\,IS + (0.20)\,BC + (0.10)\,SC$ | • Composite score |
| 11. **return** *S(q), D(q), CP, CT, IS, BC, SC, Composite* | • Output example sets & proposed metrics. |

## 2.3 Case Retrieval Framework

**Query Case.** Each test image $q$, together with its associated structured metadata and model-derived outputs, was treated as a single case to be explained by retrieving comparable reference cases from the training set. Reference images from the same subject were excluded. Candidates were first matched on anatomical location and lighting conditions, with criteria relaxed if necessary. Each case was thus represented by the pair $(x_c, x_i)$, where $x_c$ defined the context-matched neighborhood and $x_i$ was used to rank similar and dissimilar cases within that neighborhood.

**Context Matching.** Context similarity between $q$ and each candidate $j$ was quantified as

$$d_c(q, j) = d(x_c(q), x_c(j)),$$

where $d_c$ denotes the selected distance metric (Sect. 2.4). A context-matched neighborhood $C(q)$ was then defined as the closest proportion of cases:

$$C(q) = \{j : d_c(q, j) \leq \tau_c\},$$

with $\tau_c$ set experimentally to the $10^{th}$ percentile of context distances. This step restricted comparisons to cases acquired under comparable conditions.

**Injury Ranking.** Within $C(q)$, injury similarity was computed as

$$d_i(q, j) = d(x_i(q), x_i(j)),$$

and these distances were used to rank and retrieve the most similar and dissimilar cases.

## 2.4 Distance Metrics

Four different commonly used distance-based metrics were tested for case retrieval (Table 2) [13]. This analysis was not designed to identify a "best" metric, but to test if the framework produced consistent conclusions across reasonable distance choices.

**Table 2.** Distance metrics used for similarity computations in the two-stage retrieval framework.

| Metric | Context Distance* | Injury Distance* |
|---|---|---|
| Euclidean | $d_c(q,j) = \sqrt{\sum_{m=1}^{d_c} \left(x_{c,m}(q) - x_{c,m}(j)\right)^2}$ | $d_i(q,j) = \sqrt{\sum_{m=1}^{d_i} \left(x_{i,m}(q) - x_{i,m}(j)\right)^2}$ |
| Cosine | Cosine similarity: $\cos_c(q,j) = \frac{x_c(q).x_c(j)}{\|x_c(q)\|\|x_c(j)\|}$, Cosine Distance: $d_{c,\ cos}(q,j) = 1 - cos_c(q,j)$. | Cosine similarity: $\cos_i(q,j) = \frac{x_i(q).x_i(j)}{\|x_i(q)\|\|x_i(j)\|}$, Cosine Distance: $d_{i,\ cos}(q,j) = 1 - cos_i(q,j)$. |
| Manhattan | $d_c(q,j) = \sum_{m=1}^{d_c} \mid x_{c,m}(q) - x_{c,m}(j) \mid$ | $d_i(q,j) = \sum_{m=1}^{d_i} \mid x_{i,m}(q) - x_{i,m}(j) \mid$ |
| Mahalanobis | $d_c(q,j) = \sqrt{(x_c(q) - x_c(j))^\top \Sigma_c{}^{-1}(x_c(q) - x_c(j))}$, | $d_i(q,j) = \sqrt{(x_i(q) - x_i(j))^\top \Sigma_i{}^{-1}(x_i(q) - x_i(j))}$, |

* Context distances were computed on standardized/encoded context features within the query-specific candidate pool. Injury distances were computed on standardized injury features within $C(q)$. Cosine distance additionally used L2-normalized vectors, and Mahalanobis distance used a shrinkage covariance estimate to obtain $\Sigma^{-1}$.

## 2.5 Similar and Dissimilar Case Retrieval

Using the injury distances $d_i(q, j)$ computed within $C(q)$, reference cases were ranked by increasing injury distance. The $k = 5$ cases with the smallest injury distances were selected as similar cases, and the $k = 5$ cases with the largest injury distances were selected as dissimilar cases. To reduce redundancy, retrieval enforced subject-level diversity by allowing at most one reference case per subject, yielding up to $k$ unique-subject reference cases. These retrieved similar and dissimilar cases constitute the explanation presented alongside the model's prediction for the query image.

## 2.6 Evaluation Metrics

Retrieval quality was evaluated based on whether the retrieved similar set $S(q)$ and dissimilar set $D(q)$ for a query image $q$ satisfied the intended properties of a desired case-based explanation. Although expert review would be ideal, evaluation was conducted indirectly using quantitative criteria reflecting four properties: (i) context control, (ii) injury separation, (iii) behavior/explanation contrast, and (iv) similar-set cohesion. Metrics were computed for each test query and summarized across the test set.

1. **Context parity (CP)** assesses whether $S(q)$ and $D(q)$ are equally close to $q$ in context space. Lower values indicate balance between the sets:

$$\mathrm{CP} = \left| \overline{d_c(q,S)} - \overline{d_c(q,D)} \right|$$

2. **Context tightness (CT)** assesses average context distance of the sets from $q$ in context space. Lower values indicate tighter context matching:

$$\mathrm{CT} = \frac{1}{2}\left(\overline{d_c(q,S)} + \overline{d_c(q,D)}\right)$$

3. **Injury separation (IS)** measures separation between sets in injury space within the same context neighborhood. Positive values indicate that the dissimilar set is farther from the query than the similar set, reflecting stronger separation:

$$\mathrm{IS} = \overline{d_i(q,D)} - \overline{d_i(q,S)}$$

4. **Behavior contrast (BC)** assesses whether $D(q)$ differs more from $q$ than $S(q)$ on model outputs and explanation summaries. Positive values indicate stronger behavioral contrast, meaning the dissimilar set differs more from the query than the similar set. Negative values indicate that the dissimilar set was not more distinct under these features. For features F = {IoU, confidence, CFS, SRS},

$$\mathrm{BC} = \frac{1}{|F|}\sum\nolimits_{f \in F}\left(\overline{|f(D) - f(q)|} - \overline{|f(S) - f(q)|}\right),$$

5. **Similar-set cohesion (SC)** assesses within-set consistency of key behavior/explanation features in $S(q)$:

$$\mathrm{SC} = \frac{1}{|F|}\sum\nolimits_{f \in F} SD\{f(x) : x \in S(q)\}$$

Because SC reflects dispersion, values were standardized so that higher scores indicated stronger cohesion. Negative values indicated lower-than-average cohesion relative to the test set.

**Composite Score.** Since the metrics operate on different scales, each was transformed into a unitless score where higher values indicate better retrieval quality. CP and CT were reverse-coded so that lower raw values (tighter context control) map to higher scores, IS and BC were scored so that higher values reflect stronger separation and contrast, and SC was scored so that higher values reflect greater cohesion. The composite score was then computed as:

$$Composite = 0.30\ (CP) + 0.15\ (CT) + 0.25\ (IS) + 0.20\ (BC) + 0.10\ (SC)$$

**Skin Tone Subgroup Analysis.** Skin tone was grouped as Very Light/Light (Light), Intermediate/Tan (Medium), and Brown/Dark (Dark). Composite scores were compared across groups using a Kruskal–Wallis test with pairwise Mann–Whitney U post-hoc comparisons. This analysis assessed whether retrieval quality was consistent across skin tone groups, as bruise visibility and injury features may vary by tone and affect retrieval stability and interpretability [8, 14].

## 3 Results

Figure 1 exemplifies a representative case-based explanation for a single test query under Euclidean distance, displaying the top $k = 5$ similar and $k = 5$ dissimilar cases alongside structured descriptors and model-behavior summaries. A query was considered complete if both $S(q)$ and $D(q)$ contained $k$ unique-subject cases after applying the diversity constraint. Across the test set, complete explanations were generated for 97.5% of queries. As an example, for the Euclidean distance setting, CP ranged from 0.00 to 0.49, and CT ranged from 0.31 to 0.98. IS ranged from 0.12 to 0.85, BC ranged from −2.17 to 3.83, and SC ranged from −2.14 to 2.83.

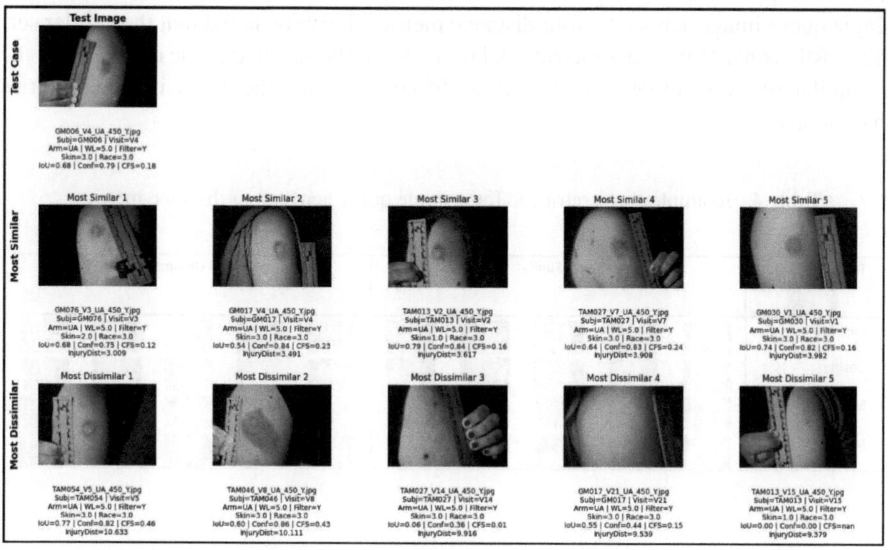


**Fig. 1.** Example case-based explanation for a single test query using Euclidean distance.

### 3.1 Retrieval Metrics Across Distance Functions

Table 3 summarizes the median retrieval metrics across the four distance functions. Median CP ranged from 0.08–0.12 and median CT ranged from 0.69–0.81 across distance metrics. Median IS ranged from 0.52–0.78 and median BC ranged from −0.23–0.24. For similar-set cohesion, values ranged from −0.26-0.13. Raw SC values closer to zero indicate greater cohesion. Median composite scores were similar across distance functions (on a 0–1 percentile-transformed scale).

**Table 3.** Retrieval metrics by distance function (values are reported as median).

| Distance metric | Context Parity (CP) | Context Tightness (CT) | Injury Separation (IS) | Behavior Contrast (BC) | Similar-set Cohesion (SC) | Composite* |
|---|---|---|---|---|---|---|
| Euclidean | 0.08 | 0.80 | 0.66 | 0.18 | −0.20 | 0.51 |
| Cosine | 0.12 | 0.69 | 0.78 | −0.05 | 0.07 | 0.50 |
| Manhattan | 0.10 | 0.73 | 0.70 | 0.24 | −0.26 | 0.50 |
| Mahalanobis | 0.08 | 0.81 | 0.52 | −0.23 | 0.13 | 0.50 |

* Composite scores use percentile-transformed metrics and do not directly reflect raw values.

### 3.2 Qualitative Comparisons

While Table 3 provides quantitative summaries, Table 4 presents a side-by-side qualitative comparison of the top five similar and top five dissimilar cases retrieved for a single query image across the four distance metrics. It can be noted that the similar sets are mostly consistent across metrics and remain closely matched to the query, while the dissimilar sets vary more and show clear differences from the query in some metrics than in others.

**Table 4.** Example cases retrieved for a single query across four distance metrics.

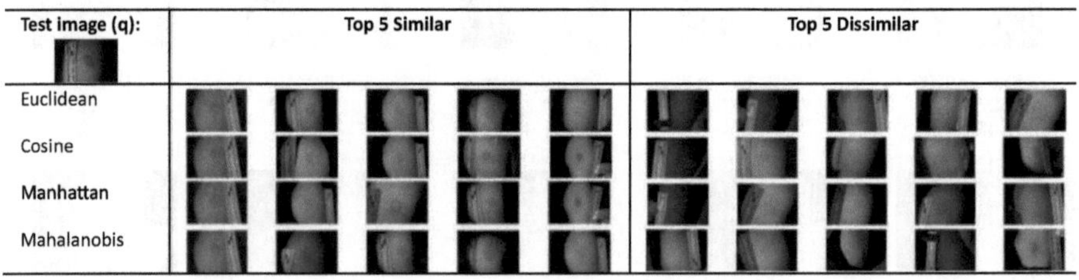

### 3.3 Composite Retrieval Quality by Skin Tone Group

Composite retrieval quality differed by skin tone group (Fig. 2). Median composite scores were 0.505 for Light, 0.494 for Medium, and 0.493 for Dark skin tone groups. A Kruskal–Wallis test indicated a significant overall difference ($p < 0.05$). Pairwise comparisons showed significant differences between Light vs. Dark ($p = 0.02$) and Light vs. Medium ($p = 0.02$), but not between Medium vs. Dark (p = 0.72).

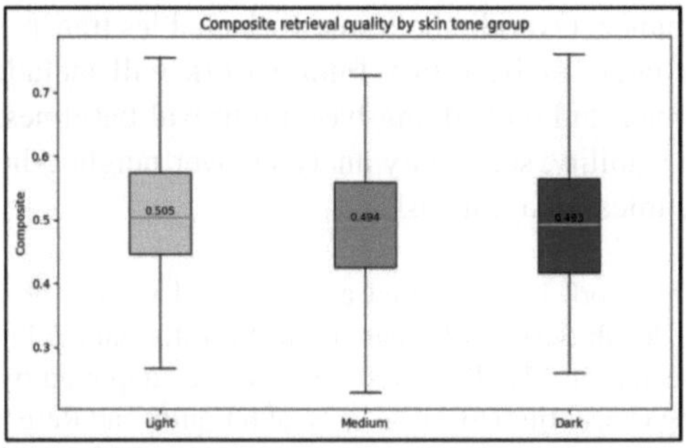


**Fig. 2.** Composite retrieval score distributions by skin tone group (Light, Medium, Dark)

## 4 Discussion and Conclusion

This study introduced a model-agnostic, structured case-based explanation framework for bruise object detection that retrieves context-matched similar and dissimilar reference sets to enable controlled comparison of detector behavior. Explanations were generated for 97.5% of test queries, indicating that the matching and diversity rules were feasible in practice. Retrieval metrics showed effective separation between context control and injury-level contrast. Median composite scores were nearly identical across distance metrics (0.50–0.51), suggesting that overall retrieval quality was consistent with respect to distance choice. Individual component metrics, however, revealed tradeoffs. Cosine distance produced the largest injury separation (0.78), Manhattan the strongest behavior contrast (0.24), and Mahalanobis the most balanced context matching (CP = 0.08), indicating that different distances emphasize different explanation properties. Reporting both composite and component metrics therefore provides a more complete view of retrieval behavior, and a particular distance metric can be selected to align with the intended use case.

The median composite scores for skin tones suggest that the framework produced lower composite retrieval scores for darker skin tones under the current similarity definition and matching rules. Several mechanisms could contribute. First, strict context matching can reduce the effective reference pool for some queries, especially after stratifying by wavelength and filter. Second, some injury descriptors, particularly color-derived variables, may be less discriminative across skin tones, reducing stability of injury-space ranking and thus separation and cohesion. Third, subgroup differences may reflect differences in model behavior itself, including variation in confidence and localization across tones, which could affect behavior contrast and retrieval ranking.

Several limitations shape how these results should be interpreted. First, retrieval quality was assessed using quantitative criteria rather than expert review, and domain evaluation is needed to confirm clinical or forensic usefulness. Second, results depend on the completeness and accuracy of structured metadata, and noise in SHAP-derived summaries may affect distance calculations. Finally, design choices such as the $10^{th}$-percentile context cutoff and $k = 5$ set size reflect practical defaults and may influence retrieval performance. Overall, the framework enables transparent, example-based explanations without latent embeddings. Future work will include expert evaluation, comparison with simpler and embedding-based retrieval baselines, feature refinement to improve subgroup stability, sensitivity analyses over neighborhood parameters, and application to other clinical imaging tasks.

**Acknowledgments.** This work is a modified and extended version of the first author's doctoral field exam in the Health Services Research (Health Informatics) PhD program at George Mason University. Research on SHAP-derived metrics was supported by the Artificial Intelligence/Machine Learning Consortium to Advance Health Equity and Researcher Diversity (AIM-AHEAD), funded by the National Institutes of Health (Grant # 1OT2OD032581-02-811). Overall project activities were supported by an anonymous gift. The authors also thank members of Mason's Injury Analytics Lab for their indirect contributions.

**Disclosure of Interests** The authors have no competing interests to declare that are relevant to the content of this article.

## References

1. Gupta, L.K., Koundal, D., Mongia, S.: Explainable methods for image-based deep learning: a review. Arch. Comput. Methods Eng. (2023) SpringerLink. https://link.springer.com/article/10.1007/s11831-023-09881-5
2. Aamodt, A., Plaza, E.: Case-based reasoning: foundational issues, methodological variations, and system approaches. AI Commun. **7**(1), 39–59 (1994). https://doi.org/10.3233/aic-1994-7104
3. Schoenborn, J.M., Weber, R.O., Aha, D.W., Cassens, J., Althoff, K.-D.: Explainable case-based reasoning: a survey. In: Madumal, P., Tulli, S., Weber, R.O., Aha, D.W. (eds.) Proceedings for the Explainable Agency in AI Workshop at the 35th AAAI Conference on Artificial Intelligence, 2021. https://www.dfki.de/fileadmin/user_upload/import/11918_AAAI___Explainable_Agency_in_Artificial_Intelligence_Workshop17.pdf. Accessed 28 Dec 2025
4. Pradeep, P., et al.: A practical exploration of the convergence of case-based reasoning and explainable artificial intelligence. Expert Syst. Appl. **255**, 124733 (2024). https://doi.org/10.1016/j.eswa.2024.124733
5. Salimi, P.: Addressing trust and mutability issues in XAI utilising case-based reasoning. In: Reuss, P., Schönborn, J. (eds.) Proceedings of the 30th Doctoral Consortium of the International Conference on Case-Based Reasoning (ICCBR-DC 2022), Co-located with the 30th International Conference on Case-Based Reasoning (ICCBR 2022), pp. 22–27, Nancy, France (2022) CEUR Workshop Proceedings, vol. 3418. CEUR-WS, Aachen (2022). https://ceur-ws.org/Vol-3418/ICCBR_2022_DC_paper19.pdf

6. Crupi, R., et al.: Counterfactual explanations as interventions in latent space. (2021). https://doi.org/10.48550/arxiv.2106.07754
7. Kelta Z. YOLO object detection explained: a beginner's guide. (2022). https://www.datacamp.com/blog/yolo-object-detection-explained
8. Scafide, K.N., Sheridan, D.J., Downing, N.R., Hayat, M.J.: Detection of inflicted bruises by alternate light: results of a randomized controlled trial. J. Forensic Sci. **65**(4), 1191–1198 (2020). https://doi.org/10.1111/1556-4029.14294
9. Tyr, A., Heldring, N., Zilg, B.: Examining the use of alternative light sources in medico-legal assessments of blunt-force trauma: a systematic review. Int. J. Legal Med. **138**(5), 1925–1938 (2024). https://doi.org/10.1007/s00414-024-03262-8
10. Redmon, J., Divvala, S., Girshick, R., Farhadi, A.: You only look once: unified, real-time object detection. arXiv.org. (2015) https://arxiv.org/abs/1506.02640
11. Object Detection Metrics: A Complete Guide with mAP, IoU. Securade.ai. (2025). https://securade.ai/blog/technology/object-detection-metrics-guide.html.
12. Desai, D., Nayebi, A., Ghyabi, M., Lattanzi, D., Scafide, K., Wojtusiak, J.: The effect of skin tone classification on bias in bruise detection. (2025), PREPRINT (Version 1) available at Research Square). https://doi.org/10.21203/rs.3.rs-6875703/v1
13. Gupta, S., Thakar, U., Tokekar, S.: A comprehensive survey on techniques for numerical similarity measurement. Expert Syst. Appl. **277**, 127235 (2025). https://doi.org/10.1016/j.eswa.2025.127235
14. Desai, D., et al.: Model quality in AI-based bruise detection: rethinking IoU and confidence thresholds. 2025 AMIA Annual Symposium. (2025). Retrieved December 29, 2025, from https://pmc.ncbi.nlm.nih.gov/articles/PMC12919542/.

# Documentation Gaps are the Primary Barrier to Reproducing Clinical ML Literature: Automated Replication with VERA

Andre Chu[1,2] and Warren Woodrich Pettine[1,2,3(✉)]

[1] Department of Psychiatry, University of Utah, Salt Lake City, USA
[2] Department of Biomedical Informatics, University of Utah, Salt Lake City, USA
[3] Department of Biomedical Engineering, University of Utah, Salt Lake City, USA
warren.pettine@hsc.utah.edu

**Abstract.** Machine learning models are increasingly embedded in clinical decision support systems (CDSS) for triage, risk stratification, and precision medicine, where patients' lives depend on model reliability. Yet the scientific literature underpinning these tools is rarely verified independently, and recent evidence reveals that even FDA-authorized AI devices may lack adequate clinical validation. We present VERA (Verification Engine for Reproducible Analysis), an automated system that takes a research paper PDF and attempts end-to-end replication, enabling systematic trust verification of the clinical ML literature. VERA integrates hybrid PDF extraction, dual-path dataset resolution (UCI Repository and dynamic MIMIC-III cohort construction), deterministic execution, and quantitative scoring.

We evaluate VERA on 19 papers: 4 UCI benchmarks and 15 clinical studies spanning sepsis, heart failure, cancer, and general ICU mortality prediction. VERA executed end-to-end without runtime failure on all 19 papers, constructed clinically plausible cohorts for all MIMIC-III papers without per-paper hardcoded logic, and executed 81 models. On the UCI benchmark subset, extracted datasets, models, and benchmark values matched manual review completely. Across 38 AUC comparison pairs from clinical papers, 24% match within 5% points and 42% within 10% points. Failure analysis attributes 67% of gaps to undocumented feature engineering, 21% to questionable reported values, and 32% to identifiable VERA limitations, demonstrating that the majority of replication gaps originate in how papers are written, not in the verification tool. These findings have direct implications for practice guidelines and adaptive clinical workflows that rely on published model performance claims.

**Keywords:** Automatic replication · Machine Learning · Clinical decision support systems · Reproducibility · Triage · Practice guidelines

© The Author(s), under exclusive license to Springer Nature Switzerland AG 2027
P. Andreev et al. (Eds.): AIME 2026, LNAI 16748, pp. 412–422, 2027.
https://doi.org/10.1007/978-3-032-30710-1_49

# 1 Introduction

Machine learning models are increasingly deployed in clinical decision support systems (CDSS) that directly affect patient outcomes: triage tools prioritize emergency department patients, sepsis prediction models trigger early interventions, and risk stratification algorithms guide treatment decisions in precision medicine workflows. When clinicians and patients trust these tools, they trust the scientific literature that validates them. That trust demands reproducibility: the ability to independently verify that reported model performance is achievable from the described methodology. Yet Baker [1] found that over 70% of researchers have failed to reproduce others' work, Gundersen and Kjensmo [6] found that most AI papers lack sufficient experimental detail, Chekroud et al. [2] demonstrated "illusory generalizability" in clinical prediction models, Mahmood [10] identified a benchmarking crisis in biomedical ML, and Chouffani El Fassi et al. [3] showed that not all FDA-authorized AI health tools are clinically validated.

The consequences are not academic: an inflated AUC for a sepsis triage model may lead to premature deployment or clinical decisions informed by unreliable predictions.

Clinical ML papers face an additional paradox: they study sensitive, access-controlled data (e.g., MIMIC-III [8]), making even code-and-data sharing insufficient; researchers with data access still cannot easily verify whether reported results are achievable from the described methodology. Existing work addresses reproducibility through *infrastructure* (experiment tracking [15]) and *standards* (checklists [12]), but neither addresses what happens when the paper itself is the only artifact. We propose a third axis, **automated replication**: VERA takes a PDF as sole input and autonomously extracts the experimental protocol, resolves datasets, instantiates models, executes experiments, and compares results against reported values. This paper makes three contributions:

1. **Feasibility of automated replication.** On 4 UCI papers (32 models), VERA matched manual review on extraction and achieved mean RM of 0.82 (Sect. 3).
2. **Scaling to clinical papers.** VERA's CohortBuilder translates prose study-population descriptions into executable MIMIC-III cohort queries across 14 papers in four clinical domains (Sect. 3).
3. **Systematic failure analysis.** We attribute every replication gap to a specific cause: insufficient documentation (67%), questionable values (21%), or VERA limitations (32%), showing that feature engineering documentation, not hyperparameter reporting, is the primary bottleneck (Sect. 4).

# 2 System Architecture

VERA processes a PDF through five sequential stages: extraction, dataset resolution, model instantiation, execution, and comparison.

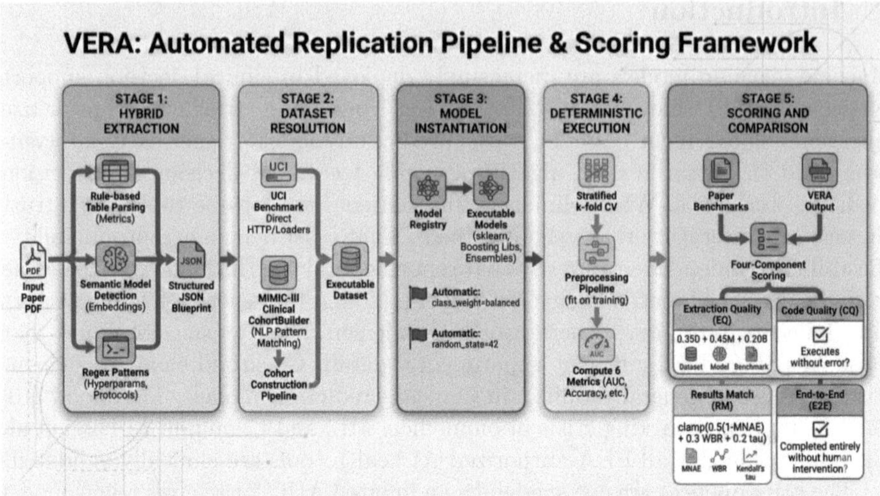


**Fig. 1.** System overview of VERA's end-to-end replication pipeline.

## 2.1 Hybrid Extraction

The extraction stage transforms a PDF into a structured **blueprint**, a machine-readable specification of the paper's experimental protocol. VERA applies three complementary strategies.

*Table Extraction.* For each PDF table detected via rule-based parsing [14], VERA identifies header rows containing metric keywords, maps columns to canonical metric names via an alias dictionary, extracts model-metric-value triples, and normalizes values to a consistent percentage scale. Multi-header tables (e.g., "Training" vs. "Test") are handled by scanning all header rows to build a composite column map. A separate text-table detector handles results presented as visually aligned text.

*Semantic Model Detection.* VERA maintains a registry of 63 canonical ML model names, spanning classifiers, boosting libraries, ensembles, and discriminant methods, each paired with a 384-dimensional embedding from all-MiniLM-L6-v2 [13]. Candidate spans are extracted via nine regex pattern groups (capitalized phrases, acronyms, CamelCase tokens, letter-number combinations, ensemble operators), then filtered through a citation-context filter ($\geq$50% citation ratio), a 23-term domain blacklist, and an ML-substring filter. Surviving candidates are matched against the registry using cosine similarity with a 0.60 threshold, resolving non-standard names (e.g., "SMO" $\rightarrow$ SVM, "IBk" $\rightarrow$ KNN). Deduplication collapses multiple surface forms to a single canonical entry.

*Protocol Extraction.* Regex patterns extract hyperparameters (27 patterns across 10 categories including tree depth, learning rate, $k$, $C$, $\gamma$, kernel type, and hidden layer sizes), evaluation protocols ($k$-fold CV, train/test splits), and preprocessing specifications. The output is a JSON blueprint specifying dataset, models, hyperparameters, protocol, and benchmark values.

### 2.2 Dataset Resolution

*UCI Path.* For papers referencing UCI datasets [4], VERA provides automated loading for 21 benchmark datasets via direct HTTP download, scikit-learn built-in loaders, or OpenML. Alias-based detection resolves variant dataset names to canonical identifiers.

*MIMIC-III Path.* VERA's **CohortBuilder** translates prose-based study descriptions into executable cohort construction pipelines using NLP pattern matching to detect: diagnosis filters (keyword matching maps conditions to ICD-9 code groups, including sepsis with six codes following Angus/Sepsis-3 criteria, heart failure, cancer, and nine diagnosis groups total), outcome definitions (in-hospital, $n$-day, or ICU mortality), age criteria, observation windows, laboratory values (28 labs from LABEVENTS), vital signs (9 vitals from CHARTEVENTS), and clinical severity scores (SOFA, APACHE, SAPS, GCS).

The pipeline follows a fixed join sequence: ICUSTAYS $\bowtie$ ADMISSIONS $\bowtie$ PATIENTS, then diagnosis filtering, outcome computation, chunked lab/vital extraction (500K and 1M-row chunks), severity score computation, and final assembly with median imputation. Critically, CohortBuilder contains **zero hardcoded logic per paper**; all decisions are driven by NLP detection. Across 14 MIMIC-III papers, it produced executable cohorts with clinically plausible characteristics (2,361–32,575 patients, 7.9–43.5% mortality).

### 2.3 Model Instantiation and Execution

VERA's model registry maps canonical names to implementations across scikit-learn [11] (14 model types), native boosting libraries (XGBoost, LightGBM, CatBoost), ensemble compositions, and clinical score baselines. Native boosting libraries are preferred over scikit-learn's `GradientBoostingClassifier` due to algorithmic differences (4–5pp higher RM). Ensemble compositions are parsed semantically (e.g., "AdaBoost + LR" → `AdaBoostClassifier(estimator=LogisticRegression())`). Clinical score baselines (SOFA, APACHE, SAPS) are thresholded by Youden's $J$ statistic on the training fold. All models use `random_state=42`; `class_weight='balanced'` is applied when the minority class falls below 30%.

Execution uses stratified $k$-fold cross-validation with a preprocessing pipeline (median imputation followed by `StandardScaler`) fit exclusively on training folds to prevent information leakage. Six metrics are computed per model: AUC (from predicted probabilities via `roc_auc_score`), accuracy, precision, recall, F1, and specificity. All random seeds are fixed for determinism.

### 2.4 Comparison and Scoring

The scoring framework has four components.
**Extraction Quality (EQ)** $= 0.35 \cdot D + 0.45 \cdot M + 0.20 \cdot B$, where $D$ is dataset detection, $M$ is model mapping fraction, and $B$ is benchmark extraction completeness. **Code Quality (CQ)** is binary (error-free execution).

**Results Match (RM)** is a descriptive composite score.

The weights were chosen a priori for interpretability, with greatest weight on absolute error. Because RM is heuristic, we also report direct AUC agreement statistics alongside it.

$$RM = \text{clamp}_{[0,1]} \left(0.5 \cdot (1 - \text{MNAE}) + 0.3 \cdot \text{WBR} + 0.2 \cdot \tau\right) \tag{1}$$

where $\text{MNAE} = \overline{|v_i - p_i|}/100$ normalizes mean absolute error to $[0, 1]$; WBR is the fraction of cells within 5pp or ratio $v_i/p_i \in [0.80, 1.25]$; and $\tau$ is Kendall's rank correlation [9] between paper and VERA model orderings. **End-to-End (E2E)** captures pipeline completion from PDF input alone.

## 3 Evaluation

We evaluate VERA on 19 papers (4 UCI, 15 clinical) across four domains, running each paper once with no manual intervention or parameter tuning (Table 1).

**Table 1.** VERA results on 4 UCI benchmark papers (32 models total).

| Paper | Dataset | Domain | Models | EQ | CQ | RM |
|---|---|---|---|---|---|---|
| Heart Disease (MDPI 2021) | Cleveland | Cardiovascular | 10 | 1.00 | 1.00 | 0.82 |
| Breast Cancer | Wisconsin | Oncology | 12 | 1.00 | 1.00 | 0.84 |
| Cardiovascular Disease | UCI Cardio | Cardiovascular | 9 | 1.00 | 1.00 | 0.77 |
| Diabetes Prediction | Pima Indians | Metabolic | 1 | 1.00 | 1.00 | 0.84 |
| Aggregate | | | **32** | **1.00** | **1.00** | **0.82** |

### 3.1 UCI Baseline

VERA achieved perfect extraction (EQ = 1.0) and code execution (CQ = 1.0) on all 4 papers with no manual intervention. The mean RM of 0.82 reflects strong agreement; the residual gap is attributable to implementation differences (Weka vs. scikit-learn), undocumented hyperparameters, and preprocessing ambiguity.

On the Heart Disease paper (10 models, Weka vs. scikit-learn), tree-based models show small gaps (RF $\Delta = -0.01$pp) while kernel/distance models diverge more (SVM $-3.31$pp, KNN $+5.29$pp), with mean absolute accuracy delta of 1.85pp. This ordering foreshadows the same pattern on clinical papers (Sect. 3).

### 3.2 Clinical Papers

VERA executed the full pipeline without runtime failure on all 19 papers, executing 81 models (32 UCI, 49 clinical). This execution success reflects VERA's deterministic, registry-based approach: every model maps to a known implementation with validated default parameters. The 49 clinical models span 14 model types including LR (9), XGBoost (6), KNN (6), SVM (6), RF (5), LightGBM (4), and CatBoost (3) (Table 2).

**Table 2.** VERA results on 15 triage papers (14 MIMIC-III, 1 UCI[§]), sorted by RM.

| Paper | Domain | Cohort | Feat. | Mort. | Models | RM |
|---|---|---|---|---|---|---|
| Pred. In-Hosp. Mort. (General) | Gen. ICU | 32,575 | 24 | 7.9% | 1 | 0.964 |
| ML Sepsis ICU Mortality | Sepsis | 4,103 | 32 | 30.6% | 4 | 0.963 |
| Heart Failure ICU Mortality | Heart fail. | 8,000 | 27 | 14.3% | 1 | 0.949 |
| AKI in Septic Patients | Sepsis | 4,103 | 32 | 29.6% | 5 | 0.921 |
| Liver Cancer ICU Mortality | Cancer | 4,405 | 25 | 19.2% | 4 | 0.855 |
| Sepsis Coagulopathy 28d Mort. | Sepsis | 4,103 | 33 | 30.6% | 3 | 0.836 |
| Geriatric TBI Mortality | Gen. ICU | 17,492 | 21 | 17.7% | 4 | 0.782 |
| Pred. In-Hosp. Mort. (ICU) | Sepsis | 4,103 | 23 | 36.3% | 4 | 0.759 |
| AKI in ARDS Patients | Sepsis | 4,103 | 37 | 43.5% | 10 | 0.751 |
| Data-Driven Sepsis Mort. | Sepsis | 4,103 | 27 | 31.2% | 4 | 0.707 |
| AKI in Heart Failure[§] | Cardiovasc. | 297 | 13 | N/A | 9 | 0.585 |
| Clinical TS Benchmarks | Multi-disease | 20,351 | 19 | 10.0% | 0 | —[†] |
| ICU Readmission Pred. | Gen. ICU | 13,643 | 21 | 16.1% | 0 | —[†] |
| Sepsis Mort. Risk Strat. | Sepsis | 2,361 | 26 | 25.4% | 0 | —[†] |
| Sepsis-3 Definitions | Sepsis | 4,103 | 32 | 31.2% | 0 | —[‡] |

[†] No extractable benchmarks; cohort and models constructed successfully.
[‡] Clinical consensus paper, not an ML study.
[§] Uses UCI data; included in triage evaluation.

*Stratification by Documentation Quality.* The results reveal three tiers. The top tier (RM $\geq$ 0.85) contains five papers across four clinical domains, demonstrating that high-fidelity replication is achievable in diverse settings. The middle tier (RM 0.75–0.85) contains four papers with systematic gaps attributable to undocumented feature engineering. The lower tier (RM $< 0.75$) contains two papers: one with questionable reported values (RF AUC of 97% for sepsis) and one where VERA systematically outperforms all models.

*AUC Comparison Analysis.* We treat AUC as the primary direct evaluation outcome because it is threshold-independent and less sensitive to class-balancing differences. Of 38 AUC pairs, 9 (24%) match within 5pp and 16 (42%) within 10pp, spanning four clinical domains and six model types. Among the 7 close matches (5–10pp), four involve linear models, three showing consistent gaps of 5.9–6.2pp across different papers, suggesting systematic feature-space mismatch.

*Model Type Predicts Fidelity.* Tree-based models ($n = 15$) replicate best: 40% within 5pp, mean $|\Delta| = 8.8$pp. Linear models ($n = 10$) show a comparable mean gap of 8.1pp but fewer close matches (20% within 5pp), reflecting bimodal behavior. SVM ($n = 5$, mean $|\Delta| = 17.6$pp) and KNN ($n = 5$, mean $|\Delta| = 19.2$pp) replicate worst due to sensitivity to undocumented kernel, distance, and scaling parameters.

*Non-AUC Metrics Show Larger Gaps.* Across 92 non-AUC pairs, threshold-dependent metrics show substantially larger gaps: F1 (23.7pp mean $|\Delta|$), precision (20.4pp), recall (17.8pp), specificity (11.3pp), and accuracy (9.3pp). These gaps arise from class-balancing differences (`class_weight='balanced'` when minority class <30%), confirming AUC as the fairest comparison metric.

*Well-Documented Papers Replicate Well Regardless of Domain.* The five top-tier papers span all four clinical domains, confirming that domain complexity is not the limiting factor; documentation completeness is. The six best-documented MIMIC-III papers achieve mean RM of 0.915, exceeding the UCI baseline of 0.82.

## 4 Failure Analysis

We attribute every replication gap to one of three causes.

### 4.1 VERA Limitations

Six papers exposed identifiable limitations: non-standard result formats (3 papers: results in prose/figures rather than tables), training/test table ambiguity (1 paper), stacked multi-line PDF cells (1 paper), incomplete SOFA computation due to missing vasopressor data from INPUTEVENTS (1 paper), and SVM $\gamma = 0.0$ edge case (1 paper). Four of six are purely extraction-related with known engineering solutions (LLM-assisted extraction, semantic header classifiers, improved PDF parsing); none require architectural changes.

### 4.2 Questionable Reported Values

Four papers report values inconsistent with clinical benchmarks. One presented training-set metrics (XGBoost AUC = 99.9%) in a table formatted identically to its test-set table (85.5%), confusing both automated and human readers. Two papers report AUC of 97–99% for sepsis/ICU mortality, substantially above established MIMIC-III benchmarks (75–87%); VERA achieves 78–81% on comparable cohorts. One paper reports systematically low values (AUC 61–81%) where VERA outperforms all 9 models by 7–28pp. The direction of disagreement is diagnostic: VERA outperforming suggests methodological issues in the original study.

### 4.3 Insufficient Documentation

The dominant source is **undocumented feature engineering**, evidenced by a consistent cross-domain pattern: linear models show AUC gaps of 6–12pp while tree-based models show only 3–8pp on the same papers. This ordering appears across all four clinical domains, implicating feature engineering rather than paper-specific issues.

We ruled out hyperparameters via exhaustive search over regularization strength ($C \in \{0.001, 0.01, 0.1, 1, 10, 100\}$), class weight, solver, and kernel parameters on three representative papers (one sepsis, one general ICU, one cancer). The search produced **zero meaningful improvement** (max 0.3pp AUC gain), confirming that the feature space, not the hypothesis space, is the bottleneck. Papers likely applied undocumented transformations (clinical ratios, temporal aggregations, additional data sources) that VERA does not currently process.

*Implication.* A paper reporting "Logistic Regression, $C$=1.0, 5-fold CV, AUC = 0.83" has documented the least consequential aspects of its methodology while omitting the most consequential (Table 3).

**Table 3.** Failure attribution across all 19 papers (papers may fall into multiple categories).

| Category | Papers | % |
|---|---|---|
| A: Identifiable VERA limitations | 6/19 | 32% |
| B: Erroneous/questionable reported values | 4/19 | 21% |
| C: Insufficient documentation (feature engineering) | 13/19 | 67% |

**Most replication gaps appear attributable to how papers are written rather than to the verification tool. Because categories overlap, these percentages are descriptive rather than mutually exclusive.** Categories B and C account for 88% of papers with gaps. Category A is qualitatively different: every limitation has a known engineering solution.

## 5 Discussion and Conclusion

*Relation to Prior Work.* Prior work falls into *measurement* (Baker [1], Gundersen and Kjensmo [6]) and *prescription* (Pineau et al. [12], Stodden et al. [15], Harutyunyan et al. [7]). VERA occupies a third category, *automated verification*, that directly attempts replication and quantifies outcomes. This distinction is consequential: only automated replication provides empirical evidence about which documentation gaps matter most (e.g., our finding that hyperparameters account for <0.3pp while feature engineering accounts for 6–12pp). VERA builds on sentence-transformer methods [13] but uniquely closes the loop from extraction through execution to comparison, executing without runtime failure via a deterministic, registry-based approach.

*Feature Engineering is the Bottleneck.* We recommend that clinical ML papers include a "Feature Engineering" subsection listing: (1) raw features and data sources, (2) derived features with formulas, (3) temporal aggregation functions, and (4) missing-data treatment. The model-type gradient (3–8pp for trees vs. 6–12pp for linear) demonstrates that the feature space determines approximately 10× more variance than the hypothesis space (<0.3pp from exhaustive hyperparameter search).

*VERA as Quality Assurance for Clinical AI.* 21% of papers contained questionable values, all flagged by VERA's systematic disagreement. For clinical decision support systems, where practice guidelines and adaptive workflows are built on published performance claims, this screening capability is consequential. Hospital systems evaluating triage tools or decision support models could integrate automated verification as a pre-deployment checkpoint. For regulatory bodies reviewing AI/ML-enabled medical devices, automated replication offers a scalable complement to manual audit. For clinical practice guideline committees, verification could flag studies whose reported performance may not generalize. Integration with peer review workflows could reduce reviewer burden while catching problematic claims before models are deployed in triage or treatment decision tools.

*Limitations.* Our 19-paper corpus is small; attribution percentages are indicative rather than precise. We also do not compare VERA against human replicators or alternative end-to-end systems. VERA supports only tabular ML (not deep learning), requires machine-readable PDFs, and cannot reproduce undocumented feature engineering by design. Future work includes LLM-assisted extraction, expanded MIMIC-III table processing, deep learning support, and corpus scaling.

*Conclusion.* VERA demonstrates that automated, end-to-end replication of ML experiments from paper PDFs is feasible and diagnostically informative. On 19 papers (81 models), it executed without runtime failure, with mean RM of 0.82 on UCI benchmarks and 0.915 on the six best-documented MIMIC-III papers. The failure analysis, attributing 67% of gaps to documentation, 21% to paper quality, and 32% to tool limitations, shows that the barrier to verification is not technical complexity but the completeness of what papers choose to report. As automated replication tools mature, they can transform reproducibility from a rare, manual activity into a routine safeguard in the clinical AI publication workflow, strengthening the chain of trust from published research to bedside decision support.

*Code Availability.* The implementation code and environment are available on GitHub (https://github.com/mmint-lab/VERA).

*Declaration of AI Assistance.* The author(s) used Cursor IDE with Claude Opus 4.6 (Anthropic) for editing and formatting of manuscript text and writing/drafting manuscript content, following the STM Association's recommended classification of AI activities (September 2025). Additionally, the same tool was used for code generation and testing during the development of the VERA system. Google's Nano Banana Pro [5] was used to generate the system architecture diagram (Fig. 1). After using this technology, the author(s) reviewed the results and take(s) full responsibility for the contents of the manuscript.

## References

1. Baker, M.: 1,500 scientists lift the lid on reproducibility. Nature **533**(7604), 452–454 (2016)
2. Chekroud, A.M., et al.: Illusory generalizability of clinical prediction models. Science **383**(6679), 164–167 (2024)
3. El Fassi, C., Abdullah, S., Fang, A., Y.: Not all AI health tools with regulatory authorization are clinically validated. Nat. Med. **30**, 2718–2720 (2024)
4. Dua, D., Graff, C.: UCI Machine Learning Repository (2019). https://archive.ics.uci.edu/
5. Google DeepMind: Introducing Nano Banana Pro (2025). https://blog.google/technology/ai/nano-banana-pro/
6. Gundersen, O.E., Kjensmo, S.: State of the art: reproducibility in artificial intelligence. In: Proceedings of the AAAI Conference on Artificial Intelligence, pp. 1644–1651 (2018)
7. Harutyunyan, H., Khachatrian, H., Kale, D.C., et al.: Multitask learning and benchmarking with clinical time series data. Sci. Data **6**, 96 (2019)
8. Johnson, A.E.W., Pollard, T.J., Shen, L., et al.: MIMIC-III, a freely accessible critical care database. Sci. Data **3**, 160035 (2016)
9. Kendall, M.G.: A new measure of rank correlation. Biometrika **30**(1/2), 81–93 (1938)
10. Mahmood, F.: A benchmarking crisis in biomedical machine learning. Nat. Med. **31**, 1060 (2025)
11. Pedregosa, F., et al.: Scikit-learn: machine learning in Python. J. Mach. Learn. Res. **12**, 2825–2830 (2011)
12. Pineau, J., et al.: Improving reproducibility in machine learning research. J. Mach. Learn. Res. **22**(164), 1–20 (2021)

13. Reimers, N., Gurevych, I.: Sentence-BERT: sentence embeddings using Siamese BERT-networks. In: Proceedings of EMNLP-IJCNLP, pp. 3982–3992 (2019)
14. Singer-Vine, J.: pdfplumber: Plumb a PDF for detailed information about each text character, rectangle, and line (2024). https://github.com/jsvine/pdfplumber
15. Stodden, V., McNutt, M., Bailey, D.H., et al.: Enhancing reproducibility for computational methods. Science **354**(6317), 1240–1241 (2016)

# Clinical Decision Support AI Startups: Funding Disparities and Deployment Patterns

Pek Hooi Soh[1(✉)] and Zelyn Lee[2]

[1] Beedie School of Business, Simon Fraser University, Vancouver, BC V6C 1W6, Canada
psa28@sfu.ca

[2] Department of Pediatrics, University of British Columbia, Vancouver, BC V6T 1Z3, Canada
zelyn.lee@bcchr.ca

**Abstract.** Healthcare Artificial Intelligence deployment exhibits systematic patterns associated with funding scale and AI complexity. Analysis of 362 Clinical Decision Support System (CDSS) startups across the United States and Canada (2010–2024) using a five-tier AI complexity framework reveals strong associations between mega-funding (>$100 M) and operational workflow deployment; 86.7% of mega-funded startups deployed workflow systems, with 13 firms alone accounting for 39.4% ($2.49B) of the $6.31B total capital raised. Workflow-oriented startups dominated across all three technology eras: pre-deep learning (73%), deep learning boom (72%), and LLM democratization (80%), while Clinical AI startups, despite requiring substantially higher technical complexity (52% operating at High complexity or above versus 25% for Workflow), declined from 18% to 15% of the cohort. These findings carry implications for healthcare policy, investment strategy, and research prioritization: the persistent underfunding of high-complexity Clinical AI relative to its potential patient impact suggests a structural market gap; investors systematically favour scalable workflow returns over clinical innovation; and researchers should attend to the widening disparity between AI complexity demands in clinical versus operational domains across successive technology eras.

**Keywords:** Clinical Decision Support · AI Complexity · Workflow

## 1 Introduction

Artificial Intelligence (AI) in healthcare has experienced explosive growth over the past fifteen years, with applications ranging from diagnostic image analysis to operational workflow automation [1]. Despite growing interest in healthcare AI, prior research has largely examined deployment challenges in isolation, focusing on implementation barriers for specific models [2, 4], technical requirements for narrow application domains [3, 5], or key obstacles to clinical impact [6], with limited attention on how these challenges vary systematically across AI complexity levels. Similarly, industry analyses of digital health funding [7, 8] document investment trends but do not examine whether and how funding scale correlates with AI deployment strategy. This fragmentation leaves

© The Author(s), under exclusive license to Springer Nature Switzerland AG 2027
P. Andreev et al. (Eds.): AIME 2026, LNAI 16748, pp. 423–432, 2027.
https://doi.org/10.1007/978-3-032-30710-1_50

a critical gap: we lack empirical evidence on how funding maturity and AI complexity jointly shape whether startups pursue clinical decision-making applications versus workflow optimization, and how these patterns have evolved across distinct innovation periods. Understanding these dynamics is essential, as deployment choices, clinical versus workflow, can profoundly impact patient care quality, operational efficiency, and the trajectories of healthcare innovation [4].

This paper presents an analysis of 362 Clinical Decision Support Systems (CDSS) startups founded between 2010 and 2024, examining the relationship among AI complexity (from rule-based to pioneering federated learning), funding scale (bootstrap to mega-funded >$100 M), and functional deployment (clinical vs. workflow). CDSS represents a critical category of healthcare AI focused on assisting clinical decision-making [9]. Our central finding reveals strong associations between funding levels and deployment types across three distinct technology eras: pre-deep learning (2010–2014), deep learning boom (2015–2019), and large language model (LLM) democratization (2020–2024).

## 2 Methodology

### 2.1 Data Collection

We compiled a comprehensive dataset of 393 CDSS startups founded in the United States and Canada between 2010 and 2024. Data sources included PitchBook [10], LinkedIn [11], company websites, press releases, and academic publications. Data collected includes founding year, total funding raised, deal dates, company descriptions, ownership status, and founding teams. Of these startups, 31 have ceased operations. The final sample of 362 CDSS startups analyzed in this study were founded over three time periods, which aligned with major AI breakthroughs: Period 1 (2010–2014, pre-deep learning), defined by the ImageNet breakthrough in 2012 [12]; Period 2 (2015–2019, deep learning boom), characterized by transformer architectures including BERT in 2018 [13]; and Period 3 (2020–2024, LLM democratization), marked by LLMs such as GPT-3 in 2020 [14]. Recent industry reports confirm continued investment growth through 2025 [7, 8].

### 2.2 AI Classification Framework

We classified the sample firms using a five-tier AI systems complexity framework developed (with data pretrained and verified) by Zahlan, Soh, and Clarysse [15, 16] to enable consistent application of technical criteria across varying AI-driven functionalities of CDSS developed by startups. The five-tier framework is defined as follows.

- Low Complexity: Rule-based systems, no machine learning
- Moderate Complexity: Basic ML on structured data
- High Complexity: Deep learning on unstructured data
- Advanced Complexity: Multi-modal AI
- Pioneering Complexity: Autonomous and multi-agent AI, real-time adaptation

## 2.3 Functional Deployment of AI in CDSS

We developed a classification for functional deployment in three categories: Clinical (diagnosis, treatment planning, risk/prognosis, precision medicine), Workflow (documentation, billing, scheduling, compliance), and Hybrid (both clinical and workflow elements). This distinction aligns with observed patterns in AI health adoption [17, 18]. We utilized Claude (Anthropic, 2024) to perform initial classification of all 362 startups using domain-specific keywords and functional indicators, with the model providing confidence assessments for each classification. In the LLM method, we also implemented a two-stage process combining initial LLM classification with systematic boundary case verification. The LLM classification results show that 72 out of 217 workflow functions were coded with a low confidence level, 19 out of 135 clinical functions were coded with a low confidence level, but all 10 of the hybrid functions were coded with high confidence. Parallel to the LLM method, one of the authors trained in life sciences and healthcare coded the entire sample by reviewing company websites, product descriptions, including user testimonials and video demonstrations, if available. Table 1 below shows the number of cases coded differently between LLM and a human coder. A comparison between LLM and the human coder indicated 69.6% agreement (252 cases). According to McHugh (2012), many texts recommend 80% agreement as the minimum acceptable interrater agreement for clinical/medical data, and the paper also suggests that any kappa below 0.60 indicates inadequate agreement [19]. Given the low confidence in LLM classification, this study adopted the classification results by a human coder. To validate the human coding used as ground truth, a second author independently coded the 110 cases where the LLM and human coder disagreed. The two human coders reached 96% agreement on these contested cases (all differences were eventually resolved), confirming the reliability of the human coding standard against which LLM performance was assessed.

**Table 1.** Comparison between LLM and a human coder.

| Category | LLM n | LLM % | Human n | Human % | Difference |
|---|---|---|---|---|---|
| Clinical | 135 | 37.3% | 58 | 16.0% | +21.3 pp |
| Workflow | 217 | 59.9% | 270 | 74.6% | −14.6 pp |
| Hybrid | 10 | 2.8% | 34 | 9.4% | −6.6 pp |

In Table 1, the Chi-square test of distributional equality is $\chi^2(2) = 49.58$, $p < .001$. The LLM and human coder assign categories at significantly different rates. The Cohen's kappa for this initial coding exercise is $\kappa = 0.381$.

Tables 2 and 3 below show the functional roles of CDSS startups by AI development period and systems complexity level. Workflow dominates across all periods, accounting for 73.3%, 71.7%, and 79.5% of startups in Periods 1, 2, and 3, respectively. Its share increases in Period 3, suggesting that administrative and operational automation remained the primary application of AI in CDSS. Clinical applications declined modestly over time, suggesting that while clinical AI received significant research attention, it translated to a proportionally smaller share of funded startups across successive periods.

**Table 2.** Distribution of functional role category by AI development period (n = 362).

| AI Development Period | Clinical n (%) | Workflow n (%) | Hybrid n (%) | Total |
|---|---|---|---|---|
| Period 1: 2010–2014 (Pre-Deep Learning) | 11 (18.3%) | 44 (73.3%) | 5 (8.3%) | 60 (100%) |
| Period 2: 2015–2019 (Deep Learning Boom) | 29 (16.1%) | 129 (71.7%) | 22 (12.2%) | 180 (100%) |
| Period 3: 2020–2024 (LLM Democratization) | 18 (14.8%) | 97 (79.5%) | 7 (5.7%) | 122 (100%) |
| Total | 58 (16.0%) | 270 (74.6%) | 34 (9.4%) | 362 (100%) |

**Table 3.** Distribution of functional role category by AI systems complexity level (n = 362).

| AI Systems Complexity | Clinical n (%) | Workflow n (%) | Hybrid n (%) | Total |
|---|---|---|---|---|
| Low | 6 (7.4%) | 73 (90.1%) | 2 (2.5%) | 81 (22.4%) |
| Moderate | 22 (12.9%) | 130 (76.5%) | 18 (10.6%) | 170 (47.0%) |
| High | 20 (27.4%) | 40 (54.8%) | 13 (17.8%) | 73 (20.2%) |
| Advanced | 6 (20%) | 23 (76.7%) | 1 (3.3%) | 30 (8.3%) |
| Pioneering | 4 (50%) | 4 (50%) | 0 (0%) | 8 (2.2%) |
| Total | 58 (16.0%) | 270 (74.6%) | 34 (9.4%) | 362 (100%) |

# 3 Results

## 3.1 Funding Tier and Functional Deployment of CDSS Startups

Table 4 presents the total funding raised by CDSS startups since their founding years. Early-Stage (<$5 M) is the largest funding tier (n = 127, 35.1% of all startups), contains the largest absolute counts across all three role categories (22 Clinical, 91 Workflow, and 14 Hybrid), and is the most representative funding group in the dataset.

Workflow commands the majority of total capital raised ($5.11B, 81.0% of the $6.31B grand total), accounting for 74.6% of firms. The capital concentration slightly exceeds its firm share, suggesting Workflow startups attract proportionally more funding on average. Mega-Funded Workflow startups dominate capital flows, just 13 firms raised $2.49B (about 48.6% of all Workflow capital and 39.4% of the entire dataset's capital). This extreme concentration means a handful of large-scale workflow automation companies account for a disproportionate share of total healthcare AI investment.

Clinical startups raised $747 M across 58 firms, an average of ~$12.9 M per firm. The single Mega-Funded Clinical startup raised $176 M, while the 18 Growth-stage Clinical firms collectively raised $211.9 M, suggesting clinical AI funding is more broadly distributed than workflow.

**Table 4.** Distribution of functional role category by funding tier (n = 362).

| Funding Tier | Clinical n (%) | Workflow n (%) | Hybrid n (%) | Row Total (%) |
|---|---|---|---|---|
| Unfunded / Bootstrap | 10 (11.8%) | 70 (82.4%) | 5 (5.9%) | 85 (23.5%) |
| Early-Stage (<$5 M) | $30.88 M<br>22 (17.3%) | $154.47 M<br>91 (71.7%) | $22.40 M<br>14 (11%) | $207.76 M<br>127 (35.1%) |
| Growth ($5–25 M) | $211.85 M<br>18 (19.6%) | $823.04 M<br>65 (70.7%) | $109.39 M<br>9 (9.8%) | $1.14B<br>92 (25.4%) |
| Well-Funded ($25–100 M) | $328.44 M<br>7 (16.3%) | $1.65B<br>31 (72.1%) | $209.57 M<br>5 (11.6%) | $2.19B<br>43 (11.9%) |
| Mega-Funded (>$100 M) | $176.25 M<br>1 (6.7%) | $2.49B<br>13 (86.7%) | $110 M<br>1 (6.7%) | $2.77B<br>15 (4.1%) |
| Column Total | $747.43 M<br>58 (16.0%) | $5.11B<br>270 (74.6%) | $451.36 M<br>34 (9.4%) | $6.31B<br>362 (100%) |

### 3.2 Funding Raised: United States vs. Canada

U.S. startups account for $6.25B (99.0%) of the $6.31B total capital raised across the dataset. Of 335 U.S. startups, 261 have recorded funding, with an average of $23.9 M and a median of $6.6 M per firm, a disparity reflecting extreme concentration at the upper funding tiers, where all 15 Mega-Funded firms are U.S.-based. In contrast, all 27 Canadian startups remain within the Early-Stage and Growth tiers, with 16 reporting recorded funding at an average of $3.8 M and a median of $1.9 M per firm; the largest single raise being $16.7 M as of 2024. Canada's absence from the upper funding tiers reflects both a smaller domestic venture capital ecosystem and a tendency for Canadian healthcare AI startups to remain at early stages of development within the study period.

### 3.3 Funding Tier and AI Systems Complexity: Workflow vs. Clinical

Tables 5 and 6 show the distributions of Workflow vs. Clinical applications by funding tier and AI systems complexity. Early-stage is the largest funding tier for both. Workflow (n = 91, 33.7%) and Clinical (n = 22, 37.9%) have their largest cohorts at Early-Stage, confirming that both clinical and workflow startups are predominantly venture-backed early-stage companies. Moderate Complexity is the modal tier for both roles. Workflow (48.1%; 130/270) and Clinical (37.9%; 22/58) are both most concentrated at Moderate Complexity, reflecting that mainstream supervised learning and predictive ML are the dominant technical approaches across both functional categories. More generally, Clinical firms cluster at Moderate-High Complexity, while Workflow firms cluster more at Low–Moderate.

**Table 5.** Distribution of workflow applications by funding tier and AI systems complexity.

| Funding Tier | Low | Moderate | High | Advanced | Pioneering | Row Total |
|---|---|---|---|---|---|---|
| Unfunded / Bootstrap | 23 (32.9%) | 30 (42.9%) | 11 (15.7%) | 6 (8.6%) | 0 (0%) | 70 |
| Early (<$5 M) | 27 (29.7%) | 42 (46.2%) | 16 (17.6%) | 4 (4.4%) | 2 (2.2%) | 91 |
| Growth ($5–25 M) | 12 (18.5%) | 36 (55.4%) | 8 (12.3%) | 8 (12.3%) | 1 (1.5%) | 65 |
| Well-Funded ($25–100 M) | 7 (22.6%) | 17 (54.8%) | 2 (6.5%) | 4 (12.9%) | 1 (3.2%) | 31 |
| Mega-Funded (>$100 M) | 4 (30.8%) | 5 (38.5%) | 3 (23.1%) | 1 (7.7%) | 0 (0%) | 13 |
| Col Total | 73 | 130 | 40 | 23 | 4 | 270 |

**Table 6.** Distribution of clinical applications by funding tier and AI systems complexity.

| Funding Tier | Low | Moderate | High | Advanced | Pioneering | Row Total |
|---|---|---|---|---|---|---|
| Unfunded / Bootstrap | 1 (10%) | 5 (50%) | 3 (30%) | 0 (0%) | 1 (10%) | 10 |
| Early (<$5 M) | 0 (0%) | 10 (45.5%) | 10 (45.5%) | 2 (9.1%) | 0 (0%) | 22 |
| Growth ($5–25 M) | 5 (27.8%) | 5 (27.8%) | 3 (16.7%) | 3 (16.7%) | 2 (11.1%) | 18 |
| Well-Funded ($25–100 M) | 0 (0%) | 2 (28.6%) | 3 (42.9%) | 1 (14.3%) | 1 (14.3%) | 7 |
| Mega-Funded (>$100 M) | 0 (0%) | 0 (0%) | 1 (100%) | 0 (0%) | 0 (0%) | 1 |
| Col Total | 6 | 22 | 20 | 6 | 4 | 58 |

# 4 Discussion

## 4.1 Funding Scale and Deployment Patterns

Our findings demonstrate strong associations between funding scale and deployment patterns across AI complexity levels. The data suggests that market dynamics at mega-scale ($100 M+) are associated with operational ROI priorities through immediate cost savings and measurable revenue impact. Sophisticated multi-modal AI platforms at mega-funding levels tend toward documentation automation and billing optimization rather than diagnostic support or treatment planning. Companies that begin clinical missions often appear to shift toward operational applications when raising mega-capital.

Recent evidence from 2024–2025 supports these observations. Hospital adoption data shows the fastest-growing AI applications are workflow simplification and billing optimization [17], while reviews of CDSS deployment emphasize ongoing challenges with clinical implementation [3]. Clinical applications appear to face challenges justifying mega-valuations, potentially due to longer FDA timelines, physician adoption barriers, liability concerns, and smaller addressable markets. While access to proprietary datasets is essential for raising capital and demonstrating clinical value [20], trust remains a critical factor for CDSS adoption among healthcare workers [21], with recent systematic reviews emphasizing that deployment success depends on workflow integration, transparency, and clinical validation [22].

### 4.2 Selected Cases

We selected three contrasting workflow and clinical examples representing distinct positions across the AI systems complexity levels and funding tiers.

LeanTaaS, founded in 2010, is a mega-funded, moderate-complexity capacity management platform that optimizes hospital workflows, such as operating room scheduling, infusion chair utilization, and inpatient bed management across health systems. Its scheduling suite, iQueue, applies predictive analytics and machine learning to match patient demand with available clinical resources in real time, reducing idle capacity and wait times across more than 1,200 hospitals. LeanTaaS is an example of how the largest funding scales in healthcare AI are associated with operational workflow deployment, achieving enterprise-wide adoption through predictive scheduling rather than clinical decision support.

OpenEvidence, founded in 2021 under the legal name Xyla Inc., has transformed from an early-stage clinical AI startup into the preeminent AI intelligence layer for modern medicine. By evolving from an evidence retrieval tool into a high-complexity LLM-powered platform capable of synthesizing peer-reviewed literature across clinical specialties, the company bridged the gap between raw medical literature and real-time clinical action. This clinical-workflow hybrid platform, marked by a $75 million Series A in early 2025 and a $12 billion valuation by January 2026, integrated evidence-based decision-making directly into the physician's workflow, replacing manual research with a seamless AI-driven interface, with approximately 40% of U.S. physicians registered as users.

Founded in 2016, Bayesian Health deployed a pioneering-complexity adaptive AI platform integrated with hospital EHR systems for real-time detection of critical conditions, raising approximately $15 M by 2019 before growing to an estimated $40 M in total funding, a trajectory that moves it from the growth to well-funded tier, yet remains a fraction of OpenEvidence's $735 M raised. While OpenEvidence functions as a top-down information layer delivering evidence to physicians at the point of inquiry, Bayesian Health represents a bottom-up integration into the clinical infrastructure itself, embedding high-precision adaptive AI alerts directly into hospital workflows to detect life-threatening deterioration before it becomes fatal.

Taken together, these three cases illustrate that funding scale and deployment orientation are mediated not only by market forces but by the nature of the clinical problem each platform addresses. LeanTaaS demonstrates that moderate-complexity, operationally scalable AI attracts the largest capital by delivering measurable returns without clinical validation requirements. OpenEvidence shows that high-complexity AI can achieve significant funding when it removes friction from a universally applicable clinical task. Bayesian Health, representing the pioneering complexity tier, faces structural funding constraints despite having one of the most rigorous clinical evidence bases in the field. As AI complexity increases and deployment becomes more clinically consequential, capital accumulation slows and market scale narrows. This points to the need for funding mechanisms that better support high-complexity, clinically interventional platforms.

## 5 Implications for Health Policy, Investors, and Researchers

Market forces alone may not support mega-scale clinical AI innovation, and policymakers should consider enhanced NIH funding mechanisms targeting clinical AI at scale, FDA fast-track programs balancing safety and innovation speed, and reimbursement reforms that value diagnostic accuracy alongside operational efficiency; recent consensus recommendations from healthcare AI experts further emphasize the need for national-level oversight and validation frameworks for CDSS deployment, supporting our findings. For investors, investment strategies should account for funding-deployment associations observed in this study; recent analyses show that workflow-focused applications, particularly clinical documentation and revenue cycle management, attracted the largest mega-rounds in 2024–2025 [23, 24], while investor evaluation of founder teams with diverse clinical and technical expertise remains critical, as team composition significantly affects resource mobilization success [15, 20]. For AI researchers, understanding the market dynamics driving deployment is equally important. Technical sophistication alone is insufficient to maintain clinical focus at scale, and success requires a defensible clinical value proposition beyond operational ROI, a business model supporting growth, and strategic partnerships enabling deployment scale.

## 6 Conclusion

Our findings reveal a tension between market forces and healthcare mission. The overwhelming workflow preference among mega-funded companies reflects rational economic incentives but raises questions about AI's contribution to clinical care quality. The complexity paradox shows that advanced technology doesn't always lead to real-world use in clinical settings. Market forces alone might not guide AI toward the most valuable uses in healthcare. To make sure AI improves patient care and streamlines operations, intentional policy actions are necessary.

**Acknowledgments.** The AI systems complexity framework and initial dataset were developed as part of a larger research project funded by ETH4D under the direction of Dr. Bart Clarysse, with contributions from Dr. Ahmed Zahlan and the first author of this study, whose collaborative work on the original dataset and complexity assessment made this research possible. The authors gratefully acknowledge the foundational contributions of these collaborators, and direct readers to the associated publication for a full account of the research work [15, 16].

**Disclosure of Interests** The authors have no competing interests to declare that are relevant to the content of this article.

**Declaration of AI Assistance Technologies during Manuscript Preparation** The authors used Copilot and Claude for AI Activity 1 and 6, published by STM. After using these tools, the authors reviewed the results and take full responsibility for the contents of the manuscript.

## References

1. Topol, E.J.: High-performance medicine: the convergence of human and artificial intelligence. Nat. Med. **25**(1), 44–56 (2019). https://doi.org/10.1038/s41591-018-0300-7
2. Cohen, J.P., et al.: Problems in the deployment of machine-learned models in health care. CMAJ. **193**(35), E1391–E1394 (2021). https://doi.org/10.1503/cmaj.202066
3. Elhaddad, M.A., Zeid, A., Kamoun-Abid, Z.: AI-driven clinical decision support systems: an ongoing pursuit of potential. Cureus. **16**(4), e57728 (2024). https://doi.org/10.7759/cureus.57728
4. Wang, F., Boag, W.: Implementing AI models in clinical workflows: a roadmap. BMJ Evid. Based Med. **30**(5), 285–287 (2025). https://doi.org/10.1136/bmjebm-2023-112727
5. Beam, A.L., Kohane, I.S.: Big data and machine learning in health care. JAMA. **319**(13), 1317–1318 (2018). https://doi.org/10.1001/jama.2017.18391
6. Kelly, C.J., Karthikesalingam, A., Suleyman, M., Corrado, G., et al.: Key challenges for delivering clinical impact with artificial intelligence. BMC Med. **17**(1), 195 (2019). https://doi.org/10.1186/s12916-019-1426-2
7. Rock Health: H1 2025 Digital Health Funding Report (2025). https://rockhealth.com/
8. Silicon Valley Bank: Healthcare Investments and Exits Report 2026 (2026). https://www.svb.com/industry-insights/healthcare
9. Sutton, R.T., Pincock, D., Baumgart, D.C., Sadowski, D.C., Fedorak, R.N., Kroeker, K.I.: An overview of clinical decision support systems: benefits, risks, and strategies for success. npj Digit. Med. **3**(1), 17 (2020). https://doi.org/10.1038/s41746-020-0221-y
10. PitchBook: Private market data platform (2024). https://pitchbook.com
11. LinkedIn: Company profiles and employment data (2024). https://www.linkedin.com
12. Krizhevsky, A., Sutskever, I., Hinton, G.E.: ImageNet classification with deep convolutional neural networks. Commun. ACM. **60**(6), 84–90 (2017). https://doi.org/10.1145/3065386
13. Devlin, J., Chang, M.W., Lee, K., Toutanova, K.: BERT: pre-training of deep bidirectional transformers for language understanding. In: Proceedings of NAACL-HLT, pp. 4171–4186 (2019). https://doi.org/10.18653/v1/N19-1423
14. Brown, T.B., et al.: Language models are few-shot learners. In: Advances in Neural Information Processing Systems 33, pp. 1877–1901 (2020) arXiv:2005.14165
15. Zahlan, A., Soh, P.H., Clarysse, B.: Mapping AI startup investment and innovation in healthcare using a five-tier AI systems complexity framework. npj Digit. Med. (2026). https://doi.org/10.1038/s41746-026-02595-5
16. Zahlan, A., Soh, P. H, Clarysse, B. AI_Definitions_Five-Tier AI Systems Complexity Framework. (2026). https://github.com/MrGluten/LLM-category-complexity
17. American Hospital Association: Hospital Trends in the Use, Evaluation, and Governance of Predictive AI, 2023–2024. ASTP Health IT Data Brief (2024) https://www.ncbi.nlm.nih.gov/books/NBK618497/
18. Davenport, T., Kalakota, R.: The potential for artificial intelligence in healthcare. Future Healthc. J. **6**(2), 94–98 (2019). https://doi.org/10.7861/futurehosp.6-2-94
19. McHugh, M.L.: Interrater reliability: the kappa statistic. Biochem. Med. **22**, 276–282 (2012). https://doi.org/10.11613/BM.2012.031

20. Zahlan, A.: Strategic resource mobilization for AI entrepreneurship in healthcare: qualitative insights from startup founders. Technovation. **145**, 103272 (2025). https://doi.org/10.1016/j.technovation.2025.103272
21. Haddad, T.C., et al.: Trust in artificial intelligence–based clinical decision support systems among health care workers: systematic review. J. Med. Internet Res. **27**(1), e69678 (2025). https://doi.org/10.2196/69678
22. Jamshidi, E., et al.: Artificial intelligence and decision-making in healthcare: a thematic analysis of a systematic review of reviews. Health Serv. Manag. Res. **37**(2), 83–96 (2024). https://doi.org/10.1177/09514848241233502
23. Silicon Valley Bank: Healthcare Investments and Exits Report 2025 (2025). https://www.svb.com/industry-insights/healthcare
24. Carta: Industry Spotlight: Healthcare 2024 (2025). https://carta.com/data/industry-spotlight-healthcare-2024/

# RegionGate-CT: A Region-Gated Framework for Anatomy-Grounded CT Report Generation

Md Mustafizur Rahman(✉), Sana Alamgeer, and Mylene C. Q. Farias

Department of Computer Science, Texas State University, San Marcos, TX, USA
{mustafiz,sana.alamgeer,mylene}@txstate.edu

**Abstract.** Automated CT report generation aims to map volumetric imaging evidence to clinically structured text. Region-guided frameworks improve interpretability by linking text to anatomical regions, but two limitations persist. First, global and region tokens are typically fused by simple concatenation, with no explicit mechanism for global–regional interaction. Second, the same global context is applied uniformly across regions, which can inject irrelevant cues and weaken region-specific conditioning. We present RegionGate-CT, a lightweight, region-aware computational framework comprising three principal components: (i) a learnable region-gated module, (ii) a geometry-aware Feature-wise Linear Modulation (FiLM) layer that incorporates anatomical spatial priors, and (iii) a pre-large language model (pre-LLM) visual self-attention block. On the RadGenome–Chest CT benchmark, our approach achieves improvements over Reg2RG of +1.9 BLEU-4, +1.4 ROUGE-L, and +1.3 METEOR. The implementation will be made publicly available at https://github.com/MustafizTXST23/RegionGate-CT.

**Keywords:** Computed Tomography · Medical Report Generation · Vision–Language Models · Region-Level Grounding

## 1 Introduction

Computed tomography (CT) plays a pivotal role in contemporary clinical diagnostics; however, the manual interpretation of examinations comprising hundreds of axial slices is both time-consuming and heavily dependent on specialized expertise. These challenges have catalyzed increasing research interest in automated CT report generation systems [2,3,7]. Recent vision–language architectures have substantially improved image-to-text reasoning in radiology [6], and region-guided approaches further enhance interpretability by explicitly associating textual descriptions with localized imaging findings [2,7]. However, two key limitations remain.

First, many contemporary frameworks rely predominantly on global image representations or fuse global and regional features via simple concatenation, a

© The Author(s), under exclusive license to Springer Nature Switzerland AG 2027
P. Andreev et al. (Eds.): AIME 2026, LNAI 16748, pp. 433–437, 2027.
https://doi.org/10.1007/978-3-032-30710-1_51

strategy that can introduce spurious contextual information and thereby attenuate region-specific reasoning. Reg2RG [2] proposes a region–report alignment mechanism, yet the fusion between global and regional information is itself fixed rather than adaptive. In parallel, MedRegion-CT reports that pipelines based solely on global features systematically overlook fine-grained regional details [5]. Second, existing methods typically apply an identical global context to all anatomical regions, disregarding the fact that structures such as the lungs, mediastinum, and heart require different contextual priors and differential weighting of global information [2,3].

We present RegionGate-CT, a region-guided framework designed to address these two failure modes through three key components. The contributions of this work are: *(i)* a learnable region-gated fusion module that enables per-region regulation of global contextual information; *(ii)* a geometry-aware FiLM modulation mechanism that conditions regional feature representations on anatomical spatial priors; and *(iii)* a pre-LLM visual self-attention block that enhances the integration between global and regional information.

## 2 Proposed Framework

Figure 1 depicts the proposed RegionGate-CT architecture. We adopt the anatomy decomposition pipeline of Reg2RG [2]. Given a CT volume $V \in \mathbb{R}^{H_0 \times W_0 \times S_0}$ and anatomical segmentation masks $\{M_i\}_{i=1}^{N}$, the region-specific subvolumes are $V_i = \mathrm{Crop}(M_i \odot V)$, with $\odot$ denoting element-wise multiplication. A frozen volumetric encoder $\mathcal{E}_v$ (RadFM 3D ViT with a Perceiver resampler [10]) produces texture tokens $F_i^{\mathrm{tex}} = \mathcal{E}_v(V_i) \in \mathbb{R}^{T \times d_v}$, and a lightweight 3-layer 3D ViT mask encoder $\mathcal{E}_m$ produces geometry tokens $F_i^{\mathrm{geo}} \in \mathbb{R}^{T_m \times d_v}$, which are resampled to $T$ tokens by 1D linear interpolation along the token axis to give $\tilde{F}_i^{\mathrm{geo}}$. The global context is encoded from the entire volume $X = \mathcal{E}_v(V)$ and collapsed to a single global token $g = W_g\,\mathrm{GAP}(X) + b_g \in \mathbb{R}^d$, where $d$ is the LLM embedding dimension.

Geometry features are aggregated into a per-region conditioning vector, $z_i^{\mathrm{geo}} = \mathrm{GAP}(\tilde{F}_i^{\mathrm{geo}}) \in \mathbb{R}^{d_v}$, and projected to FiLM parameters $\gamma_i, \beta_i \in \mathbb{R}^{1 \times d_v}$:

$$\gamma_i = W_\gamma z_i^{\mathrm{geo}} + b_\gamma, \qquad \beta_i = W_\beta z_i^{\mathrm{geo}} + b_\beta.$$

These modulate the adapted texture tokens $\hat{F}_i^{\mathrm{tex}} = A_v(F_i^{\mathrm{tex}})$ row-wise: $F_i^{\mathrm{mod}} = \hat{F}_i^{\mathrm{tex}} \odot \gamma_i + \beta_i$, which are then pooled and projected to a region token $r_i = A_r(\mathrm{GAP}(F_i^{\mathrm{mod}})) \in \mathbb{R}^d$, where $A_v, A_r$ are linear adapters.

Each region token is gated by a sigmoid conditioned on $r_i$ and $g$:

$$\alpha_i = \sigma(W_\alpha[r_i; g] + b_\alpha), \qquad r_i' = r_i + \alpha_i \odot \mathrm{MLP}([r_i; g]),$$

where $[\cdot;\cdot]$ denotes concatenation. Multi-head attention then refines the gated tokens using region queries and keys/values augmented with $g$:

$$R'' = \mathrm{MHA}([r_1', \ldots, r_N'],\ [g, r_1', \ldots, r_N'],\ [g, r_1', \ldots, r_N']),$$

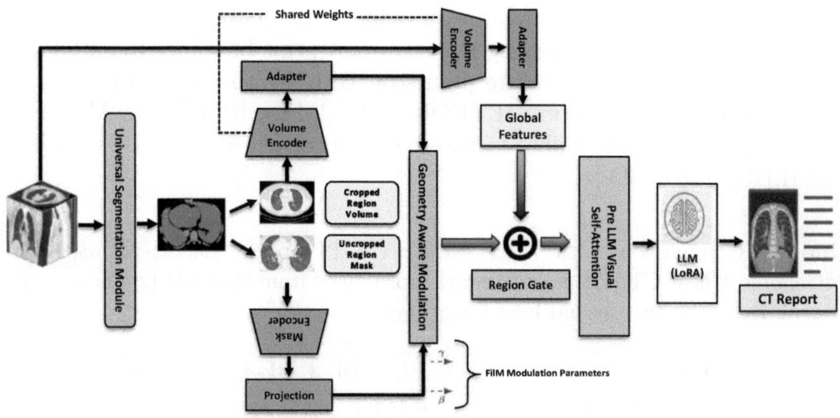


**Fig. 1.** Overview of RegionGate-CT, integrating geometry-aware modulation, region-gated fusion, and pre-LLM self-attention.

yielding $\{r_i''\}_{i=1}^N$. The global and refined region tokens form $\tilde{C} = [g; r_1''; \ldots; r_N''] \in \mathbb{R}^{(N+1)\times d}$, which a final pre-LLM self-attention block updates as

$$\tilde{C}^\star = \mathrm{MHA}(\tilde{C}, \tilde{C}, \tilde{C}),$$

before being prepended to the textual embeddings $e(y_t)$.

Consistent with Reg2RG [2], region tokens are randomly permuted during training to promote robust region–text alignment under the standard autoregressive language modeling objective $\mathcal{L}_{\mathrm{LM}}$. During optimization, only the conditioning modules, adapter layers, attention mechanisms, and LoRA parameters are updated, while the vision encoder and the underlying LLM are kept fixed.

## 3 Experimental Results

We evaluated on RadGenome–Chest CT [11] (25,692 CT volumes, $N = 10$ chest regions), following Reg2RG's preprocessing and train/test split [2].

The volumetric encoder $\mathcal{E}_v$ is initialized from RadFM [10] ($T = 32$ latent texture tokens per region), pooled into a single global token $g$; the geometry encoder $\mathcal{E}_m$ is the 3-layer 3D ViT defined in Sect. 2. The decoder is LLaMA-2-7B [8] adapted with LoRA [4] ($r = 8$, $\alpha = 32$, dropout 0.1), keeping the backbone frozen. Volumes are resized to 256×256×64; the region gate and pre-LLM self-attention each use 8 heads.

We train for 10 epochs on four NVIDIA RTX A5000 GPUs (24 GB) with AdamW (lr $5\times10^{-5}$, 20 warm-up steps, constant-with-warmup), per-device batch 1, gradient accumulation 8, bf16, and DeepSpeed ZeRO stage 2. Region prefixes are stripped before metric computation and we report BLEU, ROUGE-L, and METEOR with Reg2RG's evaluation scripts, and all baseline numbers in Table 1 are reproduced from Reg2RG [2] under their unified protocol.

As shown in Table 1, RegionGate-CT achieves the highest performance across all evaluation metrics, surpassing the strongest prior baseline, Reg2RG [2], by +1.5/ +3.3/ +3.8/ +1.9 absolute points on BLEU-1 through BLEU-4, respectively, as well as by +1.3 on METEOR and +1.4 on ROUGE-L. Moreover, it consistently outperforms global-feature-based approaches, including CT2Rep [3], RadFM [10], and M3D [1].

**Table 1.** Comparison with state-of-the-art CT report generation methods on RadGenome–Chest CT [11]. Baselines are reproduced from Reg2RG [2] under a unified protocol. Best in **bold**, second-best underlined.

| Method | BL-1 | BL-2 | BL-3 | BL-4 | MET | RG-L |
|---|---|---|---|---|---|---|
| R2GenGPT [9] | 0.433 | 0.341 | 0.282 | 0.242 | 0.399 | 0.323 |
| MedVInT [12] | 0.443 | 0.349 | 0.288 | 0.246 | 0.404 | 0.326 |
| RadFM [10] | 0.442 | 0.345 | 0.281 | 0.237 | 0.399 | 0.315 |
| CT2Rep [3] | 0.444 | 0.344 | 0.279 | 0.236 | 0.402 | 0.310 |
| M3D [1] | 0.436 | 0.345 | 0.285 | 0.245 | 0.400 | 0.326 |
| Reg2RG [2] | 0.472 | 0.365 | 0.296 | 0.249 | 0.441 | 0.367 |
| RegionGate-CT (Ours) | **0.487** | **0.398** | **0.334** | **0.268** | **0.454** | **0.381** |

Table 2 presents the contribution of each architectural component. The geometry-aware modulation yields the largest performance gain, indicating that spatial priors provide complementary information beyond that captured by the texture stream. Region gating accounts for the second-largest contribution, empirically supporting region-specific conditioning over a uniform global conditioning strategy. In contrast, removing the pre-LLM self-attention block produces the smallest degradation, suggesting that this module primarily serves as a refinement stage rather than constituting a core component of the model.

**Table 2.** Ablation on RegionGate-CT components. Best in **bold**.

| Model Variant | BL-1 | BL-2 | BL-3 | BL-4 | MET | RG-L |
|---|---|---|---|---|---|---|
| w/o Region Gate | 0.442 | 0.362 | 0.314 | 0.223 | 0.417 | 0.352 |
| w/o Geometry-Aware Modulation | 0.414 | 0.357 | 0.306 | 0.214 | 0.408 | 0.344 |
| w/o Pre-LLM Visual Self-Attention | 0.485 | 0.376 | 0.328 | 0.241 | 0.449 | 0.357 |
| RegionGate-CT (Ours) | **0.487** | **0.398** | **0.334** | **0.268** | **0.454** | **0.381** |

## 4 Conclusion

We presented RegionGate-CT, a region-guided framework that replaces static fusion with adaptive, region-conditioned components, yielding consistent gains over Reg2RG and other baselines on RadGenome–Chest CT. Two limitations remain. We evaluate only with NLG metrics on a single dataset, and the method relies on segmentation quality, which may miss small or subtle findings.

**Acknowledgments.** This work was conducted at the IMPACT Lab in the Department of Computer Science, Texas State University.

**Disclosure of Interests.** The authors declare that they have no competing interests.

**Use of AI tools.** Claude (Anthropic) was used for language refinement and LaTeX formatting. All content was reviewed and edited by the authors, who take full responsibility for the manuscript.

## References


1. Bai, F., et al.: M3D: advancing 3D medical image analysis with multi-modal large language models (2024). arXiv:2404.00578
2. Chen, Z., Bie, Y., Jin, H., Chen, H.: Large language model with region-guided referring and grounding for CT report generation. IEEE Trans. Med. Imag. **44**(8), 3139–3150 (2025). https://doi.org/10.1109/TMI.2025.3559923
3. Hamamci, I.E., Er, S., Menze, B.: CT2Rep: automated radiology report generation for 3D medical imaging. In: Medical Image Computing and Computer-Assisted Intervention (MICCAI). Springer (2024)
4. Hu, E.J., et al.: LoRA: Low-rank adaptation of large language models. In: International Conference on Learning Representations (ICLR) (2022)
5. Kyung, S., et al.: MedRegion-CT: Region-focused multimodal large language model for comprehensive 3D CT report generation (2025). arXiv:2506.23102
6. Li, C., et al.: LLaVA-Med: Training a large language-and-vision assistant for biomedicine in one day (2023). arXiv:2306.00890
7. Tanida, T., Müller, P., Kaissis, G., Rueckert, D.: Interactive and explainable region-guided radiology report generation. In: Proceedings of the IEEE/CVF Conference on Computer Vision and Pattern Recognition (CVPR), pp. 7433–7442 (2023)
8. Touvron, H., et al.: LLaMA 2: Open foundation and fine-tuned chat models (2023). arXiv:2307.09288
9. Wang, Z., Liu, L., Wang, L., Zhou, L.: R2GenGPT: radiology report generation with frozen LLMs. Meta-Radiology **1**(3), 100033 (2023). https://doi.org/10.1016/j.metrad.2023.100033
10. Wu, C., Zhang, X., Zhang, Y., Wang, Y., Xie, W.: Towards generalist foundation model for radiology by leveraging web-scale 2D and 3D medical data (2023). arXiv:2308.02463
11. Zhang, X., et al.: RadGenome-Chest CT: a grounded vision–language dataset for chest CT analysis (2024). arXiv:2404.16754
12. Zhang, X., et al.: PMC-VQA: visual instruction tuning for medical visual question answering (2024). arXiv:2305.10415

# Author Index



© The Editor(s) (if applicable) and The Author(s), under exclusive license to Springer Nature Switzerland AG 2027
P. Andreev et al. (Eds.): AIME 2026, LNAI 16748, pp. 439–442, 2027.
https://doi.org/10.1007/978-3-032-30710-1

MIX
Papier aus verantwortungsvollen Quellen
Paper from responsible sources
FSC® C105338

If you have any concerns about our products,
you can contact us on
**ProductSafety@springernature.com**

In case Publisher is established outside the EU,
the EU authorized representative is:
**Springer Nature Customer Service Center GmbH**
**Europaplatz 3, 69115 Heidelberg, Germany**

Printed by Libri Plureos GmbH
in Hamburg, Germany